Learning disability

KT-459-103

A life cycle approach to valuing people

Edited by Gordon Grant, Peter Goward, Malcolm Richardson and Paul Ramcharan

Open University Press

Open University Press
McGraw-Hill Education
McGraw-Hill House
Shoppenhangers Road
Maidenhead
Berkshire
England
SL6 2QL

email: enquiries@openup.co.uk
world wide web: www.openup.co.uk

and Two Penn Plaza, New York, NY 10121–2289, USA

First published 2005

A catalogue record of this book is available from the British Library

ISBN-13   978 0335 21439 6 (pb)   978 0335 21826 4 (hb)
ISBN-10   0 335 21439 8 (pb)   0 335 21826 1 (hb)

Library of Congress Cataloging-in-Publication Data
CIP data applied for

Typeset by RefineCatch Limited, Bungay, Suffolk
Printed in Finland by WS Bookwell

To Tracy and Olivia Paige

Contents

About the editors

Gordon Grant is Professor of Cognitive Disability at the School of Nursing and Midwifery, University of Sheffield, and Doncaster and South Humber Health Care NHS Trust. He has long-standing research interests in identities and resilience in vulnerable groups, the contributions of vulnerable groups, family care across the lifecourse, and the applications of participatory and emancipatory research in the lives of people with cognitive impairments. He has published widely in these fields. Gordon is joint editor of the *British Journal of Learning Disabilities*.

Peter Goward is a Senior Nursing Lecturer in the Mental Health and Learning Disability Department within the School of Nursing and Midwifery, University of Sheffield. His interests are predominantly in the area of identity, ethnicity and resilience with a particular emphasis on Gypsy/Traveller communities and mental health promotion.

Malcolm Richardson is currently Head of the Department of Mental Health and Learning Disabilities in the School of Nursing and Midwifery, University of Sheffield. His research interests are in the areas of disability, health, and social and political inclusion. His professional background is in learning disabilities nursing and nurse education.

Paul Ramcharan is Reader in Cognitive Disability in the School of Nursing and Midwifery at the University of Sheffield. He has maintained an interest in empowerment and people with learning disabilities. Paul's research stretches to the evaluation of aspects of the All Wales Strategy for the Development of Services for People with Learning Disabilities. Together with Gordon Grant he has also acted as coordinator of the Learning Disability Research Initiative supporting research tied to the implementation of Valuing People.

Contributors

Dorothy Atkinson, Professor of Learning Disability, School of Health and Social Welfare, Open University, Walton Hall, Milton Keynes, UK

Nigel Beail, Consultant Clinical Psychologist and Head of Psychology Services for Adults with Learning Disabilities, Psychological Health Care, Barnsley Learning Disability Service, Barnsley Primary Care Trust, 11/12 Keresforth Close, off Broadway, Barnsley, UK

Christine Bigby, Senior Lecturer and Director of Undergraduate Programmes, Department of Social Work & Social Policy, La Trobe University, Bundoora, Victoria 3083, Australia

Jane Bloom, Midwifery Lecturer, Department of Midwifery & Children's Health Nursing, University of Sheffield, Bartolome House, Winter Street, Sheffield, UK, Member of Institute of Group Analysis and the United Kingdom Council for Psychotherapy

Alison Brammer, Senior Lecturer, Department of Law, University of Keele, Keele, Staffordshire, UK

Jacqui Brewster, Lecturer, School of Nursing & Midwifery, University of Sheffield, Humphry Davy House, Golden Smithies Lane, Wath-on-Dearne, Rotherham, UK

Hilary Brown, Consultant in Social Care, Social Care & Adult Protection, Salomans Centre, David Salomans Estate, Broomhill Road, Southborough, Kent, UK

Lesley Cogher, Acting Director, Sheffield Speech & Language Therapy Agency, Sheffield Care Trust, The Ryegate Children's Centre, Tapton Crescent Road, Sheffield, UK

Helen Combes, Clinical Lecturer, Shropshire and Staffordshire Clinical Psychology Training Programme, Faculty of Health and Sciences, Staffordshire University, Mellor Building, College Road, Stoke-on-Trent, UK

Clare Connors, Research Fellow, Centre for Applied Social & Community Studies, University of Durham, UK

Eric Emerson, Professor of Clinical Psychology, Institute for Health Research, Lancaster University, Alexandra Square, Lancaster, UK

Margaret Flynn, Senior Lecturer, School of Nursing & Midwifery, University of Sheffield, Northern General Hospital, Herries Road, Sheffield, UK

Nick Fripp, Director of Business Development & Quality, The Brandon Trust, Olympus House, Britannia Road, Patchway, Bristol, UK

Linda Gething, Divisional Head of Learning Disability Studies, University of Huddersfield, HW2/14 Harold Wilson Building, Queensgate, Huddersfield, UK

Dan Goodley, Reader, School of Education, University of Sheffield, 388 Glossop Road, Sheffield, UK

Peter Goward, Senior Nursing Lecturer, School of Nursing & Midwifery, University of Sheffield, Bartolome House, Winter Street, Sheffield, UK

Gordon Grant, Professor of Cognitive Disability, School of Nursing & Midwifery, University of Sheffield, Northern General Hospital, Herries Road, Sheffield, UK

Chris Hatton, Professor of Psychology, Health & Social Care, Institute for Health Research, Lancaster University, Alexandra Square, Lancaster, UK

Sheila Hollins, Head of Department of Mental Health, Department of Mental Health & Learning Disability, St George's Hospital Medical School, Jenner Wing, Cranmer Terrace, London, UK

Jill Jesper, Nursing Lecturer, School of Nursing & Midwifery, University of Sheffield, Humphry Davy House, Golden Smithies Lane, Wath-on-Dearne, Rotherham, UK

Kelley Johnson, Senior Lecturer, School of Social Science and Planning, Royal Melbourne Institute of Technology, Level 7, Building 8, Swanston St, Melbourne 300, Australia

Gwynnyth Llewellyn, Sesquicentenary Professor of Occupation and Leisure Sciences, Occupation & Leisure Sciences, University of Sydney, PO Box 170, Lidcombe, NSW 1825, Australia

Alex McClimens, Lecturer, School of Nursing & Midwifery, University of Sheffield, Humphry Davy House, Golden Smithies Lane, Wath-on-Dearne, Rotherham, UK

Roy McConkey, Professor of Learning Disability, School of Nursing, University of Ulster, Newtownabbey, Northern Ireland, UK

David McConnell, Senior Lecturer, Occupation and Leisure Sciences, University of Sydney, PO Box 170, Lidcombe, NSW 1825, Australia

Fiona Mackenzie, Consultant Psychiatrist, Sheffield Care Trust, Sheffield, UK

Ghazala Mir, Senior Research Fellow, Centre for Research in Primary Care, University of Leeds, Leeds, UK

Ada Montgomery, Behavioural Outreach Nurse, Doncaster & South Humber Health Care NHS Trust, St Catherines, Tickhill Road, Doncaster, UK

Mark Powell, Chief Executive, IMBY, 53 Mowbray Street, Sheffield, UK

Raghu Raghavan, Senior Lecturer in Learning Disabilities, School of Health Studies, University of Bradford, Unity Building, 25 Trinity Road, Bradford, UK

Paul Ramcharan, Reader, School of Nursing & Midwifery, University of Sheffield, Northern General Hospital, Herries Road, Sheffield, UK

Malcolm Richardson, Head of Department – Mental Health and Learning Disability, School of Nursing & Midwifery, University of Sheffield, Humphry Davy House, Golden Smithies Lane, Wath-on-Dearne, Rotherham, UK

Bronwyn Roberts, Lecturer, School of Nursing & Midwifery, University of Sheffield, Humphry Davy House, Golden Smithies Lane, Wath-on-Dearne, Rotherham, UK

Philippa Russell, Commissioner with the Disability Rights Commission **and Disability Policy Adviser** to the National Children's Bureau, National Children's Bureau, 8 Wakley Street, London, UK

Jayne Stapleton, Principal Counsellor, Counselling & Psychology Services, Chesterfield Primary Care Trust, Ashgreen, Ashgate Road, Chesterfield, UK

Kirsten Stalker, Reader, Social Work Research Centre, University of Stirling, Stirling, UK

Lesley Styring, Consultant Nurse, Rivermead Unit, Sheffield Care Trust, Northern General Hospital, Herries Road, Sheffield, UK

John Taylor, Professor of Developmental Disability Psychology, Centre for Clinical Psychology & Health Care Research, Northumbria University, Coach Lane Campus, Benton, Newcastle upon Tyne, UK

Irene Tuffrey-Wijne, Palliative Care Nurse Specialist, Department of Mental Health & Learning Disability, St George's Hospital Medical School, Jenner Wing, Cranmer Terrace, London, UK

Sally Twist, Clinical Psychologist, Psychological Health Care, Learning Disability Service, Barnsley Primary Care Trust, Kendray Hospital, Doncaster Road, Barnsley, UK

Jan Walmsley, Assistant Director, The Health Foundation and Visiting **Professor in the History of Learning Disability**, Open University, 90 Long Acre, London, UK

Acknowledgements

When as editors we started to work on ideas for this textbook we were daunted by both its scope and scale. Having elected to emphasize the importance of both life cycle issues and also personal, social and environmental factors in the everyday lives of people with learning disabilities, it was clear that contributions from many people would be required. We were helped substantially in our task by the School of Nursing and Midwifery at the University of Sheffield who gave us the time and support to bring this text to fruition. The support of the university has been equalled by the goodwill and humour of the contributors to the 34 chapters in this volume, many of whom have responded with patience to our requests for editorial changes.

Many of the contributors have spent substantial amounts of time undertaking research or providing services to and for people with learning disabilities. Although the people with learning disabilities and their families, advocates, support workers and friends remain individually anonymous in this volume, we nevertheless hope that their voices can be heard throughout the text. We express our gratitude to them for sharing their knowledge and for their help and cooperation.

A project of this scale would not have been possible without the commitment and guidance of key people, first at Open University Press and later at McGraw-Hill. In this regard we are particularly indebted to Jacinta Evans, Rachel Gear and Jenni Harvey. Finally, Tracy Meredith, in her usual efficient way, has acted as design chief, coordinator and troubleshooter throughout the process and deserves more than just a medal for putting up with our sometimes unreasonable editorial demands.

PART ONE
The construction of learning disability

At the start of each Part in this book, the editors provide a content guide to the section and, by reviewing the chapters individually, identify some of the main themes and learning outcomes. In Parts Two to Five the first chapter of each is a narrative account which places the voice of people with learning disabilities across the life cycle at the forefront of our interest in their lives. By hearing their voice first the following chapters can be read against their interests and experiences. These chapters seek to establish the evidence base in terms of contemporary knowledge, as well as providing practice-based knowledge, information and advice.

To identify our subject matter for this volume as 'people with learning disabilities' may seem unproblematic. It is not.

Over the past century and a half there have been huge changes in the labelling of those people we presently categorize as having learning disabilities. In social policy terms, they have been variously labelled as 'vagabonds', 'idiots', 'mentally subnormal', 'mentally handicapped', 'learning disabled' and 'people with learning difficulties' among other names. Each of these labels has been the product of 'warranted ascription' by others – i.e. labels applied by interests who hold the power to define others and who, through their power, claim the label to be warranted. Needless to say, the 'official' label at any one point in time has harnessed and supported the development and growth of 'an industry of professionals' whose work has been based upon these varying definitions.

You will find in Part One that, historically, the separation of people with learning disabilities from the 'mainstream' (i.e. from everybody else), features among other things: placing them into the same category as other unemployable people who receive alms; seeing them as a threat to the national gene pool and hence placing them 'around the bend' (out of sight in institutions), separated by gender or sterilized to avoid procreation; medicalizing them and seeing them as 'cases' to be treated predominantly through biomedical interventions; viewing them as the focus of rehabilitation and social programmes; and only latterly defining them through their own efforts as 'people first' with the same rights as others.

The history of people with learning disabilities has not always been a pleasant one and nor have their life experiences. Their place within various categories has changed across the ages but each 'warranted ascription', though superseded, has left within contemporary policy and practice a residue of the past. In making these points it is essential therefore to see present definitions and practice as occupying just one historical point in time. It is also necessary in these respects to ask ourselves what values are driving definitions and what effect this is likely to have on the people we now label as having 'learning disabilities'.

It is the aim of the eight chapters in Part One of this book to review the varying constructions of learning disability historically and to help you think about whether the contents of the following parts of the book themselves create our present history as a 'warranted ascription'.

In Chapter 1, Dorothy Atkinson establishes why life stories and narrative accounts by people with learning disabilities matter, how such accounts have come to be told and the practical and ethical dilemmas of such work. From uncovering history through people's personal experiences to the development of a personal identity that provides a means of reclaiming their lives and planning for the future, the chapter provides a voice of hope and of reason. The life story accounts in this chapter highlight humanity at its most sublime and instruct the reader to see:

- the ways in which people with learning disabilities as expert witnesses have related the rich variety of their experience and diversity of life histories;
- resilience in the face of seemingly insurmountable odds as well as liberation from institutional practices;
- the development and maintenance of meaningful and loving relationships in the face of exclusion;
- the development of a sense of identity through storytelling that liberates people from their past and produces in them hope for their future;
- the importance of storytelling and how it can be facilitated.

The history of people with learning disabilities stretches beyond those who can give living testimony and Chapters 2, 4 and 6 provide historical evidence to fill this gap. In the first of these, Chapter 2, Alex McClimens considers the early emergence of the state's intervention in the lives of people with learning disabilities from social policy objectives under the Poor Laws of the nineteenth century to the early twentieth century. It is shown graphically how the conception of what we now term 'learning disability' established professional interests and indeed how such definitions were a product of key thinkers over the ages. Each of these 'ages of reason' was ultimately superseded. This leaves us with the conclusion that learning disability is not a 'fact' but, rather, a 'social construction'. The chapter will therefore:

- recount the history of how people with learning disabilities under the early Poor Laws and show how they came to be seen as separate from other 'indigent' and 'unemployable' groups;
- relate how the growth of scientific thinking had a crucial effect on defining people with learning disabilities and, under such definitions, the appropriate professional inputs;
- show that science and definition are not value-free, that definitions are therefore a 'social construction' based on unspoken values;
- ask the reader to reflect upon their own and present-day values that apply to the provision of services and to the place of people with learning disabilities in contemporary society.

McClimens' chapter finishes at around the time when the medical hegemony in relation to the treatment of people with learning disabilities was at its height. The biomedical approach has come a long way since that time and is arguably in a constructive debate with the emergent social model of disability about what it is to be a person with a learning disability. The movement towards a social model of learning disabilities in the past 20 years or so often seeks to dismiss the biomedical model as creating the label 'learning disability' and as being a primary source of exploitation. In Chapter 3, Fiona Mackenzie relates how a bio-psycho-social account is constructed within the medical profession. The source of different terminology in categorizing people with learning disabilities is outlined alongside the means through which diagnoses are made. Two case studies establish how, by using the medical categorizations of Down's syndrome and Prader-Willi syndrome appropriately, it is possible to improve the health and life quality of those so labelled. In an age in which the social model seems to have an ascendancy, this chapter urges the reader to:

- see the importance to social inclusion of the bio-psycho-social model in recognizing medical and health care needs;
- understand limitations in common forms of medical classification and diagnostic criteria in classifying forms and levels of impairment;
- understand the struggles at different stages of the life cycle, from neonate to late adult life, of applying a diagnosis and developing an appropriate intervention;
- develop (in non-medical practitioners) an understanding of the ways in which the bio-psycho-social model can be used to improve health and life quality.

In Chapter 4, Malcolm Richardson sets about critiquing the eugenic, segregationist perspective on disability and establishing some of the basic arguments that underlie the social model. This chapter aims to assist the reader to recognize, appreciate and understand the extent to which disability is socially determined and the role, therefore, of ideology in shaping either enabling responses to people with impairments, or responses that can disable to the point of death. More specifically, the chapter asserts that:

- disability and incapacity are not the inevitable products of an impairment such as a learning disability but, rather, of a society's ideological responses to people with an impairment;
- there have been, over history, inappropriate and segregationist ideologies that have led to models of containment and eugenics;
- forms of insidious eugenics and segregation remain within contemporary society;
- there has been a recent move towards a human rights model and that the disabled people's rights movement is playing a major role in the struggle for socioeconomic, health, educational and recreational inclusion of people with learning disabilities;
- disabling aspects of service delivery need to be transformed into services that enable and empower people.

The chapters in Part One show a substantial movement in the ways we think about people with learning disabilities and their place as citizens. In Chapter 5, Alison Brammer brings to our attention the various ways in which the law is changing in its view of people with learning disabilities. The relevance of the law is applied by Brammer to legal definitions of learning disability and to issues concerning capacity, decision-making and the relevance of human rights. The reader will:

- learn the exceptions to the rule that people with learning disabilities are treated no differently under the law;
- learn the definitions applied to people with learning disabilities for the purposes of the law;
- understand the importance of 'capacity' and how it is applied in decision-making;
- become conversant with articles of the newly-implemented Human Rights Act and how it can be applied.

The place of professionals over the past 150 years occupies the interest of Eric Emerson in Chapter 6, with a focus on their accommodation. The chapter offers an account of the patchy and extreme conditions in which some people with learning disabilities were housed under the Poor Laws of the nineteenth century, the development of the 'educational' model within large institutions up to the 1960s and the incremental move towards deinstitutionalization and community care that has culminated in the UK policy of closing all long-stay hospitals by 2006. In reviewing empirical evidence about contemporary community residential options a note of caution is sounded about how we might best assess different community residential options, pointing to the contingent relation between service provision and outcome. In this chapter we are guided to:

- understand our present service delivery and residential options as products of a long history;
- explore the real degradation, exploitation and misery of many people

with learning disabilities pre-institutionalization and then within the emergent hospital sectors;

- question, using the evidence, the assumptions we presently hold about how service design and delivery affect outcomes and impact;
- make judgements, on the basis of empirical data, about the relative merits of different residential options for people with learning disabilities in contemporary society.

Taken consecutively the chapters in Part One demonstrate substantial moves in services. In Chapter 7, Lesley Styring and Gordon Grant summarize the ways in which services now organize to establish the quality of service that is provided. The contemporary focus is on quality of life, the intended outcome, standards, equity and quality of service provision. These intentions are not unproblematic, so the authors outline some of the questions that remain about these models and the balance between outcomes, risk and the interests of service providers. The reader will:

- learn to use critically the concept of 'quality of life' as a measure for judging service inputs;
- see the ways in which government policy has led to a preoccupation with risk and with clinical governance;
- understand how services operationalize and measure service quality;
- learn how quality of life and service quality might be related to each other within practice settings.

In Chapter 1, Dorothy Atkinson made a strong case for hearing the voice of people with learning disabilities through narratives. Moving from narrative to 'voice' as a 'political' tool, Dan Goodley and Paul Ramcharan review in Chapter 8 the development of advocacy over the past 40 years. Identifying the different forms of advocacy and the limits of professional involvement in this arena, they argue that advocacy itself has a history that has increasingly moved from professional and service orientations towards one in which the voice of people with learning disabilities is fully reclaimed. This is best represented in the growing campaigning role that has, they argue, emerged over time out of the self-advocacy movement. Having read this chapter the reader will:

- be able to distinguish different forms of advocacy;
- understand the limits to professional involvement within advocacy;
- have a clear idea about how the historical development of advocacy demonstrates a consistent move towards people with learning disabilities reclaiming their voice as 'people first';
- see how campaigning represents a relationship between interests shared by people with learning difficulties and other groups.

We hope you will enjoy Part One of this book. At the end you might ask yourself what values you feel underlie your view about people with learning disabilities and the extent to which the chapters have influenced that view.

1

Narratives and people with learning disabilities

Dorothy Atkinson

Introduction

Everyone has a story to tell. However, an *entire* life story is rarely told. Instead, it is recounted in a series of oral narratives, or stories, told throughout the life as it is lived (Linde 1993). Only rarely is the full account written down as a life story or autobiography. The written and published autobiography is, of course, mostly the preserve of the rich and famous. And yet other lives matter too, especially where they shed light on otherwise neglected or hidden areas of social life. This chapter aims to switch the focus away from celebrity stories to celebrating and understanding the life stories of people with learning disabilities.

Not surprisingly, perhaps, there are relatively few published life stories, or autobiographies, written or commissioned by people with learning disabilities. Perhaps the best known is Joey Deacon's story, *Tongue Tied* (1974), which was also made into a television play. This is a particularly good example of someone who decided to write his own life story. As he was unable to write, and had difficulty in speaking, Deacon could only produce his book with the help of three friends who were also long-stay residents in St Lawrence's Hospital in Caterham, Surrey. They formed a writing team and the autobiography was written in a slow, laborious and painstaking way. In spite of Deacon's personal and social circumstances at the time, his account is primarily about the nice and ordinary things in life – family, friends, holidays, birthdays and so on – and not about the segregated world of the long-stay hospital.

There are other examples of life stories, or autobiographies, by people with learning disabilities: *The World of Nigel Hunt* (1967); *My Life Story* (1991) by Malcolm Burnside; *A Price To Be Born* (1996) by David Barron; and Mabel Cooper's 'Life Story' (1997). In addition to the single life stories are the collected narratives and autobiographies in anthologies, such as '*Know Me As I Am*' (Atkinson and Williams 1990) and *Positive Tales* (Living

Archive 1996). The first of these was an important landmark because it contained the life stories, many originally in oral form, of around 200 people with learning disabilities. The anthology, '*Know Me As I Am*', demonstrated through its unique size, scope and diversity that people with learning disabilities could, with support, tell their stories in their own words or images.

In the book, people with learning disabilities portrayed themselves as fully rounded and complex human beings. In their own accounts, they were people with distinct personal histories and a wealth of experiences to talk about. Together the anthology contributors brought out the differences and the commonalities between their lives and the lives of other people in society, and they included the ordinary, the everyday and the mundane as well as stories of loss, separation and segregation.

This chapter explores more fully why life stories matter, especially to people with learning disabilities. It also traces the influences that have come together to make life stories important now, and reviews the ways in which life stories come to be told. Finally, the chapter draws out some of the ethical and practical issues of life story work, and considers what implications they may have for practice.

Exercise 1.1

Think about times when you tell other people about your life. Why is that important to you? Why is it important to the people you are telling?

Why life stories matter

Life stories matter to everyone – they enable us to express our sense of self, conveying to others who we are and how we got that way (Linde 1993; Widdershoven 1993). Life stories, and the narratives that make them up, are oral stories, told to another person or audience at various points in time. They may be rehearsed and refined and, over time, may be revised. Life stories, and the opportunity to tell them, are particularly important for people with learning disabilities because often they have been silent, or silenced, while other people – families, practitioners, historians – have spoken on their behalf. Life stories begin to redress that balance as they become a means by which people with learning disabilities have a voice that is theirs. Chapters 9, 14, 22 and 30 of this volume provide such narratives. The narratives provide the 'voice' against which the following chapters can be read. But life stories can do more, as discussed below.

The life story conveys a sense of identity, enabling the teller or author to experience and convey a sense of who they are. When the life story is written down it becomes something to show other people, a point made by Mabel

Cooper in reflecting on hers: 'You've got something to show for your life. You've got something so that you can say, "That's what happened to me". It will keep history in my mind for years to come, what's happened to me and a lot of others like me' (Atkinson 1998: 115). Mabel Cooper's life story is no 'ordinary' story; it took me – as the researcher/facilitator – just as it takes its readers, into a separate and segregated world of children's homes and long-stay institutions. The process of telling the story was important to Mabel in making sense of history – not just her own personal history ('what's happened to me') but the history of many thousands of people who, like her, were labelled and excluded from everyday life. The end product, the written story, is 'something to show' for a life lived to a large extent in a separate world.

Following Mabel Cooper's introductory statement, it is possible to claim that the life stories of people with learning disabilities are important for a number of reasons. In particular, they:

- help us trace an otherwise hidden history;
- treat people as 'expert witnesses';
- enable people to represent themselves as fully-rounded human beings;
- show the beginnings of a resistance movement;
- encourage historical awareness and reflexivity.

We will now consider each of these points in turn.

Tracing a hidden history of learning disability

On the whole, people with learning disabilities have been silent and invisible in the historical accounts of learning disability policy and practice (Ryan and Thomas 1981). Indeed, most people with learning disabilities were silent and invisible in real life too, to such an extent that the degradation of their lives in the long-stay hospitals went unrecorded for many years. That such inhumanity was possible was attributed to their very invisibility and silence (Oswin 1978; Ryan and Thomas 1981; Shearer 1981). In a sense, these were forgotten people, leading forgotten lives, so that the telling of their stories became a social and historical imperative (Atkinson *et al.* 1997; Potts 1998).

The fact that much of the history of people with learning disabilities – prior to the coming of the life story – was hidden, put it on a par with other hidden histories such as women's history or the history of mental health survivors or black people. The argument in favour of articulating and revealing these hidden histories is that it makes possible the development of a group's sense of their own personal and collective identity – it raises awareness of what the past has meant, not just to individuals but to a whole group or category of people (Williams and Walmsley 1990).

The telling of history by historians has tended, in the learning disability field – as elsewhere – to rely on documentary sources. Such a historical account loses the 'richness and complexity' of lived historical experience as told through people's life stories (Rolph 1999). Without their own written accounts and, until recently, their own oral accounts, people with learning disabilities were seen as a people with 'no history' (Prins 1991). The development of methods that support people in the telling of their life stories (such as oral history techniques) has meant that 'more history' (new insights into history) and 'anti-history' (another set of stories or understandings which challenge conventional perceptions) (Frisch 1990) can now be told and recorded.

Treating people as expert witnesses

Life stories can act as 'a counterbalance' to other accounts (Williams 1993). Often these other accounts have focused on pathological differences or deficits/defects or, through case records, have given a very limited view of people's lives. The life story, or autobiography, allows for a richer and more rounded account. Williams also suggests that life stories act as a counterbalance in other directions too – tempering the professional orientation of normalization, for example, and 'the "victim" approach of many of the well-intentioned revelations of the worst aspects of institutional life' (1993: 57).

In public life more generally, people with learning disabilities are seen as people who have to be cared for – they are the disregarded and excluded, 'the other' (Walmsley 2000: 195). However, in telling their life stories they are historical witnesses and, as stated earlier, they portray themselves as complex and complete human beings. In telling their own stories, and representing their own lives, people with learning disabilities are also engaged in the telling of a shared and collective history of an oppressed group in society.

Life stories are the means by which people with learning disabilities are able to recall, recount and review their lives, often in depth (Booth and Booth 1998). Such an approach treats people as 'expert witnesses' in the matter of their own lives (Birren and Deutchman 1991). This is in contrast with a more usual view of people with learning disabilities as 'sources of data' for researchers' own narratives, rather than people with personal stories to tell (Booth and Booth 1996). Being the author of their own story can be especially important for those people with learning disabilities who, because of their segregated lives, have none of the usual 'stock of stories' – from family, friends and community – nor the everyday documents, photographs and memorabilia of family life, from which to draw in order to make sense of their lives (Gillman *et al.* 1997). This makes the telling of their own story even more compelling and empowering. What is needed is the time, space and context in which life stories can be told because, when that happens, the process not only enables people to regain their past but it 'also helps them towards a future' (Thompson 1988: 265).

Enabling people to represent themselves as fully-rounded human beings

It has been argued that people who lack a history are at risk of having a history, and an identity, imposed upon them (Sutcliffe and Simons 1993;

Gillman *et al.* 1997). The objectification of people with learning disabilities as 'other' is due in part to this lack of history (Ramcharan *et al.* 1997). Seen as an homogenous group, they are defined by their learning disability and their behaviour in their case records, in a 'ritual of exclusion' (White and Epston 1990).

By way of contrast, the life story that is initiated and told by the person concerned holds the greatest potential for self-representation. It allows people with learning disabilities to represent themselves as human beings above all and to develop their own accounts of family life, schooldays, relationships and so on. The telling of the stories, or narratives, that make up the life story that has and is being lived involves a life review, and enables the storyteller to emerge as a person rather than a 'case'. This enhances the sense of personal identity and is an empowering process. The capacity of people to remember, and recount, who they have been, and to know where they have come from, helps shape their sense of self or identity in the present (Thomson 1999). Life stories can be seen as 'explanatory narratives' which play a crucial role in shaping everyday life (Giddens 1991). People with learning disabilities who have been involved in telling their story attest to the positive affirmation of identity which this has given them: 'We are self-advocates who are running workshops on "telling your life story" for people with learning disabilities. We have both been supported to write our own life stories and want to help others to do theirs' (Able and Cooper 2000: 7).

Beginning a resistance movement

How can life stories be part of a resistance movement? There are two ways in which this becomes a possibility. One is that people, when telling their own stories, actually demonstrate their resistance in the face of adversity (Goodley 1996). In the telling of their stories, they do not portray themselves solely as victims but as people who had – in some situations – a measure of resistance against the forces of oppression. From their own accounts, they resisted, they fought back and they mocked the people, and the systems, which sought to control them (Potts and Fido 1991; Sibley 1995; Goodley 1996; Stuart 1998, 2002; Rolph 1999). Fighting back is one way to become a 'border crosser' from a segregated life to an inclusive one in the mainstream of society (Ramcharan *et al.* 1997; Rolph 1999).

The other way for life stories to be part of a resistance movement (Gillman *et al.* 1997) is where individual and collective accounts connect to tell a different, and more complex, story of people's lives. Put together, life stories become historical documents, between them mapping the events of the twentieth century. The authors emerge, in their accounts, not only as victims of an oppressive system but as people who survived it, and were actors in their own lives. They showed resilience in the face of adversity; agency in the shaping of their lives; and a capacity to reflect on how, and why, they survived (see Chapter 15 for further discussion of resilience).

Encouraging historical awareness and reflexivity

Life stories can bring with them historical awareness – an understanding of one's own history and the history of others. This involves developing a greater personal awareness of history, and of how past policies and practices have shaped people's lives. The telling of the life story also allows the narrator to stand back and develop reflexivity, to begin to explicate their own history as part of the wider history of people with learning disabilities.

These are points echoed by Mabel Cooper in reflecting on the importance of her (written and published) life story:

> I think it was nice for me to be able to do something, so that I could say 'I've done it'. It made me feel that it was something I had done. You've got something so that you can say, 'This is what happened to me'. Some of it hurts, some of it's sad, some of it I'd like to remember. My story means a lot to me because I can say, 'This is what happened to me', if anyone asks. So it's great, and I will keep it for the rest of my life. I will keep the book.
>
> (Atkinson *et al.* 1997: 11)

The suggestion here is that working on her life story has enabled Mabel to start to make sense of her life, and to put past events into perspective (life review). In addition, she is able to tell other people what it was like to live a separate and segregated life – to be a historical witness. The written word is important in this context: it is enduring, and it is 'something to show' for the life that has been led.

The telling of the individual story in the context of other people's lives, and the wider social and political history of the time has enabled some people with learning disabilities to develop historical awareness. This has brought in its wake a sense of a collective history of people with learning disabilities. The life stories, in this sense, are historical documents which tell the 'insider' story of the history of learning disability.

Exercise 1.2

Think of one or two people with learning disabilities with whom you work or have worked. What do you know of their history? From what sources does that history come? Is there anything else you might want to know that would help you in your support role?

Why life stories have come into prominence now

There are three key factors, in particular, that help explain how and why life stories have come into prominence as a late twentieth and early twenty-first century phenomenon: normalization, participatory research and self-advocacy. First, we look briefly at the influence of normalization ideas. The people who were involved in the life story research that underpins this chapter have all, at some point in their lives, been labelled and segregated, often in long-stay hospitals. The changed climate of ideas which may be attributed to normalization brought about a two-way shift in practice. On the one hand, people with learning disabilities were leaving the long-stay hospitals and, in that sense, were more accessible to researchers. On the other hand, researchers were increasingly able to see people with learning disabilities as potential participants in research. And although normalization supports citizen advocacy more directly than self-advocacy, nevertheless it helped create the conditions in which 'speaking up' became possible (Walmsley 2001). Indeed the recent development in learning disability research, where people are in 'valued' research roles, such as respondent, interviewee, oral historian and so on, has been attributed to normalization's insistence on valued social roles; similarly, the researcher in some post-normalization research is seen as an advocate, as well as a researcher, a development also attributed to the legacy of normalization (Walmsley 2001; Walmsley and Johnson 2003).

Second, the growth in popularity of participatory research in learning disability has also played a part in bringing life stories to prominence. Life story work is by its very nature participatory, as it involves a person, or a group of people, in a very active process of storytelling. Participatory research lends itself well to engaging people in the various stages of the research process, and it changes the social relations of research, making it a partnership rather than a hierarchical relationship.

Participatory research can also lay claim to bringing about change, especially when applied to researching history where it involves people who might otherwise be cast as victims in understanding and 'taking charge' of their history, becoming actors in it (Westerman 1998: 230). Participatory research, in these terms, can be seen as part of the struggle of disabled people – in this instance people with learning disabilities – to name oppression and counter it; to develop a historical awareness of their situation and the situation of others (Freire 1986). The capacity of participatory research to encourage and support the empowerment of people with learning disabilities makes it an attractive option both for researchers and participants, and helps explain how it has become an important development for learning disability research (Chappell 2000).

Third, self-advocacy can be seen as a factor in the growth of interest in life stories. This may be because it has grown alongside the development of research studies which aimed to include the views of people with learning disabilities (Walmsley 1995). This could be seen as a reciprocal link. On the one hand, it could be argued that self-advocacy influenced researchers by demonstrating not only that people with learning disabilities *wanted* to 'speak up' but that they *could do so*. On the other hand, it seemed likely that self-advocacy influenced the people who were involved in it, showing them the value of research and giving them the confidence to take part.

It is at least in part through the emergence of self-advocacy that people with learning disabilities have begun to speak up about their experiences and lives; to tell their life stories (see Chapter 8). In this context, people with learning disabilities have started to articulate their experience of being labelled, or categorized, as different. Alongside the growth of the self-advocacy movement has been the steady stream of autobiographies (already referred to) by people with learning disabilities, where people have told their own stories, with or without the help of a facilitator.

Life story research has been made possible in part through self-advocacy, and the interest of people within the movement in telling their stories. Where people tell their own stories, they are inevitably more complex than the stories told by others on their behalf. As stated earlier, they cast themselves as fully rounded human beings not as the perpetrators of social ills, as the eugenicists portrayed them (Abbot and Sapsford 1987; Williams 1989); nor as solely the victims of an oppressive system, as they are portrayed in the normalization literature (Wolfensberger 1975).

How life stories come to be told

In essence, life stories are told through a 'mixed method' approach, drawing on the techniques of oral history, life history and narrative inquiry. They may be told on a one-to-one basis, with the interviewer/researcher being the audience – or told in a group setting where the researcher and the peer group form a combined audience. The development of oral history from the 1960s provided a means by which the accounts of ordinary people could be recorded and preserved as historical documents in their own right (Thompson 1988; Bornat 1989). Oral history involves people remembering and recalling past personal and social events. It enables people to 'put a stamp on the past' – thus helping authenticate the account and the person (Bornat 1994). Oral history also provided the means by which people in oppressed groups (e.g. women, black people and disabled people) could record, document and reclaim their individual and shared histories (e.g. see Rowbotham 1973, and the rewriting of women's history). The reclaiming of history in this way can be seen as a way of resisting the accounts and interpretations of others, and celebrating a distinctive identity (Walmsley 1998).

Alongside the growth in popularity of oral history has been the re-emergence of life history research, which seeks to draw out and compile individual auto/biographies. The life history/narrative tradition in sociology can be traced back to the work of the Chicago School in the USA in the 1920s, in particular to the work of Thomas and Znaniecki (1918–20). The approach flourished in the 1920s and 1930s, then declined, but re-emerged in the 1980s and flourished again in the 1990s (Stanley 1992; Gillman *et al.* 1997; Rolph 1999). In an influential text, Plummer (1983) argued for the reinclusion of life history methods in sociological research, and Maines

(1993: 17) noted that the 'narrative's moment' had arrived in social science methods of inquiry. This reflects a more general move towards what Booth and Booth (1996) have called the 'age of biography', including storytelling and narrative methods of research.

Life story research sheds light on history by making possible the telling of insider accounts by people on the 'fringes' or margins of society, accounts which are grounded in real-life human experience (Booth and Booth 1994). In learning disability research, however, researchers needed to overcome barriers such as 'inarticulateness, unresponsiveness, a concrete frame of reference and problems with time' (Booth and Booth 1996: 55). Although life stories tell the stories of individuals, they are part of a wider social, historical and political context. In that sense, they form a bridge between the individual and society, showing up the structural features of people's social worlds (Booth and Booth 1998). Thus, life story methods allow for 'listening beyond' the words of the informant to the world around and beyond the person (Bertaux-Wiame 1981): to other people in similar situations, and to the networks of the wider society to which they belong. The common threads which emerge from life story research reveal how individual lives are shaped and constrained by the social world – and historical era – in which they are situated (Goodley 1996; Booth and Booth 1998).

Life story research (including both oral and life history methods) is now being used in the learning disability field. However, it is a recent development and the literature is relatively sparse. The slow take-up of life story research in the area of learning disability is due to the fact that it was seen to require people who could articulate and reflect on their experiences (Plummer 1983; Thompson 1988). This meant that people with learning disabilities were not included until relatively recent work began to show that barriers could be overcome and that life story research methods have much to offer in the telling and recording of learning disability history (e.g. see Booth and Booth 1994, 1996, 1998; Goodley 1996; Rolph 1999; Stuart 2002).

The role of the researcher is important in enabling people to tell history 'in their own words'. This, however, may be problematic as some people with learning disabilities may not easily find the words with which to recount their stories. What is emerging in the literature is the need sometimes to co-construct accounts with people where the words are hard to find, and where researchers have to listen to silences and proceed using 'creative guesswork' (Booth and Booth 1996) or the strategy of 'successive approximation' (Biklen and Moseley 1988). The fact that someone is inarticulate is no reason to exclude them, as that panders to the 'deficit' model of disability (Booth and Booth 1996). Instead, the challenge is to overcome the barriers to involvement through sensitivity and innovation on the part of the researcher (Ward 1997). 'Guided tours' of familiar places and 'guided conversations', using props such as photographs and drawings, may be needed in order to dismantle the barriers (Stalker 1998).

Inclusive methods involve the researcher working closely with the oral or

---

Exercise 1.3

Think about a person with learning disabilities who you work with. How would you enable that person to 'tell their story'? What approaches would you use? What places would you visit? Where else might you look for information?

---

life historian to enable them to tell their story (see Chapter 34 for a discussion of inclusive research methods). A 'feeling human observer' (Booth and Booth 1994: 36) is needed not only to facilitate the proceedings, but also to observe the consistency and coherence of the stories as they emerge. The researcher needs to be reflexive and self-aware: to facilitate stories, not to take them over; to work with people, not to exploit them; and to 'listen beyond' words, not speak for people (Goodley 1996). Echoing this, Ristock and Pennell (1996) recommend constant self-monitoring by the researcher as a safeguard against making and acting on unwarranted assumptions about the research participants.

The closeness of contact between the researcher and the oral or life historian can result in what Ramcharan and Grant (1994) have called 'reverse commodification', where the researcher becomes involved in the lives of people with learning disabilities – acting as advocate, scribe or supporter as well as researcher. Similarly, where people with learning disabilities are unable to articulate or elaborate on their experiences, the researcher may become their interpreter or biographer (Goodley 1996). Close and prolonged involvement between researcher and participants can continue long after the research has ended (Booth 1998).

Compiling individual life stories

A classic approach to co-constructing a life story is to work directly with the person who wants to tell it. This applied to my work with Mabel Cooper, some of whose words have already been quoted in this chapter. Our work together started when Mabel asked me to help her write her life story. We met at her home where she talked to me about her childhood in children's homes, her subsequent move to St Lawrence's Hospital and her later life in the community, including her work in the self-advocacy movement. We tape-recorded our conversations and I later transcribed them word for word. From those question-and-answer transcripts, I prepared a more flowing and chronological account which I then read back to Mabel for confirmation or amendment. The readings triggered more memories which were themselves woven into the emerging story. The result was initially a private publication for Mabel and her friends, but subsequently the life story was published in a book (Cooper 1997) and placed on the internet.

As suggested above, the autobiographical process enabled Mabel to make sense of her life and to see it in a wider social context. In telling her life story, she was not only reclaiming her past, she was at the same time reflecting on the social history of learning disability in the second half of the twentieth century. The extract below combines personal history with period detail. Here, Mabel recalls how and why she came to leave the children's home in Bedford to move to St Lawrence's Hospital:

> I moved to St Lawrence's when I was seven, because they only took children what went to school in this home. And I never went to school, so I had to move. In them days they give you a test. You went to London or somewhere because they'd give you a test before they make you go anywhere. It used to be a big place, all full of offices and what-have-you. Because they said you should be able to read when you're seven or eight. I couldn't read, I hadn't been to school. That was 1952, I was seven years old . . . When I first went in there, even just getting out of the car you could hear the racket. You think you're going to a madhouse. When you first went there you could hear people screaming and shouting outside. It was very noisy but I think you do get used to them after a little while because it's like everywhere that's big. If there's a lot of people you get a lot of noise, and they had like big dormitories, didn't they?
>
> (Cooper 1997: 22)

There seems little doubt that Mabel gained historical awareness and understanding through the process of compiling her life story – and there seems little doubt that the finished product brought with it a great sense of achievement. The experience of being an autobiographer has proved a rewarding one. Mabel is well aware of her role as a historical witness, a role which entails letting people know what life was like for her and others in the past. In one of our many subsequent conversations about the meaning and significance of her life story, Mabel pinpointed both the sense of personal achievement it brought for her and its importance as a historical record of the past:

> It's an achievement with me being in St Lawrence's for so many years, and not knowing anything else but St Lawrence's. I thought it would be nice to let people know what it was like, and to let people know how difficult it was for someone with a learning disability, and who was stuck away because of that. I thought that people outside should know these things because they're not aware of it at the moment and I think it would be nice.
>
> (Atkinson *et al.* 1997: 9)

The compilation of Mabel's life story, initially from memory, pinpointed many gaps. She was left with unanswered questions such as: Who was she? Who were her parents? What had become of them? Mabel's need to know led her into a search for documentary evidence from her own case records and from the archived papers of the institutions where she had spent her childhood and much of her adult life. Such a quest seemed daunting at times, and some of the language of the past proved hurtful, but the need to know became a strong driving force. Consequently, we visited together the records of the Lifecare Trust, the London Metropolitan Archives and the Bedfordshire record office, in search of case notes, diaries, photographs, newspaper cuttings and any other documentary evidence of the time. The successful location and access to personal records for Mabel (and sub-sequently the four other people who later became involved in what is now known as the Life History Project) meant that many long-forgotten – or never known – areas of life were revealed. Since those early visits with Mabel, the life story process with other people with learning disabilities invariably includes whatever written accounts of the time can be unearthed, the aim being to confirm key dates, times, places and people. It is important to note, though, that these records are not simply 'there', waiting to be perused, they have to be searched for and then accessed, mediated and understood.

Mabel's involvement in the 'telling' of the history of learning disability owes much to the development of the self-advocacy movement, which has enabled her and other people to 'speak up' about themselves and their lives. She and others in the life story research were, or are, self-advocates; their capacity to 'speak up' in self-advocacy groups has enabled them to speak up in the telling of their life stories. Just as self-advocacy is about self-representation, so too is the recounting of the life story. It enables people to make sense of their own lives but also to understand their lives in relation to those of other people. This has proved to be, for Mabel and others, an empowering process.

Using group work for storytelling

An alternative to individual work is to invite people to join a group. This was an approach I used in what came to be known as the Past Times Project – an approach which aimed to capture, if possible, the richness of individual accounts but to do so within what I hoped would prove to be the more insightful and reflective mode of a group setting. The Past Times Project involved a group of people with learning disabilities recalling and reflecting on their past lives. The group consisted of nine people; seven men and two women. The age range was 57 to 77, with most participants being in their late sixties or early seventies. Potential group members were approached, and invited to join, via the staff of the special residential and day settings of which they were currently users. The group met over a two-year period, each meeting lasting an hour and, with permission, being tape-recorded and later transcribed. This is where oral history techniques proved invaluable as I was able to use reminiscence and recall to enable group members to talk about their past lives.

At the time, this was set up as a history project which would cover not only the history of difference (exclusion, separation and incarceration) but also the history of sameness. The research participants were, accordingly, invited to remember and share the ordinary and everyday experiences of their lives; to recall happy memories as well as sad ones and to see their lives as part of the unfolding and wider history of the twentieth century. Against this backdrop, of course, emerged the histories of difference, where people's lives diverged from the ordinary and the everyday.

The Past Times Project used a group setting in order to provide a supportive and friendly atmosphere where (sometimes) painful memories could be shared, and to provide a forum where one person's memories of past events would spark off memories in other people. The group format in the end worked well in that the group eventually became that supportive-but-stimulating environment that I had anticipated. But it took time, practice and patience to reach that point. Early group meetings were characterized at times by silence and, at other times, by anarchic cross-talking and multiple side conversations. Some members loved to hold the floor and recount extended anecdotes whereas others seemed content to sit quietly, venturing little. Various memory triggers were used, ranging from the simple, 'Do you remember . . .?' to the use of professionally produced reminiscence slides and tapes, and our own authentic cigarette cards, photographs and other memorabilia of the time.

Running the group was never easy. There were problems of communication throughout our meetings, as it was often difficult for me to understand the words and content of many of the contributions, even when the tapes were replayed later at home. One or two staff members from the day and residential services, who knew group members well, helped where they could with translation and interpretation. Thus we struggled together to hear and be heard for the whole of the first year. At that point we took a break from meetings so that I could compile the numerous fragments and vignettes from the (by now) large pile of transcripts into a booklet which I entitled *Past Times*.

This booklet was, as it turned out, the first of a series of versions of 'our book' (as members preferred to call it). A series of readings from *Past Times* over a period of many weeks triggered off more and deeper memories. A second draft was compiled which incorporated these new accounts. Again, I proceeded on a series of readings from the expanded version and, again, more memories emerged. Thus a third and final version of *Past Times* was produced, reflecting the group's wish that we should produce a 'bigger and better' book rather than just a booklet (Atkinson 1993). Looking back, it seems as if the process of readings-and-amendments could have continued indefinitely with the book continuing to grow and grow. Certainly, at the time, group members were united in their wish to continue with the project rather than being persuaded to stop after two years.

As it was, the written account, *Past Times*, proved to be of immense importance to its contributors. As people with learning disabilities they had had restricted access to the written word. Yet they clearly recognized its value as a means of influencing opinion and shaping attitudes. They wanted their work to be in print because – like Mabel Cooper in another context – they wanted other people to know about them and their lives. They also saw the written word as authoritative. Their experiences were, it seemed, validated through being written down.

The book proved to be of interest to people beyond its own contributors, and their immediate circle of families and friends. No doubt this was because it offered a rich compilation of individual and shared memories. Some accounts of childhood and schooldays were quite ordinary for their time and place. Brian Sutcliffe's accounts of his northern working-class childhood in the early/mid years of the twentieth century sounded authentic for their time: 'We had a back-to-back house with a cellar and gas lights. We had a coal fire and a coal hole.'

In later years, Brian's life, and the lives of other contributors, turned out to be far from ordinary because, sooner or later, they became users of separate or segregated services. For some people, like Margaret Day, this happened in childhood, as the following extract illustrates: 'When I was a little girl I was put away. I was 14 and a half. I went to Cell Barnes to live because they said I was backward. My dad refused to sign the papers for me to go, but the police came and said he would go to prison if he didn't. I cried when I had to go with the Welfare officer.'

In addition, *Past Times* also includes shared memories of hospital life. These afford us glimpses into a hidden world hitherto described primarily in formal documents. In the following extract, George Coley recalls a well-remembered character from years ago: 'I don't know if Bert still remembers Lewis? He was a Charge Nurse. He used to have three stripes on each arm and three pips on the top of his jacket. And first thing in the morning you knew he was about. If you said anything, and he went like that [raises his arm], you knew what he meant. Bed!'

Overall, the stories told in the group had many classical 'narrative features' (Finnegan 1992: 172). They were clearly bounded and framed narratives, containing characters in addition to the narrator. They portrayed an event or episode, or a series of events and episodes, featuring a sequence of moves or actions, and were often spoken in different voices to indicate a dialogue. Sometimes the story also conveyed some sort of moral or message. In addition, the performance element of storytelling, and the audience effect, meant that the stories became more complex over time with increased exposure and practice.

Reviewing ethical and practical issues

There are, undoubtedly, important moral and ethical issues that arise in working with people with learning disabilities on their life stories. One such issue is developing a close involvement with 'vulnerable' or 'lonely' people over a period of time. In this sense, the research reported here reflects and feeds into the debates in feminist and disability literature on the dangers of exploitation in participatory research (Gluck and Patai 1991; Finnegan 1992; Ristock and Pennell 1996; Oliver 1997; Rolph 1999; Stalker 1998). Life story research also raises the complex issue of ending research, and its aftermath – the sense of loss and betrayal which may be felt by ex-participants (Ward 1997; Booth 1998; Northway 2000). In some participatory research with people with learning disabilities the option of contact continuing beyond the life of the project is built into the process. Not all participants opt for this but it is considered by some researchers to be an important safeguard, especially for people with relatively few social networks (e.g. see Booth 1998; Northway 2000).

The 'telling' of life histories involves close personal contact over time between the 'feeling human observer' and the research participants (Booth and Booth 1994). This means that self-awareness, and the capacity to be self-critical and reflective, are vital attributes in oral and life history research. The importance of researcher awareness and reflexivity is echoed in the wider literature (Goodley 1996; Ristock and Pennell 1996). The process of recording and co-constructing life histories involves telling, recording, searching (through records), revising (through 'readings') and compiling the words and fragments into a coherent whole. The researcher's role also entails 'listening beyond' the words of each life story to pick up echoes of other people's stories; to tease out the common threads which have shaped their lives; and to see the links into the networks and structures of the wider society (Bertaux-Wiame 1981; Booth and Booth 1994; Goodley 1996).

Finally, what are the implications of life story work for practice? One thing to note in this context is that nurses, care workers, social workers, occupational therapists and other people at the frontline of practice are uniquely placed to promote and support life story work not only through their existing relationships with people with learning disabilities, but also through their access to documentary and family sources. Good practice in field work emulates good practice in research. Enabling people with learning disabilities to develop a life book or multi-media profile, for example, involves the same processes of spending time and working closely with potential authors; searches for, and interrogation of, documentary sources; and the tracking down and interviewing, where appropriate, of family, friends and other significant people (Fitzgerald 1998). This is a labour-intensive process which, at its best, will feed into and influence person-centred planning (PCP). It is important to note in this context, however, that life stories are not the same as case notes or case histories, as they are told (or compiled) from the point of view of the people most centrally concerned. Case notes/histories, on the other hand, are formal and more 'distant' accounts of the person, told by others.

Exercise 1.4

You can try out the difference between a life story and case notes by (a) writing a paragraph about yourself as if it is written by a professional who knows you (but not well) and (b) by writing a paragraph directly about yourself. Compare the two – they should look very different.

The telling, and the recording, of lives in research and in everyday practice is the means by which unique accounts of individual lives are preserved. The collecting together of those life stories makes possible a compilation of shared experiences and marks the beginning of a complex and multi-layered shared history of people with learning disabilities. The research described here is part of that continuing process of telling and preserving individual life stories as part of the overall history of people with learning disabilities.

Conclusion

Life stories are not just a series of events in more or less chronological order but are narratives, shaped and structured by the author in the telling of the story. People tell their stories in order to make sense of their lives, to establish their identity, and to make connections with others (Gillman *et al.* 1997). This is where research emulates good practice in field work. The telling of the story as part of historical research can be empowering – but so too can the constructing of a life story book by people with learning disabilities with a care worker, social worker or other practitioner. A life story book gives people an opportunity to 're-author' their life history, and to bring out those bits which have been repressed and silenced (Sutcliffe and Simons 1993; White 1993). The life story book becomes an alternative or counter document which can recount the person's resilience and struggle against discrimination and exclusion (Goodley 1996; Gillman *et al.* 1997).

The research's success, or otherwise, in influencing practice still remains to be seen but it has the potential to strengthen self-advocacy through the emerging sense of a shared history among people with learning disabilities. It also has the potential to improve practice in both research and field work settings. Its contribution to research practice is likely to be through the further development of participatory research, and the continuing presence of the reflective researcher. The research, when transferred to field settings, also has the capacity to support practitioners in developing life story work with people with learning disabilities.

Life story research can harness the reflexivity of people with learning disabilities, and heighten their historical awareness. As research awareness also grows, so more people are likely to become involved in the telling of their personal histories and thus in the telling of history itself. Those accounts, separately and together, will help tell the history of learning disability in the twentieth and twenty-first centuries. The challenge that still remains is how that history is presented, and to whom – and how it properly becomes a history that is known and owned by people with learning disabilities themselves.

Exercise 1.5

If you want to follow up the possible ways of enabling people with learning disabilities to tell their stories, there are a number of things you can do next.

1   Discover more about oral history.

Look at copies of the journal, *Oral History*

Consider joining the Oral History Society (which runs oral history conferences and training workshops)

Visit the national sound archives at the British Library in London

2   Find out about doing oral history interviews. You may find the following references useful:

Bornat, J. (1993) *Reminiscence Reviewed: Perspectives, Evaluations, Achievements*. Buckingham: Open University Press.

Humphries, S. and Gordon, P. (1992) *Out of Sight: Recording the Life Stories of Disabled People*. London: Channel 4 Television.

Humphries, S. and Gordon, P. (1993) *Back to Your Roots: Recording your Family History*. London: BBC Publications.

Thompson, P. (1988) *The Voice of the Past: Oral History*, 2nd edn. Oxford: Oxford University Press.

Thompson, P. (1991) Oral history and the history of medicine: a review, *Social History of Medicine*, 4: 371–83.

Thompson, P. and Perks, R. (1993) *An Introduction to the Use of Oral History in the History of Medicine*. London: National Sound Archive.

Yow, V. (1994) *Recording Oral History*. London: Sage.

3   Look at examples of oral history and people with learning disabilities. In addition to the books and papers already listed in the references, the following are also useful:

Ashby, I. and Lewis, K. (1996) *Real Lives: Memories of Older People with Learning Difficulties*. London: Elfrida Rathbone.

Atkinson, D. (1997) *An Auto/biographical Approach to Learning Disability Research*. Aldershot: Avebury.

Atkinson, D., McCarthy, M., Walmsley, J. *et al.* (2000) (eds) *Good Times, Bad Times: Women with Learning Difficulties Telling their Stories*. Kidderminster: BILD Publications.

Brigham, L., Atkinson, D., Jackson, M., Rolph, S. and Walmsley, J. (2000) *Crossing Boundaries. Change and Continuity in the History of Learning Disability*. Kidderminster: BILD Publications.

Fido, R. and Potts, M. (1989) 'It's not true what was written down!' Experiences of life in a mental handicap institution, *Oral History*, 17: 31–4.

Traustadottir, R. and Johnson, K. (2000) *Women with Intellectual Disabilities: Finding a Place in the World*. London: Jessica Kingsley.

Walmsley, J. (1990) Group work, research and learning difficulties, *Groupwork*, 3(1): 49–64.

4   Consider using training resources to help you get started:

A New Life: Transition Learning Programmes for People with Severe Learning Difficulties who are Moving from Long-stay Hospitals into the Community (1992). Available from FEDA, Citadel Place, Tinworth Street, London SE11 5EH.

Working as Equal People (1996). A study pack (K503) for staff, families and people with learning difficulties to study together. The course includes how to find out about the past and how to do interviews. Available from School of Health and Social Welfare, The Open University, Walton Hall, Milton Keynes MK7 6AA.

Peterborough Voices: Extraordinary People, Extraordinary Lives (1997). Edited by Sarah Hillier. Available from Peterborough Council for Voluntary Service.

Looking Forward, Looking Back: Reminiscence with People with Learning Difficulties (1998). A training resource developed by Mary Stuart. Available from Pavilion Publications, Brighton.

References

Able, J. and Cooper, M. (2000) Mabel Cooper's and John Able's stories, *Self Advocacy Stories*. London: Mencap.

Abbot, P. and Sapsford, R. (1987) *Community Care for Mentally Handicapped Children*. Milton Keynes: Open University Press.

Atkinson, D. (1993) *Past Times*. Milton Keynes: private publication.

Atkinson, D. (1998) Reclaiming our past: empowerment through oral history and personal stories, in L. Ward (ed.) *Innovations in Advocacy and Empowerment for People with Intellectual Disabilities*. Chorley: Lisieux Hall Publications.

Atkinson, D. and Williams, F. (1990) *'Know Me As I Am': An Anthology of Prose, Poetry and Art by People with Learning Difficulties*. London: Hodder & Stoughton.

Atkinson, D., Jackson, M. and Walmsley, J. (1997) *Forgotten Lives: Exploring the History of Learning Disability*. Kidderminster: BILD Publications.

Barron, D. (1996) *A Price To Be Born*. Huddersfield: H. Charlesworth & Co. Ltd.

Bertaux-Wiame, I. (1981) The life history approach to the study of internal migration, in D. Bertaux (ed.) *Biography and Society: The Life History Approach in the Social Sciences*. Beverly Hills, CA: Sage.

Biklen, S. and Moseley, C. (1988) 'Are you retarded?' 'No, I'm Catholic': qualitative methods in the study of people with severe handicaps, *Journal of the Association of Severe Handicaps*, 13: 155–62.

Birren, J. and Deutchman, D. (1991) *Guiding Autobiography Groups for Older Adults*. London: Johns Hopkins University Press.

Booth, T. and Booth, W. (1994) *Parenting under Pressure: Mothers and Fathers with Learning Difficulties*. Buckingham: Open University Press.

Booth, T. and Booth, W. (1996) Sounds of silence: narrative research with inarticulate subjects, *Disability and Society*, 11(1): 55–69.

Booth, T. and Booth, W. (1998) *Growing Up With Parents Who Have Learning Difficulties*. London: Routledge.

Booth, W. (1998) Doing research with lonely people, *British Journal of Learning Disabilities*, 26(4): 132–4.

Bornat, J. (1989) Oral history as a social movement, *Oral History*, 17(2): 16–24.

Bornat, J. (1994) Is oral history auto/biography? *Auto/Biography*, 3(1) and 3(2) (double issue).

Burnside, M. (1991) *My Life Story*. Halifax: Pecket Well College.

Chappell, A.L. (2000) Emergence of participatory methodology in learning disability research: understanding the context, *British Journal of Learning Disabilities*, 28(1): 38–43.

Cooper, M. (1997) Mabel Cooper's life story, in D. Atkinson, M. Jackson and J. Walmsley (eds) *Forgotten Lives: Exploring the History of Learning Disability*. Kidderminster: BILD Publications.

Deacon, J. (1974) *Tongue Tied*. London: NSMHC.

Finnegan, R. (1992) *Oral Traditions and the Verbal Arts: A Guide to Research Practice*. London: Routledge.

Fitzgerald, J. (1998) It's never too late: empowerment for older people with learning difficulties, in L. Ward (ed.) *Innovations in Advocacy and Empowerment for People with Intellectual Disabilities*. Chorley: Lisieux Hall Publications.

Freire, P. (1986) *Pedagogy of the Oppressed*. Harmondsworth: Penguin.

Frisch, M. (1990) *A Shared Authority: Essays on the Craft and Meaning of Oral History*. New York: SUNY Press.

Giddens, A. (1991) *Modernity and Self-Identity: Self and Society in the Late Modern Age*. Cambridge: Polity Press.

Gillman, M., Swain, J. and Heyman, B. (1997) Life history or 'case' history: the objectification of people with learning difficulties through the tyranny of professional discourses, *Disability and Society*, 12(5): 675–93.

Gluck, S.B. and Patai, D. (1991) *Women's Words: The Feminist Practice of Oral History*. London: Routledge.

Goodley, D. (1996) Tales of hidden lives: a critical examination of life history research with people who have learning difficulties, *Disability and Society*, 11(3): 333–48.

Hunt, N. (1967) *The World of Nigel Hunt*. Beaconsfield: Darwen Finlayson.

Linde, C. (1993) *Life Stories: The Creation of Coherence*. Oxford: Oxford University Press.

Living Archive (1996) *Positive Tales*. Milton Keynes: Living Archive Press.

Maines, D.R. (1993) Narrative's moment and sociology's phenomena: toward a narrative sociology, *The Sociological Quarterly*, 34(1): 18–38.

Northway, R. (2000) Ending participatory research? *Journal of Learning Disabilities*, 4(1): 27–36.

Oliver, M. (1997) Emancipatory research: realistic goal or impossible dream? in C. Barnes and G. Mercer (eds) *Doing Disability Research*. Leeds: The Disability Press.

Oswin, M. (1978) *Children Living in Long Stay Hospitals*. London: Heinemann.

Plummer, K. (1983) *Documents of Life*. London: Allen & Unwin.

Potts, M. and Fido, R. (1991) *'A Fit Person To Be Removed': Personal Accounts of Life in a Mental Deficiency Institution*. Plymouth: Northcote House.

Potts, P. (1998) Knowledge is not enough: an exploration of what we can expect from enquiries which are social, in P. Clough and L. Barton (eds) *Articulating with Difficulty: Research Voices in Inclusive Education*. London: Paul Chapman Publishing.

Prins, G. (1991) Oral history, in P. Burke (ed.) *New Perspectives on Historical Writing*. Cambridge: Polity Press.

Ramcharan, P. and Grant, G. (1994) Setting one agenda for empowering persons with a disadvantage within the research process, in M.H. Rioux and M. Bach (eds) *Disability is not Measles: New Research Paradigms in Disability*. Ontario: Roeher Institute.

Ramcharan, P., Roberts, G., Grant, G. and Borland, J. (1997) Citizenship, empowerment and everyday life, in P. Ramcharan, G. Roberts, G. Grant and J. Borland (eds) *Empowerment in Everyday Life: Learning Disability*. London: Jessica Kingsley.

Ristock, J. and Pennell, J. (1996) *Community Research as Empowerment: Feminist Links, Postmodern Interruptions*. Oxford: Oxford University Press.

Rolph, S. (1999) *The history of community care for people with learning difficulties in Norfolk 1930–1980: the role of two hostels*. Unpublished Ph.D. thesis, Milton Keynes, Open University.

Rowbotham, S. (1973) *Hidden from History*. London: Pluto Press.

Ryan, J. with Thomas, F. (1981) *The Politics of Mental Handicap*. Harmondsworth: Penguin.

Sibley, D. (1995) *Geographies of Exclusion*. London: Routledge.

Shearer, A. (1981) *Disability: Whose Handicap?* Oxford: Blackwell.

Stalker, K. (1998) Some ethical and methodological issues in research with people with learning difficulties, *Disability and Society*, 13(1): 5–19.

Stanley, L. (1992) *The Auto/biographical I*. Manchester: Manchester University Press.

Stuart, M. (1998) *Mothers, sisters and daughters: an investigation into convent homes for women labelled as having learning difficulties*. Unpublished Ph.D. thesis, Milton Keynes, Open University.

Stuart, M. (2002) *Not Quite Sisters: Women with Learning Difficulties Living in Convent Homes*. Kidderminster: BILD Publications.

Sutcliffe, J. and Simons, K. (1993) *Self-advocacy and Adults with Learning Difficulties*. Leicester: NIACE.

Thomas, W.I. and Znaniecki, F. (1918–1920) *The Polish Peasant in Europe and America* (5 vols). Chicago: University of Chicago Press.

Thompson, P. (1988) *The Voice of the Past: Oral History*, 2nd edn. Oxford: Oxford University Press.

Thomson, A. (1999) Moving stories: oral history and migration studies, *Oral History*, 27(1): 24–37.

Walmsley, J. (1995) *Gender, caring and learning disability*. Unpublished Ph.D. thesis, Milton Keynes, Open University.

Walmsley, J. (1998) Life history interviews with people with learning disabilities, in R. Perks and A. Thompson (eds) *The Oral History Reader*. London: Routledge.

Walmsley, J. (2000) Caring: a place in the world? in K. Johnson and R. Traustadottir (eds) *Women with Intellectual Disabilities: Finding a Place in the World*. London: Jessica Kingsley.

Walmsley, J. (2001) Normalisation, emancipatory research and inclusive research in learning disability, *Disability and Society*, 16(2): 187–205.

Walmsley, J. and Johnson, K. (2003) *Inclusive Research with People with Learning Disabilities: Past, Present and Futures*. London: Jessica Kingsley.

Ward, L. (1997) *Seen and Heard: Involving Disabled Children and Young People in Research and Development Projects*. York: Joseph Rowntree Foundation.

Westerman, W. (1998) Central American refugee testimonies and performed life histories in the sanctuary movement, in R. Perks and A. Thomson (eds) *The Oral History Reader*. London: Routledge.

White, M. (1993) Deconstruction and therapy, in S. Gilligan and R. Price (eds) *Therapeutic Conversations*. New York: Norton.

White, M. and Epston, D. (1990) *Narrative Means to Therapeutic Ends*. New York: Norton.

Widdershoven, G. (1993) The story of life: hermeneutic perspectives on the relationship between narrative and life history, in R. Josselson and A. Lieblich (eds) *The Narrative Study of Lives*. London: Sage.

Williams, F. (1989) Mental handicap and oppression, in A. Brechin and J. Walmsley (eds) *Making Connections: Reflecting on the Experiences of People with Learning Difficulties*. London: Hodder & Stoughton.

Williams, F. (1993) *Social policy, social divisions and social change*. Unpublished Ph.D. thesis, Milton Keynes, Open University.

Williams, F. and Walmsley, J. (1990) *Transitions and Change* (K262, Workbook 3). Milton Keynes: Open University.

Wolfensberger, W. (1975) *The Origin and Nature of our Institutional Models*. Syracuse, NY: Human Policy Press.

2

From vagabonds to Victorian values

The social construction of a disability identity

Alex McClimens

> Discourses allow dominant groups to tell their narratives about the past in order to justify the present and prevent those who use subjugated discourses from making history.
>
> (Parker 1992: 20)

Introduction

In 1601 Queen Elizabeth I was nearing the end of her reign. The Spanish Armada had been defeated and Shakespeare was working on the tragedies. He had just completed his longest and most complex work, *Hamlet*. In this he has a character reflect, 'What a piece of work is man! How noble in reason! How infinite in faculty!' Here he demonstrates familiarity with the issues that are incorporated in our ideas of what constitutes humanity. Now, 400 years later, Shakespeare remains as relevant as ever. In an earlier play, *As You Like It*, he even appears to adopt a life cycle approach as the character Jacques contemplates existence with these words: 'All the world's a stage, and all the men and women merely players. They have their exits and their entrances, and one man in his time plays many parts'.

The idea of life as performance art was mirrored in the French asylum of Charenton where the patients took part in plays, and also in the Bicetre in Paris and at Bedlam in London where visitors could pay to observe the inmates. Bedlam began as The Priory of St Mary of Bethlem, and is probably better known now by association with the images by Hogarth in *A Rake's Progress* (1733). The small priory was built in the early fourteenth century but gradually altered its function to care for people with mental disorders, and by 1601 was operating as a neglected institution (Russell 1997: 6–9).

It was also in 1601 that the first Poor Laws came into effect. Administered through parish overseers, this legislation was an attempt to unify a collection of previous responses to the increasing problems associated with poverty. Properly titled 'An Act for the Relief of the Poor' the intention was to offer some assistance to those in reduced circumstances due to failed harvests or a struggling local economy. The 1590s had seen many poor harvests followed by severe winters, and bread riots had occurred in major cities.

Three categories of individual were identified as being suitable to receive the benefits of the Poor Laws: sturdy beggars or vagabonds, the infirm, and the deserving unemployed. This legislation is an early example of social policy with the state taking some account of the reduced circumstances of the populace. It is in this crude classification that we can trace the beginnings of legislation targeting specific social groups. Those individuals who were later to be classified as having some form of developmental/intellectual disability were not then apparent, but the origins of targeted care were beginning to emerge in the provision of poor relief.

That it became necessary to write legislation for this purpose was due to the changing patterns of charity evident in religious reforms of the previous century, when the suppression of the monasteries by Henry VIII in the 1530s reduced the amount of charitable care available. By the time of the Elizabethan Poor Laws social conditions had degenerated, with vagrant poor roaming the land feigning sickness in order to receive charity. Those Christians who felt bound to perform what were known as the seven corporal works of mercy 'feed the hungry, give water to those who are thirsty, accommodate strangers, clothe the naked, visit the sick and the imprisoned and bury the dead' were finding it increasingly difficult to distinguish genuinely deserving cases.

The purpose of the preceding historical overview is to situate the argument that follows. The group of people we know now as having learning disabilities clearly was not always in existence as a distinct entity. Neither is this group a recent creation, brought about by some twentieth-century combination of health and social care thinking. Society has always had its margins and if we look back at the early seventeenth century we can see that these margins were broader then than they might appear to be now. The process of social stratification that separates people into statistically convenient boxes was only just beginning. The social processes that separated the vagabonds from the law-abiding parishioners of the time also separated the many as yet unclassified individuals who were afflicted with physical and intellectual impairments, unidentified disabling conditions and undiagnosed illnesses. Today, the vagabonds are no longer with us: today we have new names for the old social problems. The dole queue that some readers may have stood in began in the Britain of Queen Elizabeth I as the poor of the parish stood in line to have alms doled out to them. Now, in the twenty-first century, under Queen Elizabeth II, the dole queue has a new incarnation in the form of the job centre.

The social construction of a disability

The social construction of a disability identity is a process of naming. By this I mean it refers to a way of seeing the world and generating knowledge from a particular perspective. The perspective I have in mind here is a scientific one, with science understood as a project that aims to predict and control. For many of those involved currently in professional social and health care services this has often been characterized by a privileged position that names things in order to own them – for example, to name oneself a vagabond or beggar (or unemployed) to receive alms (or the dole).

In the next section I will identify specific examples of how historical naming processes have shaped our present understanding of what it means to be labelled with a disability identity. In this exploration I will argue that science, with all its power to liberate human beings from the sharper edges of the world has, in the case of individuals with intellectual disabilities, enslaved them instead. The old-style vagabonds at least had some licence to roam within the parish. Their modern-day equivalents are constrained by the local authority. This enslavement is sanctioned by the medical profession who 'own' the knowledge necessary to operate in this fashion.

If what counts for knowledge is what receives scientific approval in the society of the day, then it is clear that the medical professions exercise power over many people by virtue of the way their knowledge is organized; this manifests itself in very unequal power relations. Of particular relevance to this chapter is the case of people who are classified by the medical professions as inhabiting the spectrum of learning disability. This diagnosis, as Burr argues, renders such individuals liable to be treated in certain ways, sanctioned by society (1995: 63–4).

Here the role of the medical expert is in exercising disciplinary power which is made manifest via social control exercised through the education system, through employment law and through the courts. Such a regulatory system exerts a huge influence over the lives of the people that fall under its jurisdiction. How this came about will be explained partly with reference to historical events and partly through an examination of what social construction offers us by way of understanding how knowledge, language and power manufactured the circumstances that created a separate social grouping of people with learning disabilities.

Social constructionism, like the history of learning disability, evolved over time and even now, like the idea of learning disability itself, attracts diverse opinions. It is more of a theoretical orientation than an explanation and revolves around a core cluster of ideas. These are the relationship between thought and language, the operation of power in society, the place of scientific knowledge and, in a nod to poststructuralist thinking, an attitude of contested meaning. When applied to a marginal social grouping such as individuals with learning disabilities there is room for much debate. What social constructionism does is to open up such debate.

In this analysis I have opted to spend a lot of time exploring another central tenet of a social constructionist approach: that knowledge is situated in both time and place. By taking this line I want to try to trace the beginnings of some current, though contested, views of what learning disability is and so try to argue a view for how this has brought us to our current appreciation. Much of the chapter will be historical as I look at medical scientific work in the formative decade of the 1860s in England and mainland Europe. It was during this time that many of the discoveries and attitudes that dictated future responses to deviance and difference were formed. I will highlight these as they occur, directing the reader to their full significance in a later commentary where the value of a social constructionist perspective should become evident.

We have, for example, already been introduced to the early social policy of the Poor Laws. Even here, as Saraga (1998) has observed, some of the principles of a social constructionist perspective were already in operation. The principle of 'less eligibility' (i.e. that alms should always be less than potential earnings) was not based on naturally occurring differences between people. The divisions between the 'deserving' and 'undeserving' poor were never natural, intrinsic or even inevitable. They were applied externally as part of a mechanism to assist the administration of policy. The meaning of such terms changes over time because the social conditions change over time. In twenty-first century Britain, to be employable is seen as a social rather than a personal characteristic (Saranga 1998: 3–4). Can we say the same for the term 'disability'?

This example highlights the situatedness of the debate. It also introduces another strand of the social constructionist perspective: that there is no essential meaning behind the labels we use to describe people. And yet labels stick. How they are made to stick and how they can be unstuck will be examined later in the chapter.

The care and treatment of individuals with a disability (understood here in its broadest sense) is traced to prehistoric times by Rudgley (2000) (see also Chapter 4 in this volume). But the fact that it was a product of legislative and administrative efforts requires us to look to more recent chapters in history. Medieval times saw the caring function (for individuals with a variety of 'disabilities') performed by families, the Church or the local aristocracy (Neugebauer 1978). This ad hoc system was eventually superseded by the Poor Laws. The original Poor Laws were deliberately broad in their application and were not aimed at any particular strata of society save for those whose circumstances were reduced. Thus, the inclusion of those individuals who might now be classified as having a learning difficulty within the remit of social care was then an unnecessary distinction. Their gradual inclusion within the orbit of social care was a slow and cumulative process.

The Victorian reforms of the early to mid-nineteenth century presaged the first attempts at a recognizable, modern welfare system (Marcus 1981: 53). Disability seen as deviance was a peculiarly nineteenth-century creation, arising out of the Poor Law Reforms of 1834 and the burgeoning medicalization and subsequent professionalization of health and social care. The amendments to the Poor Laws were made largely due to the far-reaching effects of the Industrial Revolution. By the early nineteenth century, the social landscape had changed radically and although the state still retained some measure of responsibility for the disadvantaged of society the debate about how far the needs of those on the margins should be met by the efforts of those at the centre had begun in earnest.

What is interesting to note is how the individual in society came to be the focus of legislation. In particular, it is pertinent to observe how the individual with a disability became part of that focus and further, how that person was created as a case and then treated as such. By this time, the mesh of scientific discovery, of increasing industrialization, of medicine and political theory were all combining to alter the relations of the individual to the society they inhabited. As has previously been noted 'there is a clear relationship between prevailing social structures, dominant ideology and the way society handles its deviants' (Abbot and Sapsford 1987: 7). This can seldom have been more apparent than in the treatment of those who attracted the dubious benefits of the amended Poor Laws. Symonds and Kelly (1998: 19) note that 'It was the passing of the Poor Law Amendment Act 1834 which acted as the spur to much of the work of the voluntary sector; it meant that a tripartite system of provision of social and health care was created: institutionalisation in the workhouse, relief by charitable organisations, and self-help'.

The then Prime Minister, Earl Grey, set up the Poor Law Commission in 1833 to overhaul a failing system that had been overrun by the new demands of an industrial society.

The infamous principle of 'less eligibility' meant that the rate calculated for the receipt of benefit had to be set lower than the lowest wage available. By this method it was hoped to discourage those who were not genuinely in need of poor relief. In effect this created an invidious distinction between the 'deserving' and 'undeserving' poor, with the latter being 'pauperized' in the process (Dalley 1992: 105). Further to this, it was the categories of people who became eligible for poor relief that became the basis for defining disability. Stone (1985: 40) puts it this way:

> In the regulations of the Poor Law administration and thus in the eyes of the Poor Law administrators, five categories were important in defining the internal universe of paupers; children, the sick, the insane, 'defectives', and the 'aged and infirm'. Of these, all but the first are part of today's concept of disability. The five groups were the means of defining who was able-bodied; if a person didn't fall into one of them, he was able-bodied by default. This strategy of definition by default remains at the core of the current disability programs.

The further sorting of social categories continued and was formalized by legislation such as the Lunacy Act (1845), the Lunatic Asylums Act (1853) and the Idiots Act (1886) (Pilgrim 1993: 168). Thus it was that the management of society was done on an economic basis. Scull (1993: 29) approves this line of thinking with his comments that 'the main driving force behind a segregative response to madness (and other forms of deviance) can much more plausibly be asserted to lie in the effects of a mature capitalist market economy and the associated ever more thoroughgoing commercialization of existence'.

It was against this background that the Victorian zeal for classification made itself felt within the medical system. Simultaneously, the impact of the changing economy on society was being investigated. Oliver (1990: 44) cites Marx as he introduces an argument for the production of disability. According to Marx (1913: 267):

> The further back we go into history, the more the individual, and, there-fore, the producing individual seems to depend on and constitute a part of a larger whole: at first it is, quite naturally, the family and the clan, which is but an enlarged family; later on, it is the community growing up in its different forms out of the clash and the amalgamation of clans.

The isolation of the individual economically then leads to a corresponding separation of the individual on pathological lines. Oliver (1990: 47) summarizes the argument:

> The idea of disability as individual pathology only becomes possible when we have an idea of individual able-bodiedness, which is itself related to the rise of capitalism and the development of wage labour. Prior to this, the individual's contribution had been to the family, the community, the band, in terms of labour, and while, of course differences in individual contributions were noted, and often sanctions applied, individuals did not, in the main, suffer exclusion.

Oliver then suggests how this can be linked to the emergent perspective on disability that was developing in the nineteenth century. He cites three authors who have used a similar division to account for attitudes to deviance. With particular reference to learning difficulty it can be described as first a moral, then a legal and now a medical problem. This view can be summarized as sin, crime and sickness (Conrad and Schneider 1980: 27). Soder (1984) sees the care and treatment of individuals with learning difficulties as being founded firstly on religious/philanthropic ideals, then on the protection of society and the individual through asylums and colonies, and then on treatment based on new drug therapies and rehabilitative regimes. Finally, Finkelstein (1980) suggests that society developed according to divisions characterized by feudalism, followed by industrialization and the rise of capitalism before entering the present era.

The paradox for people categorized as disabled arises in stage two, when disability is separated out from the general mass of the population. The economic influences have been discussed, but these are only half the story. The growth of the care industry and the place of medical intervention suggest that while the social construction of disability may well have begun under economic conditions, its full expression only came about with the incorporation of disabled individuals within the framework of social care. In turning to the accommodation and treatment of those classified variously as defective, retarded and disabled it should be noted that increasing specialization reflects a move away from a focus on the masses to a consideration of the individual. The modern-day practice of the named nurse and the person-centred care plan are current expressions of this perspective.

But there was more than an economic basis for the changing relations of the individual to society and their classification within it. Science was providing other frameworks by which to explain what was seen as a growing social problem. Against this political backdrop, and with the reverberations of the Industrial Revolution still fading in the background, the social circumstances that had brought about the first Poor Laws had altered utterly. The Poor Law (Amendment) Act of 1834 was the official policy response. As a piece of social legislation this ranks as one of the most important of the entire century. Properly called An Act for the Amendment and Better Administration of the Laws Relating to the Poor in England and Wales it was an extreme act. Where sturdy beggars and vagabonds had once been the socially constructed faces of the day, it was now the time of the pauper.

At the core of the new regime the parish was reconfirmed as the administrative centre and within each parish there was to be a workhouse and the workhouse was to be the sole distribution centre of poor relief. All of this was overseen by the Poor Law Commission.

Can you remember the 60s?

In the 1860s Queen Victoria was approximately mid-way through her 64-year reign and in 1861 Prince Albert died. Adult male suffrage was still incomplete, even after the 1867 Reform Act. Charles Dickens was nearing the end of a career that would establish him as one of the most famous novelists of all time. In America, a civil war was tearing the country apart while further afield the French were colonizing a small Asian republic called Vietnam.

While the British Empire turned the globe pink there were changes closer to home as the Red Cross, the Salvation Army and the Football Association were all founded. Politically it was an active decade with first Russell, then Derby and finally Gladstone leading the country.

During this period several influential writers and thinkers made a very direct contribution to the way that ideas concerning disability were constructed in the society of the time. To situate the discussion we have to remember that the scientific world was still trying to get to grips with Darwin. His ideas on natural selection published in 1859 were hugely controversial. Properly entitled *On the Origin of Species by Means of Natural Selection*, Darwin's observations in the Galapagos Islands offered limitless scope for debate when these ideas were applied to human populations.

Auguste Comte (1798–1857) also called for positivism, which he describes as an approach to knowledge construction that is premised on quantifiable methods as practised by the natural sciences but which, he claimed, was equally applicable to social sciences. Positivism works by the principle of induction. This means accumulating evidence over a period of time through observation of experimental or naturally occurring phenomena. This 'scientific method' was developed by people like Newton and Gassendi in the eighteenth century. Comte's main work, *The Positive Philosophy* ([1853] 1971) reflects his concerns with the society he lived in. Since the French Revolution of 1792 and up to the year 1848, during which there was rioting in many major European cities, society was in a volatile condition. Comte wanted to be able to explain social processes with the same certainty that existed in the natural sciences and so he termed his approach 'social physics'.

The significance of his contribution is in the way that the objective approach of the so-called 'hard sciences' was adopted as suitable for studying people. The implications are made manifest in the way that positivism established and legitimized a medical model for viewing crime, delinquency and deviance. It wasn't long before this view came to dominate the way society in general (and medicine in particular) viewed disability. At this point we will examine some of the major works of the 1860s to discover how this came about.

Gregor Johann Mendel (1822–84) was an Austrian. He joined an Augustinian monastery as a monk and there studied the fertilization of green peas in the monastery garden. This work was eventually developed into a comprehensive account of genetic inheritance. He published his findings in 1866 in the *Journal of the Brno Natural History Society* but, as with Darwin's account of natural selection, the full significance of Mendel's work was beyond the immediate understanding of the scientific community of the day. It was only with the work of Galton and the Eugenic Society in the early days of the twentieth century that the implications of genetics were grasped.

Mendel's work in grafting different strains of peas reflected the concerns of the scientific method which proceeds by meticulous attention to detail and a constant reworking of experiments in order to arrive at a reliable and replicable method of inquiry. Just as Newton had proceeded methodically in his experimental work with prisms to ascertain the composition of the visible spectrum, so Mendel made slow but careful progress, charting, recording and observing the growth of peas. The pea is a relatively simple plant and it was partly this botanical accident that guaranteed the success of Mendel's experiments. It was as a result of this painstaking work that Mendel was able to isolate the likelihood of certain characteristics being passed on from one generation of the plant to the next. To do this he used the terms 'dominant', to describe a trait or characteristic that is present in the new generation and 'recessive' to describe a trait or characteristic that is obscured by a dominant gene. He did this by noting the colour, shape, size and even the taste of the plants, as the following extract reveals: 'In 1859 I obtained a very fertile descendant with large, tasty seeds from a first generation hybrid. Since in the following year, its progeny retained the desirable characteristics and were uniform, the variety was cultivated in our vegetable garden, and many plants were raised every year up to 1865' (Mendel 1950). This indicates that it was Mendel who developed the F1 hybrid, well known to amateur gardeners today. By carefully controlling the variables he was able to predict the outcome of his cross-fertilization. That this approach was successful is evident in the way that ideas of dominance and recession continue to explain hereditary principles. However, the methods of the natural sciences are not always easily translated into the social sciences and it was in seeking to make this connection that medicine (seen here as an applied branch of the physical sciences) appears to be culpable in the way that it initially began a process of classification that attempted to account for human characteristics in a way that mirrored Mendel's work with peas.

In a series of lectures begun in 1843, entitled a 'Course of Lectures on Deformity of the Human Frame' William Little described 'a peculiar distortion which affects new born children which has never been elsewhere described . . . the spasmodic tetanus-like rigidity and distortion of the limbs of new-born infants' (Schifrin and Longo 2000). The disorder became known as 'Little's Disease' and related to what we now know as 'spastic diplegia'. This is one of many types of cerebral palsy, a condition characterized by motor dysfunction due to brain damage and frequently, but not always, accompanied by a degree of intellectual impairment.

Little began, again following the regime of the scientific method, to examine the relationship of the disorder to premature and complicated births. By 1861 he had gathered evidence from more than 200 observations. He presented his findings to the Obstetrical Society in London and proposed that potential causes might include premature birth, complications in the perinatal stage and direct trauma (Shifrin and Longo 2000). It is worth noting that Little himself was born with an obvious impairment: he had a club-foot. He had this surgically corrected and from this we might surmise that he would have agreed with Wendell's later observation that 'How a society defines disability and whom it recognizes as disabled also reveal a great deal about that society's attitudes and expectations concerning the body, what it stigmatizes and what it considers "normal" in physical appearance and performance' (1996: 32).

If Little's name and fame is relatively obscure this should be contrasted with the next contribution. John Langdon Haydon Down was a medical student in London in the 1850s where he studied under Little at the London Hospital (Wright 2001). His career moved fast and in 1858 he was appointed Medical Superintendent of Earlswood Asylum for the care and treatment of idiots. It was both here and at his earlier appointment in the London Hospital that Down completed his work on classifications. Once again the mould of the scientific method is present in Down's work, as is clear from his own description: 'I have for some time', he wrote, 'had my attention directed to the possibility of making a classification of the feeble-minded, by arranging them around the various ethnic standards – in other words, framing a natural system to supplement the information to be derived by an inquiry into the history of the case' (Down 1866: 260). His essay, published in 1866, was entitled 'Observations on the Ethnic Classification of Idiots' in which he put forward the theory that it was possible to classify different types of condition by ethnic characteristics. He concentrated his investigation on what he termed the 'Mongolian type of idiocy' that he calculated at approximately 10 per cent of his case load (Down also identified 'Malay', 'Aztec', 'Ethiopian' and 'Caucasian' in his classification). He also made an important link to the origins of the condition when he noted its congenital nature. But his more lasting contribution to the field, which survived him by a century, is in the name by which such cases came to be known.

Names as labels generally alter with the social mood of the day: consider how the word 'gay' was transformed in the late twentieth century. Mongol, however, despite its purely scientific origins, soon became odious and it took public intervention to secure the adoption of the more neutral 'Down's syndrome' (Stockholder 1994: 167). In this detail the labelling process highlights one of the main challenges to a social constructionist approach. Down's work was clearly important in that it made space for the later identification by Lejeune of the genetic component implicated in the condition. This discovery in 1959 of a mutation on the twenty-first chromosome clearly points to a physical/biological cause. There appears to be no way that we can usefully describe Down's syndrome as socially constructed in these terms. The microscopic evidence seems to refute any notion of language as a contributing factor. Individuals who have an extra chromosome (trisomy 21) have Down's syndrome and inevitably inherit a degree of intellectual impairment.

And yet the very act of attaching a name (and this gets to the heart of the system of classification, whether it be peas or people), will just as inevitably expose the dichotomy that surrounds the disability identity. That disability identity, with Down's syndrome as the current exemplar, appears to be stuck between the biological foundationalism apparent under the microscope and the social constructionism that says there can be no differences that are innate.

Calhoun (1994: 17) offers a way out of this impasse when he remarks that one suitable response might be that 'the argument suggests that where a particular category of identity has been repressed, delegitimated or devalued in dominant discourses, a vital response may be to claim value for all those labelled by that category, thus implicitly invoking it in an essentialist way'. The reader will have to decide for themselves whether elective facial surgery for people with Down's syndrome is an example of using biological solutions to address social problems or social solutions to address biological problems (Fox and Giles 1996: 231). What is perhaps more certain is that, as Calhoun argues, 'every collective identity is open to both internal subdivision and calls for its incorporation into some larger category of primary identity' (p. 27).

Down was working at a time when the developing sciences were heavily involved with classification and statistics. In their desire to sort the world into neat parcels, scientists lost sight of the importance of the labels that they attached to these parcels. One of the challenges to social scientists and to health care professionals in the field of disability studies is to find an order of words that will simultaneously describe the phenomenon under investigation without exerting undue influence over its subsequent interpretation. In the UK these labels tend to have been derived from the professions who took over the care of such individuals and as such the labelling process can be seen as an administrative function.

The medical colonization of disability began as part of the establishment of boundaries to the overall condition. What we now refer to as the 'medical model' of disability (one that locates disability as the property and concern of the individual) is premised on expertise and a business-like appropriation of knowledge. This knowledge is protected by professional cartels and a virtual monopoly over the crucial element of diagnosis.

Hughes (1998) charts the irresistible progress of medicine, suggesting that the ownership of illness culminated in a takeover bid for disability and all related conditions with the 1913 Mental Deficiency Act. This takeover was undoubtedly made easier by the background influence of the eugenic movement (see Chapter 4). But Hughes takes the argument further when he observes that psychology was introduced as a 'permitted knowledge' by the Wood Committee (1929: 72). While psychologists didn't replace doctors their influence in disability issues can be confirmed with a cursory glance at the literature and roll-call of the profession.

Exercise 2.1

Why did Little's disease disappear as a name and why did Down's name later become attached to the syndrome he identified?

In the case of both Down's syndrome and cerebral palsy, affected individuals will appear 'different' to the rest of the population. Think about how this affects efforts to be inclusive.

Work on identifying what we now refer to as learning disability was not confined to practising London doctors. In continental Europe, Jean Itard (1775–1838) wrote of his 'experiments' with Victor, the eponymous *Wild Boy of Aveyron* ([1806] 1972), and Gugenbhul's establishment of a specialist residential school for persons with learning disability in Switzerland in 1842 demonstrated the increasing international interest in identifying and 'treating' disability. America in the 1820s was beginning to experience the increased urbanization that followed the Industrial Revolution in England. When combined with immigration, a policy of institutionalization was adopted to cope with fast-growing population and changing demography (Braddock and Parrish 2001: 30, 31).

In the same year that Down published his paper on classification the Frenchman, Eduoard Seguin (1812–80), wrote *Idiocy and its Treatment by the Physiological Method* (1866). Seguin's contribution differs from those previously discussed in as much as he did not 'discover' or 'invent' anything new. He was an educationalist. A pupil of Itard, he developed a programme of remedial training that was used in the schools he ran. He left Paris in 1848 to escape the political turmoil of that time to set up similar training schools in the USA. During his time there he founded the Association of Medical Officers of American Institutions for Idiots and Feeble-Minded Persons, later renamed the American Association on Mental Deficiency (Parmenter 2001: 272). By the 1880s, however, the influence of eugenics (see Chapter 4) was conspiring against rehabilitation and the emphasis changed to one of custodial care (Braddock and Parish 2001: 37).

Seguin established that by training and education many 'idiots' could be successfully rehabilitated into society. He also argued a case for the use of the term 'idiocy' to describe the individuals he treated and for a standard terminology to be adopted with 'idiot' as his preferred descriptor.

What should be increasingly apparent is that the language used to describe a phenomenon under study is largely responsible for the way society views that phenomenon. With this insight we come to appreciate the social constructionist perspective that is concerned with the way language is used. But for now just note that the language used in disability studies is never value-free, is always somehow associated with bias and always reflects the concerns of the author as much, if not more than, it represents the population that is being described.

Francis Galton (1822–1911) the cousin of Charles Darwin, was elected a fellow of the Royal Society in 1860, knighted in 1909, was an explorer, anthropologist, inventor of the fingerprinting process and an innovative statistician: all of these things are largely forgotten now, although any one might have made his reputation. But it was as founder of the Eugenic Society that he ultimately secured his place in history. His work on the hereditary associations and measurement of intelligence had a massive influence on the way disability was viewed in both Europe and America. Social policy on both sides of the Atlantic was for decades driven by the segregationist principles that informed this perspective. Readers will probably recoil from such a world view now but it had many adherents in public life in the early decades of the twentieth century. Eugenics was not some esoteric cult movement. It attracted interest and approval from many sections of society. This interest waned significantly in the 1940s as the Nazi Party gave a graphic illustration of what an extreme policy of prejudice looked like when executed to its fullest extent. But the horrors of the concentration camps were really just a logical extension of the eugenic principle that sought to control breeding by those sections of the population deemed to be unsuitable. And so as the 'disabled' joined the Jews and the Gypsies in the queues for the gas chambers the civilized world turned away from eugenics. For the time being.

Exercise 2.2

Denying treatment is not just about not delivering the available health, medical or nursing service. Think historically about what other ways have been used to deny (the right) to treatment for people with learning disabilities.

Hereditary Genius, published in 1869, sets out Galton's vision. In essence he was concerned that low intelligence would, if breeding were to be allowed to go unchecked, reduce the overall quality of the national stock. And this, remember, was at a time when the British Empire was a live proposition and needed to be maintained largely through the efforts of large numbers of bodies. If the language sounds more appropriate for racehorse pedigrees, this is entirely in keeping with the eugenic view. If we look back to Mendel and Darwin there is some evidence to suggest that selection of positive characteristics can be manipulated at least in botanical and biological terms. Could this be applied to human traits such as intelligence and impairment? The same questions today define the ethical debate over the Human Genome Project and the concomitant tabloid debate on 'designer babies'. In the nineteenth century, the social engineering tools were more blunt. Segregation and sterilization were available and widely used but Galton was about to refine the statistical techniques that would, he surmised, lend more scientific credence to the eugenic project.

The 'normal distribution' curve was formerly the property of astronomers where it was known as the error curve. They used this to account for the errors made due to inaccuracy ascribed to their materials and instruments. Sometimes known as the bell curve, for its shape, it is, put simply, the plotted line on a standard x-y axis of the distribution of almost any measurable naturally occurring variable. Height or weight are two good examples. With a large enough sample the curve will be very smooth and peak around the mean (average) with fewer people at the very tall (heavy) or very short (light) ends of the graph.

There is still a ferocious argument in social scientific circles about the legitimacy of the psychometric basis of intelligence measurement and the application of statistical tests, particularly as it applies to IQ, though they are still used today (see Chapter 3). We will try not to get involved in the crossfire but the reader is directed to the work of Herrnstein and Murray (1994) and Gould (1981) for some guidance.

Galton was well aware of the potential of the bell curve. He was influenced here by his cousin's work and by Malthus' *An Essay on the Principle of Population* ([1872] 1971). His main contention, however, was that any variation away from the mean, expressed as 'standard deviation' would, in purely statistical terms, be the same whether the deviation was to the left or to the right of the mean. Therefore, someone whose intelligence was rated as above average would deviate from the mean just as someone with lower than average intelligence would deviate below it (see Figure 2.1). This did not suit Galton's purposes. He needed to demonstrate that higher intelligence was of more 'value' to society and so suggested a ranking that favoured the right-hand edge of the curve.

Now the apparent arithmetical neutrality of the design had given way to a new moral order. Davis (1995: 34–5) explains the significance of this:

What these revisions by Galton signify is an attempt to redefine the concept of the 'ideal' in relation to the general population. First, the

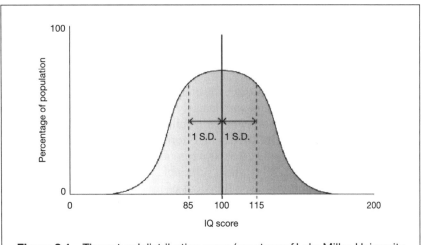

Figure 2.1   The natural distribution curve (courtesy of Luke Miller, University of Sheffield)

idea of the application of a norm to the human body creates the idea of deviance or a 'deviant' body. Second, the idea of a norm pushes the normal variation of the body through a stricter template guiding the way the body 'should' be. Third, the revision of the 'normal curve of distribution' into quartiles, ranked order, and so on, creates a new kind of 'ideal'. This statistical ideal is unlike the classical ideal which contains no imperative to be ideal. The new ideal of ranked order is powered by the imperative of the norm, and then is supplemented by the notion of progress, human perfectibility, and the elimination of deviance, to create a dominating, hegemonic vision of what the human body should be.

Galton's influence lasted well into the twentieth century. From the overcrowded pauper asylums of the 1860s (Wright 2001: 176) a policy change in the 1862 Lunatics Amendment Act recognized that too many harmless idiots were contained in the asylums and these were to be released back to the Poor Law institutions. The 1860s was the fulcrum point: the 1840s saw reform and optimism, borrowed in part from Seguin's experiments in education in France, and by the 1880s this was replaced with custodial care and control. Eugenics was becoming more influential. In the remaining decades of that century there was a gradual disenchantment with liberal philanthropic efforts to deal with the social problem of idiocy and a turn towards the more menacing ideas of the eugenic movement, focused on the dangers of the newly-identified category. The hope that had led Seguin to believe in the redemptive powers of training was waning. The promise of the Earlswood Asylum to educate was not obvious (Wright 2001).

Previously, society had to contend with a variety of idiots. Now there was a new category. In America, Goddard, a psychologist, was clear in his taxonomy. He said: 'For many generations we have recognized and pitied the idiot. Of late we have recognized a higher type of defective, the moron, and have discovered that he is a burden; that he is a menace of society and civilization; that he is responsible to a large degree for many, if not all, of our social problems' (1915: 307). This terminology was to prove useful to eugenic-inspired administrators in early twentieth-century England.

In this summary of the 1860s the influence of science is clear. It was scientists, and particularly medical scientists, who were responsible for the way that people with disabilities were classified. This emphasis on categorization, on producing taxonomies, all reflects the influence of the natural sciences on what was and remains essentially a social phenomenon. With these influences it is understandable that early ways of seeing disability focused on the individual as the locus of that disability. In this way the medical model of disability came to be a dominant perspective. It took on this hegemonic status by the main avenues, described by Berger and Luckman (1967) as externalization, objectification and internalization. By this they mean that ideas (such as the nineteenth-century notion that people with intellectual disabilities would breed voraciously and populate the country with children of low intelligence) would, by being broadcast, published and generally debated in society, gradually acquire a momentum. The next stage of the process was that such ideas then became 'objectified' until they officially represented as fact what was formerly a value position. Finally, faced with this new set of 'facts', any newcomers to the debate would readily accept the status quo and so promote the idea that people with intellectual disabilities would breed voraciously and populate the country with children of low intelligence.

By such a process was learning disability constructed. However, one of the key claims of any socially constructed position is that it should be contestable, and here we can see the difficulty of contesting the emergent definition of learning disability. In the 1860s the precise relationship of thought to language was still being considered. But clearly the language of science had influence over the way people with learning disabilities were described and so thought of by wider society. And as people with a learning disability were so obviously disadvantaged they had neither the knowledge nor the means to offer a critique of their own circumstances, so embedded was the public perception of them.

At this point it is necessary to introduce another strand to the debate as we encounter the notion of discourse. Saraga (1998) argues, borrowing from Foucault, that discourse shapes what can be talked about and this in turn determines social responses. In this view, discourse is defined as a way of organizing knowledge, which is precisely what I have argued the medical profession was doing. The medical discourse then moved on to become codified and written as social policy. The policy was enacted by the major social institutions, principally the courts, hospitals and asylums, while the agents who staffed these institutions – the doctors, nurses, asylum attendants, police and legal officers – all ensured its smooth operation at ground level.

Cooper (1997), again borrowing from Foucault, takes this further with the suggestion that it is professionalization that is in some way implicated in this process. He argues that professionals (and here we can think of doctors and nurses) use their knowledge to objectify and classify the people in their care. In so doing, the professions 'discipline' (i.e. keep in line) the people they care for through techniques which require the subject to be categorized. As Gergen (1999: 45) puts it, 'The problem . . . is not simply the essentializing carried by group characterizations. There is further the tendency of such categories to destroy differences, to suppress the enormous variations in values, sexual preferences, tastes and ways of life among those classified within a group'. From this the reader might recognize the tendency to talk about people who have a learning disability as if they were all one homogenous group, with no distinguishing or individual features. If this description were true (and within the culture of the time it was hard to resist) then a custodial model of care as delivered by the asylums would be deemed suitable.

We have now moved away from a consideration of the individual to a concern with aggregate effects. Social policy is not concerned with individuals *per se*, but addresses the perceived needs of groups, and it is as a social grouping and as a social problem that individuals with a learning disability were perceived, treated and ultimately constructed.

The social model of disability

The so-called social model of disability shares some of the central concerns of a social constructionist perspective. Both, for example, focus on meaning and power as ways of analysing the situation of people with learning disabilities. For example, the vocabulary of disability is not widely shared, as can be seen by the many epithets available for general use as different groups try to exercise political power through their choice of language in the debate. This is particularly evident in the dispute over the implications of the terms 'disability' and 'impairment'. Here both the definitions and the meanings are contestable. Marks (1999: 17) argues that 'The social model of disability draws upon a realist philosophical approach which argues that some things (such as impairments) exist independently of the way in which they are socially constructed'. If this is true for impairment then what of the term 'disability'? This interpretation suggests that there might be a split between the physical reality of impairment and the social construction of disability. Impairment might then be said to belong in the 'real' world while disability occupies a less certain space somewhere beyond language.

I suggested at the beginning of this chapter that social construction is just one way of viewing the debate. I like this way of looking, seeing and interpreting for the following reasons (and here I'm siding with Burr 1995):

*   psychology likes to deal in 'facts' and social constructionism challenges this;
*   by focusing on the context of disability, social constructionism shifts attention away from the individual as a locus and so offers a way of challenging oppressive practice;

- social constructionism accepts that there are always alternative perspectives and in this detail it refuses to conform to any big theory that attempts to explain everything – this helps to promote diversity of thought.

Of course, there are problems. Social constructionism is criticized for denying social agency. For if knowledge is socially constructed then how can we as individuals take control of the direction of our lives, given that all of the influences over us – the education and legal systems, the political machinery, the powerful discourses of medicine and the law – deny any biological imperatives? Calhoun (1994: 16) summarizes this when he says that 'Social constructionist approaches could be just as determinist as naturalizing approaches, for example, when they denied or minimized personal and political agency by stressing seemingly omnipresent but diffuse social pressures as the alternative to biology causation'.

Conclusion

In conclusion then, the phrase 'learning disability' can only have any meaning when it is set within a particular context. This context, as I have argued, was developed over a long period of time and although the terms of the debate have altered, the meaning has remained fairly constant. A disability identity is therefore one consequence of a denial by certain sections of society of the rights and responsibilities necessary to belong to that society to individuals who are relegated to the margins by a perceived inability to conform to socially anticipated norms. The task for social and health care professionals is therefore to question the circumstances that condone this sort of action while simultaneously acting in alliance with learning disability organizations and their supporters to redress the social imbalance.

References

Abbot, P. and Sapsford, R. (1987) *Community Care for Mentally Handicapped Children*. Milton Keynes: Open University Press.

Berger, P.L. and Luckmann, T. (1967) *The Social Construction of Reality: A Treatise in the Sociology of Knowledge*. Harmondsworth: Penguin.

Braddock, D.L. and Parrish, S.L. (2001) An institutional history of disability in G. Albrecht, K.D. Seelman and M. Bury (eds) *Handbook of Disability Studies*. London: Sage.

Burr, V. (1995) *An Introduction to Social Constructionism*. London: Routledge.

Calhoun, C. (ed.) (1994) *Social Theory and the Politics of Identity*. Oxford: Blackwell.

Comte, A. ([1853] 1971) The positive philosophy, in K. Thompson and J. Tunstall (eds) *Sociological Perspectives*. Harmondsworth: Penguin.

Conrad, P. and Schneider, J. (1980) *Deviance and Medicalisation: From Badness to Sickness*. St Louis: Mosby.

Cooper, R. (1997) The visibility of social systems, in K. Hetherington and R. Munro (eds) *Ideas of Difference: Social Spaces and the Labour of Division*. Oxford: Blackwell.

Dalley, G. (1992) Social welfare ideologies and normalization: links and conflicts, in H. Brown and H. Smith (eds) *Normalization: A Reader for the 90s*. London: Routledge.

Davis, L.J. (1995) *Enforcing Normalcy: Disability, Deafness and the Body*. London: Verso.

Down, J.L.H. (1866) Observations on an ethnic classification of idiots, *London Hospital Reports*, 3: 259–62.

Finkelstein, V. (1980) *Attitudes and Disabled People: Issues for Discussion*. New York: World Rehabilitation Fund.

Fox, S.A. and Giles, H. (1996) 'Let the wheelchair through!': an intergroup approach to interability communication, in W.P. Robinson (ed.) *Social Groups and Identities (developing the legacy of Henri Tajfel)*. Oxford: Butterworth-Heinemann.

Galton, Sir F. (1869) *Hereditary Genius: An Inquiry into its Laws and Consequences*. London: Macmillan.

Gergen, K.J. (1999) *An Invitation to Social Construction*. London: Sage.

Goddard, H.H. (1915) The possibilities of research as applied to the prevention of feeble-mindedness, *Proceedings of the National Conference on Charities and Corrections*, 307–12.

Gould, S.J. (1981) *The Mismeasure of Man*. Harmondsworth: Penguin.

Herrnstein, R.J. and Murray, C. (1994) *The Bell Curve*. New York: The Free Press.

Hughes, G. (1998) A suitable case for treatment: constructions of disability, in E. Saraga (ed.) *Embodying the Social: Constructions of Difference*. London: Routledge.

Itard, J. ([1806] 1972) *The Wild Boy of Aveyron*, trans. E. Fawcett, P. Ayrton and J. White. London: New Left Books.

Malthus, T.R. ([1872] 1971) *An Essay on the Principle of Population*. New York: A.M. Kelley.

Marcus, S. (1981) Their brothers' keepers: an episode from English history, in W. Gaylin, I. Glasser, S. Marcus and D. Rothman (eds) *Doing Good: The Limits of Benevolence*. New York: Pantheon Books.

Marks, D. (1999) Disability: *Controversial Debates and Psychological Perspectives*. London: Routledge.

Marx, K. (1913) *A Contribution to the Critique of Political Economy*. Chicago.

Mendel, G. (1950) Gregor Mendel's letters to Carl Naegeli, 1866–1873, trans. L.K. Piternick and G. Piternik, *Genetics*, 35(5), part 2 (supplement: 'The Birth of Genetics').

Neugebauer, R. (1978) Treatment of the mentally ill in mediaeval and early modern England: a reappraisal, *The Journal of the History of the Behavioural Sciences* 14: 158–69.

Oliver, M. (1990) *The Politics of Disablement*. London: Macmillan.

Parker, I. (1992) *Discourse Dynamics*. London: Routledge.

Parmenter, T.R. (2001) Intellectual disabilities – quo vadis, in G. Albrecht, K.D. Seelman and M. Bury (eds) *Handbook of Disability Studies*. London: Sage.

Pilgrim, D. (1993) Anthology: policy, in J. Bornat, C. Pereira, D. Pilgrim and F. Williams (eds) *Community Care: A Reader*. London: Macmillan.

Rudgley, R. (2000) *Secrets of the Stone Age*. London: Century.

Russell, D. (1997) *Scenes from Bedlam*. London: Bailliere Tindall.

Saraga, E. (ed.) (1998) *Embodying the Social Constructions of Difference*. London: Routledge.

Schifrin, B.S. and Longo, L.D. (2000) William John Little and cerebral palsy: a reappraisal, *European Journal of Obstetrics & Gynaecology*, 90: 139–44.

Scull, A. (1993) *The Most Solitary of Afflictions (Madness and Society in Britain, 1700–1900)*. London: Yale University Press.

Seguin, E. (1866) *Idiocy and its Treatment by the Physiological Method*. New York: William Wood.

Soder, M. (1984) The mentally retarded: ideologies of care and surplus population, in L. Barton and S. Tomlinson (eds) *Special Education and Social Interests*. London: Croom Helm.

Stockholder, F.E. (1994) Naming and renaming persons with intellectual disabilities, in M. Rioux and M. Bach (eds) *Disability is not Measles: New Research Paradigms in Disability*. North York, Ontario: Roeher Institute.

Stone, D. (1985) *The Disabled State*. London: Macmillan.

Symonds, A. and Kelly, A. (eds.) (1998) *The Social Construction of Community Care*. Basingstoke: Macmillan.

Wendell, S. (1996) *The Rejected Body*. London: Routledge.

Wood Committee (1929) *Report of the Joint Departmental Committee on Mental Deficiency*. London: Board of Education and Board of Control.

Wright, D. (2001) *Mental Disability in Victorian England*. Oxford: Clarendon Press.

3

The roots of biomedical diagnosis

Fiona Mackenzie

Introduction

There have been significant advances in the lives of people with learning disabilities in the three decades since the White Paper *Better Services for the Mentally Handicapped* (Department of Health and Social Security 1971) legislated for the closure of large institutions and the development of community services (see Chapter 6). The end of the era of institutions in which many people with learning disabilities, whose needs were largely social, lived in a hospital setting cared for by doctors and nurses has been associated with what has been called a 'demedicalization' of learning disabilities. Concern about the overuse of drugs to manage behavioural problems and the involvement of doctors in the eugenics movement has added impetus to the move away from a medical model. Learning disabilities have come to be understood as a socially constructed condition to which the most helpful response is social inclusion.

One important aspect of social inclusion, which has been neglected for people with learning disabilities, is health. Political changes set in motion by the human rights movement and now legislated for in the Disabilities Discrimination Act 1995 have given us a principle of equality of access to health services. People with learning disabilities have greater health needs than the general population (e.g. Moss and Patel 1993; McGrother *et al.* 2002; Kerr *et al.* 2003) but make less use of health services. The White Paper *Valuing People* (Department of Health 2001) recognizes that there are substantial unmet health care needs in the learning disabled population. In the chapter 'Improving Health for People with Learning Disabilities', one stated objective is to give such people access to health care designed around their individual needs.

The high level of unmet health needs recognized in people with learning disabilities (see Chapters 12, 27 and 33) also occurs among other socially and economically disadvantaged groups such as the homeless, and the solution may, for the large part, be social. However, in addition to the health needs that they share with the general population, some people with learning disabilities, particularly those with severe disabilities that may be multiple, have special health needs associated with the biomedical cause of their disability. In this chapter I will discuss how the diagnosis of the biomedical cause of an individual's learning disabilities can facilitate identification and appropriate management of these health needs over their life span, which is likely to have a significant impact on an individual's quality of life.

The bio-psycho-social model

A simplistic view of the medical model is that it implies the presence of pathology in an individual, which the doctor has the skills to identify and cure. The patient's role, once they have provided the doctor with the information required in order to make a diagnosis, is that of a more or less passive and compliant recipient of treatment.

This model has been heavily and rightly critiqued and is now regarded as an outmoded way of understanding and responding to the health needs of the general population. It is clearly an unhelpful and potentially devaluing way of thinking about the health needs of people with learning disabilities at either the individual or population level. The medical profession has long been aware of the complex interaction of biological, psychological and social factors in the conditions they treat and this has now been made explicit in what is termed the 'bio-psycho-social' model. This model, which is now taught in medical schools, places the patient (as a unique individual with biological, psychological and social needs) at the centre of their interaction with health services. It is within this framework that the process of diagnosis and assessment of the health needs of an individual with learning disabilities and the planning of health services to meet their needs should take place.

Terminology and definitions

There is a confusing proliferation of terms in everyday use to describe people with learning disabilities. In this section I will define the terms I use in this chapter and discuss the use of terminology in practice. In clinical situations, most doctors use the term which the patient prefers and uses to refer to their condition. In the UK this is frequently 'learning disabilities', the term adopted by the Department of Health in 1991 for use in government publications. I will use it in this chapter except where I am referring to a recognized classification of diagnosis. Such classification requires some understanding of how various categories are defined, and a summary is provided below.

The international *Classification of Mental and Behavioural Disorders*, currently in its tenth edition (*ICD-10*) (World Health Organization 1992) and the *Diagnostic and Statistical Manual of Mental Disorders*, currently in its fourth edition (*DSM-IV*) (American Psychiatric Association 1994), are the main classification systems currently in use. They assign numerical codes to the disorders they describe. The term 'mental retardation' is used in both *ICD-10* and *DSM-IV* and equates with learning disability. This term was associated with the eugenics movement (Williams 1995) and 'retard' has become a term of abuse. Hence the term mental retardation is unacceptable for use in clinical practice but because it is operationally defined in *DSM* and *ICD* it remains in use when precise communication between professionals is a priority – for example, in research publications and legal reports.

The World Health Organization (1980) defined the terms 'impairment', 'disability' and 'handicap'. Impairment is any loss or abnormality of physical or psychological function. A disability is defined as interference with activities of the whole person (often referred to in the field of learning disabilities as 'activities of daily living'). A handicap is the social disadvantage to an individual as a result of impairment or a disability. The term 'intellectual impairment' is used in the medical literature and does not necessarily equate with learning disability, as a learning disability does not necessarily result from mild degrees of intellectual impairment which do not interfere with the individual's capacity to carry out activities of daily living. Intellectual disability is sometimes preferred to learning disability because in disorders associated with intellectual impairment it is usual for other aspects of cognitive function such as attention and comprehension to be impaired as well as the ability to learn. The Mental Health Act 1983 uses the term 'mental impairment', defined as abnormal or incomplete development of mind, associated with abnormally aggressive or seriously irresponsible conduct. It implies the presence of learning disabilities and is only used in this context.

'Learning disabilities' sounds similar to 'learning difficulties', a term which can have different meanings in different contexts. Some people prefer this term, perhaps because it is inclusive (many people identify themselves as having difficulty learning in some area of their life). Learning difficulties is used in educational settings to describe children who are underachieving scholastically for a variety of reasons, which could include emotional or behavioural problems which are interfering with their ability to learn. Not all of these children have an intellectual impairment. The educational category of severe learning difficulties corresponds more closely with learning disabilities as used in health settings and many children who have been identified as having severe learning difficulties in school will need support from adult learning disabilities services. The term 'special needs' refers to children who have been given a Statement of special educational needs (SEN) by their education authority. This is based on the assessment of all professionals involved in their care and outlines the education authority's responsibilities to provide an education appropriate for the individual's needs.

ICD-10 uses the term 'disorder' to describe conditions with symptoms or behaviour associated in most cases with distress or interference with personal functions. I use it in the same way in this chapter when referring to developmental disorders. It does not imply a specific causation although there is good quality scientific evidence that many developmental disorders are associated with physical pathology in the brain.

A syndrome is the medical term for a set of clinical features which commonly occur together (e.g. in velo-cardio-facial syndrome, cleft palate, cardiac abnormalities and distinctive facial features occur together and are associated with learning disabilities). Some syndromes (e.g. Down's syndrome) are named after the researchers who first described them. Syndromes have also been named after characteristic features. Three children with learning disabilities were described in a paper entitled 'Puppet children' by Angelman (1965), who used this term to convey the children's jerky, string-puppet like movements. The term 'puppet children' is devaluing and has been replaced by 'Angelman syndrome'. Cri-du-chat syndrome is however still used to describe a syndrome in which, as a result of abnormal development of the larynx, the child has a high-pitched cat-like cry.

The term 'mental handicap' is now widely regarded as unhelpful because it implies that to be handicapped is the inevitable outcome of intellectual impairment. Nevertheless, some parents continue to refer to their learning disabled children as mentally handicapped because they feel that, for example, for a person with cerebral palsy who is incontinent and unable to walk or talk, the term 'learning disability' does not convey the extent of their care needs.

The psychoanalyst Valerie Sinason has described and critiqued the repeated change of terminology used to describe those with learning disabilities (Sinason 1992). She argues that while new terms, apparently more accurate or without unpleasant associations, are coined with good intentions, the process is driven by a defensive need to wish away the reality of actual damage and painful differences. There is a denial of the trauma which is intrinsic to having a condition in which development has gone awry. This primary trauma experienced by people with learning disabilities needs to be acknowledged and accepted.

Exercise 3.1

'I've got four handicaps. I've got Down's syndrome, special needs, learning disabilities and a mental handicap.'

(Young woman with Down's syndrome – Sinason 1992)

Discuss the use of terminology to refer to people with learning disabilities from the perspectives of a person with learning disabilities and their family.

Classification in learning disabilities

Learning disabilities are socially constructed (see Chapter 2). An individual comes to meet diagnostic criteria for learning disabilities and to be identified as learning disabled as the end point in a complex interplay of biological, psychological and social processes. As a result, who comes into the category varies over time and between societies. An individual may move in and out of the category of mild learning disabilities over their life span depending on the balance between their state of mental and physical health, and the supports and demands of the environment. A mild degree of intellectual impairment may be less disabling in a developing economy where rates of literacy are low and there is a wider range of valued social roles available. Historically, deficits in the capacity to cope with the demands of the environment, now called 'adaptive behaviour', were used to define those who would now be regarded as learning disabled (Wright and Digby 1996). Intelligence as a unitary and potentially measurable entity began to be conceptualized at the end of the nineteenth century and was then incorporated into the definition of learning disabilities.

The *ICD* and *DSM* definitions of mental retardation are broadly similar (see Boxes 3.1 and 3.2). Each is based on the presence of impairments in adaptive function in association with low IQ and both require the impairments to be present during the developmental period, which separates people with mental retardation from those who acquire intellectual impairment in adult life, for example as a result of brain injury.

Box 3.1 *DSM-IV* definition of mental retardation

A. Significantly subaverage intellectual functioning: an IQ of approximately 70 or below on an individually administered IQ test (for infants, a clinical judgement of significantly subaverage intellectual functioning).
B. Concurrent deficits or impairments in present adaptive functioning (i.e. the person's effectiveness in meeting the standards expected for his or her age by his or her cultural group) in at least two of the following areas: communication, self-care, home living, social/interpersonal skills, use of community resources, self-direction, functional academic skills, work, leisure, health and safety.
C. The onset is before 18 years of age.

Box 3.2 *ICD-10* definition of mental retardation

Mental retardation is a condition of arrested or incomplete development of mind, which is characterized by impairment of skills manifested during the developmental period, which contribute to the overall level of intelligence, i.e. cognitive, language, motor and social abilities.

ICD is the system used in the UK. It emphasizes the need to draw on wide sources of information when assessing an individual's adaptive function and to use standardized assessment schedules for which local cultural norms have been established. When comprehensive information is not available, a provisional diagnosis can be made. The limitations of IQ tests are recognized and the IQ levels specified for mild (50–69), moderate (35–49), severe (20–34) and profound (<20) mental retardation are intended only as a guide. Detailed clinical descriptions of each category of learning disability are provided.

ICD also emphasizes that while mental retardation can occur in the absence of any other disorder, the full range of mental disorders coded elsewhere in the manual can occur in people with mental retardation. The developmental disorders, including specific disorders of speech and language and pervasive disorders (autism) are of particular relevance (see Box 3.3). The manual recognizes the clinical difficulty in distinguishing for example a

---

Box 3.3   *ICD* classification of developmental disorders

Mental retardation
Mild
Moderate
Severe
Profound

Pervasive developmental disorders
Autism
Atypical autism
Asperger syndrome
Disintegrative disorder
Rett's syndrome
Other and unspecified

Specific developmental disorders
Speech and language: articulation; expressive speech; mixed expressive and receptive speech
Literacy: reading; spelling
Numeracy
Motor coordination
Mixed specific developmental disorder

---

specific disorder of speech and language from delayed speech and language in the context of global developmental delay in mental retardation. It points out that it is common for there to be an uneven profile of skills in mental retardation. For example, there may be a relative strength in non-verbal skills in comparison to language skills but when this discrepancy is marked, a specific developmental disorder should be coded in addition. *ICD* states that if the medical cause of the learning disability is known it should be coded separately.

Classification in service settings

Decisions made every day in service settings to categorize service users as having a learning disability are not generally based on the rigorous application of the operational diagnostic criteria described above (Hatton 1998). There are users of learning disability services who clearly do not meet diagnostic criteria, particularly some who were institutionalized many years ago for social reasons (see Chapters 1, 2 and 4). If they are settled and fit in well with their peer group there may be no impetus to review their classification. There are also many people who receive support from health and social services whose learning disability is not recognized as such. There is some evidence that failure to identify a learning disability may adversely affect outcomes in mental health services (Lindsey 2000).

In practice, indicators that a learning disability may be an issue, such as a history of SEN, poor language skills as well as the individual's own identity and how their needs are understood by carers, influence referral to learning disability services. Local service configurations and professional attitudes also have an impact on the decision to refer (Hatton 1998). When a referral for assessment is accepted by a learning disability service the response to immediate difficulties may appropriately take priority over the time-consuming and potentially threatening detailed assessments of adaptive behaviour. The limitations of IQ testing have been widely acknowledged. Factors such as an individual's level of motivation and state of health as well as cultural and linguistic diversity reduce the validity and utility of formal assessment of IQ in clinical practice (Jacobson and Mulick 1996). It is usual for experienced practitioners to make clinical judgements concerning whether or not it is appropriate and helpful to describe a person as learning disabled and to provide them with a service. The decision is based on information from as many sources as possible including interviews with family members and carers, health and education records, and the opinions and assessments of members of the multi-disciplinary team. Diagnostic criteria are only rigorously applied when there is disagreement, doubt or pressure to prioritize access to limited resources. Then, standardized IQ tests such as the Wechsler Adult Intelligence Scale (1981) may be used. Checklists of adaptive function are also available but these should be supplemented with direct observation (Widaman and McGrew 1996).

In medical practice little time is devoted to assigning individuals to the socially defined category of learning disabilities. The approach to diagnostic assessment of a person with an apparent intellectual impairment is similar whether or not their impairment results in them being defined as learning disabled. The priority is to identify the presence of additional mental and physical disorders, which may be contributing to the individual's impairment in adaptive function, particularly the specific developmental disorders and autism. Thought will also be given to the causes of the impairment and an attempt may be made to identify an underlying biomedical cause if this is likely to influence the individual's management plan.

Exercise 3.2

How useful are diagnostic criteria in informing decisions about who has priority of access to learning disability services? How would you go about developing eligibility criteria in a service with limited resources?

The causes of learning disabilities and their diagnosis

'Aetiology' is the word used in medical practice to refer to the cause or set of causes of a disease or condition. There is now evidence for a complex interaction of the social, the psychological and the biological in the aetiology of conditions such as cancer, which have previously been thought of as having a physical cause. The process by which an individual comes to be defined as having a learning disability also depends on this interaction of the biological, psychological and social over their life span.

Intelligence as measured using standardized IQ tests is normally distributed in the population. If a graph is drawn to plot the results of IQ tests of a representative sample of the population it is a bell-shaped curve, which is almost symmetrical around a mean of 100. Statistical methods would predict that 2.27 per cent of the population would have an IQ of less than 70, which is two standard deviations below the mean. As the definition of learning disabilities also includes the presence of associated impairments in adaptive function, fewer than 2.27 per cent of the population would be expected to be defined as learning disabled. Some people with mild learning disabilities are likely to represent the lower end of the normal distribution of intelligence in the population. Mild learning disabilities tend to be associated with social disadvantage and to cluster in families. This may be the result of adverse environmental factors ranging from lead poisoning due to traffic fumes to child abuse and neglect in the developmental period interacting with genetic determinants of intelligence. In mild learning disabilities there is likely to be an identifiable cause in about 50 per cent of people. For the remainder, low intelligence may be a qualitative variation from normality.

In practice, the number of mildly learning disabled individuals in a given population is difficult to estimate. The administrative prevalence based on numbers known to learning disabilities services varies according to the availability of services and other factors such as the degree of stigma attached to being defined as having a learning disability. The number of people in a population with severe learning disabilities is likely to be estimated more accurately as most will be known to services. It is greater than would be predicted, based on a normal distribution. The increased number of people with low IQ is seen as a bump in the curve, which has been referred to as the 'pathological tail'. This implies that this group includes people whose intellectual development is qualitatively different from normality as a result of a biological insult to their central nervous system, rather than just a quantitative variation on normality.

In 80 per cent of people with severe learning disabilities, a specific biomedical cause can be diagnosed. However, even in the presence of a disorder that has a significant impact on the development of the brain, the outcome in terms of the individual's eventual intellectual capacity and adaptive function will be significantly influenced by additional biomedical and environmental factors during the developmental period. The biomedical condition might be understood as defining the range of eventual outcomes – for example, people with Down's syndrome range from severely to mildly disabled. Factors which influence the eventual outcome include the presence of additional impairments, which might be intrinsic to the biomedical cause (e.g. motor impairment in cerebral palsy or associated with it; hearing impairment following repeated respiratory infection in Down's syndrome). These additional impairments limit the developing child's capacity to interact with and learn from their social and physical environment and may cause frustration or damage to self-esteem, which adversely affects their emotional development.

Classifying the biomedical causes of learning disabilities

A useful way of classifying the biomedical causes of learning disabilities is by the timing of the earliest factor which affected the development of the central nervous system. Diagnosis can be divided into six main groups, which are listed in Table 3.1 with common examples.

Diagnosis over the life span

The significance of a search for a main biomedical cause of learning disabilities, for the care of the individual and their family, changes over the life cycle. In this section I will discuss the relevance and implications of biomedical diagnosis at different life stages.

Perinatal diagnosis

Screening for Down's syndrome and neural tube defects (associated with spina bifida) is offered routinely in pregnancy. When risk factors are present (e.g. a family history), additional tests may be offered. Parents may interpret normal results from these tests as meaning that such disorders have been ruled out, however their sensitivity is not 100 per cent. Infants born in the UK are routinely screened for congenital hypothyroidism and phenylketonuria. Easily recognizable conditions such as Down's syndrome will be identified at birth. Parents may be informed that their child has sustained brain damage during the birth or is at risk of it as a result of prematurity.

Table 3.1 Summary of biomedical classification of causes of learning disabilities

Cause	Examples
1 Genetic	
Chromosomal disorders	Down's syndrome
Syndromes associated with microdeletions	Velo-cardio-facial, Prader-Willi syndrome
Single gene disorders	Tuberous sclerosis, fragile X syndrome, phenylketonuria
Multifactorial inheritance	Neural tube defects
2 Central nervous system malformations	
Unknown	Sotos syndrome
3 Factors in prenatal environment	
Toxic	Foetal alcohol syndrome, maternal rubella, HIV
Infectious	Prematurity, birth injury
4 Disorder acquired around the time of birth	
Various	
5 Disorder acquired postnatally	
Infections of the central nervous system	Measles, encephalitis, brain injury (e.g. traffic accidents)
Accidents	Brain injury
Toxins	Lead poisoning
6 Unknown cause	
Learning disabilities associated with other symptoms and signs of brain damage	e.g. autism, cerebral palsy
Learning disabilities where low IQ is a quantitative variant of normality	

Source: adapted from Gelder *et al.* (2000)

The identification of signs associated with developmental disabilities before or around the time of birth leads to the family being offered thorough diagnostic investigation by paediatricians. The presence of malformations may suggest that the baby has a less common genetic syndrome that will subsequently be investigated by clinical geneticists.

The impact on a family of the birth of a significantly impaired child has been likened to the grieving process (Bicknell 1983) in which what has been lost is a normative expectation, what Bicknell terms the 'fantasy' of having a 'perfect' child. There are phases of numbness, disbelief, guilt and anger followed by active adaptation. The validity of this comparison, which seems to devalue those with impairments, has since been questioned (see Chapter

10 in this volume) and an alternative model proposed. It is nevertheless a time in which families have to make considerable psychological and practical adjustments to the special needs of their child and the provision of a clear diagnosis is likely to be helpful.

The majority of parents want accurate and up-to-date information following the recognition of a disorder in their child (Philp and Duckworth 1982). A diagnosis may alleviate inappropriate guilt or anger towards health professionals that could otherwise interfere with relationships. For example, a mother was able to stop blaming herself for smoking during pregnancy when she was told that her child's severe disabilities were due the genetic disorder Cri-du-chat syndrome (Ramcharan *et al.* 2004).

Each individual is unique and it is not possible to predict exactly how a child will develop. If however the range of impairment associated with a syndrome is known it may be possible to provide parents with some information about prognosis, in reply to such questions as 'Will he ever talk?', 'Will she be able to live independently as an adult?'. Much has been written about how best to inform parents of the news that their child has a developmental disability (see Chapter 10 in this volume). When things go well the outcome will be the formation of a healthy partnership between the family and health professionals, which will enable them to work together to meet the needs of the child over its life span.

The family will be able to make contact with other families caring for children with similar disorders, to share information and support. There are well-established associations for the more common disorders such as Down's syndrome and cerebral palsy and the internet has allowed both parents and professionals involved in the care of those with rare disorders to link up and share information and support (see Box 3.4).

Box 3.4 Websites of support groups and associations

The Down's Syndrome Association	www.dsa-uk.com
The Fragile X Society	www.fragilex.org.uk
The Prader-Willi Syndrome Association	www.pwsa-uk.demon.co.uk
The Tuberous Sclerosis Association	www.tuberous-sclerosis.org

---

When an inheritable disorder is diagnosed, parents will be offered information about the probability of this reoccurring in future pregnancies and the implications for other family members. This can raise complex ethical dilemmas for families and professionals and referral to genetic counselling services, which can provide accurate information and support, may be helpful.

In some conditions associated with learning disabilities, early diagnosis and treatment can significantly improve the outcome. An example is phenylketonuria in which, due to gene mutation, the presence of the protein phenylalanine produces toxic metabolites which damage the developing nervous system. A low phenylalanine diet can prevent subsequent learning disabilities. In most other conditions there are no effective preventative treatments currently available, although there are future prospects for gene therapy in some genetic disorders, for example Duchenne muscular dystrophy, which is associated with mild learning disabilities. The value of diagnosis for the child is the creation of the potential for early identification of additional physical and psychological impairments, which are known to be associated with the condition. The optimal management of these can minimize their impact. It is well recognized that in some circumstances medical intervention can cause further problems (e.g. the treatment of epilepsy with sedating medication or the trauma of surgery to correct orthopaedic problems). A thoughtful approach based on a thorough understanding of the child's physical, psychological and social needs is needed to enable the child to develop optimally within the limits imposed by their condition.

Preschool diagnosis

For the majority of children the presence of a developmental disorder becomes apparent as, over time, delays in achieving milestones or qualitative differences from the usual pattern of development are recognized by parents or professionals. There are protocols for the developmental screening of children by health visitors and guidelines for specialist referral. The incidence of severe developmental disorders is low in primary care. A working party of the British Paediatric Association (Valman 2000) estimated that one child with a severe learning disability is born in ten years to a family on a GP's average list of about 2000 patients. It is therefore unrealistic to expect primary care teams to develop expertise in diagnosis and assessment, but the hope is that children with significant developmental delay, or whose development is qualitatively different, will be identified and referred to paediatric services for diagnostic assessment.

When a significant developmental delay is identified, whether or not a biomedical cause can be identified, the family is offered a multi-disciplinary assessment in a child development centre. The aim of this is to get a detailed picture of the child's mental and physical function and family context. Particular attention is given to identifying sensory impairments and medical conditions such as epilepsy, which might need specific intervention. There is also assessment for the presence of specific developmental disorders of speech, language and motor function, and pervasive developmental disorders such as autism. The assessment informs a care plan, which aims to optimize the child's development and prevent as far as possible the emergence of secondary impairments. The care plan may include physiotherapy to develop gross motor coordination and occupational therapy to develop fine motor skills. The parents will be given advice about how to respond to their child to promote their physical and psychological development. They will also be advised as far as possible about what to expect from their child over their life span as well being given information about services, support groups and emotional support. The care plan will be regularly reviewed and adapted.

All children with significant developmental disorder have access to free nursery placements at age 3. When the child reaches school age they will be assessed for a Statement of SEN. The aim of this is to provide educational support tailored the child's individual needs.

Diagnosis in the school-aged child

The presence of mild learning disabilities may not become apparent until the child starts to attend school and falls behind other children in their educational attainments. The group of children who fail in school is diverse and the majority will not be defined as learning disabled as adults. It includes some children who have developmental disorders with a biomedical condition, which has not been recognized in the early years. An example is foetal alcohol syndrome, which is a result of drinking in pregnancy and ranges in severity according to the timing and degree of foetal exposure to alcohol.

There are children whose ability to function and learn in the school environment is impaired by behavioural problems. These may be underpinned by attention deficit hyper-activity disorder, autism or specific learning difficulties, or be largely the result of emotional problems and social deprivation. The identification and referral for specialist assessment of children with these sorts of problems is less systematic than the screening provided by health visitors for preschool children and the availability of specialist assessment may be limited. It relies on the education of teachers in the recognition of behaviours likely to be associated with a developmental disorder. For the majority of such children a specific developmental disorder will not be identified but an assessment of strengths and needs may help inform educational approaches and may lead to a Statement of SEN.

Diagnosis in adulthood

At the time of transition from children's to adult services individuals with learning disabilities are, under present policy in England, to be offered a Health Action Plan which forms a basis for planning to meet their health needs in adult life. It will include assessments of any special health needs which are associated with the biomedical cause of their learning disability and associated conditions.

Although the majority of those with severe learning disabilities entering adult services will now have an identified biomedical cause, there are a significant number of adults already in services who do not, and for whom developments in scientific knowledge mean that a biomedical diagnosis is now possible. Children with developmental delay are seen at intervals by paediatricians and if a specific cause has not been identified the issue of diagnosis will be reviewed in the light of any emerging signs and developments in medical knowledge. Such specialist medical care is not routinely provided for adults with learning disabilities. Most adults will be known only to social and primary health care services, which may not be familiar with the less common biomedical causes of learning disabilities and associated specific developmental disorders. In some learning disabilities services there has been a reluctance to use diagnosis of any sort as this is felt to label the individual in such a way as to create negative expectations of them and deny their individuality. A counter argument is that if we live in an inclusive society in which individual differences are recognized and valued, there may be something to be gained from understanding as much as possible about the nature of those differences through the assessment of the biological, psychological and social aspects of learning disabilities.

The diagnostic assessment of adults with learning disabilities raises clinical and ethical dilemmas. Family members or professionals involved with an adult with a learning disability may request diagnostic assessment because they think it may provide useful information about how to care for the individual or access to services – for example, those for people with autism. A family member may request investigation for a genetic syndrome to inform an assessment of their risk of having a child with a developmental disorder. In each of these circumstances, the first issue to be considered is the person with a learning disability's capacity to consent to investigation. This will require assessment of their understanding of the nature and possible outcomes of such an investigation.

When an individual lacks the capacity to consent to investigation it is the responsibility of the clinician carrying out the investigation to proceed on the basis of the individual's best interests, involving them as far as possible and those family members and professionals that know them best in the decision. (Issues of capacity and consent are dealt with more fully in Chapter 5.) A useful question to consider is how likely is there to be an identifiable biomedical cause for this individual's learning disability. For example, the presence of congenital malformations or a family history suggestive of an inheritable condition makes this more likely. Factors then to be considered are the likely benefit to the individual's health, for example through a better understanding of their condition. The discomfort and distress likely to be associated with an investigation (e.g. blood tests) also needs to be taken into account.

When an adult with learning disabilities is referred to specialist health services because they have developed a problem with their physical or mental health (see Chapter 27) the investigation of the aetiology of their intellectual impairment may in some situations help in the understanding of this and therefore inform its management. Another situation in which the diagnostic investigation of an adult with learning disabilities may be considered is when they have not had access to specialist health care in childhood – for example, immigrants or refugees from economically disadvantaged countries. Again, the individual's capacity to consent and the likely impact on them of a diagnostic assessment need to be considered. When a developmental disorder, which is known to be associated with serious health problems such as tuberous sclerosis, is suspected, diagnosis is likely to be of benefit so that the health issues can be identified and treated promptly. In other developmental disorders not known to be associated with serious health problems the benefit for the individual may be less clear.

A related area is that of behavioural phenotypes, a concept first used by William Nyhan (1972) in relation to Lesch-Nyhan syndrome in which he described self-mutilating behaviour. He emphasized the role of biomedical factors in producing this behaviour and defined the behavioural phenotype as 'behaviours which are an integral part of certain genetic disorders'. Since then, behavioural phenotypes have been described for a number of conditions and it can be argued that an understanding of the pattern of motor, cognitive, linguistic and social behaviour which is characteristic of a condition can help inform the planning of education and support. There is however debate about the quality of the evidence for behavioural phenotypes and concern about the risk of creating negative expectations in conditions in which there is much individual variation. A description of the behavioural phenotype and a case example of a young woman with Prader-Willi syndrome is given below. It is followed by a description of Down's syndrome which is a common biomedical cause of learning disabilties.

Prader-Willi syndrome

Prader-Willi syndrome is caused by a deletion in chromosome 15. There are two copies of chromosome 15, one inherited from each parent. The deletion usually affects the chromosome inherited from the father. A similar deletion in chromosome 15 inherited from the mother results in Angelman syndrome, which has very different characteristics. Prader-Willi syndrome does not usually (but can occasionally) reoccur in families. It is now normally diagnosed by genetic testing in infancy when it is associated with low muscle tone and poor feeding, with failure to gain weight at the expected rate. There is developmental delay in childhood and most but not all adults have mild to moderate learning disabilities. At around the age of 3, children begin to overeat and this tendency continues throughout the life span. Other features include delayed and incomplete puberty and behavioural problems, some of which may be linked to carers' attempts to restrict their eating. People with Prader-Willi syndrome have difficulty restricting their food intake, and there are no specific treatments that are effective in preventing resultant obesity. Unless carers restrict access to food, life span is limited by the complications of obesity including Type II diabetes and respiratory problems. There has been debate about the ethical basis for the control of access to food for adults with Prader-Willi syndrome (Holland and Wong 1999).

Case study 1

Sarita is a 38-year-old woman with moderate learning disabilities who has lived in a staffed group home for two years since the death of her mother. Her GP referred her to the health support team GP because of concerns about her weight, which has increased from 16 to 21 stone over two years. Her carers have noticed her tendency to overeat and think that this is due to boredom. They have supported her to gain the confidence to go out into the local town unaccompanied but this has led to an increased food intake as she often buys sweets and chips. With her agreement her carers have encouraged her to follow a healthy eating plan but she has become angry whenever she felt under pressure to cut back on food. Sarita does not understand the health risks associated with obesity, but is aware that she is not able to walk uphill without becoming breathless and finds this distressing. She is not able to say very much about her weight and eating patterns before her move to the home and there is limited information from records apart from the fact that she has been obese since starting at primary school. Her brother describes how her mother consistently limited Sarita's access to food and even obtained a lock for the fridge. He believes that this was the only way of ensuring that his sister did not massively overeat.

Exercise 3.3

Should genetic investigation of Sarita for Prader-Willi syndrome be considered and if so how should an assessment of her capacity to consent to this be approached? If Sarita were found to lack the capacity to consent, would it be in her best interests to carry out the investigation? If Sarita is found to have Prader-Willi syndrome, how would this influence the response to her obesity?

Down's syndrome

Approximately 4.6 in 10,000 people have Down's syndrome (Steele 1996). Down's syndrome results when an individual has extra genetic material in the form of an additional copy of chromosome 21 (Lejeune *et al.* 1959). It is usual for human cells to contain 23 pairs of chromosomes, one of each pair being inherited from each parent. The majority of people with Down's syndrome have an additional copy of chromosome 21 and the condition may be referred to as 'trisomy 21'. In 3 per cent of cases the extra genetic material is joined to another chromosome (this is referred to as a translocation) and in these cases the condition may be inherited, usually from the mother, who has a one in six chance of conceiving a child with Down's syndrome.

People with Down's syndrome have a variety of physical characteristics, which include short stature, skin folds at the inner corners of their eyes, broad hands and a large tongue. People with Down's syndrome are easily identified as learning disabled by the general public which may impact on the formation of their identity. About half of babies born with Down's syndrome have heart defects. The motor and intellectual development of infants with Down's syndrome is delayed in comparison with the general population, and people with the syndrome have reduced muscle tone, which contributes to delay in the average age of walking unsupported to between 19 and 29 months. The average IQ of a young adult with the syndrome is around 50 and the majority of sufferers have severe learning disabilities. There is however a large range of IQ (from 17 to 75) and of ability in daily living skills in the population of people with Down's syndrome. The most severely disabled people with the syndrome require a high level of care, whereas the most able people with Down's syndrome acquire literacy and numeracy skills, are able to live and work without special support and do not necessarily have a learning disability as socially constructed.

Down's syndrome has historically been associated with a decreased life expectancy. This has changed dramatically in recent years from an average age of 12 years in 1947 (Penrose 1949) to at least 45 years at present (Carr 2000) as a result of health care interventions, particularly surgery to treat heart defects. One consequence of this is that parents of middle-aged people with Down's syndrome who may have been led to expect that they would outlive their children now have to readjust their expectations.

Although the majority of people with Down's syndrome enjoy good physical and mental health for much of their life span they are at an increased risk of a number of conditions, the prompt detection, accurate diagnosis and appropriate treatment of which is likely to be of benefit (see Box 3.5).

Box 3.5   Health problems associated with Down's syndrome

Congenital heart defects
Respiratory infections
Hearing and visual impairments
Hypothyroidism
Skin problem
Gum disease and tooth loss
Obesity
Depression
Alzheimer's disease

Conditions of particular note are Alzheimer's disease, which occurs at an earlier age in people with Down's syndrome, and hypothyroidism which occurs in 40 per cent of adults with Down's syndrome (Anneren and Pueschel 1996) and can mimic the early stages of Alzheimer's disease. The physical health and development of children with Down's syndrome is routinely monitored by community paediatric services. There is an argument for this monitoring to continue into adult life (Prasher 1994), although the majority of conditions should be identified in well-person clinics in primary care.

Exercise 3.4

Using a bio-psycho-social model, discuss how you would approach the construction of a Health Action Plan for a 19-year-old man with Down's syndrome who is leaving school and moving into adult services.

Conclusion

By applying the bio-psycho-social model it is possible to attach a label, a diagnosis, to a person with a learning disability. This is not done gratuitously. It is not done with the intention of labelling a person as having less value than anyone else. It is, rather, a means of ensuring that access to appropriate health and medical interventions through the lifecourse is achieved. The name or label is the most efficient way of knowing what to look out for in terms of health and medical needs. It may be a way of understanding behaviours and the ways in which people communicate. It can also be of huge value to professional staff seeking to ensure that major health needs are understood and met (see Chapter 12). And if this is the case it can be argued that the role of biomedical diagnosis, used in the appropriate way, is central to improving the quality of life of people with learning difficulty throughout their lifecourse.

References

American Psychiatric Association (1994) *DSM-IV Diagnostic and Statistical Manual of Mental Disorders*. Washington, DC: The American Psychiatric Association.

Angelman, H. (1965) Puppet children: a report on three cases, *Developmental Medicine and Child Neurology*, 7: 681–3.

Anneren, G. and Pueschel, S. (1996) Preventive medical care, in B. Stratford and P. Gunn (eds) *New Approaches to Down Syndrome*. London: Cassell.

Bicknell, J. (1983) The psychopathology of handicap, *British Journal of Medical Psychology*, 56: 167–78.

Carr, J. (2000) Intellectual and daily living skills in 30 year olds with Down's syndrome: a continuation of a longitudinal study, *Journal of Applied Research in Intellectual Disabilities*, 13: 1–6.

Department of Health (2001) *Valuing People: a New Strategy for Learning Disability for the 21st Century*. London: Department of Health.

Department of Health and Social Security (1971) *Better Services for the Mentally Handicapped*. London: DHSS.

Gelder, M.G., Loez-Ibor Jr., J.J. and Andreasen, N.G. (2000) *The New Oxford Textbook of Psychiatry*. Oxford: Oxford University Press.

Hatton, C. (1998) Intellectual disabilities – epidemiology and causes, in E. Emerson, C. Hatton, J. Bromley and A. Caine (eds) *Clinical Psychology and People with Intellectual Disabilities*. Chichester: Wiley.

Holland, A.J. and Wong, J. (1999) Genetically determined obesity in Prader-Willi syndrome: the ethics and legality of treatment, *Journal of Medical Ethics*, 25: 230–6.

Jacobson, J.W. and Mulick, J.A. (1996) Psychometrics, in J.W. Jacobson and J.A. Mulick (eds) *Manual of Diagnosis and Professional Practice in Mental Retardation*. Washington, DC: American Psychological Association.

Kerr, A.M., McCulloch, D., Oliver, K., McLean, B., Coleman, E. and Law, T. (2003) Medical needs of people with intellectual disability require regular assessment, and the provision of client- and carer-held reports, *Journal of Intellectual Disability Research*, 47: 134–45.

Lejeune, J., Gautier, M. and Turpin, R. (1959). Les chromosomes humaine en culture de tissus, *Compte rendu de l'Academie Science*, 248: 602.

Lindsey, M. (2000) Services for people with learning disabilities and mental health problems, *Mental Health Review*, 5: 5–18.

McGrother, C., Bhaumik, S., Thorp, C., Watson, J. and Taub, N. (2002) Prevalence, morbidity and service need among South Asian and white adults with intellectual disability in Leicestershire, UK, *Journal of Intellectual Disability Research*, 46: 299–309.

Moss, S. and Patel, P. (1993) The prevalence of mental illness in people with intellectual disability over 50 years of age, and the diagnostic importance of information from carers, *Irish Journal of Psychology*, 14(1): 110–29.

Nyhan, W. (1972) Behavioural phenotypes in organic genetic disease: presidential address to the Society for Paediatric Research, May 1, 1971, *Paediatric Research*, 6: 235–52.

Penrose, L.S. (1949) The incidence of mongolism in the general population, *Journal of Mental Science*, 95: 685–8.

Philp, M. and Duckworth, D. (1982) *Children with Disabilities and their Families: A Review of Research*. Windsor: NFER-Nelson.

Prasher, V.P. (1994) Screening of medical problems in adults with Down syndrome, *Research and Practice*, 2(2): 59–66.

Ramcharan, P., Whittell, B. and Grant, G. (2004) *Advocating for Work and Care: The Experience of Family Carers Seeking Work: A Report to the Community Fund*. Sheffield: University of Sheffield.

Sinason, V. (1992) *Mental Handicap and the Human Condition*: London: Free Association Books.

Steele, J. (1996) Epidemiology: incidence, prevalence and the size of the Down's syndrome population, in B. Stratford and P. Gunn (eds) *New Approaches to Down's Syndrome*. London: Casseu.

Valman, H.B. (2000) *The ABC of One to Seven*. London: BMJ Books.

Widaman, K.F. and McGrew, K.S. (1996) The structure of adaptive behaviour, in J.W. Jacobson and J.A. Mulick (eds) *Manual of Diagnosis and Professional Practice in Mental Retardation*. Washington, DC: American Psychological Association.

Williams, C. (1995) *Invisible Victims*. London: Jessica Kingsley.

World Health Organization (1980). *International Classification of Impairments, Disabilities and Handicaps*. Geneva: WHO.

World Health Organization (1992) *The ICD–10 Classification of Mental and Behavioural Disorders*. Geneva: WHO.

Wright, D. and Digby, A. (eds) (1996) *From Idiocy to Mental Deficiency: Historical Perspectives on Learning Disabilities*. London: Routledge.

4

Critiques of segregation and eugenics

Malcolm Richardson

Introduction

This chapter considers the various ideological responses to people with impairment within a number of societies throughout history. The history of how any society regards and treats people with impairments is a history of ideology. Ryan (1971) describes how ideologies develop from the 'collective conscious' of a group, or a class-based interest in maintaining the status quo. Ideologies have several components: the ideology itself; systematic distortion of reality in those ideas; the condition that the distortion must not be a conscious, intentional process; and that the ideas encompassed must specifically function to maintain the status quo in the interests of a specific group.

Consideration of these ideological bases reveals the conceptual distortions that underpin our responses to those people we term as having learning difficulties today, and so better informs us in order that we may challenge such distortions within modern services.

Exercise 4.1

Write down as many words (up to ten) as you can recall that you have heard used to refer to people with a disability or impairment.

How do you think about people with learning difficulties? Write down ten phrases or adjectives that you think apply.

Care in the community

In the UK most people probably think of community care as of recent origin in relation to people with learning difficulties, but care in the community is probably as old as human society. At Skhul, in Israel, the 95,000-year-old remains of an 11-year-old boy showed evidence of a healed cranial injury, demonstrating that his community must have looked after him for a considerable time. Similarly, at Shanidar cave in Northern Iraq, the 46,000-year-old skeleton of a 40-year-old man revealed a congenital underdevelopment of his right side of such a nature that he would have needed support from his society throughout his life. Additionally, his right arm had been amputated just above the elbow; he had arthritis and he had survived other injuries, one of which had probably blinded his left eye. Both of these finds reveal that the individuals had severe impairments, yet their survival had the commitment of their respective societies. These findings challenge some modern assumptions about the survival only of the 'fittest' in what we disparagingly call 'primitive' societies (Rudgley 2000).

But not all societies are the same and hence their ideological responses to impairment differ. For example, at the Neolithic settlement of Catalhoyuk (c.10,000 BC), in Turkey, from the thousands of skeletons excavated only one was not afforded the traditional family burial, that of an individual with a hunched back which was discovered 'unceremoniously dumped on a rubbish tip, perhaps because he was . . . perceived as an outsider' (Rudgley 2000: 74). This might be one of the earliest evidences of someone with a physical impairment being excluded from society. As such it is part of a pattern to be repeated in more recent times.

In historical records the personal accounts of people society perceived to be different in mind or body are largely absent. This is not particularly surprising since, in pre-industrial societies, only the wealthy and ruling classes were likely to be educated and literate. Surviving accounts, therefore, represent that part of society. Nevertheless, some historians have salvaged persuasive evidence suggesting that in each epoch of history, western society has generated its own particular, often dissimilar, ideological ways of responding to people who are physically or mentally different. What is of interest is the extent to which these responses were either more or less accepting of people with physical, sensory or mental impairments and therefore the different lifecourses that followed. For example, one extreme holds life-threatening exclusion, while the other extreme holds veneration. Heddell (1980) describes how the practice of exposure, by which an infant was left exposed to the elements overnight, was used to encourage the survival of healthy offspring in the ancient civilizations of Greece, Scandinavia and Sparta. Roman law permitted infanticide in order to dispose of any unwanted infant. However, McLaren (1990) points out that the extent of these practices is far from clear. Bredberg's (1999) analysis of disability history points to evidence that the ancient Greeks practised infanticide infrequently and that reports to the contrary stem from historical misinterpretation. Clearly, however, in these societies an element of social stigma was attached to impaired infants and society's social policy allowed extreme social exclusion to be utilized by those choosing to impose it.

However, Bredberg (1999) also points to evidence that not all societies were possessed of this ideology and hence disabled people throughout history have held roles other than those resulting in stigmatization. For example, in an analysis of Nordic and Celtic mythology Bragg (1997) describes how physical exceptionalities (including impairments) were associated with the gift of supernatural capacities such as great wisdom, being a 'seer', having a memory for stories, poetry and so on. The belief was that by giving up an attribute, such as speech, the use of a limb or sight, in a contract with the supernatural, the person became endowed with special powers. Hence, the possession of an impairment was often associated with being exceptionally potent in some other way, not despite the impairment, but because of it.

Yet Bragg (1997) also shows that people were cautious of impairment. For example, mythology warns against the misuse of any associated powers, as with the mythological 'blind' archer who never misses his target, but is unwittingly fooled into shooting a friend. Additionally Bragg points to a general disinterest in impairment with regard to a person's competence. People did seek cures but there was no evidence for the attribution of demonic possession, little recognition that impairment might be a medical or a personal tragedy and little if any marginalization, pity or charity. Hence, practices such as exposure and infanticide, though evident historically, may not have been quite so widespread. They slowly declined, partly due to the spread of Christian philosophy, although McLaren (1990) points out that infanticide probably remained common well into the eleventh century. The penalties for it remained lenient into the eighteenth century. An alternative, abandonment (leaving an infant in a conspicuous place in the hope that it would be 'taken in'), probably increased.

Infanticide is presumed to continue today in various parts of the world as, for example, in testimonies from Latin America, India, China, Africa and the Far East (Infanticide 2003).

Exercise 4.2

Think about the ten words or phrases you have already noted in Exercise 4.1. How well do they match the views related above? Why are these views different?

The pre-industrial age

With respect to the reign of Edward II, Race (1995a) points to a statute of 1325, *De Praerogativa Regis*, by which the lands of an 'idiot' or 'natural fool' (terms then in use for people with learning difficulties) were protected, their necessities provided for and their lands passed to their heirs after death. 'Lunatics', the term then used to refer to people to whom we would today ascribe a mental illness, had their lands protected until their recovery. Hence, the difference between the two was judged to be one of permanence (i.e

Edward's concern was for the land-owning upper classes). At village level, there was no provision and the medieval 'village idiot' (in common parlance) remained the responsibility of the family or parish.

Some historians suggest that in western pre-industrial, pre-capitalist societies people with learning difficulties (and many other physically or mentally impaired people) generally coped, sometimes in the role of 'village idiot'. For many, the ability to perform simple manual work would make them indistinguishable in a society where literacy and numeracy were comparatively rare. People classed as mad or deranged were not usually separated as deviants, but assimilated into an amorphous class comprising the poor, the morally disreputable, vagrants, minor criminals and the physically impaired. Consequently, during the Middle Ages there were very few institutions for the insane, such as Bethlem Hospital (also known as Bedlam). Demand for places at Bethlem was low and the hospital contained no more than ten beds until well into the seventeenth century, when it was rebuilt on a larger scale and renamed the Royal Bethlehem Hospital. In the 1650s, the managers of Bedlam tried to make a distinction between the 'curable mad', 'those dangerous to be abroad', who should be in a hospital, and 'harmless idiots', who they deemed should not be hospitalized. A subcommittee was established to identify and eject those who were 'idiots' and not 'lunatic' (Scull 1979; Slater 2004). Clearly, therefore, learning difficulties were not regarded as medical and not, therefore, in need of a 'cure'.

However, if Christianity frowned upon infanticide, its attitudes towards people with impairments were inconsistent. Disabled people were deemed by St Augustine of Hippo (AD 354–430) to be possessed by devils, and people with learning difficulties were suffering a punishment for Adam's original and other sins. Later, Martin Luther (1483–1546) recommended the killing of impaired infants, believing them to be 'changelings' (the devil having stolen the human child, substituting a demon). Mothers of such infants were sometimes accused of intercourse with the devil and so might be put to the stake for 'witchcraft' (Scull 1979; Clarke 1983; Race 1995b). Periods of religious zeal might, therefore, have proven problematic for people with impairments.

Yet despite the pronouncements of St Augustine and Luther, social policy was more often one of toleration and inclusion rather than stigmatization and exclusion. During periods when work was scarce and the family unable to provide, begging alms, charity, the use of almshouses, and hospitals (originally places of hospitality) offered some protection. Monasteries also played a part in caring for the sick and infirm, at least until their dissolution in the sixteenth century (Scull 1979; Clarke 1983; Baly 1995). Ryan and Thomas (1991) point to the doctrine of a Swiss physician in the sixteenth century, who made a plea for recognition that people with learning difficulties were equals and possibly even betters: 'his [humankind's] wisdom is nothing before God, but rather that all of us in our wisdom are like fools . . . Therefore the fool, our brother, stands before us . . .' (sixteenth-century physician cited in Ryan and Thomas 1991: 86).

The Elizabethan Poor Laws of 1568 and 1601 also offered some protection. But these laws constituted the beginning of social legislation aiming to contain provision within each respective parish and thereby deter the mobility of the poor. The laws therefore resulted in some degree of stigmatization being attached to the poor, which clearly comprised many people with impairments.

Generally speaking, therefore, throughout the Middle Ages a policy of social inclusion pervaded society. As Foucault (1965) put it, 'insanity' and 'idiocy' walked the streets of everyday life.

Exercise 4.3

Write two short paragraphs concerning the imaginary experiences of a person with learning difficulties during the Lutheran era and during the Elizabethan era.

Industrialization

Significant changes in the lot of people with learning difficulties came with eighteenth- and nineteenth-century industrialization, its associated land enclosures and the commercialization of agriculture. Prior to industrialization, working practices were largely rural. Gradually, work turned from small peasant labour or craftwork to village artisan or smallholder cottage industry (Hobsbawm 1962, 1968; Thompson 1968). For a period, the timing and pace of work continued to be largely self-determined and therefore favourable to people with impairments (Ryan and Thomas 1980). However, as these processes became more industrialized, the pace and timing of work altered significantly.

Industrialization created a new bourgeoisie and what many regarded as a jungle anarchy based upon a purely utilitarian, individualist system of social behaviour that theoretically justified one's position in society according to one's individual attributes. This was typified by the motto, 'every man for himself and the devil take the hindmost' (Hobsbawm 1962: 239).

Industrialization brought about the ending of centuries-old legislation that had protected workers' standards of living. This, combined with urbanization and employers bearing no responsibilities for their employees beyond payment of wages, shattered the traditional social contract between the labourer and the master (Scull 1979). The new master and servant laws threatened jail for workers who did not conform and allowed the imposition of low wages that forced workers into unremitting and uninterrupted toil in order to survive (Hobsbawm 1968). This contributed to a volatile rise in vagrancy and an unprecedented increase in the social exclusion of people with physical or mental impairments (Scull 1979).

Hobsbawm's (1962) analysis saw capitalist ideology ascribing one's position in society according to one's individual attributes. Similarly Ervelles' (1996) cross-cultural analysis demonstrates how attitudes to disability (as with race, gender, class and sexual orientation) spring from the needs of capitalism:

> the ideological category of disability is essential to the continued exist-ence of the capitalist enterprise because it is able to regulate and control the unequal distribution of surplus through invoking biological differ-ence as the 'natural' cause of all inequality, thereby successfully justify-ing the social and economic inequality that maintains social hierarchies.
>
> (Ervelles 1996: 526)

Capitalism therefore sought to remove, control and discipline those who would not or could not conform to new working practices by demanding greater secular controls. The result was an unprecedented rise in the building of houses of correction, jails and 'madhouses' (Scull 1979). Between 1720 and 1825, 150 hospitals were built in England to cater for the rising numbers of the sick poor (Baly 1973, 1995).

Despite this, Walton's (1980) study of asylum admissions from 1848 to 1850 demonstrates that supportive networks were not inevitably destroyed by industrialization, at least for those living away from the industrial con-urbations. Nevertheless, a major increase in state intervention had begun that significantly impinged upon people with learning difficulties. It can there-fore be argued that state intervention compounded the economic exclusion created by industrialization with a state policy of social exclusion, a by-product of which was the charity and welfare systems, the remnants of which still prevail. The outcomes of institutionalization against other residential provision are further considered in Chapter 6 of this volume.

For adults with learning difficulties a number of 'idiot' asylums were built. Heddell (1980) points to the opening, in 1847, of Park House at Highgate, by the philanthropist Andrew Reid. This was followed by an annex at Col-chester, later to become the Royal Counties Hospital. Earlswood asylum opened with 500 beds in 1855 and was regarded as the model institution of its time. The 1886 Idiot's Act allowed local authorities to build asylums for 'idiots' (Scull 1979).

The scandalous exposure of inhumanitarian regimes within these institutions now began to emerge. Profit before care and the excessive use of restraints fuelled alarm over wrongful and unscrupulous incarceration among the new middle classes. Feeling threatened by the same exclusionary measures that they had introduced, the ruling classes instigated controls to protect themselves. These included the so-called humanitarian reforms as exemplified by Quakers such as William Tuke, founder of the Retreat at York. Similarly, the Insanity Act of 1845 established new controls and, sig-nificantly, ensured that all asylums procured the safeguard of a medical superintendent (Clarke 1983; Scull 1979; Baly 1995).

Medicalization

The appointment of these medical superintendents hastened the medicali-zation of 'mental disorder' which became established under the legal control of the newly-emerging profession of psychiatry (Scull 1979; Potts and Fido 1991; Fennell 1996). Borsay (1997) points out that nineteenth-century physicians had largely rejected the principle of original sin, adopting instead Locke's (1632–1704) philosophy of the mind as a *tabula rasa* – i.e. susceptible to manipulation. The physicians therefore regarded mental disorder rather as they did physical disease, as something located within the individual and potentially treatable.

Early attempts at education

Similarly, eighteenth-century educational ideology reflected the work of philosophers such as Rousseau (1712–78) and his contemporary, Saint-Simon (1760–1825). These thinkers helped promulgate the belief that people with learning difficulties could be educated and society would, thereby, be opened to them (the complete opposite of the eugenic philosophy that was to come). Such ideas inspired new ways of thinking about education and prompted some attempts at treatment for people with mental disorders, including those with learning difficulties.

Accordingly, Itard and Seguin established a working philosophy in relation to people with learning difficulties, principled upon the belief that, given sensory, physical and social training, the innate potential of their pupils would flourish enabling them to be better accepted within society (Clarke 1983): 'An idiot is endowed with a moral nature and is influenced by the same things as the rest of the community' (Seguin 1846 cited in Potts and Fido 1991: 1).

Itard's widely published developmental work with the 'wild boy' found living in the woods near Aveyron (Itard [1806] 1972), and later that of his pupil Seguin, encouraged similar 'schooling' throughout Europe and America. Saxony was the first state to make training for people with learning difficulties compulsory.

Subsequently, in England, small schools for so-called 'idiots' opened, the first in 1822 at Leicester (Clarke 1983). By 1896, London had 900 pupils in 24 such schools (Heddell 1980). The 1870 Education Act made elementary education compulsory for all children. While the reasons, then as now, largely concerned the need for a literate and numerate workforce, people with learning difficulties were not excluded from schooling (Heddell 1980; Clarke 1983).

Shortly after 1870, the Victorians realized that some children were not mastering the 'three Rs'. For these 'feeble-minded' children a separate system of schooling emerged in which basic living and self-help skills replaced the 'three Rs'. Hence, the beginnings of separatist educational systems for disabled children began as soon as it became evident that the elementary education system could not fit these children for the capitalist workplace.

As Heddell (1980) points out, this utilitarian approach to the education of all children, but particularly those identified as 'feeble-minded', however paternalistic, was neither without compassion, nor without the desire to do the best possible for the children. It is worth bearing in mind that during the nineteenth century many children of normal intelligence were exploited or died in poverty. Others found themselves in the workhouse. People with learning difficulties clearly represented some of the deserving poor. The various forms of state intervention such as separate schooling and 'shutting away' in an asylum reflected the relatively new assumptions about the incapacities of people with impairments. These assumptions underpinned the ideology of protective paternalism, in turn underpinned by charity. Hence, segregation was regarded as protection rather than imprisonment.

In summary, the arrival of the industrial epoch heralded a virulent extension of social legislation (see Chapters 1 and 2). After a thousand or more years mainly characterized by tolerance and inclusion, people with impairments, newly excluded from the now commercialized agricultural and industrial workplaces, were assigned to the stigmatized class of the poor, albeit the deserving poor. Humanitarianism was evident, but largely served the interests of the capitalist class from which it sprung. Focusing upon the poor who were 'deserving' generated the charity and welfare systems that helped create and sustain a new myth of personal tragedy and individual incapacity. The appointment of medical superintendents can be seen as a step towards institutionalizing the medicalization of mental disorder.

Exercise 4.4

Adapt the stories you wrote in Exercise 4.3 to the period discussed above. How do the stories differ?

Early eugenics

Based upon their interpretation of genetic inheritance, the late Victorians feared that learning difficulty, or feeble-mindedness as they termed it, was a genetically inherited disease that would eventually reduce the nation's intelligence. Wolfensberger (1972) demonstrates at least eight myths that support eugenic and segregative ideologies within contemporary services to people with learning difficulties. These myths are the learning disabled person as sub-human organism, diseased organism, menace to society, unspeakable object of dread, object of ridicule, object of pity, holy innocent and eternal child.

To prevent the populace from 'degenerating', the eugenicists persuaded many western nations, including the UK, to segregate thousands of people identified as 'feeble-minded within asylums or colonies in order to prevent them from multiplying' (Mittler 1979; Heddell 1980; Clarke 1983; Race 1995b). The eugenicists, led by Sir Frances Galton (see Chapter 2), pressured the Home Office to make special provision for people with learning difficulties, resulting in the 1913 Mental Deficiency Act. This Act created four categories: 'feeble-minded', 'idiots', 'imbeciles' and 'moral defectives'. The feeble-minded were given education but idiots and imbeciles were not (Beacock 1992). Moral defectives were those people whom society wished to exclude, such as unmarried mothers in receipt of poor relief. It is not surprising that the 1913 Act recognized 'feeble-mindedness' as a social rather than a medical issue. After all, the eugenic aims of the Act were, in effect, to 'clear the streets' of undesirables. Hence, so-called 'moral defectives' were caught under the Act, regardless of their IQ. The admission of patients as a medical case was a formal process with no scope for any to be admitted informally (Heddell 1980).

Borsay (1997) points out that the twentieth-century institutionalization of people with learning difficulties overwhelmed nineteenth-century notions of treatment. Instead, care and control mediated by costs became the order of the day. Effectively this meant placing resources under 'one roof'. Medical interest in the causes of crime, immorality and poverty ascribed blame to people with learning difficulties (Scull 1979; Heddell 1980). Mary Dendy, writing in 1920 on 'Feeblemindedness in Children of School Age', represented that view, writing that these children should be 'detained for the whole of their lives' in order to 'stem the great evil of feeblemindedness in our country' (cited in Potts and Fido 1991: 1). Similarly, Fernald, promoting the eugenic standpoint in 1912, wrote:

> The feeble minded are a parasitic, predatory class, never capable of self-support or of managing their own affairs. The great majority ultimately become public charges in some form. They cause unutterable sorrow at home and are a menace and danger to the community. Feeble minded women are almost invariably immoral, and if at large usually become carriers of venereal diseases or give birth to children who are as defective as themselves. The feeble minded woman who marries is twice as prolific as the normal woman. Every feeble minded person, especially this high-grade imbecile, is a potential criminal, needing only the proper environment in which to express such. The unrecognised imbecile is a most dangerous element in the community.
>
> (Fernald 1912 cited in Beacock 1992: 405)

Recent accounts from former detainees under the 1913 Act (Potts and Fido 1991) describe children suspected of feeble mindedness being scooped off the streets by the hospital's officer, and taken before the hospital panel to be assessed, often with no allowance for the child's tender years, emotional state or educational opportunities. The judgement and subsequent labelling ascribed were frequently arbitrary. At the end of the first and second years, and five-yearly thereafter, the asylum panel reviewed each case. Parents were normally present, but formality was such that only the views of the medical superintendent carried influence. Often the damning character references from the original admission papers were used years later to warrant continued detention.

Consequently, few detainees obtained release. Indeed 'high grades', as able detainees were called, provided valuable unpaid work within the colonies. Not only did they help care for detainees with multiple impairments and children, they also helped the colonies to be largely self-sufficient, working the farms, gardens and laundries and with the carpenters, cobblers and so on (Potts and Fido 1991). Ironically, therefore, a class of people ideologically deemed unfit to live, or bear children, and incapable of productive employment, worked within and helped to sustain the very institutions that confined them.

During the 1920s and 1930s the eugenicists campaigned for compulsory sterilization of what they termed the 'unfit to breed' (Clarke 1983; Fennell 1996). Legal opinion since the 1880s advised that to sterilize a person, even with their consent, would amount to maiming under Section 18 of the Offences Against the Person Act 1861, unless there were clear medical (health) reasons. In the 1920s, legal opinion had not changed (Fennell 1996).

During the 1930s, the British government commissioned the Brock Committee to examine the sterilization issue. The committee recommended the authorization of sterilization only with consent, rejecting compulsion (Fennell 1996). Neville Chamberlain, as Minister for Health, deferred to allow the formation of public opinion. Meanwhile, Nazi Germany legislated for compulsory sterilization of people with learning difficulties. By the end of the 1930s the Nazis had murdered more than 70,000 people with physical and mental impairments. Newspaper reports during 1934 alarmed the British public, who were advised that visitors to Germany might be considered 'aliens' and sterilized. News also came from the USA that 900 American children were mutilated to prevent their breeding. Some 60,000 to 70,000 American citizens with learning difficulties were sterilized against their will during this period (Fennell 1996). Consequently, support for sterilization dwindled in the UK.

During the 1950s sterilization returned to the agenda, but this time based upon the right to a life free from the burden of childbearing. In 1960 the Medical Defence Council, seeking counsel's opinion, were advised that sterilization would be legal as a means of birth control. This could be enforced without consent if the woman concerned was deemed to be incapable of caring for offspring due to learning difficulties. Subsequently, the 1967 Abortion Act reflected liberal public opinion giving women greater control by allowing termination of pregnancy up to 26 weeks. This limit did not apply to 'handicapped' foetuses, which could be aborted up to the full term of gestation. Therefore the 1960s bore acceptance of what, 100 years previously, could not take place: the sterilization of a woman with learning difficulties without her consent (Fennell 1996).

Certainly, marriage and parenting were discouraged, as the following accounts by Pam testify. Pam, a lady now in her fifties, spent much of her life in an institution for people with learning disabilities. Pam is speaking to a group of former institutional residents and the writer about her elder non-disabled sister who, unlike Pam, married and had children:

Pam: . . . my sister . . . she's grown-up and married. Got kids of her own. Nice house. Left school, she were only 14 then.

Writer: What happened when you got to 14, did you have to leave school?

Pam: Oh we left school at 14 years old. Monica was 14. My sister . . .
            she was 14. She fell in love with a young man . . . and they
            got happily married and have children of their own and a nice
            house.
Writer: What happened to you when you were 14? Did you leave school
            and get a job?
Pam: Er not exactly . . . When me mum was alive she brought us here
            [the institution] . . . because they couldn't cope. So me and Jane
            came here.
Writer: Where did you go to live?
Pam: Up at . . . I was on Field View.
Writer: . . . what was it like in those days?
Pam: Well it, staff were bossy and that.
Writer: They were bossy?
Tim: They were too bossy! . . . [indistinct].
Writer: Was it scary when you went there to begin with?
Pam: Ooh I was frightened. I was morbid.
Jane: Yes, yes I was!
Writer: You were, you were frightened were you, Jane?
Jane: Yes.
Pam: But now we've grown up . . . We used to wear institution clothes
            then . . . but we don't wear institution clothes now.
Jane: Boots like football boots.
Barry: Institutional dresses . . . Others are left now what were bossy . . .
            Now there's some more people that's nice now.
Robin: That's old [insitution]. They were old nurses.
Pam: The old ones are left . . . It was a long time ago!

Pam's account clearly indicates that the regime within the institution, built
for eugenic purposes, was strict. Later, Pam told her story about some
parts of her life; this is what she had to say: 'It's true what I said, my life
has been different to that of my sister Margaret. My mum and dad told me
when I was younger that children and marriage were not for me. But I have
never wanted children. I did enjoy my nephews when they were children
and it is lovely to visit staff and see their children . . .'. Like the vast majority
of people with learning disabilities in Pam's generation, the idea that
'children and marriage are not for them' took a deep hold within their
concept of self.

At the start of the twenty-first century, eugenics remains potent; its
death-making 'it's better to be dead than disabled' essence has diversified
into eugenic abortion, euthanasia, voluntary euthanasia, sterilization and
genetic screening – all aimed at eradicating those likely to be stigmatized
for their difference (Stanworth 1989; Swain 1989; Williams 1989). Eugenics
today operates by stealth.

In summary, social policy within the early eugenic epoch stigmatized
specific groups of individuals, and denied their basic human rights, in order
to maintain the genetic 'purity' of the rest of society.

Exercise 4.5

If you had a condition such as Down's syndrome and you knew that people were aborting pregnancies carrying Down's babies, how might this affect you?

The road to deinstitutionalization

Just as the first half of the twentieth century moved towards institutionalizing people with learning difficulties, the second half of that century began the process of deinstitutionalizing them.

The UK National Health Service (NHS) Act 1946 handed responsibility for these colonies from the local authorities to the new hospital authorities. Local authorities, however, continued to provide for people with learning difficulties living at home. The 'mental deficiency' colonies thus became hospitals and their transfer to the NHS represented the pinnacle of the medicalization of people with learning difficulties. Hospitals for people with learning disabilities continued to be built into the early 1970s. However, forces were gathering that would challenge the supremacy of the medical model.

The late 1950s saw the emergence of a new social policy in which hospitals were no longer the servant of eugenics, but recast as rehabilitation centres preparing people for community living (see Chapter 6). From the 1950s a period of slow change was to be set in motion (Heddell 1980; Beacock 1992; Race 1995b).

Parental pressure groups

The 1944 Education Act placed responsibility for the education of 'handicapped' children with the local authorities. However, on eugenic grounds it had excluded children with severe forms of learning difficulties from schooling and this was unacceptable to many parents. In 1946 the National Association of Parents of Backward Children (later the National Society for Mentally Handicapped Children) was established, becoming a forerunner for many similar pressure groups. It aimed to change the law to provide community care and proper education for such children (Heddell 1980). The removal of state-funded schooling prompted many parents and volunteers to establish their own 'schools', usually referred to as junior training centres (JTCs), often in church halls. By the late 1960s many were funded or aided by the local health authority or local authority in purpose-built centres (Heddell 1980; Clarke 1983).

These JTCs helped to disprove Sir Cyril Burt's eugenic assertion that children with severe learning difficulties were ineducable. The 1970 Education Act reinstated education for these children within special schools provision (Heddell 1980; Clarke 1983). In the decades since then, debates have ensued about the pros and cons of including all children with learning difficulties within mainstream education (e.g. Clough and Barton 1995).

Social research

While the medical model resulted in research into the medical roots and genetic causes of impairments and their treatments, hence determining the lifecourses of people with learning disabilities in accordance with this model, non-medical research explored different avenues that would, ultimately, propose different life paths.

For example, educational and clinical psychologists demonstrated the potential of people with severe learning difficulties to benefit from education and training for skills and employment (e.g. Tizard and O'Connor 1952; Clarke and Clarke 1954; Clarke and Hermelin 1955). Research was also pointing out the importance of social and environmental factors in the creation of learning difficulties, as opposed to genetics or disease. One example, the Brooklands experiment (Tizard 1964), demonstrated the disabling effects of institutional care upon children, while also illuminating the clear advantages of child-centred practices in alternative community-based care environments. In the same period, Goffman's *Asylums* (1957) exposed the mechanisms of institutionalization and stigmatization. Morris' *Put Away* (1969) and Miller and Gwynne's *A Life Apart* (1972) further exposed the detrimental consequences of institutionalizing people with learning difficulties, and King *et al.* (1971) demonstrated how institutionalized patterns of care were detrimental to those living within them.

By 1959, public opinion had been sufficiently influenced to prompt a change in the law. The 1959 Mental Health Act was the first major revision since 1913. Under the new Act, degrading certification ended. 'Mental deficiency' was replaced by what many considered a more disablist term, 'mental subnormality'. Most patients were technically free to leave or remain in the hospitals as voluntary patients. Some left, mainly those who had worked as unpaid staff, but for most there was simply nowhere else to go (Clarke 1983; Potts and Fido 1991).

Additionally, the hospital scandals of the 1960s and 1970s (DHSS 1969, 1971, 1978) revealed degrading conditions and abuses within institutions. These scandals helped spur government policy in the direction of community care for the 52,000 people with learning difficulties then in hospital. Peter Mittler (1978: 1) summarized the situation:

> 50,000 citizens of this country are living in hospitals for the mentally handicapped. 20,000 of them . . . for 20 years or more . . . Many thousands of them do not need to be in hospital at all. Some look upon the hospital as their home . . . But for others, hospital is a prison without walls . . . where they must remain because there is nowhere else for them to live and nothing for them to do outside the hospital . . . Anyone who looks at mental handicap hospitals today cannot fail to be struck by the discrepancy between the quality of life for the general population and

that of mentally handicapped hospital residents. The physical conditions under which mentally handicapped people are expected to live and work for year after year have long been regarded as unacceptable for the rest of society. Wards of over 50 adults and over 30 children are not only unpleasant places in which to live but are totally incompatible with good standards of professional practice.

However, upon the removal of such adverse factors the potential for personal growth and development becomes evident within the lives of people with learning difficulties. In a retrospective review of their own and contemporaries' research Ann and Alan Clarke (2003) bring to light extensive evidence that survival, development and adaptation in this population are normative and subject to the same interactions between nature and nurture that affect the rest of society, especially when adverse social and environmental factors, such as institutionalization and social exclusion, are removed. In contrast to eugenics, this reveals the importance of recognizing the capacity and resilience of people with learning disabilities, their strengths and resourcefulness together with their personal potential.

The voices of people with learning difficulties

A review of social research publications (Whittlemore *et al.* 1986) demonstrated that early social research in this area was aimed, primarily, at the problems faced by parents and guardians in coping with their impaired child or adult. Therefore, perhaps in the belief that they knew best, parents and professionals usually planned the lifecourses for people so labelled (Ryan and Thomas 1991; Race 1995a, 1995b; Atkinson and Walmsley 1999).

But from a small start in the late 1960s the voices of people with learning difficulties have been adding their perspectives and making an increasing and significant mark upon research agendas (see Chapter 34). Those perspectives are too numerous and wide-ranging to address in detail here, but they do vividly convey the common humanity of people with learning difficulties trying to get by in their daily lives, much like the rest of society (Edgerton 1967; Hunt 1967; Edgerton and Bercovici 1976; Edgerton *et al.* 1984; Flynn 1986; Jahoda *et al.* 1988). For example, adults with learning difficulties generally prefer to live in the least restrictive places, usually separate from their parents (Flynn and Saleem 1986), in a hostel rather than hospital, in a group home rather than a hostel and in independent living rather than a group home (Passfield 1983; Conroy and Bradley 1985; Heal and Chadsey-Rush 1985; Richards 1985; Booth *et al.* 1990; Gold 1994). They are often excluded from respected social positions and not allowed the same rights, privileges or obligations afforded the rest of society, and nor are they accredited with the same emotional capacities (Flynn 1989; Potts and Fido 1991; Cheston 1994; Cambridge *et al.* 1994; Etherington and Stocker 1995; Collins 1996; Holland and Meddis 1997). Many are coping within impoverished circumstances yet, despite these adversities, they are often making the best of community living, and complaining less than they might (Flynn 1989; McVilly 1995).

Their stories are, therefore, largely reflective of the resilience of the human spirit, revealing that people with learning disabilities, in contrast to eugenic assumptions, develop throughout their life span, adapting to changing circumstances much like the rest of society. They contribute to society in a variety of ways such as through their diverse social presence, the work they do and, in some cases, the way they provide for others. Too often their network of friendships and relationships is underdeveloped and the support and assistance to develop and maintain such relationships is lacking.

Human rights and normalization

In response to the Holocaust and other atrocities of the Second World War, the United Nations made a universal declaration of human rights, Article 1 stating, 'All human beings are born free and equal in dignity and rights' (Beacock 1992: 406). Later, the 1971 *United Nations Declaration on The Rights of Mentally Retarded Persons* defined specific rights to education, citizenship, health and work. During these same decades, humanist concepts of person and being (e.g. Maslow 1943, 1954; Rogers 1951), combined with the principles of basic human rights, were beginning to influence the ideologies of a broad spectrum of professionals in health and educational fields. Beacock (1992) identifies how these were combined within the principles of normalization (Bank Mikkelsen 1969; Nirje 1972; Wolfensberger 1972, 1983; O'Brien and Tyne 1981).

Normalization began formally in the Danish Mental Retardation Act of 1959. It aimed to create normal living conditions for people with learning difficulties (Bank-Mikkelson 1969). Hence it stood in stark contrast to both eugenics and the medical model. Normalization influenced a generation of professionals, generating a mini epoch of social policy. While it did not significantly influence government policy over the closures of the old 'mental handicap' hospitals, it did help to win hearts and minds in favour of deinstitutionalization (Race 1999).

Exercise 4.6

List ten ways in which the presence of people with learning disabilities helps improve society.

The social model

With industrialization, western capitalist ideology created a world solely adapted for people who conformed to a narrowed perception of humanity.

Those falling outside this perception were thereby disabled through social and economic exclusion and disablist practices embedded within the culture. For example, the very act of recognizing learning difficulty and naming it became a self-fulfilling prophesy because it contained within it the assumption of incapacity. This inaccurate assumption led to the person being treated as though incompetent, and thereby denied opportunities to learn and develop skills. However, as many argue, it is not competence that is at issue, but rather the social and physical barriers faced by disabled people being so pervasive that they are prevented from ensuring themselves a reasonable quality of life (Manion and Bersani 1987; Bynoe *et al.* 1991). This sustains the charity-led approach to disabled people. It still usurps that place in the minds of the wider public which more rightfully belongs to the recognition of social justice and human rights by which all people could find access to an interesting and satisfying life.

Not surprisingly, the socially constructed nature of disability (see Chapter 2) has become a rallying call to disabled people. By the early 1990s Disabled Peoples International comprised 70 national assemblies with the British Council of Organizations of Disabled People (BCODP) representing 90 organizations comprising over 300,000 disabled people (De Jong 1979; Finkelstein 1980; UPIAS 1981; Stone 1985; Davies 1993; Finkelstein 1993). How many of these comprised people with learning difficulties is hard to judge. Certainly People First, a London-based group, and a small number of similar self-advocacy groups in other parts of the UK were operational by the early 1990s (see Chapter 8 for a review of the development of self-advocacy). Hence a growing number of disabled people have adopted a disability identity that rejects charitable status and classification by impairment-led labels because such labels locate disability within the person rather than within the barriers that disable them (Harris 1995).

Disabled people seek, therefore, to establish new social policy in which they produce and control their own services – for example, through centres for independent living (Oliver 1993). The traditional disability professions, however, tend to hold on to power. Hence, the disabled rights movement argues for powerful legislation to place the control of disability services in the hands of disabled people and, in the UK, establish a Bill of Rights (Davies 1993; Oliver 2000).

The success of the disability rights movement will depend, in large part, on the extent to which disabled people and their allies can rid themselves and society of oppressive practices. For example, within the disability movement people with cognitive impairments have experienced marginalization. Additionally, not all disabled people have signed up to the social model, and many wield their impairment as their lived reality and cite social and economic exclusion as secondary factors. Similarly, there are detractors within the academic sphere.

Eugenics today

Of course, despite improvements in community services, eugenics has not gone away. It remains an insidious part of our culture where the popular ideal of beauty covets perfection without blemish. This ideology can be seen on supermarket shelves where only 'unblemished' fruit is allowed, right through to the human genome. For example, we have laws that make eugenic abortion for impairments as 'trivial' as a club foot or cleft palate possible up to the full term of pregnancy. People with Down's syndrome have to live with the knowledge and consequences for their own self-esteem that foetuses with Down's syndrome are often aborted. And, although people are no longer hospitalized because of their learning difficulties, this is not to say that deprivation and institutional practices have disappeared (see Table 4.1).

Other chapters in this book reveal how people with learning difficulties continue to face physical or sexual abuse, often because their lives continue to be restricted and excluded and therefore somewhat 'hidden' from view. Fortunately, those chapters point to workable strategies for minimizing abuse. Typically, adults with learning difficulties have to remain living with their parents because there is little prospect of obtaining alternative supported living. Others experience 'containment' within a group home, where choices about how and with whom they live are limited. Poor-quality supported living means that opportunities for gainful employment (see Chapter 26), meaningful activities and personal relationships (see Chapters 23 and 29) are unsupported and hence lacking. Segregated schooling and day services persist, as does the view that people with learning disabilities need to be segregated for their own protection. Therefore, RESCARE, a mainly parental pressure group, campaigns against community living, preferring the creation of 'protective' village communities (Cox 1995).

For those people with a learning difficulty who also have a psychiatric disorder, diagnosis and treatment of their illness is often overlooked or misunderstood (Clarke 1999; Moss *et al.* 2000; Hatton 2002). Similarly, for those with a physical or medical condition, dehydration, pressure sores, chronic life-threatening constipation, not being washed or changed after soiling, not receiving correct medication, being over-sedated, lack of communication, having too many carers and not having your plan of support consistently delivered are, too often, additional life experiences due to unrecognized or unmet health requirements (Mencap and MLD Link 2002; Kozma and Mason 2003; NPSA 2004).

Conclusion

This chapter has critiqued the eugenic perspective by examining a range of ideological perspectives from different cultures and epochs. It has been

Table 4.1 Some examples showing traces of eugenics in contemporary services

Health services throughout the life span	*Social and educational services throughout the life span*
Screening and abortion of 'impaired' foetuses up to full-term of pregnancy	Segregated housing for disabled people
Withholding life-saving/health enhancing treatments to children, adults and elderly people with Down's syndrome, and other syndromes associated with learning difficulties	Segregated schooling and barriers to accessing mainstream schools
	Poor building design that does not accommodate wheelchairs
Persuading non-disabled people that acquiring a major physical or mental disability is always so ghastly that it's a good idea to have a 'living will' telling the authorities to let you die if this happens to you	Barriers – physical, social and attitudinal – to accessing youth clubs and youth facilities
	Barriers to accessing public facilities such as community centres, sports stadiums, recreational facilities, clubs, restaurants, nurseries, educational facilities, colleges, universities
Disabled people with a terminal illness having to seek judicial review to obtain the right to have their lives prolonged	Pressure from society to have 'the perfect body'
Plastic surgery to make people with Down's syndrome look 'normal'	Barriers to work and employment
If you are admitted to hospital, being put in a bed away from the ward simply because you have Down's syndrome	Lack of consistency in availability of financial, social and health care support to families of a disabled person
Having your health care needs unnoticed despite chronic constipation, dehydration, epilepsy, medication side-effects, brittle bones and difficulty swallowing being conditions associated with your cerebral palsy	Being told you are 'irresponsible' for wanting to marry and have children
	Not being taken seriously when you express your thoughts or opinions
	Under-resourcing of services to support people with newly-acquired severe impairments such as head/brain injury, paralysed or damaged limbs or spinal injury
	Low wages for disability support workers and home care staff
	Lack of training for disability support staff/carers
	Having to travel in the 'Sunshine Charity Bus' for disabled children/adults/elderly
	Having a benefits system that forces you to wear second-hand clothes in a society where people 'show off' their 'designer' wear

Exercise 4.7

This chapter began by identifying that ideology has several constituents: the ideology itself; the systematic distortion of reality in those ideas; the condition that the distortion must not be a conscious, intentional process; and that the ideas encompassed must specifically function to maintain the status quo in the interests of a specific group. The myths that Wolfensberger (1972) identified (see below), or each subtle permutation thereof, continue to support contemporary eugenics. Examples of this are shaded in grey. Use the space in the central column to add further examples that you recognize.

Myths (Wolfensberger 1972)	Contemporary eugenic outcomes (examples shaded grey) Use the centre column to add some more. How often do the outcomes involve segregation, abuse, neglect, lack of personal safety and/or a disregard for capacity and talent?	Whose interests are served? (examples shaded grey) Add some more that you identify
Subhuman organism	Deny human rights; treat like animals; abortion of disabled foetuses	Scientific experiments, use as guinea pigs; house in substandard accommodation; no need to provide education
Diseased organism	Hospitalize; find a 'cure' or accept 'diseased status'	Jobs for medical staff; medical research
Menace to society	Lock up somewhere away from society to protect society from danger	Institutions/administrators/ workforce
Unspeakable object of dread	Do not associate yourself with 'them'; euthanasia	Institutions/administrators/ workforce
Object of ridicule	Bullying; harassment; teasing	Bullies
Object of pity	Charity	Welfare system, 'do-gooders'
Holy innocent	Protect in segregated pseudo-religious communities; seek miracle cures	Charlatans
Eternal child	Incompetence; incapacity	Protection and welfare services

demonstrated that disability and incapacity are not the inevitable outcomes of mental or physical impairments, but that the outcomes differ according to any given society's underpinning ideological standpoint.

Thus, the relatively recent institutionalization of people with learning difficulties was a product of capitalist ideology aiming to control the 'sick poor' and, subsequently, misguided eugenic concerns. Institutionalization began during a period when the medical profession was expanding and led to the medicalization of learning difficulties. The first half of the twentieth century saw upwards of 60,000 people in the UK institutionalized. The second half of that century witnessed increasing recognition of the misguided nature of institutionalization and the commencement of programmes of deinstitutionalization.

More recently, social research, the voices of parents and people with learning difficulties and the disabled rights movement have alerted service providers to the significant disabling potential arising from the medicalization of disability and social and economic exclusion.

In recognizing the important advances that are supporting people with learning difficulties to live in their communities, we must also recognize that for many the reality remains one of insidious segregation, mini institutions, the legacy of institutional practices, contemporary but segregated day occupation, adults 'trapped' in their parents' homes, the monotony of poor quality independent living and inadequately met health needs.

Progress in resolving these issues will remain hampered without legislation based upon human rights, by which disabled people will have a right to a decent level of income, social, educational and work access and inclusion. These are things that the disabled rights movement wishes to promulgate, and to which health and social professionals may pledge their allegiance.

References

Atkinson, D. and Walmsley, J. (1999) Using autobiographical approaches with people with learning difficulties, *Disability and Society*, 14(2): 203–16.

Baly, M.E. (1973) *Nursing and Social Change*. London: Routledge.

Baly, M.E. (1995) *Nursing and Social Change*, 3rd edn. London: Routledge.

Bank-Mikkelson, N.E. (1969) A metropolitan area in Denmark: Copenhagen in R. Kugel and W. Wolfensberger (eds) *Changing Patterns in Residential Services for the Mentally Retarded*. Washington, D.C.: President's Committee on Mental Retardation.

Beacock, C. (1992) Triggers for change, in T. Thompson and P. Mathias (eds) *Standards and Mental Handicap: Keys to Competence*. London: Bailliere Tindall.

Booth, T., Simons, K. and Booth, W. (1990) *Outward Bound: Relocation and Community Care for People with Learning Difficulties*. Buckingham: Open University Press.

Borsay, A. (1997) Review article – language and context issues in the histography of mental impairments in America, c. 1800–1970, *Disability and Society*, 12(1): 133–41.

Bragg, L. (1997) From mute God to the lesser God: disability in medieval Celtic and Norse literature, *Disability and Society*, 12(2): 165–77.

Bredberg, E. (1999) Writing disability history: perspectives and sources, *Disability and Society*, 14(2): 189–201.

Bynoe, M., Oliver, M. and Barnes, C. (1991) *Equal Rights for Disabled People: The Case for a New Law. IPPR Welfare Series, 1991/1992*. London: Institute for Public Policy Research.

Cambridge, P., Hayes, L., Knapp, K., Gould, E. and Fenyo, A. (1994) *Care in the Community Five Years On: Life in the Community for People with Learning Disabilities*. Aldershot: Ashgate.

Cheston, R. (1994) The accounts of special education leavers, *Disability and Society*, 9(1): 59–69.

Clarke, A. and Clark, A. (2003) *Human Resilience – A Fifty Year Quest*. London: Jessica Kingsley.

Clarke, A.D.B. and Clarke, A.M. (1954) Cognitive changes in the feeble-minded, *British Journal of Psychology*, 45: 173–9.

Clarke, A.M. and Hermelin, B.F. (1955) Adult imbeciles, their abilities and trainability, *Lancet*, 2: 337–9.

Clarke, D. (1983) *Mentally Handicapped People: Living and Learning*. London: Bailliere Tindall.

Clarke, D. (1999) Functional psychosis in people with mental retardation, in N. Bouras (ed.) *Psychiatric & Behavioural Disorders in Developmental Disabilities & Mental Retardation*. Cambridge: Cambridge University Press.

Clough, P. and Barton, L. (eds) (1995) *Making Difficulties – Research and the Construction of SEN*. London: Paul Chapman Publishing.

Collins, J. (1996) Housing, support and the rights of people with learning difficulties, *Social Care Research*, 81: March.

Conroy, J. and Bradley, V. (1985) *The Pennhurst Longitudinal Study: A Report of Five Years of Research and Analysis*. Philadelphia, PA: Temple University Developmental Disabilities Centre.

Cox, Baroness (1995) The case for village communities for people with learning difficulties, *British Journal of Nursing*, 4(19): 1130–4.

Davies, K. (1993) On the movement, in J. Swain, V. Finkelstein, S. French and M. Oliver (eds) *Disabling Barriers – Enabling Environments*. London: Sage.

De Jong, G. (1979) *The Movement for Independent Living: Origins, Ideology and Implications for Disability Research*. Michigan: University Centre for International Rehabilitation, Michigan State University.

DHSS (1969) *Report of the Committee of Inquiry into Allegations of Ill-treatment of Patients and Other Irregularities at the Ely Hospital, Cardiff*. Cmnd 3975. London: HMSO.

DHSS (1971) *Report of the Farleigh Hospital Committee of Inquiry*. Cmnd 4557. London: HMSO.

DHSS (1978) *Report of the Committee of Inquiry into Normansfield Hospital*. Cmnd 7357. London: HMSO.

Edgerton, R.B. (1967) *The Cloak of Competence: Stigma in the Lives of the Mentally Retarded*. Berkley, CA: University of California Press.

Edgerton, R.B. and Bercovici, S. (1976) The cloak of competence: years later, *American Journal of Mental Deficiency*, 80: 485–97.

Edgerton, R.B., Bollinger, M. and Hess, B. (1984) The cloak of competence after two decades, *American Journal of Mental Deficiency*, 88: 345–51.

Ervelles, N. (1996) Disability and the dialectics of difference, *Disability and Society*, 11(4): 519–37.

Etherington, A. and Stocker, B. (1995) Moving from hospital into community: an evaluation by people with learning difficulties, *Social Care Research*, 64.

Fennell, P. (1996) *Treatment Without Consent: Law, Psychiatry and the Treatment of Mentally Disordered People Since 1845*. London: Routledge.

Finkelstein, V. (1980) *Attitudes and Disabled People*. New York: World Rehabilitation Fund.

Finkelstein, V. (1993) The commonality of disability, in J. Swain, V. Finkelstein, S. French and M. Oliver (eds) *Disabling Barriers – Enabling Environments*. London: Sage.

Flynn, M. (1986) *A Study of Prediction in the Community Placement of Adults who are Mentally Handicapped*. Final report to ESRC, Hester Adrian Research Centre, University of Manchester.

Flynn, M. and Saleem, J. (1986) Adults who are mentally handicapped and living with their parents: satisfaction and perceptions regarding their lives and circumstances, *Journal of Mental Deficiency Research*, 30: 379–87.

Flynn, M.C. (1989) *Independent Living for Adults with Mental Handicap: A Place of My Own*. London: Cassell.

Foucault, M. (1965) *Madness and Civilisation*. London: Tavistock.

Goffman, I. (1957) *Asylums*. New York: Doubleday.

Gold, D. (1994) We don't call it a circle: the ethos of a support group, *Disability and Society*, 9(4): 165–9.

Harris, P. (1995) Who am I? Concepts of learning disability and their implications for people with learning difficulties, *Disability and Society*, 10(3): 341–57.

Hatton, C. (2002) Psychosocial interventions for adults with intellectual disabilities and mental health problems: a review, *Journal of Mental Health*, 11(4): 357–74.

Heal, L. and Chadsey-Rush, J. (1985) The Life Style Satisfaction Scale (LLS): assessing individual satisfaction with residence, community setting and associated services, *Applied Research in Mental Retardation*, 6: 475–90.

Heddell, F. (1980) *Accident of Birth*. London: British Broadcasting Corporation.

Hobsbawm, E.J. (1962) *The Age of Revolution*. New York: Mentor.

Hobsbawm, E.J. (1968) *Industry and Empire*. Harmondsworth: Penguin.

Holland, A.C. and Meddis, R. (1997) People living in community houses: their views, *British Journal of Learning Disabilities*, 25(2): 68–72.

Hunt, N. (1967) *The World of Nigel Hunt*. Beaconsfield: Darwen Finlayson.

Itard, J. ([1806] 1972) *The Wild Boy of Aveyron*, trans. E. Fawcett, P. Ayrton and J. White. London: New Left Books.

Infanticide (2003) www.womankind.org.uk/8gwhiteribbon.htm, accessed 1 October 2003; www.aidindia.net/deskfemale.htm, accessed 1 October 2003.

Jahoda, A., Markova, I. and Cattermole, M. (1988) Stigma and self concept of people with a mild mental handicap, *Journal of Mental Deficiency Research*, 32: 103–15.

King, J., Raynes., N.V. and Tizzard, J. (1971) *Patterns of Residential Care: Sociological Studies in Institutions for Handicapped Children*. London: Routledge & Keegan Paul.

Kozoma, C. and Mason, S. (2003) Survey of nursing and medical profile prior to deinstitutionalization of a population with profound mental retardation, *Clinical Nursing Research*, 12(1): 8–22.

McLaren, A. (1990) *A History of Contraception*. Oxford: Blackwell.

McVilly, K.R. (1995) Interviewing people with a learning disability about their residential service, *British Journal of Learning Disabilities*, 2(25): 138–42.

Manion, M. and Bersani, H. (1987) Mental retardation as a western sociological construct: a cross-cultural analysis, *Disability, Handicap and Society*, 2(3): 231–46.

Maslow, A. (1943) A theory of human motivation, *Psychological Review*, (50): 370–96.

Maslow, A. (1954) *Motivation and Personality*. New York: Harper & Row.

Mencap and MLD Link (2002) No ordinary life, *PNLD-LINK*, 14(2): 12–16.

Miller, A. and Gwynne, R. (1972) *A Life Apart*. London: Tavistock.

Mittler, P. (1978) *Helping Mentally Handicapped People in Hospital: A Report to the Secretary of State for Social Services*. London: DHSS.

Mittler, P. (1979) *People not Patients*. Cambridge: Methuen.

Morris, P. (1969) *Put Away*. London: Routledge & Keegan Paul.

Moss, S., Emerson, E., Kiernan, C., Turner, S., Hatton, C. and Alborz, A. (2000) Psychiatric symptoms in adults with learning disability and challenging behaviour, *British Journal of Psychiatry*, 177: 452–6.

Nirje, B. (1972) The right to self determination, in W. Wolfensberger (ed.) *The Principle of Normalization in Human Services*. Toronto: National Institute on Mental Retardation.

NPSA (2004) *Understanding Patient Safety Issues for People with Learning Disabilities*. London: National Patient Safety Agency.

O'Brien, J. and Tyne, A. (1981) *The Principle of Normalisation: A Foundation for Effective Services*. London: Campaign for the Mentally Handicapped.

Oliver, M. (1993) Disability and dependency: a creation of industrial societies? in J. Swain, V. Finkelstein, S. French and M. Oliver (eds) *Disabling Barriers – Enabling Environments*. London: Sage.

Oliver, M.J. (2000) Capitalism, disability, and ideology: a materialist critique of the normalization principle, in R.J. Flynn and A.L. Lemay (eds) *A Quarter Century of Normalization and Social Role Valorization: Evolution and Impact*. Ottawa: University of Ottawa Press.

Passfield, D. (1983) What do you think of it so far? A survey of 20 Priory Court residents, *Mental Handicap*, 11(3): 97–9.

Potts, M. and Fido, R. (1991) *A Fit Person to be Removed: Personal Accounts of Life in a Mental Deficiency Institution*. Plymouth: Northcote House Publications.

Race, D. (1995a) Classification of people with learning disabilities, in N. Malin (ed.) *Services for People with Learning Difficulties*. London: Routledge.

Race, D. (1995b) Historical development of service provision, in N. Malin (ed.) *Services for People with Learning Difficulties*. London: Routledge.

Race, D.G. (1999) Hearts and minds: social role valorization, UK academia and services for people with a learning disability, *Disability and Society*, 14(4): 519–38.

Richards, S. (1985) A right to be heard, *Social Services Research*, 14(4): 49–56.

Rogers, C. (1951) *Client Centred Therapy*. London: Constable.

Rudgley, R. (2000) *Secrets of the Stone Age*. London: Century.

Ryan, W. (1971) *Blaming the Victim*. London: Orbach & Chambers.

Ryan, J. and Thomas, F. (1980) *The Politics of Mental Handicap*. Harmondsworth: Penguin.

Ryan, J. and Thomas, F. (1991) *The Politics of Mental Handicap*, revised edn. London: Free Association Books.

Scull, A. (1979) *Museums of Madness: The Social Organisation of Insanity in Nineteenth Century England*. London: Penguin.

Slater, C. (2004) *Idiots, Imbeciles and Intellectual Impairment – A History of Mental Handicap/Learning Difficulties from 1000*AD *to 2000*AD. http://caslater.freeservers.com/disability3.htm, accessed 30 July 2004.

Stanworth, M. (1989) The new eugenics, in A. Brechin and J. Walmsley (eds) *Making Connections: Reflecting on the Lives and Experiences of People with Learning Difficulties*. London: Hodder & Stoughton.

Stone, D.A. (1985) *The Disabled State*. London: Macmillan.

Swain, J. (1989) Learned helplessness theory and people with learning difficulties: the psychological price of powerlessness, in A. Brechin and J. Walmsley (eds) *Making Connections: Reflecting on the Lives and Experiences of People with Learning Difficulties*. London: Hodder & Stoughton.

Thompson, E.P. (1968) *The Making of the English Working Class*. Harmondsworth: Penguin.

Tizard, J. (1964) *Community Services for the Mentally Handicapped*. Oxford: Oxford University Press.

Tizard, J. and O'Connor, N. (1952) The occupational adaptation of high grade defectives, *Lancet*, 2: 620–3.

UPIAS (1981) *Disability Challenge, No.1*. London: Union of the Physically Impaired Against Segregation.

Walton, J.K. (1980) Lunacy in the Industrial Revolution: a study of asylum admissions in Lancashire, 1848–50, *Journal of Social History*, 13: 1–22.

Whittlemore, R., Langness, L. and Coegel, P. (1986) The life history approach to mental retardation, in L. Langness and H. Levint (eds) *Culture and Retardation*. London: Reidel.

Williams, F. (1989) Mental handicap and oppression, in A. Brechin and J. Walmsley (eds) *Making Connections: Reflecting on the Lives and Experiences of People with Learning Difficulties*. London: Hodder & Stoughton.

Wolfensberger, W. (1972) *The Principle of Normalization in Human Services*. Toronto: National Institute on Mental Retardation.

Wolfensberger, W. (1983) Social role valorization: a proposed new term for the principle of normalization, *Mental Retardation*, 21(6): 234–9.

5

Learning disability and the law

Alison Brammer

Introduction

The focus of this chapter is how law relates to people with learning disabilities. 'Law' refers to both legislation (e.g. the Disability Discrimination Act 1995), and case law, (e.g. *R (on the application of A)* v. *East Sussex CC* (no. 2) (2003) EWHC 167). Most of the time, people with learning disabilities (particularly where mild or moderate) are treated no differently in law than any other citizens. The law assumes that all individuals have the capacity to make their own decisions unless proven otherwise. The provisions of the Human Rights Act 1998 apply equally to all citizens regardless of disabilities or other characteristics. There are exceptions however and in each area where the law differentiates it defines the characteristics of those individuals to whom it applies. For example, if a crime is committed, the criminal law will operate to identify and punish the perpetrator and protect the victim. If a person with a learning disability is involved then the law provides additional safeguards to the individual, recognizing that they might otherwise be disadvantaged in the legal system. If it is alleged that a learning disabled adult has committed a crime an 'appropriate adult' will be present during police questioning to advise, observe and facilitate communication (see Chapter 19). If a learning disabled person is a witness in criminal proceedings, as a victim or otherwise, 'special measures' may apply to enable them to give evidence more effectively. In other circumstances the learning disabled adult may benefit from support services.

The gateway to an assessment of need for services is the National Health Service and Community Care Act 1990 (see also Chapter 24). People with learning disabilities are sometimes considered with people with physical disabilities in legal terms and definitions may extend to incorporate both, as for example in the Disability Discrimination Act 1995. Elsewhere, particularly if capacity is relevant, learning disability may be addressed separately as under the Sexual Offences Act 2004.

In law, for the purpose of clarity, categories are drawn based on different individual characteristics (e.g. age, mental illness, physical or learning disability). Such clarity is not reflected in reality. It is important to recognize that some individuals will cut across categories and may for example be aged and have learning and physical disability. Generalized assumptions should be avoided and diversity fully recognized. A practice response to the limitations of legal definitions has been to utilize the term 'vulnerability'. This term is not without criticism and carries some negative connotations, but it is one which is increasingly used to refer to an individual who may require support or protection due to a variety or combination of characteristics including age and disability.

In considering the role of law there is an apparent conflict. It may be empowering. There are provisions that may be employed to promote the four principles contained in *Valuing People* (Department of Health 2001), namely civil rights, independence, choice and inclusion. Further support is provided by the *United Nations Convention on the Rights of Mentally Retarded Persons 1971* (which the UK government is morally bound to follow), which states that all mentally retarded persons (the term used in the *Convention*) shall enjoy the right to proper care; education; rehabilitation; guidance; economic security; work to the fullest extent possible; family life; protection from exploitation and abuse; and proper procedure to be adopted before any deprivation of rights.

Despite the existence of anti-discrimination legislation, the law itself may also be discriminatory in both its terminology and its application. The term 'subnormality' was in use until 1983 in mental health legislation and until 2003 'defective' was the term used in sexual offences legislation. It remained in the Sexual Offences Act 1956 until the introduction of the Sexual Offences Act 2003 and was defined as a 'person suffering from a state of arrested or incomplete development of mind which includes severe impairment of intelligence and social functioning'. There is evidence to suggest that perpetrators of offences against people with learning disabilities are less likely to be brought to justice, due to failure to initiate proceedings and failure to understand the nature of learning disability and its relevance to competence in giving evidence, as will be illustrated later in this chapter (see also Chapter 19).

The first section of this chapter will consider definitions in current use and their significance in terms of service provision and other measures, including protection. This is followed by a closer examination of the legal status of individuals with learning disabilities where capacity is impaired. Legal aspects of competence and informed consent are then considered, including an overview of the provisions contained in the Mental Capacity Bill which will reform the law on capacity. The second half of the chapter considers application of the law to three case studies.

Definitions

The status and needs of children and young people with learning disabilities are specifically addressed in the Children Act 1989, as children in need, and in a variety of pieces of education legislation, the most notable of which is the Special Educational Needs and Disability Act 2001.

The philosophy of the Children Act 1989 was to position children with disabilities as 'children first' (Department of Health 1991), though there are some references to disabled children in the Act (e.g. Schedule 2, Part 1, Para. 6). A child who is disabled is defined in the Act in the same terms as contained in the National Assistance Act 1948 in relation to adults, as one who is blind, deaf or dumb (or suffering from mental disorder of any description), substantially and permanently handicapped by illness, injury or congenital deformity or other such disabilities as may be prescribed. In effect, this provides a statutory definition of disability including both learning and physical disability. The terminology is that adopted in 1948.

In respect of adults, Section 21 of the National Assistance Act 1948 contains the duty of local authorities to provide residential accommodation for persons who, by reason of age, illness, disability or any other circumstances are in need of care and attention not otherwise available to them. Local authorities are required to inform themselves of the number of people who fall within the definition contained in Section 29 of the National Assistance Act 1948 (above) and to make arrangements for them (see Section 1 of the Chronically Sick and Disabled Persons Act 1970). Under Section 2, local authorities are required to assess individual needs and provide services to meet the needs of disabled persons. The definition in Section 29 is also employed in the National Health Service and Community Care Act 1990, the legislation which provides for the assessment of eligibility for services established under a range of other pieces of legislation.

The most recent piece of anti-discriminatory legislation, the Disability Discrimination Act 1995, makes it unlawful to discriminate against a person on the grounds of disability in relation to employment and the provision of goods and services. Disability in this context is defined as 'a physical or mental impairment which has a substantial and long-term adverse effect on ability to carry out normal day-to-day activities'.

Mental health legislation applies to people with a mental disorder, defined as 'mental illness, arrested or incomplete development of mind, psychopathic disorder and any other disorder or disability of mind' (Mental Health Act 1983). This generic category which applies to short-term orders and emergency intervention is further divided into four specific categories, namely mental illness, severe mental impairment, mental impairment and psychopathic disorder. Longer-term detention and guardianship under the Act are only available in respect of individuals within one of the four categories and where it is necessary in the interests of the patient. People with learning disabilities are most likely to fall within the categories relating to mental impairment. The term 'severe mental impairment' replaced 'severe subnormalities' in previous legislation. The term refers to handicap rather than illness, conditions which are less likely to be cured and which would now be referred to as 'learning disabilities'.

The arrested or incomplete development of mind must be associated with abnormally aggressive or seriously irresponsible conduct to come within the terms of the Mental Health Act 1983. This provision was introduced in response to concern that compulsory detention would not normally be appropriate for people with learning disabilities and could be stigmatizing. Incorporation of the requirement for abnormally aggressive or seriously irresponsible conduct was intended to include only those people with mental impairment who need hospital detention for their own safety or that of others. The same definition is provided for mental impairment as for severe impairment, except that it talks about significant rather than severe impairment. Again there is no legal guidance as to the factors that would distinguish 'severe' from 'significant'; it is a question of degree.

There are ongoing plans to reform mental health law and a new Mental Health Bill has recently been published. Among other things it contains a single (very broad) definition which would include mental illness and learning disabilities, and proposals for compulsory treatment in the community (Department of Health 2004).

Capacity

The question of capacity or legal competence is central to any consideration of the law and learning disability. It is a complex area of practice, involving significant ethical dilemmas, made more complex by the absence of a clear framework for substitute decision-making. Law proceeds on the basis that adults are deemed capable of making their own decisions until the contrary is established – a presumption in favour of capacity. It is pertinent first to question what the law defines as 'capacity'.

Elements of capacity were set out in *Re C (Adult: Refusal of Treatment)* [1994] 2 WLR 290. To be deemed 'competent', following this case, a patient must comprehend and retain treatment information; believe it to be true; and weigh it in the balance to arrive at a choice. It is a functional approach. This case also made it explicitly clear that mental incapacity and mental illness are separate issues in law. The adult concerned in *Re C* was detained for treatment in a mental hospital suffering from schizophrenia. He nevertheless had the capacity to refuse proposed treatment for a physical condition.

There are different standards of capacity in law – it is not a fixed concept. For example, the capacity required to enter into a sexual relationship is different to that required to manage property and financial affairs. The level of capacity required attempts to reflect the complexity of the issue at stake. In practice this means that no one should be considered incapable in a total sense as most people, including those with severe learning disabilities, will have the capacity to make some decisions for themselves. Assessment of capacity, though a legal concept, is often a matter for the medical profession. An individual's capacity to make a decision may fluctuate and it is therefore obviously good practice to take steps to enhance capacity and to enable decision-making during lucid periods.

Difficulties arise where an individual does not have the capacity to make a particular decision. Under current law, proxy decision-making is only recognized in respect of legal and financial matters and takes effect through the operation of the Court of Protection (an arm of the High Court with jurisdiction to manage the property and financial affairs of people who lack that capacity), Enduring Powers of Attorney (documents which provide for an attorney to deal with the finances of a person if that person loses that capacity in the future), and use of a litigation friend (a person appointed to commence or defend legal proceedings on behalf of an individual who lacks capacity). There is an absence of formal machinery to delegate decision-making in other areas, including health and welfare matters.

Medical treatment without consent actually constitutes the tort of battery (i.e. a civil wrong which comprises infliction of physical force, such as a punch, for which damages (compensation) may be payable). A defence to this is provided by the principle of necessity which allows a doctor to give treatment when it is in the patient's best interests (*F* v. *West Berkshire HA* [1989] 2 All ER 545). A series of cases have dealt with the sterilization of mentally handicapped women, based on this principle. Critics have argued that this line of case law demonstrates a paternalistic application of law which gives great credence to medical evidence in the absence of a full consideration of social circumstances (Keywood 1995). For example, in *Re M (A Minor) (Wardship: Sterilization)* [1989] 1 FLR 182, the court accepted the view of doctors regarding sterilization as a form of contraceptive and was persuaded that sterilization was justified as there was a 50 per cent chance that the woman would conceive a mentally handicapped child.

The case of *Re A (Mental Patient: Sterilization)* [2000] 1 FLR 549 CA, where an application to authorize sterilization of a learning disabled man was refused, implicitly supports this reasoning. In these cases an application was made to the court for a 'declaration' that the proposed treatment was not unlawful, eliminating the risk of a legal action for battery afterwards. In recent years the use of 'declaratory relief' has extended beyond medical cases to some 'welfare' areas. This is discussed further in case study 1.

In practical terms, decisions are made on behalf of people lacking capacity as a matter of routine on a daily basis. There may be little objection raised where decisions are made in the best interests of the individual. However, there is a gap in the law in terms of responding to disputes about 'best interests' or providing a clear framework for decision-making. In response to this unclear position the Law Commission began a process of examination of the law relating to mental incapacity in 1991 which highlighted deficiencies in the law and the need for reform, stating:

It is widely recognised that, in this area the law as it now stands is unsystematic and full of glaring gaps. It does not rest on clear or modern foundations of principle. It has failed to keep up with social and demographic changes. It has also failed to keep up with developments in our understanding of the rights and needs of those with mental disability.

(Law Commission 1995)

There was a lengthy period of consultation that resulted in the publication of a Mental Capacity Bill in July 2004 which, at the time of writing, has begun its passage through Parliament. A draft Mental Incapacity Bill was published in June 2003, and subjected to scrutiny by a Parliamentary Joint Committee which reported at the end of November 2003. The Bill broadly reproduced the proposals outlined in the 1999 document *Making Decisions: The Government's Proposals for Making Decisions on Behalf of Mentally Incapacitated Adults* (Lord Chancellor's Department 1991). The government published its response to the Scrutiny Committee recommendations early in 2004, and a revised Bill was published in July 2004, renamed the Mental Capacity Bill. It provides a comprehensive legal framework for decision-making on behalf of those who lack capacity. It is significant that similar legislation has already been introduced in Scotland in the form of the Adults with Incapacity (Scotland) Act 2000.

In summary, the key elements of the proposed legislation are as follows:

- The Bill applies to those over the age of 16. It introduces a statutory definition of incapacity, and restates the common law presumption *against* lack of capacity. It encourages 'all practical steps' to be taken to help an individual to make decisions for himself or herself.

- A person lacks capacity if at the material time he or she is unable to make a decision for himself or herself in relation to the matter because of an impairment or a disturbance in the functioning of the mind or brain. It does not matter whether the impairment or disturbance is permanent or temporary. Being unable to make a decision means that the person is:

    unable to understand the information relevant to the decision, unable to retain the information;

    unable to use the information as part of the process of making the decision; or

    unable to communicate the decision. An 'unwise' decision will not be treated as inability. 'Relevant information' includes the reasonably forseeable consequences of deciding or failing to make a decision.

- The Bill introduces a 'general authority to act reasonably' which provides security for those people making day-to-day decisions for a person who lacks capacity. It cannot be used to justify use of force, or restrict a person's liberty.

- For the avoidance of doubt the common law best interests principle will be enshrined in new legislation. Factors to be taken into account when determining best interests include:

the ascertainable past and present wishes and feelings of the person concerned;

the need to permit and encourage participation in decision-making; the views of others it is considered appropriate to consult (such as family members);

achieving the desired purpose in the least restrictive manner;

whether there is a reasonable expectation of recovery in the future.

- Where an individual has capacity but anticipates possible loss of capacity in the future he or she may execute a Lasting Power of Attorney (referred to in the consultation process as a Continuing Power of Attorney). This replaces and extends beyond the currently used Enduring Power of Attorney and can apply to decisions relating to health and welfare as well as property and affairs. A Lasting Power of Attorney (LPA) will have to be registered with the Public Guardian to take effect.

- A new Court of Protection will be established with regional offices. The Court will have jurisdiction to determine disputes relating to capacity and make single orders about particular issues, such as contact or residence. The Court may also appoint a 'deputy' to make welfare and financial decisions for a person who either has not made an LPA and subsequently loses capacity, or could not have made an LPA because of a long-term disability. This system will replace and extend the use of receivership currently operating from the Court of Protection.

- Finally, the Bill introduces a new offence. A person is guilty of an offence if she or he has the care of a person who lacks capacity or is reasonably believed to lack capacity, or is the donee of an LPA or a deputy, and she or he ill-treats or wilfully neglects the person. The offence carries a maximum sentence of two years' imprisonment.

In practice this list is not intended to be exhaustive and while it can help to structure decision-making, the concept of 'best interests' is likely to remain extremely difficult to apply in many cases. New legislation in the form set out in the Bill is likely to receive a broad welcome. The legislation restates important common law principles, significantly the presumption in favour of capacity, and encourages first-hand decision-making. In instances of incapacity there are a range of options for substitute decision-making, via the general authority, LPA and orders of the Court of Protection, including the appointment of a deputy. The reconstituted Court of Protection should provide an accessible forum for adjudication of disputes on the question of individual capacity and 'best interests' decisions.

Case study 1

This case study illustrates how the courts have innovated and extended the use of the High Court power to rule whether proposed action is lawful, by making a declaration (also referred to as declaratory relief) to make decisions in respect of adults who lack mental capacity, in the absence of a clear statutory mechanism for substitute decision-making. This line of case law has its origins in medical treatment cases based on the doctrine of necessity. As an example, in *Airedale NHS Trust* v. *Bland* [1003] 1 All ER 821, a declaration was made that it was unlawful to discontinue life-sustaining treatment for a person who was in a persistent vegetative state. The law has developed in a piecemeal fashion with issues being determined on a case-by-case basis. On more than one occasion the courts have signalled the need for Parliament to introduce legislation. Until that happens, declaratory relief has been developed by the courts to fill the legal loophole that exists whereby it is not possible to formally delegate decision-making to another individual concerning social and welfare matters.

Extension of declaratory relief beyond medical cases was first noted in *Re S (Hospital Patient: Court's Jurisdiction)* [1996] Fam 1. Here, the court indicated that declaratory relief might be available wherever a 'serious justiciable issue' arose and with flexibility in order that the court could respond to social needs as they are manifested on a case-by-case basis. A few years later in *Re D-R (Adult: Contact)* [1999] 1 FLR 1161 the court considered a claim by a father for access to his adult daughter who had a learning disability. The Court of Appeal confirmed that, for an adult with a disability, the question the Court must address was whether it was in her best interest to have contact, relying on *Re F (Sterilization: Mental Patient)* [1990] 2 AC 1. To determine best interests where there was family conflict, it was necessary to look at all the circumstances, which included the history and former relationship of the father and daughter, the current situation and the prospects for the future. The comments of Lord Justice Butler-Sloss in this case are significant:

> I would add however that this case discloses the inadequacy of the procedure adopted by the father, which, even if he had succeeded, might well not have been likely to have given him an effective contact. Ever since the lapse of the *parens patriae* jurisdiction over the mentally incompetent on the coming into force of the Mental Health Act 1959 and its successors there has been a huge gap in the non-mental care of those who cannot care for themselves. That gap has been bridged to some extent by the House of Lords and this court in *Re F* and succeeding cases. But it is a poor substitute for a statutory framework to provide proper health both to incompetent adults and to their families.

Susan

Susan is aged 33. She has a moderate to severe learning disability. She was cared for by her parents in the family home until 1995 when, following her mother's death, she was cared for by her father with support from care assistants. An allegation was received from the district nurse that Susan was punched in the face by her father (while drunk). Susan lacks capacity to choose where to live. Her father's love is not disputed but his health is deteriorating. He does not allow contact with her siblings. The local authority sought a declaration that it would be lawful for them to remove Susan from the family home, place her in specialist residential accommodation and restrict access between her and her father.

Exercise 5.1

How should Susan's needs be met?

The facts outlined are drawn from a further case in the development of declaratory relief, *Newham London Borough Council* v. *S* [2003] EWHC 1909 Fam.

In cases where a declaration is sought the court describes the decision-making process in terms of 'four essential building blocks':

- Is mental incapacity established?
- Is there a serious justiciable issue relating to welfare?
- What is it?
- With welfare of the incapable adult as the court's paramount consideration, what are the balance sheet factors which must be drawn up to decide which course of action is in a person's best interests?

The factors that weighed against the authority's application in Susan's case were the father's love and sense of duty towards her, the fact that he had cared adequately for her since her mother's death and the fact that the allegations against him were not substantiated. Factors in favour of the application included the relevance of the father's age and health which meant his ability to care would diminish. Contact between Susan and her siblings had ceased due to a rift between the father and his other children and this contact could resume if Susan were accommodated by the council. Also, the proposed accommodation was purpose-built for Susan and would enable her to socialize with people of her own age. Finally, independent evidence of a consultant psychiatrist supported Newham's plans as the best way of meeting her needs.

The father's argument that a 'significant harm' threshold needed to be satisfied (analogous to that in the Children Act 1989) before Newham could intervene was rejected. The court stated that as long as the adult concerned lacked the capacity to make decisions about future care and there was a serious justiciable issue requiring resolution, the court's inherent jurisdiction was available to it.

Prior to this decision it had been assumed that declarations would only be sought by local authorities where they had concerns about possible abuse. That was precisely the case in *Re F (Adult: Court's Jurisdiction)* [2000] 3

WLR 1740 CA, where the local authority sought a declaration as to the place of residence and contact arrangements for a mentally handicapped woman who was unable to care for herself. It was accepted that the woman lacked capacity to make decisions as to her future. She did not fall within the guardianship provisions of the Mental Health Act 1983, and as she was aged over 18, the wardship jurisdiction could not be utilized. The family circumstances were complex but evidence was provided of chronic neglect, a lack of minimum standards of hygiene and cleanliness in the home and possible sexual abuse. The court confirmed that where there was a risk of possible harm in respect of an adult who lacked the capacity to make decisions as to their own future the court had power, in the best interests of that person, to hear the issue involved and to grant the necessary declarations.

In a subsequent case, *A* v. *A Health Authority & Others* [2002] Fam 213, the court provided a clear statement on eligibility to apply for declarations: 'The jurisdiction can be invoked by anyone whose past or present relationship with the incompetent adult, whether formal or informal, gives him a genuine and legitimate interest in obtaining a decision, in contrast to being a stranger or an officious busybody. Thus proceedings can be brought by a local authority.'

The Newham case (Susan) apparently opens the way for declarations to be sought to resolve any 'best interest' decision regarding an incapacitated adult. This pre-empts the role envisaged for the new Court of Protection under the proposed mental capacity reforms. Declaratory relief does, however, carry the disadvantage of being a High Court based remedy which is expensive and less accessible than the new proposed Court of Protection.

Case study 2

While the vast majority of people with learning disabilities live in the community, often with members of their family, for some people accommodation in a residential home is appropriate. It is well documented that residential accommodation, whether providing homes for children, adults with disabilities or very elderly people, has provided opportunities for abuse of individual residents and for abusive practices to develop (see Chapter 16).

This case study illustrates the need for close regulation of residential accommodation.

Alan

Alan, who had a severe learning disability, lived in a home in Northamptonshire which was registered to accept 16 people with physical disability, or mental handicap and mental disorder. Registration of the home was cancelled for reasons including failure to care for Alan and recognize his care needs. Alan had been kept in conditions of squalor and degradation, deprived of his liberty. His dignity was ignored, his right to property compromised, and he was in pain with a dental abscess and no action was taken to treat him. One of the inspection officers commented that she had never seen an animal kept in that way. He was effectively abandoned by Essex County Council 12 years before and kept in conditions reminiscent of those which led to the closure of many large mental institutions. He spent time sitting on a plastic chair dressed in only a ripped T-shirt, surrounded by urine in a cold room with no bed linen and a high handle on the door to prevent escape. Of the 15 residents, only 4 had a care plan. The human rights implications were noted in the judgement of the Registered Homes Tribunal:

> We had in mind that local authorities now have a duty under the Human Rights Act 1998 to safeguard the rights of those, like Alan, for whom they are responsible. We consider that both Essex and Northampton as public authorities by virtue of section 6 of the Act, behaved in a way, which was incompatible with Alan's convention rights. Inspection units and Registered Persons should consider that it may be appropriate to look at how convention rights are promoted and protected in Registered Homes when questions of registration and fitness arise. [Essex was the placing authority and Northamptonshire was the registration authority.]

This case is reported as *Freeman and Goodwin* v. *Northamptonshire CC* 2000, Decision 421. The case reached the Registered Homes Tribunal while the Registered Homes Act 1984 was in force. A similar scenario would now be dealt with under the Care Standards Act 2000, before the Care Standards Tribunal.

The framework for regulation (which implicitly includes prevention of abuse) of residential care homes and domiciliary care agencies is now provided by the Care Standards Act 2000 (in force from 1 April 2002), supported by National Minimum Standards. Any concerns of possible abuse, which the home is aware of, should be notified to the registration authority, now a national body, the Commission for Social Care Inspection (CSCI). The CSCI was created by the Health and Social Care (Community Health and Standards) Act 2003. It incorporates the work done by the Social Services Inspectorate (SSI), the SSI/Audit Commission Joint Review Team and the National Care Standards Commission (NCSC) (see Chapter 7).

This case study presents an opportunity to discuss the application of the Human Rights Act 1998 in relation to people with learning disabilities. It has already been noted that the Act applies equally to all citizens, and people with learning disabilities may rely on its provisions to secure a guarantee of their basic human rights. The Act incorporates the *European Convention on Human Rights* 1951 and enables individuals for the first time to enforce compliance with the articles in the UK courts. Previously cases could only be brought against the UK in the European Court of Human Rights in Strasbourg, a costly and time-consuming process. Under the Human Rights Act 1998 it is unlawful for a public authority to act in a way which is incompatible with a convention right (Section 6). The term 'public authority' includes the courts, central and local government, social services, police, health authorities, the CSCI and others carrying out functions of a public nature. The effect of this provision is that the placing and receiving authority in Alan's case and the inspection body (the CSCI) would be obliged to ensure that Alan's rights under the *Convention* were not violated. In Alan's case it could be argued that aspects of the regime could amount to inhuman or degrading treatment under Article 3 of the *Convention*. Application of this article hinges on definition of the terms used. In *Ireland* v. *UK* 1978–5 techniques, wall standing, hooding, subjection to noise, sleep, food and drink deprivation were found to be degrading treatment. 'Torture' was defined as deliberate inhuman treatment causing very serious and cruel suffering; 'inhuman treatment' as intense physical and mental suffering and acute psychiatric disturbances; and 'degrading' as behaviour which aroused in the victim feelings of anguish and inferiority capable of humiliating and debasing them and possibly breaking their physical or moral resistance. The case also said that ill treatment must attain a minimum level of severity. That is a relative issue and will depend on all the circumstances of the case, including duration of treatment, its physical and mental effects, and the age, sex and state of health of the victim.

Alan's right to respect for private and family life, contained in Article 8, may also have been violated. Much of existing human rights case law has focused on application of Article 8, the right to respect for private and family life, which has been described as:

> a broad term not susceptible to exhaustive definition. It covers the physical and psychological integrity of the person. Elements such as gender identification, name & sexual orientation & sexual life fall within the personal sphere protected by Art. 8. Art. 8 also protects a right to personal development, & to establish & develop relationships with other human beings & the outside world.
>
> (*Pretty* v. *UK* [2002] 35 EHRR 1)

Article 8 is a qualified article. This means that there are some permitted exceptions to the rights protected by it. A breach or interference with the right may be permissible where it is in accordance with law, necessary in a democratic society and in the interests of named justifications including public safety, prevention of disorder or crime, or the protection of the rights and freedoms of others. In the latter circumstances this may involve a balancing exercise between the competing rights of two or more parties. For example, a resident in a home might argue that his right to freedom of expression permits him to make offensive comments about people with learning disabilities. A resident with a learning disability, however, might well argue that this behaviour infringes their right to respect for private and family life. It is also important that any interference under Article 8 is a 'proportionate' response, and that proper procedural safeguards are followed. As an example, closure of a home following a minor incident of poor record-keeping by the owners would not seem to be a proportionate response to the need to safeguard the residents.

The case of *R (on the application of A)* v. *East Sussex CC* (no. 2)

(2003) EWHC 167 which centred on a dispute about manual handling for two severely disabled sisters includes a number of statements about the application of Article 8 to disabled people:

> The other important concept embraced in the 'physical and psychological integrity' protected by article 8 is the right of the disabled to participate in the life of the community and to have what has been described as 'access to essential economic and social activities and to an appropriate range of recreational and cultural activities'. This is matched by the positive obligation of the State to take appropriate measures designed to ensure to the greatest extent feasible that a disabled person is not 'so circumscribed and so isolated as to be deprived of the possibility of developing his personality'.

The Human Rights Act 1998 offers an opportunity to ensure best practice in respecting the human rights of people with learning disabilities and provides an effective route to challenge any violations by public authorities.

It is significant that Alan suffered mistreatment at the hands of a professional carer. One of the most effective ways of reducing abuse must be to ensure that unsuitable adults do not come into contact with vulnerable adults in a caring role. The Care Standards Act 2000 introduces the Protection of Vulnerable Adults (POVA) index, a list of individuals who are considered unsuitable to work with vulnerable adults (Section 81). All care providers must check whether a person they propose to employ in a care position is included on the list. Employment in a care position is given a broad interpretation to include those in paid or unpaid work, and to include anyone who has regular contact with a person receiving care services. As well as care staff this could also include cooks, gardeners and administrative staff in care homes, and regular visitors, such as hairdressers or clergy, for example. An individual's name will be added to the list where the Secretary of State considers the worker to be guilty of misconduct which harmed or placed at risk of harm a vulnerable adult.

Case study 3

Research suggests that people with learning disabilities may be particularly vulnerable to sexual abuse. The operation of the criminal law is the focus of this case study. It should also be remembered that such behaviour would be covered by adult protection guidelines and joint investigation by the police and social services would be appropriate at least in the initial stages. Multi-agency guidelines are in place nationally following publication of *No Secrets: Guidance on Developing and Implementing Multi-agency Policies and Procedures to Protect Vulnerable Adults from Abuse* (Department of Health 2000). *No Secrets* defines abuse as follows: 'Abuse is a violation of an individual's human and civil rights by any other person or persons'. Beyond that broad definition the guidance continues to describe abuse:

It may be physical, verbal, or psychological. It may be an act of neglect or an omission to act, or it may occur when a vulnerable person is persuaded into a financial or sexual transaction to which he or she has not consented or cannot consent. Abuse can occur in any relationship and may result in significant harm to, or exploitation of, the person subjected to it.

(Department of Health 2000: para. 2.6)

Abusive acts may embrace more than one category so, for example, it would be unusual for sexual abuse to occur in isolation, without any psychological abuse. The issue of consent is central to the determination of whether sexual behaviour is abusive. This approach is also taken in the criminal law. However, as this case study details, there has been a lack of legal clarity as to what constitutes consent in this context.

Jenkins

David Jenkins, aged 61, worked at a project providing supported housing for people with learning disabilities, as a support worker. He admitted a sexual relationship with a woman resident after she was found to be pregnant and a DNA test proved paternity. She was described as having a mental age of 2 years and 8 months and had no concept of sexual relationships nor of their consequences. He was charged with rape. An alternative charge would have been 'sexual intercourse with a defective' under the Sexual Offences Act 1956. This however carries a maximum sentence of only two years compared to rape which carries a life sentence. The key question before the court was whether she had given her consent. Expert evidence was provided to the court based on the Law Society and British Medical Association (BMA) guidelines on capacity. It was argued that in order to consent to sex a woman must be able to understand what is proposed and its implications and must be able to exercise choice. On this analysis the woman could not have given consent.

The court rejected this evidence preferring to rely on a judgement from the 1800s which suggested that consent could be given by following 'animal instinct'. In the circumstances the prosecution was not able to offer any further evidence on the rape charge and Jenkins was acquitted.

Clearly in the above case the law failed to offer protection to an alleged victim of sexual abuse in circumstances involving abuse of trust. The law on sexual offences, including those where the victim is unable to consent, has been reformed and is now contained in the Sexual Offences Act 2003. The act includes a range of sexual offences relating to people with mental disorder, where the mental disorder impedes choice. For example, under Section 30 a person (A) commits an offence if he (or she) intentionally touches another person (B) in a sexual way, B is unable to refuse because of or for a reason related to a mental disorder, and A knows or could reasonably be expected to know that B has a mental disorder and that because of it or for a reason related to it B is likely to be unable to refuse.

A person is unable to refuse if he or she lacks the capacity to choose whether to agree to engaging in the activity whether because he or she lacks sufficient understanding of the nature or reasonably foreseeable consequences of the activity, or for any other reason, or he or she is unable to communicate such a choice to A.

There are further offences where a person uses inducement, threat or deception to procure sexual activity with a person with a mental disorder, or engages in sexual activity in the presence of a person with a mental disorder, or causes a person with a mental disorder to watch a sex act (including one on film).

The Act also introduces a new 'breach of a relationship to care' offence, where a 'care worker' who has face-to-face contact through employment (paid or unpaid) in a care home, National Health Service body, or independent health setting engages in sexual activity with a person with a mental disorder. With the exception of rape, all offences contained in the Act are 'gender neutral'. Maximum sentences range from ten years to life imprisonment. The new legislation provides a range of offences that may be charged where some form of sexual behaviour takes place that a person with a learning disability did not or could not consent to.

It is important to remember that the aim of this legislation is to protect individuals from inappropriate and abusive sexual acts. It is not in any way intended to give the message that people with learning disabilities should be prohibited from enjoying an appropriate and consenting sex life. Guidance to the Act reminds us that 'It is important to appreciate that where a person with a mental disorder is able to consent freely to sexual activity, they have the same rights to engage in sexual activity as anyone else' (Home Office 2003).

It was encouraging in the Jenkins case that the Crown Prosecution Service was committed to pursuing the case and charging rape. It has been suggested that many sexual (and other) offences are not prosecuted for reasons associated with actual or perceived lack of credibility of the person with a learning disability when giving evidence (Mencap 1997). Provisions in the Youth Justice and Criminal Evidence Act 1999 recognize that giving evidence may be particularly stressful for some vulnerable witnesses and allow for special measures to be employed. A vulnerable adult witness is defined as a person suffering from mental disorder or otherwise having a significant impairment of intelligence and social functioning or a physical disability (Section 16 (2) (b). Further, a witness may be entitled to special measures if the court is satisfied that the quality of their evidence is likely to be diminished by reason of fear or distress in connection with testifying (Section 17). Special measures available include screening the witness from the accused, giving evidence via a live link, removal of formal wigs and gowns during testimony, giving evidence in private (particularly in sexual cases), video-recording of evidence in chief, cross-examination and re-examination, use of an intermediary and use of communication aids.

Conclusion

At all times, the law starts with the premise that an adult with a learning disability has the same rights to participate fully in society as any other adult. This is supported by legislation which prohibits discrimination. Exceptions to this principle have been incorporated into law. Where individuals with learning disabilities may benefit from support services, legislation contains powers to provide such services. Sadly, we know that adults with learning disabilities may be abused in different ways in different contexts and by a range of individuals, who may or may not have a professional relationship with the adult. The law provides certain avenues to secure protection of the individual. The criminal law may prosecute perpetrators, punish them and act as a deterrent to others. Some specific sexual offences recognize that learning disability may impede genuine choice to enter into sexual relations and prohibits others from taking advantage of invalid consent.

Case studies have been used in this chapter to illustrate the application of law to different scenarios concerning adults with learning disabilities. In each area, actual and potential law reforms present the option of more positive outcomes. The major criticism which may be targeted at the law and learning disability centres on capacity. The law starts with a positive presumption in favour of capacity but fails currently to deliver a clear framework applying to cases where individuals lack capacity to make their own decisions. In the absence of such a statutory framework the courts have been proactive and have extended the application of declaratory relief to cases where capacity is impaired. The Mental Capacity Bill, when implemented, will provide this statutory framework. Supported by provisions of the Human Rights Act 1998 the law in 2005 is developing positively to uphold the rights of individuals with a learning disability.

Exercise 5.2

Consider the potential violations of human rights an individual with learning disabilities might experience, living at home with family members or in a supported living environment.

When an individual lacks the capacity to make a particular decision, who can make the decision and on what basis?

What should be the role of law where a person with a learning disability suffers abuse by a carer?

Consider the range of legal definitions relating to learning disability which are in place. Are there any you would replace and if so what alternatives would you propose?

Should the primary purpose of law be to uphold the human rights of adults with learning disabilities, provide support services, or offer protection from abuse?

Further reading

Bartlett, P. (2003) Adults, mental illness and incapacity: convergence and overlap in legal regulation, *Journal of Social Welfare and Family Law*, 341.

Brammer, A. (2000) Human Rights Act 1998: implications for adult protection, *Journal of Adult Protection*, 3(1): 43. The *Journal of Adult Protection* includes a range of practice, law and research articles concerned with vulnerable adults including adults with learning disabilities.

Brammer, A. (2003) *Social Work Law*. Harlow: Pearson Education.

Lord Chancellor's Department (1999) *Making Decisions: The Government's Proposals for Making Decisions on Behalf of Mentally Incapacitated Adults*. London: The Stationery Office.

Resources

www.carestandardstribunal.gov.uk/index.htm. This website provides details about decisions of the Care Standards Tribunal and archive decisions of the Registered Homes Tribunal.

www.csci.gov.uk. The CSCI is the new inspectorate for all social care services in England.

www.doh.gov.uk/learningdisabilities. The section of the Department of Health website that addresses learning disability issues.

www.drc-gb.org/. The Disability Rights Commission (DRC) is an independent body established by an Act of Parliament to stop discrimination and promote equality of opportunity for disabled people.

www.voiceuk.org.uk/. Voice UK is an organization that supports people with learning disabilities, their families and carers, who have experienced crime or abuse. The organization campaigns for changes in law and practice.

References

Department of Health (1991) *The Children Act 1989 Guidance and Regulations*, vol. 6. London: HMSO.

Department of Health (2000) *No Secrets: Guidance on Developing and Implementing Multi-agency Policies and Procedures to Protect Vulnerable Adults from Abuse*. London: The Stationery Office.

Department of Health (2001) *Valuing People: A New Strategy for Disability in the 21st Century*. London: The Stationery Office.

Department of Health (2004) *Improving Mental Health Law – Towards a New Mental Health Act*. London: The Stationery Office.

Keywood, K. (1995) Sterilising the woman with learning difficulties, in S. Bridgman and S. Mills (eds) *Law and Body Politics: Regulating the Female Body*. Aldershot: Dartmouth Publishing Co.

Home Office (2003) *Guidance on Part 1 of the Sexual Offences Act 2003*, circular 021/2004. London: Home Office.

Law Commission (1995) *Mental Incapacity* (No. 231). London: HMSO.

Lord Chancellor's Department (1991) *Making Decisions: The Government's Proposals for Making Decisions on Behalf of Mentally Incapacitated Adults*. London: HMSO.

Mencap (1997) *Barriers to Justice*. London: Mencap.

6

Models of service delivery

Eric Emerson

Introduction

The last 150 years, and in particular the last 30 years, has witnessed a revolution in the way in which public agencies have sought to provide 'care' or 'support' for people with learning disabilities. The period has seen a revolution in models of service delivery. These changes have been most noticeable in the way in which 'care' or 'support' has been provided for people with learning disabilities who do not live with their family.

A hundred and fifty years ago, England's first publicly-funded 'asylum' for people with learning disabilities was opened. The number of such institutions and the number of people with learning disabilities who were placed in them rose steadily through the last quarter of the nineteenth century and the first half of the twentieth century (see also Chapters 2 and 4). Only 30 years ago over 50,000 people with learning disabilities were living in these large institutions (by then renamed 'hospitals'). These numbers dropped precipitously during the 1980s and 1990s. In 2001 the government announced in the White Paper *Valuing People* that all remaining learning disability hospitals would close (Department of Health 2001). This target should be achieved by April 2006.

While these changes in models of service delivery have been most noticeable in the way in which 'care' or 'support' has been provided for people with learning disabilities who do not live with their family (i.e. people who require some form of 'supported accommodation'), similar changes have taken place in the realm of education and employment (see Chapters 14, 20 and 26).

In this chapter I will use supported accommodation as a case study through which we can describe the nature of the changes that have taken place, begin to understand what has driven these changes and assess the impact of the changes on the lives of people with learning disabilities.

But what exactly do we mean by 'models' of service delivery? For example, while the term 'institution' is often associated with images of Dickensian deprivation, it is important to keep in mind that this term is used by different people at different times to refer to:

- the physical structure of services (e.g. large socially isolated accommodation arrangements);
- administrative categories of services (e.g. learning disability hospitals);
- practices and social arrangements (e.g. 'institutional' regimes);
- the ideological underpinnings of approaches to providing support.

As we will see, while these dimensions of what constitutes a 'model' may often overlap, the fit between them is often far from perfect.

Changing patterns and practices in supported accommodation

Throughout history the majority of children and adults with learning disabilities have always lived with their families or have lived independently. Historical information has been extracted from a range of secondary sources including Wolfensberger (1975, 1981), Malin *et al.* (1980), Simmons (1982), Scheerenberger (1983), Scull (1984, 1993), Ryan and Thomas (1987), Alaszewski (1988), Race (1995) and Wright and Digby (1996). An important question for societies and their public agencies, however, has been what type of accommodation should be provided to those people with learning disabilities for whom neither independent living nor family support is an option. The answer to this question has been shaped by (and itself served to shape) several factors including:

- public and professional conceptions of the nature of 'learning disability';
- public and professional expectations regarding notions of 'common decency';
- pre-existing mechanisms for the delivery of welfare support.

The rise of institutions for people with learning disabilities

Prior to the mid-nineteenth century, no supported accommodation was available specifically for people with learning disabilities. Instead, such people who needed 'out-of-home' support had to rely on the range of generic options available to people who were destitute. Since the Poor Law Act of 1601, local parishes had been empowered to raise taxes for the support of the indigent poor. Up until the nineteenth century most aid was provided in the form of household relief with an effort to maintain the 'worthy poor' within their community. There were, however, other options. These included the 'binding out' of pauper children by parish authorities to factory owners (these arrangements sometimes involving the negotiated arrangement for

1 in 20 'idiots' to be included in each batch) and early 'institutions': medieval hospitals, foundling homes, workhouses, prisons and the early 'lunatic asylums'.

Conditions were often appalling. Higgins (a magistrate at York) made the following observation on conditions in the York Asylum in 1815. The cells were:

> in a very horrid and filthy condition . . . the walls were daubed with excrement; the air holes, of which there was one in each cell, were partly filled in with it . . . I then went upstairs . . . into a room . . . 12 feet by 7 ft 10 inches, in which there were thirteen women who . . . had come out of the cells that morning . . . I became very sick, and could no longer remain in the room. I vomited.

As we have seen, this pattern of provision was soon to change. In 1842 Guggenbuhl opened the Abendberg in Switzerland, the first recorded institution specifically for people with learning disabilities. In 1848, Park House Asylum for Idiots (a private asylum) opened in Highgate, London. In 1855 this became England's first publicly-funded institution for people with learning disabilities. Within the next 20 years, specialized 'idiot asylums' were established in, among other places, Caterham, Leavesdon and Lancaster, and Europe's first asylum specifically for children with learning disabilities had been established at Darenth in Kent.

What led to these changes? At least three interlinked factors appear to be important. First, the nineteenth century saw a major revision in professional conceptions of the essential nature of 'learning disability'. Compare the following two quotes, both by leading French medical reformers of the nineteenth century.

> We have at last reached the utmost limit of human degradation. Here, the intellectual and moral faculties are almost null . . . Their senses . . . are incapable of exercising a corrective influence over each other; nor can education prove a substitute to so many disadvantages . . . Incapable of attention, idiots can not control their senses. They hear, but do not understand; they see but do not regard. Having no ideas, and thinking not, they have nothing to desire; therefore have no needs of signs or speech.
>
> (Esquirol, early nineteenth century)

> most idiots . . . may be relieved in more or less complete measure of their disabilities by . . . education . . . idiots have been improved, educated, and even cured: not one in 1,000 has been entirely refractory to treatment; not one in 100 who has not been made more happy and healthy.
>
> (Seguin 1866)

The belief in the power of education as voiced by Seguin stands in stark contrast to the view of Esquirol, for whom to have a learning disability appears to be an immutable condition that (almost) deprives the person of their humanity. These two opposing views would, of course, have radically different implications for guiding societal responses to people with learning disabilities. In fact Seguin's optimism reflected a more widespread trend. Belief in the general power and possibilities of education grew markedly in Europe and North America in the mid-nineteenth century, probably as a result of the requirement of increasing industrialization to create a more malleable workforce (see Scull 1984).

Second, the mid-nineteenth century was also a time of social upheaval and social reform. Slavery was abolished in England in 1833. Engels published his investigation of the condition of the working class in England in 1845. These changes are likely to have been associated with shifts in public notions of what was 'acceptable' or 'decent' in the care or treatment of the destitute and (among them) people with disabilities.

Third, a 'model' was available that could possibly provide a solution to the perceived need to improve the care and support provided to people with learning disabilities. The model was that of the 'lunatic asylum'. The first charitable asylums had been established in the early eighteenth century (Norwich in 1713, a ward at Guy's Hospital in 1728). The first purpose-built private asylum opened in 1806 (Brislington House in Bristol). By 1850 (five years before the establishment of the first asylum for 'idiots' in England) there were 24 county or borough asylums in England and Wales with an average size of 298 residents. There were at that time also over 120 private asylums in operation in England.

This combination of factors set the scene for the construction of educationally-oriented institutions for people with learning disabilities. By 1887, 55 specialized institutions had been established in Europe and while most were relatively small (supporting less than 100 people), the Asylum for Idiots at Earlswood was by then supporting 594 people. It is important to keep in mind that these institutions were founded with a clear commitment to education. Wolfensberger (1975) has described this phase in the life of institutional provision as one of 'making the deviant undeviant'. Admission was often restricted to people with less severe learning disabilities (i.e. those who would be likely to benefit most from education). It was also often (at least to begin with) time limited. The underlying notion was that, following a period of effective education, people would be equipped to return to and occupy a position within their local communities. As we shall see, the educationalist model of service delivery was to reappear nearly 100 years later.

The evolution of institutional provision

Wolfensberger (1975) describes four phases in the evolution of institutional models: making the deviant undeviant; protecting the deviant from society; protecting society from the deviant; and finally a 'loss of rationale'. Unfortunately, the early optimism of the power of education to 'solve' the problem of out-of-home support for people with learning disabilities proved unfounded.

First, such options were only available to a minority of people with learning disability. The 1908 Royal Commission estimated that most people with mild learning disabilities were paupers under no authority, or in generic institutions for the destitute. The Commission estimated that 18 per cent of the population in workhouses had learning disabilities, 10 per cent of those in prison and 2 per cent of those on outdoor relief. Second, it proved highly problematic to return people to their communities after several years in an isolated asylum. In the light of these difficulties, professional pronouncements of appropriate models of support began to gradually shift from those that emphasized education to those that emphasized long-term care and protection. Consider, for example, the following two quotes, both from past presidents of the American Association on Mental Retardation and both quite remarkable for their paternalistic/maternalistic tone:

> A well fed, well cared for idiot, is a happy creature. An idiot awakened to his condition is a miserable one.
>
> (Butler 1885)

> They must be kept quietly and safely away from the world, living like the angels in heaven, neither marrying nor given in marriage.
>
> (Johnson 1889)

The shift from short-term education to a more paternalistic/maternalistic ethos was accompanied by a rapid expansion in the number of institutions and the number of people living in them. For example, the Royal Albert Asylum was founded in Lancaster in 1870 as a charitable institution for young people with less severe learning disabilities. In 1873, 141 people lived there. By 1893, this number had grown to 600. It would eventually rise to over 1000.

This paternalistic/maternalistic ethos was, however, to prove to be another relatively short-lived phase (although again, we shall see the resurgence of such ideas a century later). The early twentieth century saw a fundamental shift in public discourse about people with learning disability. No longer were they to be seen as part of the 'worthy poor'; instead they came to be seen as a significant threat to the current and future social order.

Three sets of beliefs were combined by eugenicists (see Chapter 4) to argue that people with learning disabilities (and in particular people with less severe learning disabilities) posed a significant threat to English society. First, it was believed that intelligence and ability were inherited (a belief supported by the growing 'science' of psychology). Second, it was believed that people with learning disability were 'breeding' faster than the rest of society (Tredgold, an influential psychiatrist, for example reported that while 'normal' parents had an average of four children, 'feeble-minded' parents had an average of seven children). Third, it was believed that there were strong links between 'feeble-mindedness' and most of the major social problems of the day. On the basis of these three beliefs, eugenicists argued that without 'appropriate action' the gene pool would gradually but inevitably become corrupted and the extent of associated problems would increase.

These ideas were taken seriously. The findings of the 1908 Royal Commission on the Care of the Feeble Minded stressed the importance of hereditary factors and the association between feeble-mindedness and promiscuity, delinquency, alcoholism and illegitimacy. In 1898, Lord Hershel moved a resolution at a meeting of the National Association for the Care of the Feebleminded (NACFM) that: 'the existence of large classes of feeble minded persons is a danger to the physical and moral welfare of society and calls for immediate attention both on the part of public authorities and charitable enterprise'. What would constitute such 'immediate attention'? The 1908 Royal Commission recommended the segregation of people with learning disabilities, while rejecting the Eugenics Education Society's call for 'genetic purification'. In 1909, Tredgold argued that:

> I have come to the conclusion that, in the case of the majority of the feebleminded, there is one measure, and one measure only . . . which is practically possible, namely the establishment of suitable farm and industrial colonies . . . Society would thus be saved a portion, at least, of the cost of their maintenance, and more important, it would be secure from their depredation and danger of their propagation.

In 1910, the NACFM met with Prime Minister Asquith and Home Secretary Winston Churchill. Following this, Churchill stated that people with learning disabilities should 'be segregated under proper conditions [of sexual quarantine] so that their curse dies with them'. In the 1910 general election the NACFM petitioned all candidates to support measures that would 'tend to discourage parenthood on the part of the feebleminded and other degenerate types'. In 1912, a Mental Deficiency Bill was introduced into Parliament with a clause prohibiting marriage among people with learning disabilities. This Bill was later withdrawn.

These ideas were taken to their logical conclusion in Germany. In October 1939, Hitler authorized a euthanasia programme targeted at people with disabilities. It is estimated that approximately 100,000 people with learning disabilities and 200,000 people with other disabilities were killed in this programme, primarily administered in medical institutions. For example, of the 16,300 inmates of psychiatric institutions in Berlin, only 2400 (15 per cent) survived the euthanasia programme.

While no parallel to these atrocities actually occurred in England, support for the 'mercy killing' of people with learning disabilities was (and continues to be) voiced. Consider the following quote taken from the eighth edition of Tredgold's *Textbook on Mental Deficiency* that was published in 1952:

> The 80,000 or more idiots and imbeciles in the country . . . are not only incapable of being employed to any economic advantage, but their care and support, whether in their own homes or in institutions, absorbs a large amount of time, energy and money of the normal population which could be utilised to better purpose. Moreover, many of these defectives are utterly helpless, repulsive in appearance, and revolting in manners. Their existence is a perpetual source of sorrow and unhappiness to their parents, and those who live at home have a most disturbing

influence upon other children and family life . . . In my opinion it would be an economical and humane procedure were their existence to be painlessly terminated.

These ideas did, however, help to support a system of 'care' or 'support' that was based on the establishment of large physically segregated institutions in which men and women with learning disabilities led regimented and separate lives. Gray (1997), for example, assisted Herbert (Bertie) Lawford to tell his story of life in Church Hill House Hospital. Bertie was admitted to Church Hill House in August 1934 when he was 9 (he was told he was going for a day at the seaside). He lived there for the next 60 years. His memories include hard physical work on the farm or scrubbing and polishing the wards, and the 'boys' (who were grown men by then) always having to walk two by two whenever out of the institution's grounds, a practice which persisted until the 1960s.

Deinstitutionalization

In 1976, there were just over 50,000 people with learning disabilities living in large-scale segregated institutions (by now renamed 'mental handicap hospitals') in England. Over the next 25 years this number dropped to around 4000 (Emerson 2004a). In 2001 the government announced in the White Paper *Valuing People* that all remaining 'learning disability hospitals' would close (Department of Health 2001). This target should be achieved by April 2006. Within 30 years the approach which had completely dominated the way we have sought to provide 'supported accommodation' for 100 years will have been dismantled. What drove these remarkable changes and what has replaced these institutions?

At least three factors were important in bringing about these changes. First, the 1960s was a period of significant economic growth, growth that was reflected in increasing living standards and a more liberal approach to social policy. The atrocities of the Second World War had contributed to an increasing international focus on defining and defending people's 'human rights' (e.g. the *Universal Declaration of Human Rights* of 1948, the *European Convention on Human Rights* of 1951). In the late 1960s attention began to focus on extending the notion of rights to more 'marginal' groups within societies, including people with disabilities. This move culminated in 1971 with the United Nations General Assembly adopting the *Declaration on the Rights of Mentally Retarded Persons*. Four years later in 1975 they adopted the wider *Declaration of the Rights of Disabled People*.

Second, the backdrop of increasing living standards for the majority, and an increased focus on human rights, threw into stark contrast the regimes operating in large-scale state-operated institutions in the UK and North America. In the UK, a series of public scandals and inquiries highlighted the degrading conditions under which people with learning disabilities (and people with mental health problems and elderly people) were being 'cared for' or 'supported' by the state (Martin 1984). Similar scandals were occurring across North America (e.g. Blatt and Kaplan 1966); scandals that prompted John F. Kennedy in 1963 to call upon Congress for action 'to bestow the full benefits of our society on those who suffer from mental disabilities [and] to retain in and return to the community the mentally ill and mentally retarded, and there to restore and revitalize their lives'.

Third, there were already in existence models of alternative approaches to providing supported accommodation. The 1950s saw the beginnings of the re-emergence of an interest by professionals in the possibilities of education for people with learning disabilities. Jack Tizard, for example, suggested in 1952 that: 'Young feebleminded adults are the greatest single group in mental deficiency hospitals. There seems no reason why most of them cannot be restored to the community after a period of education and training' (Tizard 1954: 164). In the 1960s and 1970s, behavioural psychologists demonstrated time after time the ability of people with learning disabilities (including people with severe learning disabilities) to acquire new skills and competencies (Remington 1991). Furthermore, Scandinavian services had during the 1950s and 1960s begun to develop a range of much smaller living arrangements whose aim, in the terms used in a 1959 Danish Act, was to 'create an existence for the mentally retarded as close to normal living conditions as possible' (Bank-Mikkelsen 1980).

The policy response was contained in the White Paper *Better Services for the Mentally Handicapped* (Department of Health and Social Security 1971). While not calling for the abandonment of institutional provision, *Better Services* did place considerable emphasis on developing alternative, smaller-scale, community-based residential services for people with learning disabilities. By 1980, however, a policy commitment had been made to ensure that children with learning disabilities would not be placed in 'mental handicap hospitals'. It was not until 2001, however, that the Department of Health explicitly stated that all 'learning disability hospitals' should close.

So what has replaced 'learning disability hospitals'? The answer to this question is complex as deinstitutionalization has not been a unified policy in England. Responsibility for developing alternative forms of supported accommodation fell to two main agencies, the social services departments of local authorities, and health authorities (and more recently Trusts) operating under the auspices of the National Health Service (NHS). There was very little central guidance available to these agencies regarding what exact form these alternatives should take. As a result, there was (and continues to be) extensive variation across England with regard to how the policies of deinstitutionalization were transacted. There were, however, some common themes.

In the 1970s, deinstitutionaliztion primarily involved the movement of people with mild learning disabilities (the old 'feeble-minded') into a range of often pre-existing services including hostels, semi-supported group homes, family placement (adult 'fostering') schemes, bed and breakfast arrangements and independent living. During this period, however, attention also began to turn to developing community-based support for people with more severe disabilities.

Initially, this often involved the development of medium-sized locally based hospital (or community) units. These were developed and operated by health authorities (who also operated the mental handicap hospitals). Simon, a highly influential psychiatrist, described them thus:

> community units that already exist vary in size from 12 to 30 beds. The most convenient and economic size has been found to be 24 beds, 8 catering for long-term residents, 8 providing residential care with training for up to a two-year period and 8 being retained to meet the need for short-term, on demand services. Community units of this size should serve a population of about 80,000.
>
> (Simon 1981: 24)

These services were the focus of considerable interest, attention and research (e.g. Felce *et al.* 1980). Interestingly, Simon also suggested that the learning disability 'hospital of the future will be a great deal smaller, 200 beds or less' (1981: 26).

During the 1980s, however, the development of these medium-sized medicalized facilities was subject to increasing challenges. As noted above, an Act passed in Denmark in 1959 had suggested that the aim of services was to 'create an existence for the mentally retarded as close to normal living conditions as possible' (Bank-Mikkelsen 1980). From this movement the notion, or more accurately notions (see Emerson 1992) of normalization were born. The most influential definition of normalization was provided by a North American psychologist, Wolf Wolfensberger. He defined it (and has since renamed it as social role valorization) (Wolfensberger 1983) as the 'utilization of means which are as culturally normative as possible, in order to establish and/or maintain personal behaviors and characteristics which are as culturally normative as possible' (Wolfensberger 1972: 28). In the UK, notions of normalization found their voice in an influential series of publications from the King's Fund (King's Fund Centre 1980, 1984). Grouped under a banner proclaiming 'An Ordinary Life' these papers argued that services should aim to provide the level of support necessary to enable *all* people with learning disabilities to live in ordinary domestic housing and to be employed in ordinary jobs. These ideas now underpin official health and social care policy for people with learning disabilities in England (Department of Health 2001).

During the 1980s a number of pilot schemes involving small group living arrangements for people with severe learning disabilities in 'ordinary' domestic housing (group homes or staffed houses) had been developed and evaluated (e.g. Felce 1989; Lowe and de Paiva 1991), including pilot schemes for people with extremely disturbed or 'challenging' behaviour (Mansell *et al.* 2001). By the end of the 1980s, use of staffed domestic housing for people with learning disabilities had become the dominant approach in many localities. In others, however, deinstitutionalization was accomplished (at least in part) by the development of cluster housing or large campus-style facilities, or by the development of relatively large 'residential care homes'.

Current provision

Figure 6.1 illustrates the patterning of provision across different sectors in England in 2001 (the last year for which full data are available).

NHS provision

The NHS provides both long-stay 'beds' and residential 'places' for people with intellectual disability, accounting for 12 per cent of total recorded provision in 2001. Long-stay 'beds' represent provision in which the person has the legal status of being a patient within the NHS. There has been a marked and continuing reduction in the number of NHS long-stay beds since 1976. In 2001 there were just over 3500 NHS long-stay beds for people with intellectual disability in England (representing 50 per cent of NHS residential provision for people with intellectual disability). Of these, approximately 1000 are spread across the 22 remaining NHS long-stay hospitals for people with intellectual disability. The nature of the remaining 2500 long-stay beds is unclear. It is likely, however, that they are primarily composed of either 'campus-style' or 'cluster housing' arrangements or long-term 'treatment' facilities. Recent research has seriously questioned the cost-effectiveness of such services (Emerson *et al.* 2000a, 2000b; Emerson 2004b). As a result, the Department of Health has made a commitment to review the situation

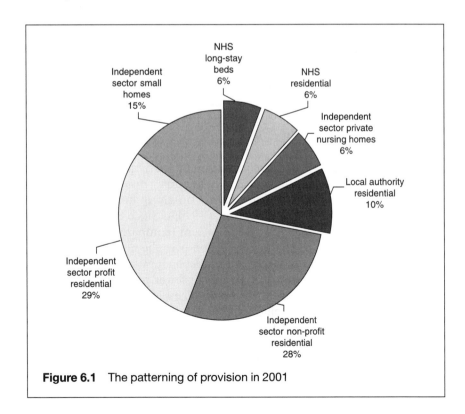

Figure 6.1   The patterning of provision in 2001

of all people living in 'campus-style' arrangements (Department of Health 2001).

The NHS also provides residential 'places' for people with intellectual disability. This includes all forms of residential provision operated by the NHS in which residents have been legally 'discharged' from hospital care. Again, the nature of this type of provision is unclear. It is likely, however, that they are composed of either 'campus-style' or 'cluster housing' arrangements, dispersed group homes or staffed housing schemes. Information on NHS residential places has only been collected since 1996–7.

Local authority provision

In England, local authorities are responsible for arranging social care (but not health care). The initial phases of deinstitutionalization saw the amount of residential services that were directly managed by the local authorities rise from just under 7000 in 1976 to over 12,500 in 1988/9. As a direct result of legislative change introduced in 1990 to create 'internal markets' in social care the extent of local authority provision has now fallen back to under 6000 and is expected to continue to fall. Local authority provision currently accounts for 10 per cent of all provision. Thus, provision directly managed by statutory sector organizations accounted for 22 per cent of all residential provision for people with learning disabilities in England in 2001. The average size of local authority provision fell between 1994 and 2001 from 15.4 to 13.0 places per home.

Independent sector provision

Deinstitutionalization (and the more recent pressure to reduce residential services directly managed by local authorities) has been associated with a significant increase in provision managed by independent sector organizations. Total provision by the independent sector has risen nearly 15-fold from just over 3000 in 1976 to over 50,000 in 2001. The majority of this provision is in group homes for four or more people (independent sector 'residential' currently accounts for 57 per cent of all provision). Provision is equally split between 'voluntary' non-profit and 'private' profit-making organizations. Information on group homes for fewer than four people has only been collected since 1993/4. Since that time, provision in small homes has risen by over 200 per cent (compared with 63 per cent for independent sector 'residential' provision over the same period).

The average size of independent sector non-profit provision (excluding all 'small homes' for three or fewer people) fell between 1994 and 2001 from 9.3 to 8.4 places per home. The average size of independent sector for-profit provision (excluding all 'small homes' for three or fewer people) fell between 1994 and 2001 from 10.7 to 9.5 places per home.

Community-based residential support is not, however, the only alternative to traditional forms of institutional care. Other options include intentional or village communities (Cox and Pearson 1995). There is little reliable information available on this form of provision. However, it appears that: (1)

all such services are operated by independent sector non-profit organizations; (2) they account for approximately 2 per cent of supported accommodation services for people with intellectual disabilities in England (Department of Health 1999); (3) the majority of people who live in such communities are relatively able and moved there from their family home or from residential schools. As such, the village community movement has developed independently of deinstitutionalization.

Overall levels of provision

The currently recorded overall level of provision is equivalent to 129 places per 100,000 of the general population. This level of provision is markedly lower than that reported in the USA (155) and markedly higher than that reported in Australia (100) (Braddock *et al.* 2001). Our best estimate is that there has been no change in the overall level of provision over the last 25 years. This is a matter of concern since it is widely recognized that the extent of provision in the UK is insufficient to meet demand (Department of Health 1971).

The impact of changing patterns and practices in supported accommodation

Deinstitutionalization was perceived as a contentious and risky policy. While there was general agreement that existing institutional provision was often of an unacceptable quality, there was no consensus on what the most appropriate alternatives would be. As a result, deinstitutionalization came under close scrutiny and generated a significant volume of applied research (Emerson and Hatton 1994; Hatton and Emerson 1996). Initially, most of this research tried to answer the question: are people with learning disabilities better off in community-based services than they were in institutions? But what was and is meant by 'better off' and who decides what 'better off' means? The answer to the latter question is quite clear. With very few exceptions indeed, researchers and the policy-makers who commission research were the people who decided what 'better off' means. People with learning disabilities themselves and their relatives had virtually no say at all in deciding what outcomes research should focus on. As a result, the definition and measurement of being 'better off' tended to reflect the biases and preoccupations of academics (like myself) and senior policy-makers. Fortunately, these interests were sufficiently wide and varied for some generally robust conclusions to be drawn.

Hatton and Emerson (1996) systematically reviewed all research that had been undertaken in the UK between 1980 and 1996 on the impact of different types of supported living arrangements for people with learning disabilities. They identified a total of 70 separate research studies that involved the participation of 10,000 people with learning disabilities. Table 6.1 provides a summary of the results of their research synthesis.

Table 6.1   Summary of research evidence on differences between learning disability hospitals, hostels, group homes and independent living schemes

Domain	Main conclusions
Social indicators	Group homes provide a more pleasant and less institutional physical environment than either hostels or hospitals, although there was wide variation in the quality of physical environment in group homes. People living in group homes or hostels have more personal possessions than people living in hospital. Rates of employment across all settings was uniformly low.
Medication	People in hospital are more likely to be prescribed psychoactive medication than people in community-based settings, although levels of prescription in all settings was high.
User satisfaction	People living in community-based settings (and in particular those living in group homes) report greater satisfaction with their place of residence and life in general than people living in hospital. The majority of people living in hospital express a preference to live in more independent settings, while the majority of people living in community-based settings express a preference for staying where they are.
Choice	People living in community-based settings (and in particular those living in group homes) have greater privacy and choice over everyday aspects of their lives, although the differences are often marginal. However, people across all settings appear to have little influence over major life decisions.
Competence and personal growth	*Adaptive behaviour:* people moving from hospital to community-based settings may show some modest gains in adaptive behaviour which are likely to be maintained (but not built upon) over time. *Challenging behaviour:* overall, no change in the rated severity of challenging behaviour is apparent on moving from hospital to community-based services. There is a trend, however, for observed levels of challenging behaviour to decrease on the move from hospital to community-based settings.
Participation: domestic and other activities	Rated and observed levels of the participation of users in domestic activities are higher in community-based services (and in particular in group homes) than in NHS mental handicap hospitals. There is, however, marked variation in the extent to which users participate in everyday activities.

Table 6.1   (*continued*)

Participation: friends and families	There are few, if any, differences in levels of friendships or contact with families between service models. Where differences have been reported, they suggest greater levels of friendship and contact with families in community-based settings. Levels of contact with friends appear uniformly low across all types of services.
Community presence	People living in community-based services (and in particular in group homes) make more use of ordinary facilities in the community than people living in hospital.
Status and acceptance	Neighbours and local business people report few concerns about living next to or serving people with learning disabilities. People with learning disabilities living independently do, however, report victimization.
The views of parents and relatives	Parents express greater satisfaction with community-based services than with hospitals. Only a small minority of parents express overall negative views about the support their son or daughter is receiving in community-based services, although specific concerns were noted by a larger proportion of parents.
Service practices	Community-based services (and in particular group homes) are more resident-oriented and less institutional than hospitals. There is, however, wide variation in the 'social climate' of community-based services. People living in community-based settings make greater use of 'ordinary' health services than people in hospital.
Staff contact	People living in community-based services (and in particular those living in group homes) can expect to receive more contact from care staff than people living in hospital. There is, however, marked variation in the levels of contact received by people in all settings.
Costs	Studies which have examined the comprehensive costs of residential services have all reported marked variation in costs within models. There are no clear differences between the comprehensive costs of community-based services and mental handicap hospitals.

Source: Hatton and Emerson (1996)

More recently, the Office of the Deputy Prime Minister and the Department of Health have been developing new guidance for housing and support services. The consultation document (released in 2003) summarized the existing evidence base in three brief statements:

- Smaller community-based housing and support services provide higher quality support and better outcomes for people with learning disabilities than larger more 'institutional' forms of provision.

- The quality of support and outcomes provided by community-based housing and support services is often unacceptable when judged against the aspirations of *Valuing People*.
- There are few robust relationships between measures of resource input and either the quality of support or outcomes for people with learning disabilities. Quality is determined by how resources are used.

The evidence, therefore, suggests that deinstitutionalization has been a qualified success. It is clear that while smaller community-based supports are associated with better outcomes, there still exists a marked gap between what is being delivered and the aspirations of social inclusion and empowerment that underlie current policy.

This gap has led to increasing criticism of the reliance of public agencies on staffed housing or group homes as the dominant model of provision. Some commentators have argued that this model did not go far enough in addressing issues of inclusion and choice and have promoted the notion of 'supported living' (e.g. Kinsella 1993; O'Brien 1994; Simons 1997). Others have suggested that it has gone too far and have promoted the notion of 'village communities' (Cox and Pearson 1995; Grover 1995).

Proponents of 'supported living' argue that the role of services should be to provide the support necessary to enable people with learning disabilities to live in their own home, rather than in a residential facility (whether large or small) that is owned and operated by a welfare agency. O'Brien (1994) draws attention to some of the key aspects of 'home' in terms of providing a secure sense of place over which the person living there exerts considerable control. As a result, approaches to supported living have sought to provide people with legal security regarding their accommodation (e.g. by ensuring that people hold legal tenancies) and to maximize the degree of control they have over where and with whom they live. To date, there have been few formal evaluations of the impact of supported living. The little evidence that is available suggests that the gains associated with supported living are relatively modest when compared against group homes of similar size (Emerson *et al.* 2001).

The guiding ethos behind village communities is that, by paralleling the operation of rural villages, they can provide a relatively self-contained, rich and varied life for people with learning disabilities in a setting that is to a certain extent physically separate from mainstream society. As such, village communities demonstrate continuity in ideas with romantic notions of village life and the rationale for institutions for people with intellectual disabilities that emerged at the end of the nineteenth century.

A number of village communities have a clear religious or philosophical foundation. The latter include Camphill communities that are based on life-sharing arrangements between people who do and who do not have disabilities (see www.camphill.org.uk). As Fulgosi (1990: 43) describes:

> As the word 'village' implies, each Camphill village centre endeavors to create and maintain an environment where the economic, social and spiritual life of the community complement each other. Villagers [people

with intellectual disabilities] and co-workers live and work side-by-side, running their homes, and sharing what needs to be done. Some villages have a village store, a gift shop, café, and even a post office ... The rhythm of the farming year, the seasons and the celebration of the Christian festivals play an important part in the life of each community.

Again, there have been few formal evaluations of the impact of village communities. The little evidence that is available suggests that they offer a different, though not necessarily inferior, quality of life to community-based approaches (Emerson *et al.* 2000a).

Conclusion

As we have seen, the last 150 years, and in particular the last 30 years, has witnessed a revolution in the way in which public agencies have sought to provide 'care' or 'support' for people with learning disabilities who live outside the family home. Overall, the changes of the last 30 years appear to have been to the benefit of people with learning disabilities. Different 'models' have been associated with different outcomes, although the magnitude of these differences is often quite modest. As the Office of the Deputy Prime Minister and Department of Health suggested in 2003, the quality of support and outcomes provided by community-based housing and support services is often unacceptable when judged against the aspirations of *Valuing People*.

What are we to make of this? First, it suggests that there is often a significant gap between rhetoric and reality. All too often, the aims of different models prove remarkably difficult to realize in practice. Perhaps part of the problem here has been our tendency to think about different 'models' of support, models that are often promoted as radical departures from the status quo (e.g. King's Fund Centre 1980; Kinsella 1993). Such an approach emphasizes discontinuity and change. Maybe we need to turn our attention to understanding the basis for continuity in supported accommodation and use this knowledge to attempt to close the gap between policy aspirations and reality.

Recently, a number of research studies have adopted this focus. That is, instead of asking whether people are 'better off' in model A or B, they have attempted to identify what it is that leads to better outcomes in some circumstances than in others (see Felce 2000; Hatton 2001). The results of these studies have indicated that:

- Considered on their own, resources (e.g. costs, staffing levels, staff values, skills or qualifications) are, at best, only weakly associated with the quality of support or outcomes for people with learning disabilities.
- There is strong evidence that in all 'models' people with less severe learning disabilities are likely to enjoy a better quality of life than people with more severe learning disabilities.
- There is growing evidence that certain aspects of the internal organiza-

tion and management of support are key to assuring quality outcomes for people with learning disabilities. Institutional working practices have been consistently associated with a wide range of poor outcomes. The use of systematic individualized working practices has been associated with the provision of increased and more effective support, increased participation, increased social inclusion and increased user satisfaction.

These findings suggest that attention needs to be paid to aspects of the day-to-day operation of services, rather than broad aspects of the 'model' of provision.

Then again, perhaps we should not be surprised about the often modest progress made toward promoting full inclusion and an equitable quality of life for people with learning disabilities. To be surprised, in effect, subscribes to a simple 'idealist' view of history which sees gradual progress as a result of benevolent implementation of changes resulting from new ideals, theories, visions and advances in knowledge. In this view, the development of services is seen as a victory of humanitarianism/science over irrational prejudice. Failure is seen in terms of remaining irrationality, poor communication, public prejudice and lack of resources.

There are, however, alternative (and some would say more pessimistic) views. In some, intentions are seen as solutions to conflicts arising from social change and change is considered to result from the complex interdependence of 'conscience and convenience'. In this model, unholy alliances between benevolent rhetoric and operational needs lead to the symbolic rather than actual implementation of 'advances' in knowledge (e.g. Rothman 1980). Still other approaches argue that all we are seeing are changing patterns of social control in response to changes in the social order. In this approach, ideals and intentions are seen as mystifying rhetoric concealing the true nature of the control process (e.g. Scull 1984).

Understanding the nature and impact of 'models of service delivery' requires us to address these broader issues concerning the nature of change in social responses to people with disabilities.

Exercise 6.1

Consider the types of supported accommodation described in this chapter. Think about what type of accommodation you would most like to live in and why.

From the evidence (Table 6.1) about types of supported accommodation, and from your wider reading, compare what you consider to be the most desirable features of community-based types of accommodation for people with learning disabilities.

Given the weak association between staffing levels and user/resident outcomes across types of supported accommodation, consider what staff-related and organization-related factors are most likely to make a difference to the quality of a person's everyday life in those settings. Discuss your views and evidence with one of your peers and a person with learning disabilities.

References

Alaszewski, A. (1988) From villains to victims, in A. Leighton (ed.). *Mental Handicap in the Community*. Cambridge: Woodhead-Faulkener.

Bank-Mikkelsen, N.E. (1980) Denmark, in R.J. Flynn and K.E. Nitsch (eds) *Normalization, Social Integration and Community Services*. Austin, TX: Pro-Ed.

Blatt, B. and Kaplan, H. (1966) *Christmas in Purgatory: A Photographic Essay on Mental Retardation*. New York: Allyn & Bacon.

Braddock, D., Emerson, E., Felce, D. and Stancliffe, R. (2001) The living circumstances of children and adults with mental retardation or developmental disabilities in the United States, Canada, England and Wales, and Australia, *Mental Retardation & Developmental Disabilities Research Reviews*, 7: 115–21.

Cox, C. and Pearson, M. (1995) *Made to Care: The Case for Residential and Village Communities for People with a Mental Handicap*. London: The Rannoch Trust.

Department of Health (1999) *Facing the Facts: Services for People with Learning Disabilities – A Policy Impact Study of Social Care and Health Services*. London: Department of Health.

Department of Health (2001) *Valuing People: A New Strategy for Learning Disability for the 21st Century*, Cm 5086. London: The Stationery Office.

Department of Health and Social Security (1971) *Better Services for the Mentally Handicapped*. London: Department of Health.

Emerson, E. (1992) What is normalisation? in H. Smith and H. Brown (eds) *Normalisation: A Reader for the 1990s*. London: Routledge.

Emerson, E. (2004a) Deinstitutionalisation in England, *Journal of Intellectual & Developmental Disability*, 29: 17–22.

Emerson, E. (2004b) Cluster housing for adults with intellectual disabilities, *Journal of Intellectual & Developmental Disability*, 29: 187–97.

Emerson, E. and Hatton, C. (1994) *Moving Out: The Impact of Relocation from Hospital to Community on the Quality of Life of People with Learning Disabilities*. London: HMSO.

Emerson, E., Robertson, J., Gregory, N., Kessissoglou, S., Hatton, C., Hallam, A., Knapp, M., Järbrink, K., Walsh, P. and Netten, A. (2000a) The quality and costs of village communities, residential campuses and community-based residential supports in the UK, *American Journal of Mental Retardation*, 105: 81–102.

Emerson, E., Robertson, J., Gregory, N., Kessissoglou, S., Hatton, C., Hallam, A., Järbrink, K., Knapp, M., Netten, A. and Linehan, C. (2000b) The quality and costs of community-based residential supports and residential campuses for people with severe and complex disabilities, *Journal of Intellectual and Developmental Disability*, 25: 263–79.

Emerson, E., Robertson, J., Gregory, N., Hatton, C., Kessissoglou, S., Hallam, A., Järbrink, K., Knapp, M., Netten, A. and Walsh, P. (2001) The quality and costs of supported living residences and group homes in the United Kingdom, *American Journal of Mental Retardation*, 106: 401–15.

Felce, D. (1989) *The Andover Project: Staffed Housing for Adults with Severe or Profound Mental Handicaps*. Kidderminster: British Institute for Mental Handicap.

Felce, D. (2000) *Quality of Life for People with Learning Disabilities in Supported Housing in the Community: A Review of Research*. Exeter: Centre for Evidence based Social Services (www.ex.ac.uk/cebss).

Felce, D., Kushlick, A. and Mansell, J. (1980) Evaluation of alternative residential facilities for the severely mentally handicapped in Wessex: client engagement, *Advances in Behaviour Research and Therapy*, 3: 13–18.

Fulgosi, L. (1990) Camphill communities, in S. Segal (ed.) *The Place of Special Villages and Residential Communities: The Provision of Care for People with Severe, Profound and Multiple Disabilities*. Bicester: AB Academic Publishers.

Gray, G. (1997) *A Long Day at the Seaside*. Windsor: Reedprint.

Grover, R. (1995) *Communities that Care: Intentional Communities of Attachment as a Third Path in Community Care*. Brighton: Pavilion.

Hatton, C. (2001) *Developing Housing and Support Options: Lessons From Research*. Lancaster: Institute for Health Research, Lancaster University (www.lancaster. ac.uk/depts/ihr/ld/download/housing_support.pdf).

Hatton, C. and Emerson, E. (1996) *Residential Provision for People with Learning Disabilities: A Research Review*. Manchester: Hester Adrian Research Centre, University of Manchester (www.lancaster.ac.uk/depts/ihr/ld/download/res_ review.pdf).

King's Fund Centre (1980) *An Ordinary Life: Comprehensive Locally-based Residential Services for Mentally Handicapped People*. London: King's Fund Centre.

King's Fund Centre (1984) *An Ordinary Working Life: Vocational Services for People with Mental Handicap*. London: King's Fund Centre.

Kinsella, P. (1993) *Supported Living: A New Paradigm*. Manchester: National Development Team.

Lowe, K. and de Paiva, S. (1991) *NIMROD – An Overview*. London: HMSO.

Malin, N., Race, D. and Jones, G. (1980) *Services for the Mentally Handicapped in Britain*. London: Croom Helm.

Mansell, J., McGill, P. and Emerson, E. (2001) Development and evaluation of innovative residential services for people with severe intellectual disability and serious challenging behaviour, in L.M. Glidden (ed.) *International Review of Research in Mental Retardation*. New York: Academic Press.

Martin, J.P. (1984) *Hospital in Trouble*. Oxford: Blackwell.

O'Brien, J. (1994) Down stairs that are never your own: supporting people with developmental disabilities in their own homes, *Mental Retardation*, 32: 1–6.

Office of the Deputy Prime Minister/Department of Health (2003) *Housing and Support Options for People with Learning Disabilities* (draft released for consultation). London: DoH.

Race, D. (1995) Historical development of service provision, in N. Malin (ed.) *Services for People with Learning Disabilities*. London: Routledge.

Remington, B. (1991) *The Challenge of Severe Mental Handicap: A Behaviour Analytic Approach*. Chichester: Wiley.

Rothman, D.J. (1980) *Conscience and Convenience: The Asylum and its Alternatives in Progressive America*. Boston, MA: Little, Brown.

Ryan, J. and Thomas, F. (1987) *The Politics of Mental Handicap*, revised edn. London: Free Association Books.

Scheerenberger, R.C. (1983) *A History of Mental Retardation*. Baltimore, MD: Brookes.

Scull, A. (1984) *Decarceration: Community Treatment and the Deviant – A Radical View*, 2nd edn. Cambridge: Polity Press.

Scull, A. (1993) *The Most Solitary of Afflictions: Madness and Society in Britain, 1700–1900*. New Haven, CT: Yale University Press.

Simmons, H.G. (1982) *From Asylum to Welfare*. Downsview, Ontario: National Institute on Mental Retardation.

Simon, G.B. (1981) *Local Services for Mentally Handicapped People*. Kidderminster: British Institute of Mental Handicap.

Simons, K. (1997) *A Foot in the Door: The Early Years of Supported Living for People with Learning Difficulties in the UK*. Manchester: National Development Team.

Tizard, J. (1954) Institutional defectives, *American Journal on Mental Deficiency*, 59: 158–65.

Wolfensberger, W. (1972) *The Principal of Normalization in Human Services*. Toronto: National Institute on Mental Retardation.

Wolfensberger, W. (1975) *The Origin and Nature of Our Institutional Models*. Syracuse: Human Policy Press.

Wolfensberger, W. (1981) The extermination of handicapped people in World War II Germany, *Mental Retardation*, 19(1): 1–7.

Wolfensberger, W. (1983) Social role valorization: a proposed new term for the principal of normalization, *Mental Retardation*, 21: 234–9.

Wright, D. and Digby, A. (1996) *From Idiocy to Mental Deficiency: Historical Perspectives on People with Learning Disabilities*. London: Routledge.

7

Maintaining a commitment to quality

Lesley Styring and Gordon Grant

Introduction

Maintaining a commitment to quality in the planning, design, delivery and review of services for people with learning disabilities is an important requirement in ensuring that public money is wisely spent. Equally important is the task of enabling people with learning disabilities to achieve a quality of life (QoL) comparable to that of other citizens. Unless services are locked into ways of improving the quality of people's lived experiences there are dangers that services will be working to an irrelevant agenda. In this chapter the reader is therefore introduced to some of the contemporary thinking about QoL, and how this can be used to inform quality in services. The first part of the chapter reviews QoL literature. This is followed by an examination of quality assurance mechanisms in services that are intended to create and maintain high service standards. The final part of the chapter poses some challenges about the prospects for linking quality assurance (QA) mechanisms to the achievement of a high QoL for people with learning disabilities. Vignettes are used to personalize some of the thinking behind QoL and service quality issues.

Quality of life

'Quality of life' is a term used in everyday talk but its meaning is very much dependent on context. In their review of conceptual and measurement issues about QoL, Schalock and Felce (2004) suggest that it is a multidimensional construct, used in different ways throughout the world, for example as:

- *A sensitizing notion* that provides a frame of reference from the individual's perspective, about the person and his or her environment. In this sense, 'quality' makes us think about individual characteristics such as happiness, success, wealth, health and satisfaction, whereas 'of life' suggests a concern with the essential aspects of human existence for the individual.

- *A social construct* that can be used as the basis for evaluating person-referenced outcomes and to enhance a person's perceived QoL. This ties in with ideas about service designs and how these might inform valued outcomes for individuals.

- *A unifying theme* that provides a systematic framework for understanding and applying the concept of QoL. This typically involves knowing about the linkages between the 'microsystem' (the person, family, friends, advocates and wider social network), the 'mesosystem' (neighbourhood, community or organization providing services or support) and the 'macrosystem' (overarching patterns of culture, society and sociopolitical influences).

- *A motivational construct*, meaning that a sensitivity to important and desirable outcomes in one's personal life reinforces a heightened awareness of, and commitment to, the means to achieve them.

There is a huge literature on QoL, much of it focusing on conceptualization and measurement, heralding many scales and instruments that claim to assess QoL. Historically, two underlying approaches are evident in measuring QoL. The first, the 'social indicators' approach, relies on external conditions such as health, standard of living, housing conditions, public safety and so on, using statistics about objective standards. An example of this in relation to a housing conditions measure about heating might be: central heating throughout whole dwelling; central heating in certain rooms only; fires or other heating appliances available in certain rooms only; no heating available. Responses could then be scored or ranked. The second approach is typically referred to as the 'psychological indicators' approach. This concentrates on a person's subjective appraisals of life experiences. Taking again the example of the heating measure of housing conditions, this might be evaluated as largely irrelevant if the person was living in a country with a warm climate, but even in a country like the UK two different persons are likely to weigh the importance of heating in the home from different perspectives unique to them. For example it might matter more to someone with young children at home, or to an older person with poor blood circulation, than to someone who spends little time at home. Accordingly, QoL studies often integrate objective and subjective systems of appraisal.

Though these may be regarded as starting points for getting a 'fix' on QoL, different models have emerged about ways of conceptualizing and measuring QoL.

QoL models

There are now many QoL models that have been developed and applied to varying extents to the lives of people with learning disabilities. Three of the more established QoL models are summarized in Table 7.1 so a few words of explanation about them are in order here.

In the Felce and Perry (1996) model, QoL is seen as the product of three interacting elements: personal values, life conditions and personal satisfaction. Briefly stated, QoL is defined as overall well-being comprised of objective and subjective evaluations of the domains of physical, material, social and emotional well-being, together with the extent of personal development and purposeful activity. All these evaluations are then weighted by personal values – i.e. by what is important to individuals. Objective evaluation concerns those everyday conditions in which people live their lives, such as health, income, housing quality, friendships, activities and social roles. Subjective evaluation refers to satisfaction with these life conditions. However, the key to these lies in the value or importance the individual attaches to each domain.

In this model, physical well-being is comprised of health, personal safety, fitness and mobility. Material well-being comprises finance, income, transport, security and tenure, as well as other aspects of the living environment. Social well-being includes the quality and breadth of interpersonal relationships, and community involvement. Emotional well-being is characterized by affect, fulfilment, mental state, self-esteem, status and respect, faith and sexuality. Finally, development and activity concerns the acquisition and use of skills in different arenas – at home, work, education and leisure for example.

The social well-being framework described by Bach and Rioux (1996) takes a different direction. At its core are three elements: self-determination, democratization and equality. These elements are founded on the empirical literature on well-being, philosophical literature and human rights declarations and conventions (Roeher Institute 1993).

It is claimed that self-determination can be exercised when people, communities and governments can make known their hopes and aspirations, and make plans and decisions to achieve them. Self-determination is expressed both as freedom from resistance and as freedom to do things that are worth doing. Hence it emphasizes the interdependent relations between people, communities and governments in nurturing the resources and conditions for aspirations to be realized. Put another way, it highlights the help and support people require in order to exercise self-determination, rather than assuming that self-determination is an inherent or voluntary capacity of individuals. The second element in the model, democratization, is closely linked to the idea of self-determination. The reason for this is that it is concerned with enabling the democratic participation of individuals and diverse groups in decisions that directly affect their lives and well-being. It therefore places an importance on respect for different points of view in decision-making, emphasizing the key role of a principled approach to

Table 7.1 QoL models compared

Felce and Perry (1996): a model for people with and without disabilities	Bach and Rioux (1996): a social well-being framework	Renwick and Brown (1996): centre for health promotion model
QoL constructs:	**Social well-being constructs:**	**QoL constructs:**
Physical well-being	*Self determination:* making decisions and choices without coercion; exercising control	*Being:* who the person is as an individual
Material well-being		*Belonging:* how environments and others fit with the person
Social well-being	*Equality:* equal access to the means of self-development, coupled with freedom from political control, social pressure, economic deprivation and insecurity in order to engage in valued pursuits	*Becoming:* what the person does to achieve hopes, goals and aspirations
Development and activity		
Emotional well-being	*Democratization:* participation in decision-making that directly affects well-being	**Mediating influences:**
Measurements:		Opportunities and constraints presented both by chance and by choice
Objective assessment of life conditions, and subjective assessment of personal satisfaction		
Mediating influences:		
Personal values		

consultation (Grant 1997). Social well-being is more likely, it is claimed, where democratization becomes an integrating force. The third element, equality, is defined as the absence of barriers to mutual respect and recognition between people. It implies freedom from political control, social pressure, economic deprivation and insecurity (Lukes 1980). This is a quite different view of equality from the more conventional one that has predominated in public policy and court rulings which involves treating similar cases in similar ways.

In the social well-being model therefore, a high QoL depends upon self-determination, democratization and equality being realized at the individual, community and societal levels. It also reminds us that QoL cannot be attained by individuals alone.

The model proposed by Renwick and Brown (1996) is different again. It is based first of all on the humanist-existential tradition that acknowledges a person's needs to belong, in both physical and social terms, and to pursue personal goals, making decisions and choices along the way. Renwick and Brown also describe how they were influenced by other QoL research that stressed the importance of how individuals view their own QoL.

Three core components lie at the heart of this model: being, belonging and becoming. Being refers to an individual's physical, psychological and spiritual identities. Belonging is about the links individuals have with their physical, social and communal environments, and whether they feel 'at home' in these environments and enjoy meaningful and supportive relationships within them. Finally, becoming relates to personal aspirations in terms of purposeful activity, leisure and personal growth. Importance and enjoyment are considered to be factors determining QoL, moderated by how much control individuals can exert over the perceived opportunities they have to exploit change and enhancement in each area of life.

These models continue to be tested and to evolve. Though each has rather different philosophical roots there are nevertheless some unifying themes. Brown and Brown (2003: 30–1) suggest that five ideas about QoL need to be kept constantly in mind:

1   QoL addresses similar aspects, attributes and processes of life for all of us, disabled and non-disabled. It concerns things that are important to all, such as nutrition, health, social connections, housing and leisure, irrespective of country or region, or of historical period.

2   QoL is personal. Similarities in the processes people face (e.g. services) start to diverge when we make choices and respond according to our unique needs and circumstances. In this view, QoL is largely dependent therefore on the unique interactions between a person and the attributes of their environment – i.e the microsystem, mesosystem and macrosystem identified by Schalock and Felce (2004). Understanding these interactions therefore becomes a key in designing interventions and support to help people improve QoL. Typically, this is best understood from the individual's own perspective.

3   We can judge specific aspects of our own lives. There may be broad

agreement about the dimensions of QoL but each person will nevertheless have a view about which are most important to them. This presents a challenge for person-centred practice as it means that the personal dispositions of individuals may diverge from those of practitioners.

4   All parts of our lives are interconnected. This means that there is a premium on being able to map the interlocking relations of the microsystem, mesosystem and macrosystem for their effects on the individual and their QoL. This can make QoL quite complicated, but then it can help practitioners and others to look at individuals more holistically and to judge how well-intentioned interventions might improve QoL in one domain but perhaps undermine it in another.

5   QoL is ever-changing. As has been stressed elsewhere, people's lives are rarely if ever static given the demands, vicissitudes, unplanned events and changing circumstances that occur over the life cycle (see Chapter 11). Accordingly, QoL may change from day to day and year to year, and things that contribute to QoL at one stage may be quite different to those that contribute to it later on.

We might also add that:

6   QoL is one way of conceptualizing what might constitute valued outcomes for individuals. Hence it may be feasible to incorporate elements of QoL into the evaluation of person-centred or family-centred interventions or into appraisals of the citizenship status of people with disabilities at different stages of their lives. A QoL orientation may help to concentrate attention on the things individuals value in life and, used wisely, it can therefore act as a counterpoint to dominant professional, academic and political agendas.

7   QoL literature sometimes appears to imply that the person's life is purely a product of services. It may be better to ask first what part services play in people's lives and then ask them to rate their use and importance. Even then, evaluations need to take account of biographic, social and environmental factors beyond services that shape the quality of everyday life for individuals.

Although QoL measures have typically been applied to individuals, they have also been developed in work with families. The work of Park *et al.* (2003) is a good example.

Case study: *Ernie*

Ernie is 54 years old. He lives by himself in a bungalow that he used to share with his mother until she died five years ago. He is supported by a home help, Sue, four to five mornings a week though he rarely sees her as he is typically at work. Ernie has a family aide, Jemma, who takes him out for three to four hours at weekends, though he says that they often go to places that Jemma decides, including her own home where he sometimes has a meal with Jemma and her husband. Ernie has eyesight problems with cataracts and is awaiting surgery. He has a heart condition and is checked every six months by his GP. Ernie attends the local social activity centre but he also has some work experience where he assists with the running of a community centre. When interviewed about his everyday life, Ernie revealed how his support network and the wider environment influence the quality of his everyday experiences:

Decision-making

Ernie:	My niece came down, buy a shirt.
Interviewer:	Did she tell you you needed a shirt?
Ernie:	Yes.
Interviewer:	Did she take you out and buy one?
Ernie:	Yes.
Interviewer:	Did she choose it or did you choose it?
Ernie:	They bloody choose it!
Interviewer:	Did you like it though?
Ernie:	Lump it! It was alright.

Perceptions of safety

Interviewer:	Do you ever go to the pictures?
Ernie:	No. On the news always grabbing people.
Interviewer:	You hear on the news about grabbing people?
Ernie:	Yes.
Interviewer:	So what do you think?
Ernie:	Say to myself stay home.
Interviewer:	It's safer?
Ernie:	Yes!

Loneliness

Interviewer:	What don't you like about living alone? Can you answer that one?
Ernie:	Sometimes very lonely.
Interviewer:	You'd like someone to talk to in the evenings?
Ernie:	I go home, put the radio on. Yes.
Interviewer:	So sometimes you feel a bit lonely at home?
Ernie:	Yes, my mother died.
Interviewer:	So you feel a bit lonely without her?
Ernie:	Yes, yes, feeling loneliness.
Interviewer:	You miss her?
Ernie:	Yes.

Interviewer: So how do you fill your evenings then?
Ernie: See TV, *Coronation Street.*

Exercise 7.1

From these brief extracts about Ernie taken from a longer interview:

List which 'objective' features of Ernie's environment you consider to affect the quality of his everyday experiences.

Which 'objective' features would you identify with the microsystem, mesosystem and macrosystem in turn?

Taking any one of the three QoL models shown in Table 7.1, write down what you think are the best 'indicators' that capture Ernie's main sentiments in the above interview extracts. What do the indicators you have identified tell you about Ernie's social environment?

In collaboration with Ernie, how might you address the environmental factors that influence his QoL?

QoL: critiques and challenges

QoL has a strong allure reflected in a burgeoning international literature on the subject. Yet there remains a deal of healthy scepticism about the idea of QoL. Several points are worth bearing in mind in this respect:

- Most of the research on QoL among people with learning disabilities has been conducted with people who have speech. The validity of underlying QoL constructs in people without speech is not yet clear.

- There is a high dependency on using proxies (third parties like advocates, allies or support workers) to speak for people who cannot speak for themselves. According to Schalock and Felce (2004) little is known about concordance between self-reports and proxy accounts. The scope for disagreements between individuals and proxies is likely to be higher in relation to questions requiring people to make subjective appraisals.

- Most of the QoL models in use with people with learning disabilities, including the three highlighted in this chapter, were developed before substantive advances in oral history, life history and narrative research within this field, and before the emergence of the user movement with its increasingly powerful articulations. This means that QoL constructs have been largely imported from modes of enquiry about people rather than modes of enquiry designed and controlled by people with learning disabilities (see Chapter 34). In other words, the constructs have typically not emerged from the social constructions of people with learning disabilities themselves, but rather from others with vested interests, particularly academics.

- Improving the quality of services may not necessarily lead directly to improvements in QoL. This is because services reflect shifting policy priorities that may not be fixed around QoL dimensions; most people spend only part of their lives using services so it is easy to exaggerate the influence of services on QoL; and evidence suggests that satisfaction, as one way of measuring subjective well-being, is unresponsive to important changes in people's lives. This has left some commentators to question the relevance of QoL (Hatton 1998; Hensel 2001). In addition, some evidence suggests that people with learning disabilities judge all domains of their lives to be very important. This suggests that the relationships between judgements of importance and people's aspirations, preferences and opportunities for choice need closer attention, and may give a better sense of what is important than QoL constructs (Hensel *et al.* 2002).

- In regard to family QoL there appear to be unresolved tensions between looking upon the family as the unit of analysis as opposed to individual family members where individual differences may be important.

The final section of the chapter takes a closer look at connecting service quality with QoL. Before that it is important to say something about what is being done to raise the stakes in the quality of services.

Maintaining a commitment to service quality

We consider here how current policy and thinking integrates with practice, and how this ultimately impacts on the life of a person with a learning disability. *Valuing People* (Department of Health 2001a) seeks to accomplish a better life for people with learning disabilities by stressing the importance of inclusion, support for independence, choice-making and legal and civic rights. The reforming health agenda of New Labour (Department of Health 1997), of which *Valuing People* is a part, has emphasized three key aspirations:

- improve the overall standards of clinical practice;

- reduce unacceptable variations in clinical practice;

- ensure best use of resources – so that care is appropriate, effective, efficient and economic.

In its determination to set and monitor standards the government proposed a new framework (see Figure 7.1). Central to the framework is clinical governance, essentially an umbrella term for structures such as clinical audit, clinical effectiveness, evidence-based practice, risk assessment and performance management. While clinical governance is a relatively new term, these individual structures have been around in the National Health Service (NHS) for a number of years.

What the framework seeks to do is integrate the different elements. Linked to the governance agenda is professional regulation and lifelong

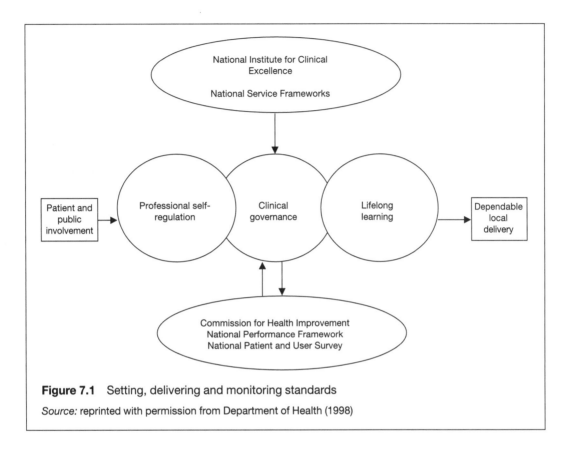

Figure 7.1 Setting, delivering and monitoring standards

Source: reprinted with permission from Department of Health (1998)

learning, both of which are integral components designed to improve standards and quality of care. While the onus is on all staff in the NHS to be accountable for their practice, the government made its commitment to improve standards at local and national level by introducing the National Institute for Clinical Excellence, National Service Frameworks and the Commission for Health Improvement (Department of Health 1998).

Critics of *Valuing People* argue that a National Service Framework for people with learning disabilities would have had more of an impact because it would have carried a higher profile and substantive investment. A strategy sets out a general direction for services to travel, with a value base and some guiding principles. In the case of *Valuing People* the key principles of the strategy are linked to citizenship and people with learning disabilities being valued members of society. A National Service Framework on the other hand is much more directive with action points and measurable outcomes against which services can be benchmarked. In the case of National Service Frameworks there has been considerable financial backing and a powerful evidence base to drive the agenda forward, both of which are decidedly absent from *Valuing People*. Supporters of *Valuing People* however argue that people with learning disabilities are not exempt from public health policy so that National Service Frameworks for specific conditions such as coronary heart disease apply equally to them. We wait to see exactly how this is borne out in practice.

Clinical effectiveness and evidence-based practice lie at the heart of clinical governance and it is often hard to differentiate between the two. While both terms are often used synonymously, evidence-based practice supports clinical effectiveness by ensuring that the care delivered to patients is appropriate, timely, is of the highest quality and based on the best available evidence at the time. Clinical effectiveness on the other hand is more concerned with what treatments and practices actually work and make a difference to a person's health. Structures within the clinical governance framework also contribute to clinical effectiveness and in recent years there has been a rapid growth in departments designed to enhance patient outcomes – for example, through local research, clinical audit and risk management. Clinical activity is also more open to public scrutiny than it has ever been, with the introduction of open forums and published service performance indicators.

Integrated Care Pathways and Essence of Care Benchmarking are good examples of how clinical effectiveness works in practice. There has been a proliferation of Integrated Care Pathways that are multi-professional in nature and designed to provide a structured approach to a specific problem or condition (Brett and Schofield 2002). The emphasis here is on integration and joined-up thinking – when a response to a particular illness, subsequent therapeutic interventions and rehabilitation are beyond the remit of one health care provider. Consequently an Integrated Care Pathway includes all health professionals involved in the patient's care journey and is designed to provide a holistic approach to care and reduce variations in practice. For example, a stroke Care Pathway would be activated on suspicion of diagnosis and should offer patients a standardized approach to assessment, treatment and care management of their condition both in hospital and on discharge home.

Some of the issues identified above can be illustrated within the following vignette about David.

Case study 2: *David*

David is a young man with autism. He has an outgoing personality but his autism is not well understood by his peers so he finds it difficult to maintain friendships. David also has a number of complex health problems including a heart condition, circulatory problems, epilepsy and recurrent eye infections. He has limited communication skills but high staff turnover means that few front-line staff understand what he is trying to communicate (see Chapter 13). David exhibits self-injurious behaviour by head banging as well as by throwing objects or hitting other people. He is prescribed anticonvulsant therapy overseen by his GP. He uses skin products to control his eczema.

David currently lives at home with his parents, Madge and Bill. They have their own health problems that make caring for David difficult. Bill has taken early retirement because of his angina and Madge has recurrent back problems so she has difficulties with moving and handling David safely. David has an older married brother with a young family who live in another part of the country but they are unable to offer any practical support. As a result, Madge and Bill are considering community living options so that David can lead a more independent life. They are concerned that others may not be able to provide personalized care for David to the standards they have come to expect of themselves as carers.

Exercise 7.2

Questions to consider:

How would you begin to judge the QoL of (i) David, (ii) Madge and Bill?

What difference, if any, will Integrated Care Pathways and, more generally, evidence-based practice have on the QoL of David and his parents?

In David's case an Integrated Care Pathway for epilepsy based on National Institute for Clinical Excellence guidance may be beneficial because it would ensure that his epilepsy is treated in exactly the same way as someone else with the condition. However, while this is good in principle the question remains as to whether Integrated Care Pathways are truly inclusive. Indeed there is a tension between providing standardized care and meeting targets, leading to questions about whether initiatives designed to drive quality forward are resource-driven. For example, are people with learning disabilities being excluded from falls clinics because they cannot meet rehabilitation targets?

The Essence of Care Initiative (Department of Health 2001b) reflects the government's commitment to use benchmarking as a means to improve essential aspects of care. Qualitative in nature, Essence of Care provides a toolkit for health care professionals to measure and reflect on the quality of the care provided (Chambers and Jolly 2002). It actively encourages services to share best practice that is evidence-based. Although initially concentrating on eight key aspects of care (self-care, hygiene, nutrition, continence, pressure ulcers, safety, record-keeping and privacy and dignity) the process is gaining momentum and further benchmarks are being developed, all of which are highly relevant for people with learning disabilities.

More importantly there is an expectation, or rather an insistence, that there is patient involvement at a local level to drive the quality agenda forward. The question then is how this model has been translated into practice, and how much of an impact it may have on David (see Figure 7.2).

Another key component of the clinical governance agenda is risk

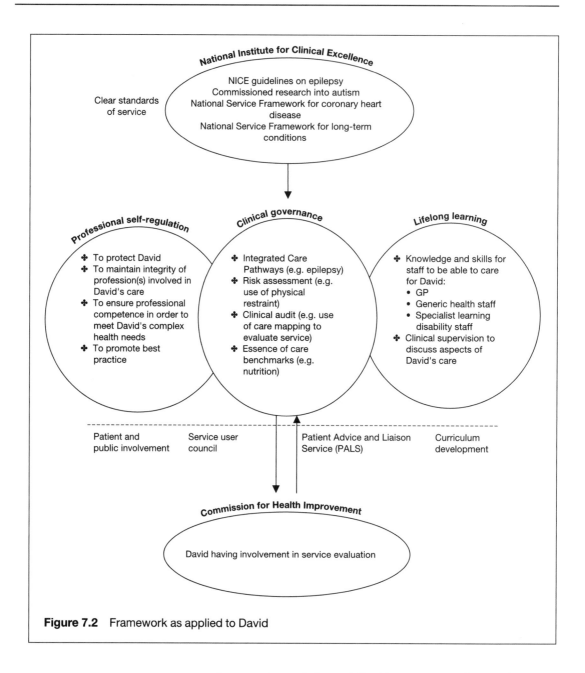

Figure 7.2   Framework as applied to David

management and protection of the public (Department of Health 1998). While the emphasis in the health service has been on improving quality and maintaining safe systems of care (Walshe 2001), there are some who argue that fear of litigation and increasing costs of compensation are the main reasons why risk management has such a high profile. Symon (2003) argues that this may have a critical effect on how health care practitioners act or react in respect of client care because they may be unduly cautious so as to prevent anything untoward from happening. Risk management then presents a challenge in terms of working with people with learning disabilities because in trying to promote independence and choice and in doing so there is always an element of risk. This creates professional tensions. For employees of an NHS organization that is fearful of litigation, there are undoubted limits about allowing David (and others with similar support needs) to take risks for themselves without affecting a professional duty of care or organizational propriety.

The National Patient Safety Agency (NPSA) recently published a document that identified some key concerns relating to people with learning disabilities, their safety and quality of care (NPSA 2004). The NPSA drew attention in particular to:

- inappropriate use of physical intervention;
- vulnerability of people with learning disabilities in general hospitals;
- dysphagia (swallowing difficulties);
- lack of accessible information;
- illness or disease being misdiagnosed or under-diagnosed.

It is worth considering aspects of these concerns in more detail as they relate directly to David. People who exhibit behaviours that challenge services often have difficulty leading valued lifestyles and having their health needs met. The use of physical interventions (British Institute of Learning Disabilities 1999) poses many ethical dilemmas but good practice dictates wherever possible the use of non-invasive interventions, as well as procedures that prevent or minimize the use of restraint (Lovett 1996). Working with David requires that we do not lose sight of related issues such as duty of care or the safety of members of the public and staff. Furthermore, such a risk assessment and care plan requires regular review. A government agency like the NPSA can raise the profile of issues like this at a national level and help to keep it in the minds of front-line staff. At the same time, families deal tacitly with risk-related issues on a daily basis, but their expertise and strategies for coping are often lost on services (see Chapter 11).

People with learning disabilities continue to be vulnerable when accessing and using general hospitals, their illnesses or diseases frequently being misdiagnosed or not diagnosed at all. *Valuing People* (Department of Health 2001a) recognizes that while people with learning disabilities have greater health needs than the general population they often have difficulty accessing health care and getting their needs addressed (see also Chapter 33). *Valuing People* supports the view that people with learning disabilities have a right to benefit from the expertise of mainstream services and recommends that more should be done to prevent discriminatory practice and reduce health inequalities. It will be interesting to see what impact the new General Medical Services contract has on primary care services because it will govern the way general practices receive funding and quality measures will be based on how many patients have had immunizations or breast screening, for example. Primary care services have a responsibility to the whole community, but in discharging this responsibility it is important that the health needs of vulnerable groups are not neglected.

Lefort and Fraser (2002) argue that once people start to equate QoL with the value of life then they could begin to endorse the idea that some people are less valuable than others. Though there is now more informed thinking, people with learning disabilities and their families can still face formidable difficulties when accessing and using mainstream services. For example, although some people with learning disabilities have conditions one would associate with pain (e.g. epilepsy, musculo-skeletal problems and osteoporosis), they are rarely referred to specialist pain services. Furthermore, David and others with similar support needs who exhibit challenging behaviour may have an untreated pain condition or an underlying physiological problem that can lead to undetected serious health conditions and avoidable deaths (NPSA 2004). Certainly some people with learning disabilities have benefited from specialist pain management services and their behaviour has improved considerably as a result, which has led to a positive change in attitude towards the person and a greater degree of understanding about the behaviour previously displayed. QA mechanisms consequently need to be sensitive to the more subtle ways that people's lives can be improved through integrated approaches to care and treatment.

Much work is being done at a local and national level to improve access to mainstream services including the development of photographic journeys around hospital departments, designated clinic time for longer appointments, and having Link Nurses with an interest in learning disability in each ward or department.

Through its *A First Class Service* report (Department of Health 1998), the government has made a commitment to improve the quality of care through continued professional development and professional self-regulation. This philosophy has been endorsed by *Agenda for Change* (Department of Health 2004b), the proposed new pay structure that incorporates a knowledge and skills framework. If people like David are to be cared for properly, more must be done in terms of workforce training and development. The Learning Disability Awards Framework (Department of Health 2001a) is designed to provide a career pathway for care workers, giving greater validation to vocational training. However, there remain questions about how best to involve people with learning disabilities and families in the design and creative delivery of continuing professional development initiatives, so as to ensure a close match between staff competencies and what people require from services.

There are increasing examples of how people with learning disabilities are getting involved in developments aimed to improve quality of care including Patients Advice and Liaison Services (PALS), Service User Councils and service reviews undertaken by the Commission for Health Improvement (2003). More needs to be done to include people with limited communication skills and people with more profound disabilities in forums like these, and to evaluate the best ways of accomplishing this.

A note of caution needs to be sounded about public involvement in services. If there is to be meaningful patient and public involvement in developing services, as with clinical audit (Secker-Walker and Donaldson 2001), it is vital to consider whether they are exempt from the clinical governance framework and whether they are bound by advice and good practice. This also raises another interesting point because if the public is in practice accountable to the organization, by default an independent voice would be lost and absorbed in the 'politics of the service'.

Quality frameworks in social care

The Health and Social Care (Community Health and Standards) Act introduced in 2003 requires NHS providers and local authorities to work together to bring about improvements in health care (Department of Health 2004a). Likewise, *Valuing People* emphasizes partnership working to bring about positive change for people with learning disabilities, evidenced by the establishment of Partnership Boards involving a wide range of service providers, service users and carers.

In future there will be greater emphasis on standards across health and social care services. The government is trying to create a situation where standards rather than national targets are the driving force for continuous quality improvements (Department of Health 2004a). It will be interesting to see how the roles of the Commission for Social Care Inspection (CSCI) and the Health Care Commission (formerly the Commission for Health Improvement) evolve, but what is clearly evident is the UK government's intention to use these bodies to address national priorities, these being:

- the health and well-being of the population;
- long-term conditions;
- access to services;
- patient/user experience.

There is an emphasis on equity of service so as to ensure that resources are distributed fairly across differing groups. Practitioners meanwhile remain concerned about being gridlocked by standards in the same way they did with targets. The CSCI assesses services against national standards and, as in the case of David, his family should be reassured by the fact that when he moves into community-based accommodation there are quality measures in place that will ensure regular monitoring, unless of course he is placed in an unregistered unit. For example, one set of standards relates to the environment and the amount of personal space each individual has, furniture and fittings, bathing and toilet facilities, communal areas, aids and adaptations and infection control. Although the standards are designed to have measurable outcomes, care home inspections should be done in collaboration with service users and their families through direct observation of practice and by scrutinizing policies and procedures. Of course there remain ever-present dangers that such measures become little more than a tick box exercise about care processes rather than a means to ensure that the processes deliver high standards of support and care.

A further cause for concern is the application of fair access to care services criteria. There are four criteria within the framework and people are judged to have either critical, substantive, moderate or low needs. Local authorities are expected to prioritize individuals whose level of risk is deemed to be critical and although the framework is intended to widen the entry gate to care services, this is not in practice the case. Local authorities that feel they only have sufficient resources to meet the needs of people falling into high risk categories can set their criteria to critical and substantive bands only. Tanner (2003) argues that although the language of assessment is 'need' it is 'risk' that takes precedence when it comes to service provision. This has major implications for people with mild learning disabilities who often have difficulty accessing appropriate services. It also creates a tension between government philosophy and resource management because new ways of working always incur hidden costs.

The principle of integrating health and social care for the benefit of service users cannot be argued against if it reduces repetitive assessments and leads to resources being used more effectively. Many practitioners still retain concerns about service integration and what effect this will have on their professional identity and role, but what is important is how services fit together in ways that make sense to the people who need to use them. Evidence on inter-agency working and inter-professional working (Hudson *et al.* 1997) suggests that effective collaboration is the product of local networks based on cooperation, mutual respect and trust rather than imposed conditions.

What does this add up to?

In offering some descriptions of regulatory and QA mechanisms it is easy to overlook what is implied by quality standards criteria. Terms bandied about tend to include:

- *Access*: are services available to people with respect to information (are services known), location (are they conveniently placed), means of access (physical barriers like steps) and eligibility criteria (some services still exclude people because of the way their needs are defined)?

- *Acceptability*: do services reflect the cultural and moral norms of a plural multi-ethnic society? Do they meet the same standards expected by service users?

- *Reliability*: are services available at the right time? Do they fit personal and family schedules? Are services dependable?

- *Coordination*: are health and social care services sufficiently well integrated so as to meet the unique needs of individuals and families? Is there a single point of access to services? Are care management and person-centred planning coordinated by a named person?

- *Efficiency*: can service users be assured of best value? Is service duplication and waste avoided or minimized?

- *Effectiveness*: is support provided on the basis of best evidence, and in ways that maximize a person's QoL or other valued personal outcomes?
- *Rights and redress*: do services respect people's individual civil rights? Do people know what recourse they have to complain and seek redress should they wish to?

Exercise 7.3

Think of a local service well known to you, then ask yourself how well it would evaluate in terms of access, acceptability and so on.

If services were improved in regard to the above criteria, in what ways might the QoL of service users change?

Put together, these benchmarks of quality in services represent a challenging agenda. It has already been demonstrated that services often fail at the first hurdle (access), and it will be seen later (Chapter 25) that users' cultural norms are not always accommodated, meaning that the acceptability of services can be left wanting. Hospital waiting times are apparently coming down but delays and interruptions still perpetuate difficulties with service reliability. Coordination, as illustrated earlier, remains an everpresent challenge for all health and social care services, yet is vital in helping people to secure seamless support. Efficiency improvements in an organization as large and complex as the NHS can always be made. In learning disability services values and visions often precede good evidence about what works, so effectiveness too is an issue to be constantly checked. Then finally, even when systems of redress are in place, people may still regard some of their rights as strictly 'non-negotiable' – there is no point trying to satisfy a vegetarian with even a Harry Ramsden serving of fish and chips!

Even were all of these criteria to be met there remain prospects of discontinuities between service quality and QoL. The reason for this is that these criteria represent service outcomes reflecting service priorities *of the day*. Moreover, they are typically pursued singly rather than as a package. It takes a leap of faith to assume that QoL improvements will come about as a result of, say, improving service access or boosting service reliability. Promoting service improvements according to these criteria is one thing; ensuring that they connect to valued QoL outcomes in service users and families is another.

Conclusion: connecting service quality with QoL

As will now be evident there is an almost bewildering array of government policies emphasizing the quality agenda through a variety of QA mechanisms, regulatory and inspection systems. Readers may be forgiven for feeling a trifle confused about what this all represents. Those taking a cynical view like Watson (2002) would suggest that all this 'quality speak' merely reinforces the power and position of managers rather than fundamentally challenging existing power structures within services that so easily disable service users. It has been suggested that benchmarking and performance measurement are less straightforward than claimed, and that front-line workers obligated into taking part in these activities frequently find therapeutic work with service users being displaced or passed on to those with lesser qualifications. Further, it is sometimes claimed that the industry of quality measurement tends to focus on those aspects of services that are more tangible – these being rather more concerned with efficiency and economy rather than effectiveness. Qureshi (1999: 264), describing a project about collecting outcome information as a part of routine practice in social care, sums up the position well:

> If the collection of outcome information is to form part of routine practice it must fit with what is already done, or staff must be convinced of its ultimate benefits to them or to service users, otherwise the information will either not be collected, or it will be subject to 'gaming' as people try to fit with the letter of requirements instead of the spirit.

In their exploration of performance measurement in sheltered housing, Foord *et al.* (2004) made similar observations, suggesting that the 'expert' knowledge required by regulatory bodies remains privileged over service user knowledge. They found, like other observers, that the voice of users should be central to measuring satisfaction or outcomes, but that in practice the methods and systems in use failed to capture issues of importance to users. For Watson (2002: 885), the solution is seen to lie in reasserting the agenda of empowerment which 'should open up all the decision-making process to provider and user involvement, including those at a day-to-day level, which impact directly on individual lives and make up the fine texture of the organization'.

Quality, in this sense, is therefore inextricably tied up with the democratization of services at a national and local level – that is, with opening up services to scrutiny in order to ensure that they are not only moulded but driven by the interests and aspirations of service users. What then does this mean in terms of the relationship between the QoL of people with learning disabilities and their families and QA mechanisms in services?

Firstly, it means that voice really matters. Hearing and attending to what people with learning disabilities say is vital. This will not happen unless they are meaningfully involved in forums where decisions affecting their lives are made. At the local level this means securing their proper involvement in person-centred planning contexts (see Chapter 24), in consultative forums like PALS, in Partnership Boards where they can help shape the planning and strategic management of local services, and in self-advocacy groups (see Chapter 8) where they can articulate and lobby in relation to shared concerns with a view to challenging the status quo.

Secondly, enabling people to give voice to their interests and aspirations means that there is a chance that the agendas of local services will be guided by what service users say. It should be hard for services to deny the validity and force of people's everyday accounts of their struggles to express their identities and hopes. A listening service organization will in this sense be guided towards meeting those outcomes that individuals see as relevant to themselves. It is here that the QoL perspectives discussed earlier are likely be important.

Thirdly, it seems obvious that the development of a performance-oriented culture with all the trappings of regulatory, standard-setting and auditing systems will come to nothing if those standards and how they are measured are not transparent, meaningful and agreed with people with learning disabilities, their families and advocates.

Fourthly, experience suggests that the appetite and enthusiasm for this from people with learning disabilities (and their families and advocates) will wane rapidly if action to maintain and ratchet up quality in services is not seen to follow. Service users and families will not commit their time and energy to being associated with endless data collection exercises if findings are not acted on in their best interests. There therefore needs to be a principled and proactive culture committed to constant improvement in the delivery of quality services in which people with learning disabilities and families are both partners and beneficiaries.

References

Bach, M. and Rioux, M.H. (1996) Social well-being: a framework for quality of life research, in R. Renwick, I. Brown and M. Nagler (eds) *Quality of Life in Health Promotion and Rehabilitation*. Thousand Oaks, CA: Sage.

Brett, W. and Schofield, J. (2002) Integrated care pathways for patients with complex needs, *Nursing Standard*, 16(46): 36–41.

British Institute of Learning Disabilities (1999) *Physical Interventions: A Policy Framework*. Kidderminster: BILD Publications.

Brown, I. and Brown, R.I. (2003) *Quality of Life and Disability: An Approach for Community Practitioners*. London, Jessica Kingsley.

Chambers, N. and Jolly, A. (2002) Essence of care: making a difference, *Nursing Standard*, 17(11): 40–5.

Commission for Health Improvement (2003) *Learning Disability Services – Bedfordshire and Luton Community NHS Trust*. London: The Stationery Office.

Department of Health (1997) *The New NHS: Modern, Dependable*. London: The Stationery Office.

Department of Health (1998) *A First Class Service: Quality in the new NHS*. Leeds: DoH.

Department of Health (2001a) *Valuing People: A New Strategy for Learning Disability for the 21st Century*. London: The Stationery Office.

Department of Health (2001b) *The Essence of Care: Patient Focused Benchmarking for Health Care Practitioners*. London: The Stationery Office.

Department of Health (2004a) *National Standards, Local Action: Health and Social Care Standards and Planning Framework 2005/06–2007/08*. London: The Stationery Office.

Department of Health (2004b) *Agenda for Change: Proposed Agreement*. London: The Stationery Office.

Felce, D. and Perry, J. (1996) Exploring current conceptions of quality of life: a model for people with and without disabilities, in R. Renwick, I. Brown and M. Nagler (eds) *Quality of Life in Health Promotion and Rehabilitation*. Thousand Oaks, CA: Sage.

Foord, M., Savory, J. and Sodhi, D. (2004) Not everything that can be counted counts and not everything that counts can be counted – towards a critical exploration of modes of satisfaction measurement in sheltered housing, *Health and Social Care in the Community*, 12(2): 126–33.

Grant, G. (1997) Consulting to involve or consulting to empower? in P. Ramcharan, G. Roberts, G. Grant and J. Borland (eds) *Empowerment in Everyday Life: Learning Disability*. London: Jessica Kingsley.

Hatton, C. (1998) Whose quality of life is it anyway? Some problems with the emerging quality of life consensus, *Mental Retardation*, 36: 104–15.

Hensel, E. (2001) Is satisfaction a valid concept in the assessment of quality of life of people with intellectual disabilities? A review of the literature, *Journal of Applied Research in Intellectual Disabilities*, 14: 311–26.

Hensel, E., Rose, J., Stenfert Kroese, B. and Banks-Smith, J. (2002) Subjective judgements of quality of life: a comparison study between people with learning disability and those without disability, *Journal of Intellectual Disability Research*, 46(2): 95–107.

Hudson, B., Hardy, B., Henwood, M. and Wistow, G. (1997) Working across professional boundaries: primary health care and social care, *Public Money and Management*, 17(4): 25–30.

Lefort, S. and Fraser, M. (2002) Quality of life measurement and its use in the field of learning disabilities, *Journal of Learning Disabilities*, 6(3): 223–38.

Lovett, H. (1996) *Learning to Listen: Positive Approaches and People with Difficult Behaviour*. London: Jessica Kingsley.

Lukes, S. (1980) Socialism and equality, in J. Sterba (ed.) *Justice: Alternative Political Perspectives*. Belmont, CA: Wadsworth.

NPSA (National Patient Safety Agency) (2004) *Listening to People with Learning Difficulties and Family Carers Talk About Patient Safety*. London: NPSA.

Park, J., Hoffman, L., Marquis, J., Turnbull, A.P., Poston, D., Mannan, H., Wang, M. and Nelson, L.L. (2003) Toward assessing family outcomes of service delivery: validation of a family quality of life survey, *Journal of Intellectual Disability Research*, 47(4/5): 367–84.

Qureshi, H. (1999) Outcomes of social care for adults: attitudes towards collecting outcome information in practice, *Health and Social Care in the Community*, 7(4): 257–65.

Renwick, R. and Brown, I. (1996) The Centre for Health Promotion's conceptual approach to quality of life: being, belonging and becoming, in R. Renwick, I. Brown and M. Nagler (eds) *Quality of Life in Health Promotion and Rehabilitation*. Thousand Oaks, CA: Sage.

Roeher Institute (1993) *Social Well-Being: A Paradigm for Reform*. North York, Ontario: Roeher Institute.

Schalock, R. and Felce, D. (2004) Quality of life and subjective well-being: conceptual and measurement issues, in E. Emerson, C. Hatton, T. Thompson and T. Parmenter (eds) *The International Handbook of Applied Research in Intellectual Disabilities*. Chichester: Wiley.

Secker-Walker, J. and Donaldson, L. (2001) *Clinical Risk Management: Enhancing Patient Safety*. London, BMJ Books.

Symon, A.G. (2003) Reactions to perceived risk defensiveness in clinical practice, *Clinical Risk*, 9: 182–5.

Tanner, D. (2003) Older people and access to care, *British Journal of Social Work*, 33(4): 449–515.

Walshe, K. (2001) The development of clinical risk management, in C. Vincent (ed.) *Clinical Risk Management: Enhancing Patient Safety*. London: BMJ Books.

Watson, D. (2002) A critical perspective on quality within the personal social services: prospects and concerns, *British Journal of Social Work*, 32: 877–91.

8

Advocacy, campaigning and people with learning difficulties

Dan Goodley and Paul Ramcharan

Introduction

After a substantial history of silence people labelled as having learning difficulties have in the last 30 years made substantial moves to have their voices heard, to reclaim their lives and to take charge of their own destiny and identity. Public records of their work (see Ramcharan and Grant 2001) have, particularly since the 1990s, included life histories, autobiographies and other personal testaments (e.g. Barron 1989; Atkinson and Williams 1990; Lundgren 1993; Cooper 1997; Souza and Ramcharan 1997), a substantial amount of media from the user movement, particularly self-advocacy groups (e.g. People First 1993, 1997; LMPF 1996; Change 1997; WWG 1999) and research texts in which their voice features strongly (e.g. Whittaker *et al.* 1990; Minkes *et al.* 1995; Williams 1998; Gramlich *et al.* 2002). Alongside these public records, people with learning difficulties have begun to campaign for their rights, largely through the self-advocacy movement and have further made their voices heard in less public domains through more personalized forms of advocacy. Indeed, it might be asserted that the written and public record of their voice represents but a small part of their efforts both individually and collectively to assert their rights – that is, to advocate for themselves.

In this chapter we begin by outlining various types of advocacy and then ask questions about the place of professionals under the 'advocacy umbrella'. Having established some of the limitations for professional service workers within the advocacy movement we then recount the historical struggle that has characterized (and continues to characterize) the growing voice of people with learning difficulties over time. The specific place of self-advocacy in leading this struggle means that it is taken in the latter sections of the chapter as a particular focus alongside the growing arm of campaigning by people labelled with learning difficulties.

Forms of advocacy

Perhaps one of the first ideas that emerges when we are presented with the words 'advocacy' and 'campaigning' is the notion of making our own views and ambitions heard through a variety of individual and collective means. We are all aware when we are not being listened to. Think of those times at home, with partners, family and friends or at work with colleagues. It is, to say the least, a particularly frustrating experience and threatens to make us feel worthless and devalued by those around us who are unprepared to take on board what we have to say. For some individuals in society not being listened to is a common, daily experience, with serious implications and is based upon particularly pernicious assumptions about those individuals.

People with mental health problems, individuals with physical and sensory impairments, those labelled with 'learning difficulties' and older adults are among the social groups that have historically been marginalized. Their experiences and ambitions have been ignored or simply not acknowledged. Often there is a pervasive idea, a commonsensical notion, that individuals within such groups have little of importance to say. They are ignored because they are considered to be somehow 'lacking' the skills, abilities or self-awareness to say anything of worth. Furthermore, they are often viewed as being 'at risk' (to themselves and others). Here professionals are positioned in ways that permit them to talk on behalf of these labelled groups: to speak for those who cannot or are taken not to be able to do so either 'rationally' or 'responsibly'.

Exercise 8.1

Think about a time when you felt your voice was not being heard, for example in your family or at work. What did you do about the situation?

Now think of a person with a learning difficulty whose voice, views or feelings were being ignored. How could this person make his/her voice heard?

You may find similarities between the two situations in Exercise 8.1. For example, it is difficult to speak up in situations where there is a power difference between yourself and others. So, while it may be difficult to question your charge nurse or manager it might similarly be as difficult for people with learning difficulties to challenge service workers or parents. In certain circumstances a person may not have a legitimate voice. They may, for example, be an asylum-seeker who does not speak the dominant language or a person in a court of law who cannot speak for himself or herself because of the specialist language involved (see Chapter 5) or, indeed, a person who communicates in ways that others find difficult to understand (see Chapter 13).

We all need someone to speak on our behalf at some times in our life. But for people whose predominant experience is of having their voice appropriated by others this has been problematic. The central idea of advocacy is that the person speaks for themselves or that an advocate speaks for that person as if that person's voice were their own.

Advocacy models

What has been termed 'advocacy' has taken many forms. It has been associated with a formal and paid role (professionals, paid advocates or lawyers) and with an informal volunteer role (e.g. friends or other self-advocates). Advocacy has also been categorized as being 'instrumentally' orientated to the resolution of an issue/problem or 'affective' in terms of long-term friendship (see Butler *et al.* 1988). Wolfensberger (1977), arguably the originator of a 'systematic' advocacy approach for people with learning difficulties, argues that the various types of advocacy might be categorized by asking a number of questions (see Ramcharan 1995): 'For whom?' (individual, group, class); 'For what?' (e.g. services, service quality, rights, life and health); 'Towards or against whom?' (e.g. institutions, functionaries, other individuals); 'By whom?' (lawyer, lobby or pressure group, voluntary sector association, unpaid citizens); and 'How done?' (persuasion, education, confrontation, litigation, demonstration, whistle-blowing). Wolfensberger refers to the countless advocacy combinations possible when asking each of these questions as producing what he terms an 'advocacy salad'.

In describing advocacy as it relates to people with learning difficulties, Atkinson (1999: 5) relates that:

> Advocacy takes many forms but is essentially about speaking up – wherever possible for oneself (self-advocacy), but sometimes with others (group or collective advocacy) and, where necessary, through others. Speaking up through others can involve another 'insider' (a peer advocate), an 'ordinary' person or volunteer (a citizen advocate), or a person paid and trained as an advocate (a paid advocate).

Simons (1992) adds to this list 'professional advocacy' where a professional seeks to support a client, for example in a planning meeting, case conference or medication review, raising a complaint or using the Patient Advice and Liaison Service (PALS). It may be that in your professional role this is the form of advocacy you are most likely to adopt. As we will demonstrate shortly, however, there are some issues with this particular role of which you will need to be fully appraised.

There are, then, a multitude of potential advocacy forms and these are summarized along with their strengths and weaknesses in Table 8.1.

Advocacy and 'best interest'

One of the key themes in the early advocacy literature was the importance of 'advocate independence'. In the column marked 'weaknesses' in Table 8.1

Table 8.1   Types of advocacy and their strengths and weaknesses

Type of advocacy	Strengths	Weaknesses
Citizen advocacy (*see* e.g. Wolfensberger 1983; Butler *et al.* 1988; Simons 1993; Williams 1998; Brooke 2002)	Unpaid volunteers offer wide-ranging one-to-one support, both instrumental and affective If the advocate partner relationship lasts it can be a highly significant one Independence from services gives them a strong voice	Maintains a distinction between 'advocate' and 'client' Difficult to recruit volunteers who have the time and motivation to commit to a long-term relationship There can be a skills gap in terms of the instrumental side of advocacy There remains a patchwork of projects because it is not cheap to run citizen advocacy programmes Advocates impart idealistic and overly-ambitious views
Peer advocacy (*see* e.g. Brandon 1994, 1995)	Advocates share experiences with similar others, not least of service experiences Advocacy is independent of the service sector Friendships can blossom and similar groups be brought together	Advocates' experiences may not be in line with those they are working for Advocates might impart idealistic and overly-ambitious views
Parent/carer advocacy (*see* e.g. FEU 1989)	Care and love define the relationship over a lifetime Advocacy located in dynamics of family Advocacy skills translated into family	Parents/carer needs may dominate at the expense of individual choices Potential for over-protection and conflict of interest over key issues Emotional involvement *may* negatively affect both relationships with professionals and decisions being taken

Table 8.1   *(continued)*

Type of advocacy	Strengths	Weaknesses
Professional advocacy (*see* e.g. Crawley 1990; Simons 1992; Atkinson's 1999 argument in relation to advocacy as social work)	Close one-to-one relationships can blossom Sophisticated and trained approach to advocacy	Professionals tied to demands of services rather than the ambitions of the individuals they are supporting Reaffirms professional expertise Professionals move on and leave a vacuum in people's lives
Individual and collective self-advocacy (*see* e.g. Dybwad and Bersani 1996; Shoultz 1997; Ward 1998; Goodley 2000)	Promotes positive self-identity and capacity for advocating for oneself Challenges professional expertise and contributes to development of the self-advocacy social movement	Issues raised about individuals unable to advocate for themselves May require substantial support from others and is not cheap Suffers from lack of professional and service resources

this issue of 'independence' appears against a number of forms of advocacy. In the early years of the development of advocacy in the UK, National Citizen Advocacy (now Citizen Advocacy Information and Training, CAIT) argued that citizen advocates should neither be service personnel nor be funded by services (Butler *et al.* 1988). Rather, the citizen advocate should be an ordinary citizen willing to partner a person 'for life', offering both instrumental help to change their lives and expressive help (i.e. friendship). Others have argued similarly strongly for the need for independence within self-advocacy (Dowson 1991) though many self-advocacy groups are both funded by statutory authorities and facilitated by service workers. There are some fundamental issues here to be considered in terms of an argument concerning 'conflicts of interest'.

Many advocates and advocacy organizations fight for more services, better quality services or can make complaints against or be critical of services. If the funding for advocacy comes from the statutory sector it is easy to see how such funding might be easily curtailed were the advocacy organization to become too critical (i.e. to bite the hand that feeds it). There is some sense in which such an advocacy organization therefore has a potential conflict of interest between the person or persons it is advocating for and its funding source.

Simons (1993) has outlined a number of further such conflicts of interest with the service sector: conflicting demands between users make it difficult to favour one; managing limited resources often means allocating a less than favourable budget for each user; socialization as a professional means there is a need to rely on clinical judgements or professional cultures at the expense of what the user wants; having to work to a professional hierarchy or the fact that professionals are apt to settle for the 'quiet life'.

The idea of a 'quiet life' is not one in which the person simply settles for such an approach but may involve 'external factors'. As Wolfensberger (1977) has pointed out, there is often a personal cost involved in advocacy. At its most extreme this may even mean losing a job and career. For example, in a now famous case, Nurse Pink, after several warnings to management complained publicly about the standards of care in a long-stay elderly ward on which he worked. In the furore that followed Nurse Pink lost his job and, indeed, his career. Chapter 16 of this volume begs questions about just how much abuse might be covered up under such circumstances and Chapter 19 describes the huge difficulties people with learning difficulties are faced with in getting their voices heard in the criminal justice system. It is, then, much easier to settle for an easy life, not to make waves, not to be seen as a 'troublemaker' – in short, to be on the side of your employer and profession where there is any disagreement with the 'user' voice.

Table 8.1 also points out potential conflicts in respect of family carers advocating for their relative where it is often difficult to disentangle the family's interest and values from those of the person with a learning difficulty (Mitchell 1997). For example, it may be that parents feel their son or daughter will never be able to live in supported accommodation or have relationships. They may be against new part-time employment for their relative to replace a full-time day service on the grounds that it affects their working week. The intricacies of family life will often cloud judgement and make decision-making that incorporates the person's voice very difficult and less than independent.

Exercise 8.2

Callista has been taking medication for epileptic seizures for a number of years but feels the tablets are making her feel both sick and very tired. Callista wants to reduce the medication since she has recently started seeing her boyfriend Joe with whom she would like to spend more time. This means she would like to feel more lively and get out more. Callista feels the medication is stopping this from happening. Her parents though, have voiced strong reservations about Callista having a boyfriend. In your role as nurse you have been told that the medical opinion is that the drugs are necessary.

What could you do to advocate for Callista? What would stop you from advocating on her behalf?

Speaking in relation to nurses, Allmark and Klarzynski (1992) go so far as to suggest that nurses cannot act as an advocate because of the number of potential conflicts of interest. Nor do the United Kingdom Central Council for Nursing (UKCC) (1996) guidelines on advocacy help in clarifying a position: 'As a registered nurse, midwife or health visitor you are personally accountable for your practice and in the exercise of your professional accountability, must . . . act always in such a manner as to promote and safeguard the interests and well-being of patients and clients' (p. 13). There is a presumption here that 'best interests' as professionally defined are the same as the 'client's wishes', and this simply compounds what is already a difficult problem. In the earlier categorization of advocacy by Wolfensberger there does seem to be a recognition that professionals can be in the position of advocate (i.e. speaking on behalf of a person as if that person's voice were their own). What seems to be vital though is that each nurse or professional recognizes where conflicts of interest arise and hence where the limits to their advocacy role lies. At this point the 'competent' advocate is likely to be able to divest themselves of the advocacy role and find another able to do so with continued independence.

Professionals are likely to experience conflicts of interest as a service provider, professionally and in terms of the demands of other formal and family carers. Knowing how to ensure that independence of voice is maintained is one of the key tasks you may have as a professional working with people with learning difficulties. However, in terms of the professional advocacy role it may be that the breadth of your role will be very limited in providing a direct advocacy input. We will revisit other roles for the professional later in this chapter, having looked a little more at the historical and future development of the voice of people labelled as having a learning difficulty. By doing this it is possible to place the professional role within a context set by people labelled with a learning difficulty themselves.

Advocacy developments and people with learning difficulties

Above we have categorized different forms of advocacy. However, over the last 30 years groups of people with learning difficulties have organized themselves, individually and collectively, with the help of allies (including professionals and volunteers), to challenge such limiting assumptions through self-advocacy and campaigning. This moves beyond previous categorizations of advocacy as providing 'instrumental' or 'affective' inputs. Note the notions of 'input' and 'providing' imply that somehow the person is not themselves in control of the situation. We argue that 'advocacy as campaigning' is therefore gaining ascendancy as the chosen means through which people with learning difficulties can use their power and voice.

Lest we think this is 'pie in the sky' it is worth noting that success in the growth of self-advocacy in particular has also been reflected in government policy in Britain. During the All Wales Strategy it has been shown that participation of people with learning difficulties in local and county planning groups during the 1980s was closely linked to the development of self-advocacy groups (Whittell and Ramcharan 1998). Similarly, such representation is seen as a vital part of the work of Partnership Boards under present policy in England.

Indeed, alongside the White Paper, *Valuing People* (Department of Health 2001a) a document termed *Nothing About Us Without Us* (Department of Health 2001b) was produced by self-advocates after consultation with members of the self-advocacy movement. *Valuing People* committed £3m per annum over three years to the development of both self and citizen advocacy. Moreover, seven Regional Forums of self-advocates have been set up and representatives from each sit on the task force at the Department of Health which reports on the implementation of *Valuing People* and plans for its further development.

The voice of people with learning difficulties is being heard at all levels of practice and policy in health and social care services as well as in relation to their lives 'in the community'. There is a close relationship between these emergent voices and the growth of both self-advocacy groups and of campaigning by people with learning difficulties. In understanding the further development of voice it is therefore to the history and future development of self-advocacy and campaigning by people with learning difficulties that we now turn.

The rise of self-advocacy

It is fitting to start this section by pointing out that in this chapter we have adopted the term 'learning difficulties' (rather than 'mental handicap', 'mental impairment' or 'learning disabilities'), because it is the term preferred by many in the British self-advocacy movement. As one member of the movement puts it, 'If you put "people with learning difficulties" then they know that people want to learn and to be taught how to do things' (quoted in Sutcliffe and Simons 1993: 23). As one of the best known aphorisms of the People First self-advocacy movement puts it, 'Label jars, not people'.

The implication made by people with learning difficulties is one that has a resonance with theorizing by disabled people that has been developing over the past decade or so. These approaches take issue with administrative definitions of 'learning difficulties' that appear to locate disability within the impaired individual: a learning disability is an impairment of intellectual functions, which occurs before adulthood and results in significant disabilities in day-to-day life (The West Midlands Regional Health Authority's definition 1993 cited in Ford 1996: 57). Similarly, the 1995 Disability Discrimination Act defines disability as: 'Either a physical or mental impairment, which has a substantial and long-term adverse affect on a person's ability to carry out normal day-to-day activities' (HMSO 1995: Section 1.1). These administrative definitions are crucial in locating a group of individuals who are particularly at risk in a disabling society. However, they are incredibly problematic, not least in viewing disability as causally related to some form of individualized impairment. These definitions say something very simple – that impairment, whether it be physical or 'of mind' results in and creates disability. Hence impairment and disability are synonymous, inseparable concepts (Goodley 1997).

Following this, 'impaired thought' leads *to* a myriad of disabilities – disabled thinking, disabled educational potential, disabled relationships with others, disabled sex lives and disabled parenting. Noteworthy too is that professional and service interventions are geared towards providing inputs that are based on these assumptions. The emerging image of the person with learning difficulties then, is not one of autonomy but of a loss of wholeness and a personal tragedy that renders the individual the focus of a specialist professional intervention. Barnes (1990) argues that this results in disabled people being assigned a position in a culture of dependence. Their social 'ineptitude', reified by the dominant discourse, renders them as burdens to their families and to society at large. They are conceptualized as any other minority group and treated and reacted to as a category rather than as people. They represent a challenge, a problem at the level of everyday interaction.

In contrast, campaigns by people with learning difficulties have emphasized their views of themselves as 'people first'. This posits a key tenet of new social movements to re-present another vision of humanity that may have been ignored by dominant discourses of the health and social welfare professions. Hence, self-advocacy, as we shall see, taps into a more critical view of disability and impairment (see also Goodley 1997) as exemplified through the following argument: 'Mental retardation is, in fact, a socio-political not a psychological construction. The myth, perpetuated by a society which refuses to recognise the true nature of its needed social reforms, has successfully camouflaged the politics of diagnosis and incarceration' (Bogdan and Taylor 1982: 15).

Self-advocacy has the potential to publicly revisit and challenge the very political processes that position people with the label of learning difficulties as a different, 'othered' social group. In this sense then, advocacy and campaigning are crucially involved in challenging the very processes of diagnosis, incarceration and treatment, on a variety of private and public, individual and group, short- and long-term levels.

Exercise 8.3

Explain to a good friend or colleague why the term 'people with learning difficulties' has been adopted. Can you do this without mentioning a previous collective description? What response did you get?

The beginnings of the self-advocacy movement

'Empowerment is a process. Power is not given to people nor is it earned. It happens as a result of a constructive, meaningful activity that leads people to be more knowledgeable, skilful, informed and aware than they were before' (Worrell 1988: 7).

Following Goodley (2000), the self-advocacy movement is a living testament to the group activity of people with learning difficulties in challenging institutionalized prejudice within society (Williams and Shoultz 1982). As Potts and Fido (1991) put it, people with learning difficulties have consistently had their histories written for them by others – 'from careworker and psychologist to historian and social scientist'. The origins of the self-advocacy movement can be traced back to the late 1960s and have, not surprisingly, moved from a professional/practice based approach initially to one that is now led by people with learning difficulties themselves. Following the historical overview provided in Goodley (2000), a small group of people with learning difficulties in Sweden developed a list of requests about how their services should be provided. They gave this list to the parent organization that supported them. Whether or not the requests were acted on remains unknown, but something unprecedented and previously undocumented had occurred. Perske (1996: 20–1) describes another similar episode:

> STOCKHOLM, SWEDEN, November 8, 1969. Ten persons with mental retardation and six university students – all good friends – came together for a special adventure . . . [They met in a club and intended to go to the theatre] . . . The sixteen went to a coffee shop and discussed all that they had experienced. Everyone decided that they wanted to see the play at a later date. So, they began making a checklist of preparations. As they left, the group decided not to return to the club. They agreed to break up at this new and strange location and each find his or her own way home.

Perske (1996) suggests that Bengt Nirje, a prominent writer of normalization principles, used the scenario presented above in formulating ideas about 'risk-taking' for people with learning difficulties. Normalization marked a radical departure in terms of professional ideology and policy values in relation to learning difficulties. Bengt Nirje, Wolf Wolfensberger and John O'Brien called for the empowerment of people so labelled to lead as 'normal' a life as possible in relation to housing, community membership, education, work and leisure.

Exercise 8.4

The early 1970s saw a number of attempts to make available to people with learning difficulties patterns of life and conditions of everyday living that were as close as possible to the regular circumstances of life in society. Can you think of ways of making available such patterns of life for people with learning difficulties through your professional work?

Normalization was championed as a method for assessing service systems that were in tune with the needs of disabled people (via the PASS Programs, see Wolfensberger and Glenn 1975) by comparing services to a 'culturally valued analogue' (i.e. to the life one would expect for any person within mainstream society). Later, O'Brien's 'five major service accomplishments' aimed to provide a starting point for putting normalization into practice (O'Brien 1987). O'Brien's philosophy was that if services were to 'empower' they must have ensured that their users were:

- present in the community;
- supported to make choices;
- participants in community environments;
- that they enjoyed respect;
- participation within the community.

As Wolfensberger (1972: 238) asserted: 'We should assist a person to become capable of meaningful choosing for himself among those normative options that are considered moral and those that are not. If a person is capable of meaningful choice, he must also risk the consequences'.

Advocacy in this sense was therefore associated with 'professional-practice' models of normalization. The move to 'ordinary' or 'socially valued' lifestyles was at once liberating for those whose lives had previously been wholly subsumed under the professional aegis. In this light, professional and citizen advocacy played a key role through the 1970s. However, a further development, in moving beyond the professional-practice model to one in which people with learning difficulties themselves reclaimed their own voice, was also beginning to take shape.

Self-advocacy and civil rights

'Once upon a time I wouldn't speak out at all. I used to be told to shut up. Now that I've been around a self-advocacy group I have learned to say what I want to say' (the views of a member of People First Liverpool quoted in Goodley 2000: 6).

We would argue that, though associated more with civil rights and new social movements than with service consumerism, self-advocacy's beginnings can be traced back to the first and second Swedish National Conferences of Retarded Adults in 1968 and 1970. The staging of these conferences reflected a social climate, inside and outside of services, wherein the views of people with learning difficulties were starting to be formally recognized. Around the same time, two conferences in America contributed substantially to public visibility of adults with learning difficulties (Dybwad 1996). The first, the 35th Spring Conference at a school in Massachusetts, entitled Outlook for the Adult Retarded, debated the social impact of the increasing life spans of people with learning difficulties. The other, the Golden Anniversary White House Convention on Children and Youth, saw one of the first questions to be publicly raised over the legal status of adults and children with learning difficulties.

These were among the earliest documented conferences at which the experiences of people with learning difficulties was the primary interest. In 1969 at the third National Youth Conference on Mental Retardation in Miami, a panel of young adults with learning difficulties discussed their personal reactions to work programmes. This kind of overt participation represented a radical departure from advocacy to something which appears to have seriously embraced the experiences of people with learning difficulties as a public account by those so-labelled.

These events in Sweden and America inspired what became known as participation events in the UK. The first one, 'Our Life' (in June 1972), organized by the Campaign for Mentally Handicapped People (CMH), brought together a number of residents from long-stay hospitals to talk about where they would like to live in the future. When written up (Shearer 1972) it was the first publication in the UK to be wholly made up of the comments by 'mentally handicapped' people about the services they received. The following year another conference took place called 'Listen' (see Shearer 1973). This considered relationships, choices and independence, with another workshop on participation occurring soon afterwards (see Williams 1973). The next two in 1974 and 1975 had delegates discussing experiences of employment.

Hersov (1996) states that these events had an immeasurable impact upon the UK self-advocacy movement. 'Listen', for example, cites delegates articulating views on aspects of life including relationships (with each other, family and staff), and choice and independence. For Shearer (1973), the CMH meetings sensitized those professionals and researchers who were present to the sharp perceptions held by delegates with learning difficulties. The delegates demonstrated their entirely realistic desire to share experiences and to challenge society's preoccupation with impairment. Delegates expressed scepticism about staff reactions in hospitals ('The staff won't do anything like that . . . every time you do it [speak out] they don't like it'), and in hostels ('I wouldn't bet on it . . . very few speak . . . people don't want to listen'). Furthermore, many delegates felt that the one-off nature of the CMH conferences was inadequate: 'we should have a meeting once a month'. On writing up the 'Listen' conference report, Shearer's (1973: 34) concerns and ambitions typify many feelings prominent in the early days:

> 'Listen' and 'Our Life' have shown the potential for development and have indicated the waste if this potential is neglected. It is now up to others to ensure that the future is one of development and not neglect. It is up to everyone . . . to do them justice and show that something lasting was achieved at the conference.

Fortunately, CMH's American links culminated in Paul Williams and Bonnie Shoultz co-writing *We Can Speak for Ourselves* (1982), reviewing international developments. This highlighted the variety of groups that were taking off in the UK and the USA, fitting the United Nations *Declaration of the Rights of Human Persons* (1975, cited in Campbell and Oliver 1996: 19), which asserted that 'organisations of disabled persons may be usefully consulted in all matters regarding the rights of disabled persons' (Section 3447.12).

Self-advocacy and people first

'Until I started going to a self-advocacy group, which set me free, I couldn't put my views across, tell people what I thought of them, tell the DHSS, tell anyone. I couldn't tell the staff where they were going wrong' (Patrick Burke, self-advocate, quoted in Goodley 2000: xii).

Self-advocacy groups continued to grow in dance companies, sport and recreational clubs, through to adult training centres and hospitals. According to Hersov (1996), in the UK, two of these, the MENCAP London Division's Participation Forum and City Lit, grew in stature in the early 1980s (reflecting strong financial support gained through charity funds). In 1984, they sent representatives to the First International Self-advocacy Leadership Conference in Tacoma, North America. By this time the movement had grown markedly in the USA, with the People First organization holding its first convention for North American members as early as 1974 (Dybwad 1996). By 1975 there were 16 People First chapters formed in 12 cities (Crawley 1982). According to O'Brien and Sang (1984) the links between English and American self-advocates continued to be productive. Things were starting to take off.

At the First International People First Conference in 1984, a number of English delegates were inspired to set up People First of London and Thames. This self-advocacy group was independent of a service base, with members attending voluntarily, and by 1997 had a number of paid independent supporters. It has continued to be one of the most influential collectives within the movement. In 1988 the Second International People First Conference was held in Twickenham, entitled 'A Voice of Our Own – Now and in the Future', followed in 1993 by the Third International Conference which took place in Toronto, Canada, with many UK People First groups attending. The fourth was held in Alaska in 1998.

While the UK movement has grown in strength internationally, it has also made some links with the larger disability movement in the UK. Hersov (1996) records how the well-known self-advocate Gary Bourlet represented London People First on the 1992 national council of the British Council of Organizations of Disabled People as it was then known (now the British Council of Disabled People, BCODP). More recently, Simone Aspis, previously campaigns officer at People First London, has maintained links with the BCODP, and was the self-advocacy movement's only representative in Campbell and Oliver's (1996) account of the British disability movement. Moreover, self-advocates have become involved in formal studies of services (see e.g. Whittaker *et al.* 1990: Gramlich *et al.* 2002), published widely, produced video materials and other learning packages (see Ramcharan and Grant 2001), appeared on TV, in the broadsheets and taken part in civil rights demonstrations: 'In the last decade, there have been important landmarks in the growth of self-advocacy throughout the country . . . There is every reason to believe that the [movement] . . . will continue to gain new members and widespread support, and that it will reach even greater heights in the future' (Hersov 1996: 139).

In introducing this chapter we highlighted the ways in which the public voice of people with learning difficulties had been heard. As this history shows, this movement has, over time, fought hard to unshackle itself from ownership by professionals and service workers and to gain independence.

The history leads us to recast our thoughts about the place of self-advocacy within the professional and support services and, indeed, the role of professionals in that movement. A central principle that arises from this is that while self-advocates require support, that support should not affect the 'freedom of expression' of the self-advocates. Below this principle is formalized in terms of the professional role within self-advocacy.

Self-advocacy and services

'I think there's a problem with advisors who are staff because you see them every day . . . She was always watching you' (Joyce Kershaw, self-advocate, quoted in Goodley 2000: 127).

For some the People First movement is the self-advocacy movement. However, the foundations of the British movement are not found solely in People First (nor the London groups focused on by commentators like Hersov). The movement's origins can be traced back not only to 'independent' (People First) groups but also to the growth over the last three decades of trainee committees in adult training centres, social education centres, hospitals, long-stay institutions and group homes. Crawley (1982, 1988) has documented the rush of self-advocacy issues into centre curricula while Whittell and Ramcharan (1998) have reported on the growth of self-advocacy in Wales during the 1980s and early 1990s. Similarly, Paul Williams' paper on participation and self-advocacy reflects some small-scale translation of self-advocacy issues into service decision-making (participation). He argued that:

> Handicapped people have a lifetime of experience of being controlled and dominated by others. They are denied experiences of equality with others and control over their own affairs . . . Participation seeks to provide handicapped people and others with experiences of equality and sharing. Self-advocacy enables handicapped people to take their own decisions and exercise control over their own affairs.
>
> (Williams 1982: 3)

In terms of recognizing diversity, it is clear that the doing of self-advocacy in service bases fits the user participation and community care discourses in government policy that have proliferated since the mid-1980s in Britain. As learning difficulties services experience a transition from public sector organizations to private sector management, and a shift from residential to community bases, self-advocacy appeals to those promoting service innovation in a market economy. Service personnel may therefore have a role in supporting the development of a 'consumer voice'. How then might this be accomplished?

Setting up a self-advocacy group

For those of you interested in being involved with the continued growth of the movement it will be necessary for you to know how best to provide the support necessary to help people with learning difficulties start such a group. Box 8.1 provides advice. Point 4 about the role of the adviser raises some issues in relation to supporting the self-advocacy of people with learning difficulties. Indeed, one could view this relationship as rather paradoxical: that people with learning difficulties need to be supported in their own self-advocacy. In this sense support and advocacy appear to be very different things: the role of the supporter is not to advocate but to support others to advocate for themselves.

Box 8.1   Setting up a successful self-advocacy group

1   *Get people interested* – tell clients, centre users, hostel flatmates and work colleagues what they will get out of being in the group, either by word of mouth, leaflets or posters.

2   *Find a meeting place* – get those involved to choose someone's house or a community centre, while an adult training centre could be used if nowhere else is available.

3   *Organize transport* – so that members can get to meetings. This is made easier if a self-advocate takes on the role of 'transport officer'.

4   *Find an adviser* – this is a person (usually without learning difficulties) who helps the group, 'Someone who gives support especially in the early days', but who, '*Shouldn't* run your group but help *you* to run it'. *Speak for Ourselves* suggest getting in touch with the National Council for Voluntary Organisations (www.ncvo-vol.org.uk). It is as they say, 'Better to find someone who doesn't work at the day centre'. Later, 'You will have to decide if your adviser is to be paid or a volunteer'.

5   *Elect a committee* – officers should include chairperson, secretary, treasurer and transport officer. Officers may be chosen on a nomination and election basis or members may take turns in the various positions.

6   *Raise money* – through sources such as charitable trusts, health authorities and local councils. Alternatively, payment may be accrued if self-advocates help train people who work with people with learning difficulties.

7   *Make the group aware of what it can do* – members of *Speak for Ourselves* give their own experiences: 'Talking about improving services, write letters to the council, plan conferences, invite guests, right to get engaged, have a boyfriend and get married, have parties and discos'.

Source: Start! How to Set Up and Run a Successful Self-advocacy Group, a video made by *Speak for Ourselves* of Newcastle (1993)

Exercise 8.5

What constitutes 'good support' in relation to facilitating self-advocacy groups?

Are the people with learning difficulties with whom you work involved in a self-advocacy group? If so, what sort of group is it? What sort of things are they advocating for?

If they are not involved in such a group consider whether they should be, and what role you might play in supporting them.

Dowson and Whittaker (1993) conceptualize 'good support' by introducing the notion of intervention. They argue that at particular times different types of intervention are required on the part of the supporter, including ones that are:

- *prescriptive* (i.e. aim to give advice, recommend a behaviour or course of action);
- *informative* (i.e. aim to give knowledge or information);
- *confronting* (i.e. challenge attitudes, beliefs or behaviours);
- *cathartic* (i.e. provoke a release of tension);
- *catalytic* (i.e. elicit information or opinion from the group);
- *supportive* (i.e. affirm the value or worth of the group).

Any intervention that (re)creates dependency is an intervention that is at odds with the aims of self-advocacy and campaigning (Goodley 1997). As a service worker the role of supporting self-advocacy may be contentious, not only in terms of the support role. Professionals often have substantial and time-consuming responsibilities with employers not seeing such support as a priority. There are many support workers who have therefore chosen to operate in a voluntary capacity and in 'their own time'. There are also, as indicated earlier, still issues that arise in relation to potential conflicts of interest between the professional role and the commitment to supporting the voices of self-advocates. Indeed, for some self-advocates, there is a growing call for complete independence of voice through campaigning and it is to this we now turn.

Self-advocacy, politicization and campaigning: the new politics of the twenty-first century

Over the last 30 years, a rise in the amount of advocacy and campaigning by a variety of labelled groups has demonstrated the potential of such interventions in challenging societal ignorance and a lack of representation. A popular point of analysis in contemporary sociology and social policy at the start of this century is the argument that the old grand narrative political identities of class, 'race' and gender have given way to more diverse and varied political identities and aspirations.

The move towards diversity in the latter part of the twentieth century was characterized by a struggle for access to the production of knowledge. Here individuals and groups, with particular political interests, were increasingly engaged actively with the 'knowledge society's' production of information about them and others. Knowledge is power and who owns or utilizes knowledge has important consequences. A variety of political concerns have increasingly been represented through the emergence of a diverse collective of campaigning groups.

Exercise 8.6

Identify two political campaigns that have taken place over recent years.

Have you been involved in advocacy and campaigning in relation to an issue about which you feel strongly? Why did you get involved?

How might you support people with learning difficulties to become involved in something they believe in?

A number of examples can be cited. Think of those many organizations – from Trotskyists, to anarchists, to charities set up to support developing countries – that were brought together in the demonstrations against global capitalism and the World Bank in Seattle, Prague and London in 1999 and 2000. Consider political and ideological boundaries that have shifted to such an extent that the two main political parties in Britain – New Labour and Conservative – are engaged not in old debates about privatization and nationalization but about how much or little should be saved in terms of public expenditure and taxation. Finally, consider the role of globalization in identity politics, where disabled people around the globe organize themselves under the banner organization of Disabled People's International. All of these collectives can be seen as contributing to the emergence of new social movements. Such movements encompass a whole host of groups impacting upon various private, public, statutory and voluntary institutions and contexts.

What are new social movements?

Following the commentaries of Bersani (1996: 265–6) and Shakespeare (1993) on the self-advocacy movement and disability rights movement respectively, a new social movement might be characterized by a number of key ideas. These include the following:

- *Members go beyond typical roles* – here people transcend typical positions that have been assigned to them (in this case by health and social welfare professionals). So, for example, people labelled with a learning difficulty have chosen on the basis of sharing an interest to collaborate with the British Council of Organizations of Disabled People.

- *Representation of a strong ideological change* – new social movements readdress traditional ideologies that have shaped the life worlds of members. The control of the production of information by people with learning difficulties for people with learning difficulties represents a major attempt to represent their interests independently of those voices that have traditionally spoken on their behalf.

- *Emergence of a new identity* – members of a new social movement often start by refining the labels that they have assigned to them. Thus the People First movement, as its name implies, insists that each person labelled with a learning difficulty is seen as a person first and not a member of a labelled group. Another group, MK Sun, has adopted the term 'survivors of mental health services' instead of the more negative 'mentally ill person'. Here there is emphasis on an active label as opposed to a passive, pathological one.

- *Relationship between the individual and movement is blurred* – one of the key points of a new social movement is its emphasis on collective as well as individual action. People with learning difficulties have chosen the name they prefer for themselves as a collective and, through the People First movement, they have been represented in pushing for disabled people's rights.

It is possible to view the disability movement as a new social movement in four ways. Firstly, disabled people have become recognized as 'disabled activists' lobbying governments for adequate anti-discriminatory legislation, pushing for independent living. Secondly, the disabled people's movement has recast 'disability' as a social and political issue – the exclusion of people with impairments – rather than simply viewing it as the product of an individual impairment. Thirdly, disabled people have embraced this new politicization of disability and have provided alternative views of disability and impairment through, for example, disability arts where theatre companies such as 'The Lawnmowers' present people with the label of learning difficulties as skilled, competent performers rather than 'tragic' victims of 'mental impairment'. Finally, the concerns of disabled individuals and the wider disability movement overlap, for example in demands for supported living in the community and for extending access to direct payments.

Recognizing the emergence of new social movements, consisting of various groups with shared political agendas, presents a rather homogeneous and, perhaps, simplistic picture of organized campaigning and advocacy. It also, however, suggests that 'advocacy' and 'campaigning' have substantial similarities. Jackie Downer, an advocate with the label of learning difficulties who works for others who are similarly labelled, argues that diversity is crucial to any social movement. She recognizes such diversity both in terms of the multiple interests represented among people with learning difficulties (Downer and Walmsley 1997) as well as the role of the interests of people with learning difficulties in the wider disability movement (Goodley 2000). In making these points Downer is, along with other people, implicitly moving beyond the identities ascribed to them by others. They are moving towards a position as People First.

Conclusion

From what has been argued above it is fair to say that advocacy and campaigning are overlapping interventions. Both require some form of speaking for oneself and/or others in ways that put certain ambitions and aims in a public arena. Both appear to be associated with individuals and groups challenging authorities and institutions to take on board concerns marginalized by other individuals or wider society. Furthermore, both are terms and actions bound up with the notion of power. Advocacy and campaigning can both engage with powerful institutions and individuals and attempt to challenge or disrupt the distribution of power. We have also shown that advocacy itself has evolved and that in its original incarnation it was still, perhaps unavoidably, a professional and service orientated approach. Establishing power has therefore involved a struggle over time towards reclaiming voice, power and identity.

In this chapter we have argued that the development of advocacy has moved from being led by professionals to being supported by professionals, and further to being forged under the rubric of 'people first'. We might also argue, using a consumerist framework, that the development has been from a position in which people with learning difficulties were *given* a say, to one in which they were involved and in which they participated in services, to a contemporary position in which they have claimed their own voice and campaigned for their own interests. In terms of voice we might also assert that the movement started with the voice of people with learning difficulties being heard for the first time through professional support, then became a voice in itself, and then developed into a voice that is also now being heard in unison with others with whom an interest is shared. In other words, advocacy and campaigning seem to have a natural history which, over time, relocates power to, with and for people themselves.

Such a progression is not one that is pursued by all people with learning difficulties today. There remain some questions about whose voice is being heard, at the expense of whom and representing which interests. However, if the key elements of this progression are towards 'empowerment', if they are about reclaiming equal rights to each person within society, then they are fundamental to each of us in demonstrating 'civility' in all our interactions and in wider terms accomplishing a 'civil society' and a civilization of 'people first'.

Acknowledgements

The following sections of this chapter draw on the Open University Press text *Self-Advocacy in the Lives of People with Learning Difficulties* (Goodley 2000: Ch. 2): the rise of self-advocacy; the beginnings of the movement; self-advocacy and civil rights; services and People First; and setting up. We would like to thank Open University Press for granting us permission to draw upon this text in the writing of this chapter.

References

Allmark, P. and Klarzynsky, R. (1992) The case against nurse advocacy, *British Journal of Nursing*, 1(2): 33–6.

Atkinson, D. (1999) *Advocacy: A Review*. Brighton: Pavilion Publishing.

Atkinson, D. and Williams, F. (eds) (1990) *Know Me As I Am: An Anthology of Prose, Poetry and Art by People with Learning Difficulties*. London: Hodder & Stoughton.

Barnes, C. (1990) *The Cabbage Syndrome: The Social Construction of Dependence*. London: Falmer Press.

Barron, D. (1989) Locked away: life in an institution, in A. Brechin and J. Walmsley (eds) *Making Connections: Reflecting on the Lives and Experiences of People with Learning Difficulties*. London: Hodder & Stoughton.

Bersani, H. (1996) Leadership in developmental disabilities: where we've been, where we are, and where we're going, in G. Dybwad and H. Bersani (eds) *New Voices: Self-advocacy by People with Disabilities*. Cambridge, MA: Brookline Books.

Bogdan, R. and Taylor, S. (1982) *Inside Out: The Social Meaning of Mental Retardation*. Toronto: University of Toronto Press.

Brandon, D. (1994) Peer advocacy: care in place, *The International Journal of Networks and Community*, 1(3): 218–24.

Brandon, D. (1995) Peer support and advocacy – international comparisons and developments, in R. Jack (ed.) *Empowerment in Community Care*. London: Chapman & Hall.

Brooke, J. (2002) *Good Practice in Citizen Advocacy*. Kidderminster: BILD Publications.

Butler, K., Carr, S. and Sullivan, F. (1988) *Citizen Advocacy: A Powerful Partnership*. London: National Citizen Advocacy.

Campbell, J. and Oliver, M. (1996) *Disability Politics: Understanding our Past, Changing our Future*. London: Routledge.

Change (1997) *More Access Please*. London: Change.

Cooper, M. (1997) Mabel Cooper's life story, in D. Atkinson, M. Jackson and J. Walmsley (eds) *Forgotten Lives: Exploring the History of Learning Disability*. Kidderminster: BILD Publications.

Crawley, B. (1982) *The feasibility of trainee committees as a means of self-advocacy in adult training centres in England and Wales*. Unpublished Ph.D. thesis, University of Manchester.

Crawley, B. (1988) *The Growing Voice: A Survey of Self-advocacy Groups in Adult Training Centres and Hospitals in Great Britain.* London: Values into Action.

Crawley, B. (1990) Advocacy as a threat or ally to professional practice? In G. Brown and G. Wistow (eds) *The Roles and Tasks of CMHTs.* Avebury: Aldershot.

Department of Health (2001a) *Valuing People: A New Strategy for Learning Disability for the 21st Century.* London: Department of Health.

Department of Health (2001b) *Nothing About Us Without Us: The Service Users Advisory Group Report.* London: Department of Health.

Downer, J. and Walmsley, J. (1997) Shouting the loudest: self-advocacy, power and diversity, in P. Ramcharan, G. Roberts, G. Grant and J. Borland (eds) (1997) *Empowerment in Everyday Life: Learning Disabilities.* London: Jessica Kingsley.

Dowson, S. (1991) *Keeping It Safe: Self-advocacy by People with Learning Difficulties and the Professional Response.* London: Values into Action.

Dowson, S. and Whittaker, A. (1993) *On One Side: The Role of the Advisor in Supporting People with Learning Difficulties in Self-Advocacy Groups.* London: Values into Action in association with the King's Fund Centre.

Dybwad, G. (1996) Setting the stage historically, in G. Dybwad and H. Bersani (eds) *New Voices: Self-advocacy by People with Disabilities.* Cambridge, MA: Brookline Books.

Dybwad, G. and Bersani, H. (eds) (1996) *New Voices: Self-advocacy by People with Disabilities.* Cambridge, MA: Brookline Books.

FEU (Further Education Unit) (1989) Working Together? Self-advocacy and Parents: The Impact of Self-advocacy on Parents of Young People with Disabilities FEU.

Ford, S. (1996) Learning difficulties, in G. Hales (ed.) *Beyond Disability: Towards an Enabling Society.* London: Sage.

Goodley, D. (1997) Locating self-advocacy in models of disability: understanding disability in the support of self-advocates with learning difficulties, *Disability and Society*, 12(3): 367–79.

Goodley, D. (2000) *Self-advocacy in the Lives of People with Learning Difficulties: The Politics of Resilience.* Buckingham: Open University Press.

Gramlich, S., MacBride, G., Snelham, N. and Myers, B. with Williams, V. and Simons, K. (2002) *Journey to Independence: What Self-advocates tell us about Direct Payments.* Kidderminster: BILD Publications.

Hersov, J. (1996) The rise of self-advocacy in Great Britain, in G. Dybwad and H. Bersani (eds) *New Voices: Self-advocacy by People with Disabilities.* Cambridge, MA: Brookline Books

HMSO (1995) *Disability Discrimination Act.* London: HMSO.

LMPF (1996) *Our Plan for Planning.* Manchester: People First.

Lundgren, K. (1993) *Ake's Book.* Orebo: Bokforlaget Libris Sweden.

Minkes, J., Townsley, R., Weston, C. and Williams, C. (1995) Having a voice: involving people with learning difficulties in research, *British Journal of Learning Disabilities*, 23(3): 94–8.

Mitchell, P. (1997) The impact of self-advocacy on families, *Disability & Society*, 12(1): 43–56.

O'Brien, J. (1987) A guide to life style planning: using the activities catalogue to integrate services and natural support systems, in B.W. Wilson and G.T. Bellamy (eds) *The Activities Catalogue: An Alternative Curriculum for Youth and Adults with Severe Disabilities.* Baltimore, MD: Brookes.

O'Brien, J. and Sang, B. (1984) *Advocacy – The UK and American Experiences.* London: King Edward's Hospital Fund.

People First (1993) *Oi! It's my Assessment – Why Not Listen to Me?* London: People First.

People First (1997) *Access First: A Guide on How to Give Written Information to People with Learning Difficulties.* London: People First.

Perske, R. (1996) Self-advocates on the move, in G. Dybwad and H. Bersani (eds) *New Voices: Self-advocacy by People with Disabilities.* Cambridge, MA: Brookline Books.

Potts, M. and Fido, R. (1991) *A Fit Person to be Removed: Personal Accounts of Life in a Mental Deficiency Institution.* Plymouth: Northcote House.

Ramcharan, P. (1995) Citizen advocacy and people with learning disabilities in Wales, in R. Jack (ed.) *Empowerment in Community Care.* London: Chapman & Hall.

Ramcharan, P. and Grant, G. (2001) Views and experiences of people with intellectual disabilities and their families (1) The user perspective, *Journal of Applied Research in Intellectual Disabilities*, 14: 348–63.

Shakespeare, T. (1993) Disabled people's self-organisation: a new social movement? *Disability, Handicap & Society*, 8(3): 249–64.

Shearer, A. (1972) *Our Life.* London: CMH/VIA.

Shearer, A. (1973) *Listen.* London: CMH/VIA.

Shoultz, B. (1997) *More Thoughts on Self-advocacy: The Movement, the Group, and the Individual.* Center on Human Policy, Syracuse University, New York, http://soeweb.syr.edu/.

Simons, K. (1992) *'Sticking Up For Yourself': Self Advocacy and People with Learning Difficulties.* London: Joseph Rowntree Association.

Simons, K. (1993) *Citizen Advocacy: The Inside View.* Bristol: Norah Fry Research Centre.

Souza, A. and Ramcharan, P. (1997) Everything you ever wanted to know about Down's syndrome . . . but never bothered to ask, in P. Ramcharan, G. Roberts, G. Grant and J. Borland (eds) *Empowerment in Everyday Life: Learning Disability.* London: Jessica Kingsley.

Speak for Ourselves (1993) *Start! How to Set Up and Run a Successful Self-advocacy Group.* Newcastle: Speak for Ourselves.

Sutcliffe, J. and Simons, K. (1993) *Self-advocacy and Adults with Learning Difficulties: Contexts & Debates.* Leicester: The National Institute of Adult Continuing Education in Association with the Open University.

UKCC (1996) *Guidelines for Professional Practice.* London: UKCC.

Walsall Women's Group (WWG) (1999) *No Means No.* Brighton: Pavilion.

Ward, L. (ed.) (1998) *Innovations in Advocacy and Empowerment for People with Intellectual Disabilities.* Whittle-le-Woods: Lisieux-Hall.

Whittaker, A., Gardener, S. and Kershaw, J. (1990). *Service Evaluation by People with Learning Difficulties: Based on the People First Report.* London: King's Fund Centre.

Whittell, B. and Ramcharan, P. (1998) The All Wales Strategy: self advocacy and participation, *British Journal of Learning Disabilities*, 20(1): 23–6.

Williams, F. (1973) *Workshop on Participation.* London: CMH/VIA.

Williams, P. (1982) Participation and self-advocacy, *CMH Newsletter*, 20 (spring): 3–4.

Williams, P. (1998) *Standing by Me: Stories of Citizen Advocacy*, London: CAIT.

Williams, P. and Shoultz, B. (1982) *We Can Speak for Ourselves.* London: Souvenir Press.

Worrell, B. (1988) *People First: Advice for Advisors.* Ontario: National People First Project.

Wolfensberger, W. (1972) *Normalization: The Principle of Normalization in Human Services.* Toronto: Leanord Crainford.

Wolfensberger, W. (1977) *A Balanced Multi-component Advocacy Protection Schema.* Toronto: Canadian Association for the Mentally Retarded.

Wolfensberger, W. (1983) *Reflections on the Status of Citizen Advocacy.* Ontario: National Institute of Mental Retardation.

Wolfensberger, W. and Glenn, S. (1975) *PASS 3: Program Analysis of Service Systems. Handbook and Manual.* Toronto: National Institute on Mental Retardation.

PART TWO

Childhood

Rights, risks and responsibilities

In Part One of this book, attention was given to different constructions of learning disability and the implications for service design and development. We now turn to the first of the life cycle sections. It is important to provide a space for the voice of children with disabilities themselves, and family members, parents in particular, so as to hear what they say about their own identities, social relationships and support needs. We hope that the narratives and case material will provide readers with important points of reference for weighing and evaluating professional, policy and academic perspectives about the lives of children with learning disabilities and their families.

Consideration is then given to the important issues of the birth of a child with a suspected disability, disclosure and early support to families, family adaptations to caregiving and the longer-term consequences. Chapters dealing with these issues stress the importance of understanding development, adaptation and management over time. Attention is then given to ways of supporting children with high support needs, especially those with profound and multiple learning disabilities, before examining how to assist children and young people who may experience difficulties with communication. Both these chapters provide clear indications of the kinds of expertise and skills required of front-line staff to support individuals with these challenging needs.

This section of the book begins to elaborate some of the grander themes that permeate work with categories of vulnerable people described here and elsewhere in the book, especially in relation to the balancing of rights and risks, together with an appreciation of professional responsibilities.

Chapter 9 by Kirsten Stalker and Clare Connors demonstrates that children with learning disabilities, given the opportunity and necessary support, can give interesting and insightful narrative accounts about their everyday lives. Children's talk reveals that they do not necessarily look upon themselves in terms of a disability identity. For the most part they talk about and do the things that most young children do and talk about. However, the narratives illustrate that relationships with siblings can be very mixed, and that bullying can occur at home, from siblings, and also at school. Circumstances can limit friendships with other children and boredom can be common, especially at weekends and during holidays. The chapter will help the reader to gain an appreciation of:

- the value of listening to children with disabilities talking;
- important people in children's lives;
- children's experiences of school and other services;
- theoretical frameworks from the sociology of childhood and the social relational model of disability, and how these can inform an understanding of children's narratives;
- the practice implications of working with young disabled children.

Breaking bad news, one of the most difficult tasks professionals face, is the theme of Chapter 10 by Jane Bloom. Despite the emergence of many guidelines about the practice of disclosure, it is something that continues to receive a poor press from patients and service users. In this chapter the breaking of bad news is considered in two main contexts: disclosure to parents about disability, suspected disability or serious illness in babies and young children; and conveying bad news to disabled mothers. The reader is led through evidence about what seems to support good disclosure practice, and what support professionals may themselves need in order to feel protected and empowered in carrying out this difficult practice. The chapter provides the reader with an understanding of:

- theories and frameworks for locating good practice in the disclosure of 'bad' news;
- potential effects of 'bad' news on both giver and receiver;
- disclosure as a process rather than an event;
- guidelines for disclosure, their advantages and disadvantages;
- support for professionals carrying out disclosure.

Chapter 11 by Gordon Grant considers the nature and scope of family care of children and adults with learning disabilities with respect to the lifecourse. It therefore has temporal connections with subsequent parts of this book. The reader is introduced to metaphors as a way of understanding the lifecourse and the discontinuities or breaks that can disrupt family care over the lifecourse, but also ways of anticipating them. Different 'trajectories' are introduced as ways of sensitizing the reader to shifts and changes in relationships over time between children and adults with learning disabilities, their families and services. Practice implications of supporting families as opposed to supporting individuals are reviewed. The chapter is intended to provide the reader with an appreciation of:

- who and what is the family in the twenty-first century;

- how families manage caregiving;
- theoretical perspectives about family coping and resilience;
- family lifecourse considerations;
- priorities for supporting families.

Promoting healthy lifestyles in people with learning disabilities who have additional physical and sensory impairments is the subject of Chapter 12 by Bronwyn Roberts. This chapter addresses issues about children and young people with profound and multiple learning disabilities or high support needs, concentrating in particular on youngsters with cerebral palsy, visual impairments or hearing loss. People with high support needs are enjoying longer lives than before, so it is important for professionals to acquire the skills that can help them to contribute to and enrich the lives of the growing number of people in these circumstances. This chapter will acquaint the reader with:

- conceptual and definitional issues about the identification of people with profound and multiple learning disabilities;
- ways of enriching the environments of people with profound and multiple learning disabilities;
- a detailed account of cerebral palsy, visual impairments and hearing loss;
- ways of being sensitive to the personal communication repertoires of individuals;
- evidence-based helping strategies.

Chapter 13 by Lesley Cogher is themed entirely on communication since this is something that challenges many people with learning disabilities and also those that support them – families, friends, allies and professionals. Since most language development takes place in the early years much attention is given to this life stage, though case examples also include adolescents and adults. By means of a language skills model the reader is presented with a way of taking stock of the different communication challenges that people with learning disabilities often face. Strategies for supporting people with communication difficulties are outlined, including the use of augmentative and alternative communication systems. The reader is guided towards an understanding of:

- critical features of interpersonal communication, illustrated by use of a language skills model;
- development of communication in the infant and young child, the school-aged child, and young people and adults;
- tasks of the communicator and communication partner;
- what can go wrong with communication;
- augmentative and alternative communication systems.

Some of the chapters in Part Two illustrate how personal, familial and environmental factors shape important transitions in the lives of children and young people with learning disabilities and their families, paving the way for a fuller exploration of adolescence and young adulthood which follows in Part Three.

9

Children with learning disabilities talking about their everyday lives

Kirsten Stalker and Clare Connors

Introduction

Over recent years, many studies have examined children's lives from their own perspective. A much smaller literature reports the views of disabled children, and most focuses on young people's experiences of school or support services (e.g. Lewis 1995; Morris 1998, 2001; Kelly *et al.* 2000; Skar and Tamm 2001). Few studies have sought disabled children's accounts of their everyday lives, although Hirst and Baldwin (1994), Widdows (1997) and Watson *et al.* (2000) are significant exceptions. The views of children with learning disabilities are particularly poorly represented in the literature. In this chapter, we report what children with learning disabilities involved in one study had to say about their everyday lives.

The chapter begins by identifying some theoretical frameworks which help to make sense of the children's accounts and place them in a wider context. These are drawn from the sociology of childhood and the social relational model of disability. The reader is encouraged to find out more about these ideas by following up the references given. Next, we describe the aims and methods of our study: this involved 26 disabled children, but this chapter presents an analysis of the interviews with 13 children who had learning disabilities. The bulk of the chapter reports their accounts of their lives, looking in turn at home, school, services and 'views of self', followed by case studies of two children. The final section draws out conclusions and implications for policy and practice. The real names of our respondents, and of anyone they referred to, have been changed. A full account of the study can be found in Connors and Stalker (2003).

Theoretical frameworks

Where childhood is seen as a period of predictable development leading to independence and autonomy, then, Priestley (2003) argues, disabled children are bound to 'fail'. Traditionally, research about children has focused on their biological or psychological development: viewed through adult eyes, children were seen as playing a relatively passive role, reacting in a fairly predictable way to 'natural' processes going on within them and social processes going on around them. The sociology of childhood, however, views childhood as socially constructed (James 1993; James *et al.* 1998). Being a child has carried a wide variety of meanings across different cultures and times. For example, young working-class people in early Victorian Britain enjoyed precious little 'childhood' before being sent to work down mines or up chimneys, and those in developing countries may have similar experiences today. For much of the twentieth century, children with learning disabilities were excluded from mainstream child care legislation and treated as 'small' or 'pre-' adults with learning disabilities. The sociology of childhood recognizes the cultural and historical diversity of children's lives, which are further differentiated by class, gender and disability. Children have a unique perspective which differs from that of adults and are active in shaping their own lives: thus we need to recognize the contribution which their accounts can make to a broader analysis of childhood itself.

Another set of ideas which can usefully inform our thinking about disabled children can be found in the social model of disability. This was developed by disabled people to explain, and help overcome, oppression and discrimination (Oliver 1990; Barnes 1991). The social model draws an important distinction between 'impairment', meaning the loss or limitation of functional ability (such as the inability to see, hear or walk) and 'disability' which refers to social, material and cultural barriers which exclude people from mainstream life (such as inaccessible buildings or information). This way of looking at disability, widely promoted by the disabled people's movement, has won considerable political success, for example in campaigns for anti-discrimination legislation.

At the same time, some disabled people have pointed out limitations within the social model. These include its lack of attention to the implications of living with impairment on a daily basis and its neglect of the importance of personal experience (French 1993; Morris 1993). Thomas (1999) has developed what she calls a *social relational model of disability* which addresses these issues. She suggests that disabled people face two types of barrier. First, there are 'barriers to doing' which restrict what people can do: these are the buildings with steps which prevent wheelchair users from entering, or written information leaflets which cannot be read by people with visual impairment. Secondly, Thomas identifies 'barriers to being', caused by the hurtful or hostile attitudes and/or behaviour of other people. Over time, these can undermine a person's psychoemotional well-being, restricting who they can 'be' or become by damaging their self-esteem and confidence.

Thomas also talks about 'impairment effects': these are restrictions of activity which result directly from impairment, as opposed to physical barriers or other people's attitudes. For a child with learning disabilities, for example, difficulty with reading may well be related to intellectual impairment. However, there could be other contributing factors: people may have undermined the child's confidence, and thus willingness to persevere with reading, by making thoughtless remarks about their ability or achievement.

In our study we drew on ideas from both the sociology of childhood and the social relational model of disability to help explain the children's experiences.

Study aims and methods

This was a two-year study funded by The Scottish Executive. Its aims were as follows:

- to explore disabled children's understandings of disability;
- to explore how they negotiate the experience of disability in their everyday lives;
- to explore their experiences of using services;
- to explore siblings' views about having a disabled brother or sister.

We did not set out to recruit children who would be representative of the wider population of disabled children; rather, we aimed to include youngsters with a range of ages and impairments, attending a variety of schools and so on. Families were recruited to the study through schools and voluntary organizations. These agencies were asked to send information and consent forms to parents on our behalf. Once a positive response was received, we sent information and consent forms to the disabled children and their siblings. Three or four visits were made to each family, the first meeting being an opportunity to discuss their participation in the study. Semi-structured interviews were carried out with the disabled children, spread over two or three visits. In most cases we talked to the children alone but mothers of young people with learning disabilities 'sat in' on two occasions. In one case, where the child had autism, this proved very helpful but in the other case the mother's presence had an inhibiting effect, the child being noticeably less forthcoming during the second interview when the mother was present than the first, when she was not.

Two different versions of the interview schedule were used with the disabled children, one for older children (aged 11–15) and one for younger ones (aged 7–10). The latter schedule, which included various activities and visual aids to engage the children's interest and facilitate communication, was used for all those with learning disabilities. While it is important to use age-appropriate material with children, when we piloted the schedules, it became clear that the more structured schedule worked better with this group. We offered the younger children and those with learning disabilities various activities (such as drawing or writing a story), as well as certain games and exercises, so that those who were not verbally skilled, or not very forthcoming, had alternative means of expressing themselves. Two children used British Sign Language and two used Makaton, a signing system which accompanies speech: they were interviewed by one of the authors who has these communication skills. Another child used facilitated communication: his mother went through some of the questions with him and passed on his responses to us.

Booth and Booth (1994: 36) report that their respondents – parents with learning disabilities – tended to answer questions with 'a single word, a short phrase or the odd sentence'. This sometimes happened in our study, presenting challenges in terms of analysis and writing up. Some of the data are quite 'thin'; the key points are sometimes expressed only briefly and intermittently – or they may be repeated many times over. Booth (1996) discusses possible ways of editing such material. Is it acceptable, for example, to rewrite someone's words if they will be unclear or even incoherent to the reader, if the researcher 'knows' what the respondent meant? We think not. Booth also talks about 'cutting and pasting' data from different parts of the same interview to form a coherent narrative or develop a theme. As this does not involve adding to nor changing the respondent's words, at times we have used this method in presenting the data below. Where we have run together data from different parts of the interview, we indicate this with . . . to show that some material has been omitted. Elsewhere we reproduce chunks of data including the interviewer's questions or responses, which allows the reader to follow the meaning and flow of the conversation.

A full account of the methods and materials used in the study can be found in Stalker and Connors (2003).

Exercise 9.1

Find out what legislative rights children with learning disabilities have to be consulted about their views, and to be protected from discrimination.

The sample

Of the 26 disabled children in the study, 15 had learning disabilities. Two had profound multiple impairments and here we interviewed their parents. Thus, the following sections focus on the accounts of 13 children – nine boys and four girls. Some had additional diagnoses, including attention deficit hyperactivity disorder, hearing impairment, autism and, in one case, a combination of cerebral palsy, epilepsy and 'challenging behaviour'. Six attended special (segregated) schools, including one residential establishment, four were in integrated units (special units within mainstream schools) and three were in mainstream schools. Only five lived with both parents: four were in single-parent families and four had step-parents. They lived in central or southern Scotland – three in a city, eight in towns and two in rural settings.

The rest of the chapter presents the main findings about this group of children.

Findings

Important people in the children's lives

We asked the children to tell us about important people in their lives. Their comments showed that most had close, loving relationships with their parents, especially mothers. One boy gave his mum 'ten out of ten' for helping him. Asked what was his most valuable possession, he said: 'My mum and dad, my family . . . cos they're kind.' One girl said of her mother, 'She's the best.' Most children described their brothers and sisters as important and several mentioned members of their extended family – grandparents, aunts, uncles and cousins – who played a significant roles in their lives. Several told us they were worried about a close relative who was ill, or had been upset by the death of a family member (usually a grandparent). Some named particular friends, and a couple included a teacher, as important people in their lives.

Three children seemed to have an ambivalent relationship with their parents, none including them as 'important people'. A 9-year-old girl, prompted to say something about her mother, replied, 'I'm not quite sure about my mum . . . there's not much about her.' Of her father she said, 'I like him a lot. He doesn't shout a lot . . . but he smacks a lot . . . he shouts a little bit.' A boy, also aged 9, who declined to take part in a second interview, said little about his father and nothing about his mother during the first interview. Asked who helped him at home, he replied, 'Nobody. My dad gives me my medicine and my dad makes the breakfast all the time.' This child's mother had experienced mental health difficulties leading to several hospital admissions: data collected from his siblings suggest the boy was very close to his mother and upset when separated from her. Perhaps it was too painful a subject to talk about.

Among the wider sample of 26 children, relationships with siblings were mostly positive: the children talked about the fun they had playing together and their appreciation of support offered. There was some conflict too, as would be expected among any brothers and sisters, with arguments about ownership of toys, uninvited incursions onto each other's territory or which television channel to watch. Looking just at the group of children with learning disabilities, it is evident that their relationships with siblings were generally more fraught. A couple of youngsters seemed to get on well with their brothers or sisters most of the time while some got on better with one sibling than another. However, the three children in the study who reported being bullied by their siblings all had learning disabilities, while two others only referred to their siblings in negative terms. One boy, aged 9, had brothers aged 2 and 5 of whom he complained: 'Tom always bullies me . . . he wants my toys all the time . . . he annoys me at school . . . Roy bullies me . . . he scratches me.'

The other two children who felt bullied by siblings were those who also had ambivalent relationships with their parents, perhaps indicating some wider family difficulties. The 9-year-old boy had this exchange with the interviewer about his older brother, Paul:

Child: Bully.
Interviewer: Oh, is he a bully?
Child: Yes.
Interviewer: When is he?
Child: What?
Interviewer: When?
Child: Just now he's a bully.
Interviewer: Is he? Does he bully you?
Child: He bullies every single one, even Jane and Elspeth [older sisters] . . .
Interviewer: And what does Paul do?
Child: I don't know. Punch, kick, whack.
Interviewer: Why does Paul punch you?
Child: Because he's a bully and he likes it.

A third child described being hit by her older brother. In these cases, the siblings interviewed also described physical aggression on the part of the disabled child, and the problematic sibling relationships were confirmed by parents' accounts. However, when talking to us, the disabled children all strongly denied ever provoking their brothers or sisters!

Friends and foes

Friendships were very important to the children. Seven said they had friends locally with whom they played. Shared activities included riding bikes, building dens, shopping and going to the park. However, in four cases comments about friendships were qualified by later remarks. For example, one boy began by saying he had friends round about, but later stated he did not have many 'pals' locally. An older boy named a couple of his neighbours as friends with whom he played, but it then transpired that for some time they had refused to talk to him. In the separate interviews with siblings and parents, we learnt more about the children's experiences with other youngsters in the area. They described incidents where children had been called nasty names, taken advantage of and, in one case, returned home with torn clothes, apparently as a result of physical aggression from other children. One girl had been the subject of particularly cruel harassment, not just by children but also by adults: this is described in more detail in a case study below. The children's friendships at school are also discussed later.

Activities

Between them, the children were involved in a wide range of activities, most of which were very typical pastimes for children of their age. The boys tended to like football, basketball, computers, riding bikes and swimming while the girls enjoyed drawing, dancing, drama, music and swimming. Other pastimes included going to the park, shopping, visiting relatives, and watching TV and videos. Some children attended organized activities, such as youth clubs, Brownies or Sunday School. A few proudly described holding positions of responsibility, such as being an altar server in church. In contrast, one boy said he was a member of a gang which had several secret dens locally. His exploits included the following:

Child: The best thing that happened to me during the weekend would have to be being able to climb a tree that nobody else could climb.

Interviewer: Right, and you didn't fall out?

Child: Yes, I fell down.

Interviewer: At the weekend you fell out the tree?

Child: Yes.

Interviewer: So that was the best thing and the worst thing is it?

Child: *Yes.*

Interviewer: Oh, did you hurt yourself?

Child: Yes.

Interviewer: Did you?

Child: See when I fell down it right, I was holding onto a branch then suddenly I kinda caught between bits of my arm so I fell and I didnae stop till I hit the bottom so it would be very painful.

Interviewer: I'm sure it would have been.

Child: So what do you think of that?

Interviewer: Did you tell your mum you'd hurt yourself?

Child: No. I just crawled down underneath the hedge and I went to bed.

However, a few children felt bored at times, lacking interesting occupation. One 12-year-old girl said that weekends were not better than school, while a 9-year-old boy, asked what he did at weekends, commented, 'We do nothing on thae days,' adding that he never went out to play.

Overall, the children's accounts of the time they spent in and around home suggest lives that have much in common with any other youngsters. While there is relatively little evidence of impairment effects, there are reports of other children's hurtful and hostile behaviour upsetting these children, which may lead to what Thomas (1999) calls 'barriers to being'.

At school

Ten of the 13 children said they liked school – some were very enthusiastic about it. One boy described school as 'brilliant'; one girl, asked 'what was the worst thing about school yesterday?' replied 'nothing'. One boy (who was not always happy at home) reported always being happy at school. Similarly, another child, who sometimes felt bored at home, commented 'there are a lot of things we can do. But when the weekend comes I think oh, no school, no school, I want to go back to school.'

All the children but one named at least one teacher whom they liked – often this was a class teacher who took the children for most of their lessons. They described teachers as kind and helpful: 'She helps me count . . . help me do my maths and tell me what to do'; 'Mr Murray is . . . helps me and Ross and John . . . He's very important. Because he helps the school. He helps the people, helps people that's stuck on work'; 'Sometimes nice, sometimes angry at people.'

However, as discussed shortly, although these children's overall view of school was very positive, the majority reported falling out with friends or being bullied at times.

Three children were unhappy at school. In two cases, the child had moved from a mainstream school, which they had liked, to a special school (in one case, a residential establishment) which they did not enjoy. One boy compared his new school unfavourably with the last one: 'I dinnae like getting transport to school . . . I'd rather walk it or cycle or something . . . I hate that school . . . Up at [previous school] you dinnae get detention . . . I dinnae like the school uniform and all . . . at [previous school] we dinnae wear a school uniform.' This boy had a twin who remained at the local mainstream school: being separated from his brother, perhaps coupled with the implication that he was managing less well at school, may have added to his unhappiness – although he did not say so himself. In contrast to most of the other children, when asked to name the best thing about school, he replied 'nothing' while the worst thing was 'everything'.

The child at residential school had autism and was not very vocal. Here is an extract from the interview:

Mum: What do you do at [new school]? What's that? Happy or sad?
Child: Sad.
Mum: Does Jo like that one? What's that one?
Child: [Previous school].
Mum: [Previous school]. Is that happy or sad?
Child: Happy.

The third child, who used facilitated communication, felt his current school placement was not providing him with enough challenge. Through his mother, he had written a letter to his headteacher which the child agreed could be passed on to us. It read: 'I am feeling very frustrated and annoyed as a result of attitudes to Facilitated Communication. I feel able to avail myself on a level of education far beyond what your school is providing me at the moment. I believe that I need an education more suited to my needs.'

In the last two cases, the child's parents were also unhappy with the current school placement and were seeking an alternative.

Nine of the 13 children reported difficulties with other children at school.

It was not always easy to gauge the extent of the problem, but in three cases it appeared the child had experienced a serious 'falling out' with friends. One girl, for example, reported she was sad at school: 'When my friends leave me . . . my friends normally leave me.' Two boys had been upset when their friends would not play with them for a while. Four children (including one in the last group) reported what appeared to be isolated incidents of bullying; they had been 'picked on', called names or 'punched'. Three others had been bullied on a more continuing basis. The transcript from an interview with a 12-year-old boy suggests he did not want to discuss this topic:

Interviewer: When it's playtime, who do you play with?
Child: I kicked the football right over the fence.
Interviewer: Was that at school or at home?
Child: At home.
Interviewer: So what about in school, who do you play with in school?
Child: I kicked the yellow one up over the house and [the cat] went climbing up there and ran away.
Interviewer: So that was at home too. What about in school? Who do you play with in school?
Child: I stay in the classroom. I don't play in school.
Interviewer: You don't go outside at playtime?
Child: Uhu.
Interviewer: Who stays with you in the classroom?
Child: Miss Bryson.

Later, he reported sometimes feeling sad at school:

Interviewer: What happens in school to make you sad?
Child: Bully me.
Interviewer: Who bullies you?

At this point, he changed the subject again.

Thus there is evidence of what Thomas (1999) calls psychoemotional disablism which, in the example given above, stopped the child from playing outside during breaks (a barrier to doing) but also made him sad (possibly resulting in a barrier to being). However, the children were by no means passive victims of bullying. Although these incidents were clearly distressing to them, they usually took steps to deal with them. Some reported the matter to teachers, others to their parents who passed on the information to the school. One child, who said he had not been bullied, commented: 'No, I just bully them back . . . Or if they started kicking us, I'd kick them back.' This boy had received a number of detentions for fighting. Two of the children who had been 'sent to Coventry' by their 'friends' had not told their parents about these incidents, which had now passed; a third had not told her mother about a recent name-calling incident. On the whole, however, the children's prompt action in dealing with bullying is worth noting, since this flies in the face of the more usual view of children with learning disabilities as helpless and lacking in agency.

Exercise 9.2

How far do you think the difficulties experienced by children with learning disabilities are due to their impairment, and how far are they caused by other factors? What other factors are involved?

What do you think are the benefits of inclusive education for children with learning disabilities? Are there potential drawbacks? If so, how could these be reduced or overcome?

Children's experiences of using services

The children were asked about any services they had used. They were shown picture cards depicting various professionals (doctor, nurse, social worker – although that was more difficult to convey pictorially!) and services (hospital, short breaks unit, play scheme) and asked, for example, if they had ever been to 'a place like that' and, if so, what happened and what it was like. Apart from the comments about school and teachers reported above, the children had relatively little to say about services. This could be seen as a finding in itself, showing that the children did not frame their lives in terms of using services and/or it may be that children saw this as their parents' concern, since they themselves were not directly involved in accessing and negotiating with services. This may explain why the only service which several children talked about was their experience of being in hospital, which had a direct, immediate impact on them.

Nine children spoke – or expressed feelings – about being in hospital, including six who had unpleasant memories. Here is a 10-year-old boy talking:

Child:	Um, I must have been about 5 or 6 when I got an operation on my eye . . .
Interviewer:	What was it like?
Child:	Scary at the time.
Interviewer:	Scary? What ways was it scary? Can you still remember it?
Child:	Yes.
Interviewer:	What happened? Did you go into hospital on your own?
Child:	My mum wasn't allowed to come in with me.
Interviewer:	Was she not?
Child:	Into the theatre.
Interviewer:	Into the theatre. Was she allowed to be with you in the ward?
Child:	Yes. Uh-huh.
Interviewer:	Good.
Child:	What made me scared most was, there were these tongs, they were like that with big bridges with lights on them, you know, and 'oh, oh, what are they for? What are they for?'
Interviewer:	Hmm. Hmm.
Child:	And there were things all in my mouth.

Interviewer:	Hmm hmm.
Child:	Then everybody was there.
Interviewer:	Ah ha.
Child:	Then I went 'Mum!'
Interviewer:	Hmm. So it's quite scary. Did it help?
Child:	Yeah.

None of the other children went into details about why they didn't like hospital, although one referred to being in pain and bleeding. A particularly concerning report came from a girl who said that while in hospital, a man 'had done a bad thing to her'. She went on to say that although her mother believed her, the police had not. She did not elaborate on the incident, and we did not ask her to. However, other research has reported that women with learning disabilities are not always believed when they report sexual abuse (McCarthy 1999).

Three children had more cheerful accounts of being in hospital. One awarded a doctor '20 out of 10' points for helping her, while another said his hospital consultant was 'brilliant'. He enjoyed going back to the hospital because he 'was the first tiny baby born there' and all the nurses knew him.

Overall, the families in the study had little contact with social work departments and only four had an allocated social worker. Two of the children with learning disabilities commented on a social worker. One girl, asked if a social worker had ever helped her, responded, 'No, she just makes it worse.' However, further details were not forthcoming. The other described the social worker as unhelpful (see case study below).

Only one child had a befriender and none had an independent advocate. A few attended regular youth clubs or groups run by voluntary agencies, which they seemed to enjoy.

Exercise 9.3

Imagine you are working with a family which has a child with learning disabilities, high support needs and no speech. One weekend a month, she goes to a short breaks residential unit. How would you find out what she feels about going there?

What could be done to make things easier for children with learning disabilities going into hospital for medical treatment?

Views of self

In this section, we bring together data which throws light on how the children saw themselves and in what ways they tried to make sense of their experiences of impairment and disability.

The children were asked to complete a 'word choice' exercise which involved picking out words, from a given list, which matched 'what they were like' at school. There were 12 words in all, representing a mix of positive, negative and neutral words. The findings suggest that children generally saw themselves as good friends, helpful pupils and active participants in school life. Sometimes their responses were backed up with examples: several named their best friends while one boy, who was a 'class helper', commented, 'I do letters, helping the little ones because we have new ones in the classroom because they're only little and I'm helping them.' While most denied ever being 'naughty', several did admit to being dreamy at times.

Most of the children, when asked, could name some activities they were 'good at': this ranged from achievements which had received formal recognition – one child was a member of a Junior Olympics sports team, others had trophies, medals or certificates to show off – to children describing themselves as 'good at playing' or 'good at pretending'.

However, the children could be self-deprecating at times. When asked if there was anything they found hard, several referred to particular school subjects: 'The only thing I don't like, naw, the only thing I'm not good at is money problems and that.' Another said, 'Sometimes reading big words but I try to do them myself.' Some children had been told they were not good at something: 'They tell me my spelling and reading's no good.' Conversely, one girl did not believe the praise she had been given: 'The teacher says I am really good at maths but I don't think I am.'

Some of the most interesting findings from this study relate to how the children with physical and sensory impairments saw and understood disability. Those children were all aware of their impairments, but most took a practical and pragmatic approach, encapsulated in one boy's comment: 'That's it. I'm in a wheelchair so just get on with it. Just get on with what you're doing.' These children also identified a number of disabling barriers, such as inaccessible buildings and transport, and ineffective inclusion policies. They were sometimes made to feel aware of their difference in a negative way by other people's insensitive, hurtful or hostile comments or behaviour. When such incidents occurred, they knew that they were connected to other people's response to them as a person with an impairment.

Matters were rather different for the children with learning disabilities. They made fewer references to their impairment. Only one child referred to her diagnosis. She had written a piece about herself for the researcher, with whom she had this exchange as they read it together:

Interviewer: What's that? My name is . . .
Child: Jenny Hoskin. I have X syndrome.
Interviewer: Right. Tell me what X syndrome is.
Child: Em . . . eh . . . what is it again?
Interviewer: How does it make you feel? I mean because you have that, there are certain things that . . .
Child: Different.

It is not clear how far the other children were aware of having a learning disability. Certainly there was evidence that some were aware of being treated differently by those around them, and subject to different interventions or policies from, say, their siblings. One boy, talking about his friend, said:

Child: He's the last to get dropped off the bus because he's in a . . . he's like me too.
Interviewer: Like you?
Child: In the special class.

This child's mother reported that he had once asked her what he had 'done wrong' to be placed in a special class. This question points to a lack of clear information and explanation given to the child, but also suggests that he had come to associate difference with badness. This in turn indicates that he had not been given positive messages about diversity.

The children were asked what they would be doing when they were the same age as their parents. Overall, they had very similar aspirations to any other children of their age. One boy wanted to be in the army, another wanted to be a builder and a third, a fireman ('go to fires and save people'). One girl wanted to be a singer and dancer, another a vet or nurse. Two said they would not need any help to achieve their ambitions.

The children's hopeful yet 'ordinary' aspirations might be seen as a good thing except for the fact that, whether through impairment effects, disabling barriers or a mixture of the two, we may not be optimistic about how many will go on to achieve their ambitions. There were indications that a couple of children with physical/sensory impairment believed they would outgrow their impairment. The mother of a deaf child, for example, told us she had recently discovered that her son thought that he would be able to hear when he grew up. We do not know if any of those with learning disabilities thought they would outgrow their impairment. Alternatively, research with adults with learning disabilities suggests that while some individuals are aware of those around them having a learning disability label, they may choose to distance themselves from that label, being aware of the perceived stigma (Finlay and Lyons 1998). We do not know how common this is, nor at what age the distancing process begins. Alternatively, the children's views of the future may have been shaped by the combination of (in most cases) their relatively young age and a lack of awareness of impairment effects.

The following sections present case studies of two children. They are not intended to be representative of the wider sample but they illustrate the richness and diversity of children's lives. These two children were very articulate; thus, there is more 'meat' in their stories than in some others.

Case study: *Jenny Hoskin*

Jenny, aged 13, lived with her single mother in a Scottish city. She had no contact with her father. She told the researcher she had [X] syndrome which, she said, made her feel 'different'. Jenny attended a special school.

Jenny had experienced a high level of change and disruption in her life. She had previously lived in England, where she had been subjected to some cruel treatment by other children: 'When I lived in London, nine children between the ages of 7 and 13 stood me by the garage wall and stoned me.' Jenny had drawn a picture of this incident for the researcher. She went on: 'We moved to Scotland when I was 5. First, I went to Highfield, and I got spat on and urine and, is it shit, and called a 'spazzy' . . . and my swing set got slashed and then we went to Monument Street . . . then it got worse when I lived there. Then I went to my uncle's . . . then my gran's, then my uncle's again . . .'

Jenny recounted how she and her mother eventually ended up in homeless accommodation, as well as being placed in a succession of local authority housing. This included one house where: 'We were not there three months when the man next door came to our door and rattled the letter-box and shouted "come out you cows or I will get you". So we called the police and then they did not believe us because I was a special needs.' She had drawn a picture of this frightening incident as well.

Jenny had a number of important people in her life. Her mum came first – 'Who else?' – followed by a friend and various members of her extended family who lived locally. It was sometimes Jenny and sometimes her mother who made decisions about different day-to-day aspects of Jenny's life. Sometimes they disagreed, for example, about what Jenny should wear to school. She had a wide range of interests: apart from her sporting achievements, which were clearly exceptional, Jenny enjoyed going shopping, watching videos and listening to music.

Jenny said that school was 'okay': there were six children in her class. She had various friends there and enjoyed playtime most. Jenny had had a boyfriend at school – she was the only young person to mention having a boy- or girlfriend – but was no longer talking to him because he had started going out with someone else. Although she had friends at school, Jenny reported having no friends to play with locally. She did have a befriender, who was clearly an important figure, and had taken Jenny to see her favourite pop group. Jenny was also aware of a social worker coming to the house but this person had made little impact on her:

Interviewer:	Do you know why you saw the social worker?
Jenny:	No.
Interviewer:	No? When she came, what did she talk to you about?
Jenny:	She spoke to my mum usually.
Interviewer:	So she didn't come to see you. If you were going to give the social worker a mark out of ten for how helpful she was, what mark would you give her?
Jenny:	One.
Interviewer:	One? Why was that?
Jenny:	Because she doesn't – she is always on sick leave and that.
Interviewer:	So you don't find she is very helpful?
Jenny:	No.

Jenny's ambitions for the future were to tour the world with her favourite pop group and be a swimming teacher.

Case study: *Colin Baxter*

Colin was an 11-year-old boy who lived in a Scottish town with his parents, brother and sister. He attended an integrated unit. Colin referred several times to his extended family – grandparents, aunts and uncles – but did not choose to include his parents as 'important people'. He did however describe good relationships with his siblings. He said he got on with his younger brother 'when we help each other . . . sometimes in the mornings getting ready', and with his sister, 'when we play and sometimes we have wee chats about what it's like to get a bit bigger.'

Colin had several friends living locally. He had a particular friend of whom he said, 'He's so kind, helps people and, eh, we play games.' Colin had been befriended by a teenage boy who, his mother explained, was helping Colin become accepted within the community because 'a lot of people were picking on him'.

Colin identified a number of things he was good at. He said he was 'too good' at drawing and was also proficient at swimming, typing and wood-work: 'I'm good at craft things like putting two nails into a piece of wood to put it together.' He also proudly told us that he was responsible for helping look after the family dogs, taking them for walks with his mother: 'I make sure they're fed and I check their legs and make sure they're alright.'

There were some things that Colin found less easy. He described French as 'hard and strange' and said that it was difficult 'trying to understand about things that you've no' seen and you've no' heard'. Colin had an awareness but, it seems, limited understanding of being 'different' from other children. He was the child, mentioned above, who asked his mother if he was attending an integrated unit because he had done something wrong.

At the same time however, Colin was very enthusiastic about school. He gave an engaging account of a typical school day. He began by describing who was on the school bus:

> A lot of big people, a lot of big people, and there's a driver and it's got seatbelts on the bus. There's an escort and she opens the door and she lets us in. And then we're going to pick everyone up and we go to the school and when the bell goes we go in, then the bus goes away, then we're just sitting in the desk . . . then we do our work, like hard work, hard work . . . counting all the sums up and it's hard work . . . Then, we come home and the escort says 'Have a good afternoon' and I come home and the dog jumps on me and I say, 'I see, I see you.' Then I get my jammies on and we watch telly and we go to our beds.

Colin had some intense friendships with other boys and took relation-ships with his peers very seriously. He was willing to go far to help one boy stay on track: 'He's a wee trouble-maker. I watch what he's doing because he gets into big bother and I get him out of it. When we're speaking I'll say "Martin, if you're going to be like that, I want you to go out and have a wee walk and take two deep breaths and you'll be alright".'

Colin had been 'picked on' at school by one particular boy. Although he had reported this to his teacher, who had apparently reprimanded the culprit, Colin described it as an ongoing problem. However, he was not averse to taking the law into his own hands: 'One person bullied me once . . . in school and my old school and that was Tracey but I got her back. In the girls' toilets I got her back.'

Colin had great ambitions for the future: 'I'd like to be a film expert and art too because I'm into art and film.'

Exercise 9.4

Note down your responses to these two case studies – does anything in them surprise you? Compare notes with a fellow student or in a small group. Discuss how far and in what ways children with learning disabilities are like any other children, and in what ways they might be seen as different.

Conclusion

This study demonstrates that many children with learning disabilities are able to give narrative accounts of their everyday lives which are interesting and useful, often engaging, sometimes insightful. Some young people are very articulate and will happily talk at length; others need prompting and encouragement; some will benefit from, or need to rely on, alternative forms of communication. Practitioners should assume that every child can communicate and, at the least, can express likes, dislikes and preferences. It is no longer acceptable to avoid seeking a child's views on the grounds that she or he does not have an opinion or cannot communicate it.

The findings show that in many ways these children had ordinary lives and much in common with their non-disabled peers. Most had close loving relationships with their parents and valued contact with their extended family. Overall, they were involved in a wide range of activities and had many interests, typical of their age and gender. Most enjoyed school, liked their teachers and had a sense of pride and achievement in some of their activities. In all these aspects of their lives, they were similar to any other youngsters, underlining the importance of practitioners approaching all children as children first and foremost.

At the same time, it is important to be aware of areas where difficulties may arise. The findings suggest that relationships with brothers and sisters were mixed, with three children complaining of being bullied by siblings and some reports of physical aggression. As well as giving children with learning disabilities a chance to talk about their feelings towards siblings, practitioners can offer support to brothers and sisters, which may help reduce conflict. Tozer (1996) argues that attention to siblings' needs should begin at the point of birth or diagnosis: they should be given clear age-appropriate information about their sibling's impairment, with ongoing opportunities to ask questions and discuss any concerns. They can be offered support through one-to-one counselling if required, or simply space and time to enjoy themselves through siblings' groups or other activities if they wish.

Some of the children said they were bored at weekends and in school holidays. For those attending special schools or units outside their local area, it may have been difficult both to meet up with friends outside school hours and make friends locally. However, those who reported feeling bored included some at local mainstream schools. Other research has shown a paucity of social and leisure activities for disabled children (Murray 2002). Practitioners can help by encouraging local play groups and youth clubs to become more inclusive, by recruiting befrienders and by encouraging families to apply for direct payments from the local authority, whereby they may be able to purchase one-to-one support for their child to access leisure activities.

Most children made no direct reference to their impairment, although there were a couple of exceptions. Their accounts include some experiences which may reflect impairment effects, notably difficulty with schoolwork. The children in the study who had physical or sensory impairment were brought up against difference through – among other things – inaccessible buildings or transport. These 'barriers to doing' were less evident to those with learning disabilities in this study, with most having positive aspirations for their future. It was the hurtful or hostile reactions of other people which upset them most.

Some of the disabled children said they had friends locally but sometimes they had been ignored or taunted by these 'friends'. The majority had also experienced difficulties with other children at school, ranging from 'being sent to Coventry' to fairly relentless bullying. Several had taken steps to deal with this behaviour but a lot more needs to be done to prevent bullying occurring in the first place. One boy told us he was not bullied at school 'because there's rules' showing that, in his experience at least, anti-bullying policies can be effective. Although all schools nowadays have such strategies, the children's accounts, supported by findings from other studies (Shaw 1998; Watson *et al.* 2000), show that these policies need to be regularly monitored and reviewed. Practitioners in all agencies working with children need to be alert to signs of bullying and act quickly to stop it. Some schools are introducing peer mediation schemes, whereby certain pupils are trained to mediate between the perpetrators and victims of bullying. These schemes can reduce bullying in the playground by two thirds, and can involve relatively young children as mediators.

The children had relatively little to say about formal services other than hospitals. The findings underline the need for medical staff to be aware that children with learning disabilities experience the same range of feelings as any others and are likely to feel anxious, and perhaps frightened, when admitted to hospital, especially if this involves some separation from parents. Children should be given information and explanations about the medical procedures they have to undergo. Again, this needs to be in a format appropriate to the child's age, ability and, perhaps, desire to hear (see Stalker *et al.* 2003 for more good practice suggestions regarding disabled children in hospital).

As only a couple of the children commented on their social workers, it would be wrong to draw conclusions from what they said. However, recent developments in social work have greatly reduced the time available for one-to-one counselling and 'listening' work, with increasing time spent on paperwork and care management. Research elsewhere has shown the beneficial effects of having a dedicated key worker, with an advocacy and coordinating role, who spends time building up a relationship with all family members (Beresford *et al.* 1996; Mukherjee *et al.* 1999). Reviews of services to people with learning disabilities north and south of the border have led to more posts of this kind being created although it is not clear whether these are sufficiently widespread and resourced as yet to make a difference.

Other research has found that young disabled people value exchanging information and support with young people of similar age who have the same condition, in informal social settings (Beresford and Sloper 2000). If this were to work for those with learning disabilities, they would need good support from a skilled facilitator: voluntary organizations could play an important role here. Organizations of people with learning disabilities also have huge potential, albeit limited resources, to offer positive adult role models to children with learning disabilities. Along with schools and local authorities, they could support children to participate in self-advocacy groups and learn about their right to speak up for themselves. Given adequate funding, such organizations would be ideally placed to deliver disability awareness and inclusion training to staff at all levels in schools, public authorities and voluntary agencies.

Further reading

Ali, Z., Qulsom, F., Bywaters, P., Wallace, L. and Singh, G. (2001) Disability, ethnicity and childhood: a critical review of research, *Disability & Society*, 16(7): 949–68.

Berseford, B., Sloper, P., Baldwin, S. and Newman, T. (1996) *What Works in Services for Families with a Disabled Child?* Barkingside: Barnardos.

Bethel, J. and Harrison, M. (2003) *'Our life! Our say!' A Good Practice Guide to Young Disabled People's Peer Mentoring/Support*. Brighton: Pavilion Publishing. The Companion CD-ROM *Peer Mentoring/Peer Support: A Good Practice Guide by the Young Disabled People's Forum* is available for £10 from Greater Manchester Coalition of Disabled People, 0161 273 8141/7870.

Children In Scotland (undated) *Onwards and Upwards: Involving Disabled Children and Young People in Decision Making – A Training Manual for Professionals.* Edinburgh: Children in Scotland.

Dowling, M. and Dolan, L. (2001) Disabilities – inequalities and the social model, *Disability and Society*, 16(1): 21–36.

Morris, J. (1998) *Don't Leave Us Out: Involving Disabled Children and Young People with Communication Impairments.* York: Joseph Rowntree Foundation.

Robinson, C. and Stalker, K. (eds) (1998) *Growing Up With Disability.* London: Jessica Kingsley.

Stainton, T. and Besser, H. (1998) The positive impact of children with an intellectual disability on the family, *Journal of Intellectual and Developmental Disability*, 23(1): 57–70.

Resources

Barnardos: for particulars of work with children and families, information on research and publications, also news and events. www.barnardos.org.uk/.

Children in Scotland: a special educational needs helpline, providing information about policy and legislation, participation networks and details of projects. www.childreninscotland.org.uk/.

Contact-a-Family: for information on support networks, a database of specific conditions and rare disorders, publications and a helpline. www.cafamily.org.uk/.

Council for Disabled Children: for details of projects, a parent partnership network, early support pilot programmes, events and publications. www.ncb.org.uk/.

NCH Action for Children: for help with issues such as adoption/fostering, child protection and children's rights, details of campaigns and volunteer schemes. www.nchafc.org.uk/.

The Family Fund: for information, publications and research. The Fund gives grants to families with 'severely disabled' children. www.familyfund.org.uk.

The Joseph Rowntree Foundation: for summaries of research projects, and information on current research about disabled children and their families. www.jrf.org.uk.

The Norah Fry Research Centre, University of Bristol: for summaries of research projects and information about current research on disabled children and their families. www.bris.ac.uk/Depts/NorahFry/.

Triangle: an independent organization promoting good practice in communication, inclusion and child protection for disabled children and young people. The website outlines training and consultancy available to professionals throughout the UK, and some outreach work with families; also provides details of publications and other relevant organizations. www.triangle-services.co.uk/.

References

Barnes, C. (1991) *Disabled People in Britain and Discrimination: A Case for Anti-Discrimination Legislation.* London: Hurst/BCODP.

Beresford, B. and Sloper, P. (2000) *The Information Needs of Chronically Ill or*

Physically Disabled Children and Adolescents. York: Social Policy Research Unit, University of York.

Beresford, B., Sloper, P., Baldwin, S. and Newman, T. (1996) *What Works in Services for Disabled Children?* Barkingside: Barnardos.

Booth, T. (1996) Sounds of still voices: issues in the use of narrative methods with people who have learning difficulties, in L. Barton (ed.) *Disability and Society: Emerging Issues and Insights*. Harlow: Longman.

Booth, T. and Booth, W. (1994) *Parenting Under Pressure: Mothers and Fathers with Learning Difficulties*. Buckingham: Open University Press.

Connors, C. and Stalker, K. (2003) *The Views and Experiences of Disabled Children: A Positive Outlook*. London: Jessica Kingsley.

Finlay, M. and Lyons, E. (1998) Social identity and people with learning difficulties: implications for self-advocacy groups, *Disability & Society*, 13(1): 37–52.

French, S. (1993) Disability, impairment or something in between? in J. Swain, V. Finkelstein, S. French and M. Oliver (eds) *Disabling Barriers – Enabling Environments*. London: Sage.

Hirst, M. and Baldwin, S. (1994) *Unequal Opportunities: Growing Up Disabled*. London: HMSO.

James, A. (1993) *Childhood Identities: Self and Social Relationships in the Experience of the Child*. Edinburgh: Edinburgh University Press.

James, A. Jenks, C. and Prout, A. (1998) *Theorising Childhood*. Cambridge: Polity Press.

Kelly, B., McColgan, M. and Scally, M. (2000) 'A chance to say': involving children who have learning disabilities in a pilot study on family support services, *Journal of Learning Disabilities*, 4(2): 115–27.

Lewis, A. (1995) *Children's Understanding of Disability*. London: Routledge.

McCarthy, M. (1999) *Sexuality and Women with Learning Disabilities*. London: Jessica Kingsley.

Morris, J. (1993) Gender and disability, in J. Swain, V. Finkelstein, S. French and M. Oliver (eds) *Disabling Barriers – Enabling Environments*. London: Sage.

Morris, J. (1998) *Still Missing? Vol 1: The Experiences of Disabled Children and Young People Living Away from their Families*. London: The Who Cares? Trust.

Morris, J. (2001) *That Kind of Life*. London: Scope.

Mukherjee, S., Beresford, B. and Sloper, P. (1999) *Unlocking Key Working: An Analysis and Evaluation of Key Worker Services for Families with Disabled Children*. Bristol: Policy Press.

Murray, P. (2002) *Disabled Teenagers' Experiences of Access to Inclusive Leisure, Findings 712*. York: Joseph Rowntree Foundation.

Oliver, M. (1990) *The Politics of Disablement*. London: Macmillan.

Priestley, M. (2003) *Disability: A Life Course Approach*. Cambridge: Polity Press.

Shaw, L. (1998) Children's experiences at school, in C. Robinson and K. Stalker (eds) *Growing Up with Disability*. London: Jessica Kingsley.

Skar, L. and Tamm, M. (2001) My assistant and I: disabled children's and adolescents' roles and relationships to their assistants, *Disability & Society*, 16(7): 917–31.

Stalker, K. and Connors, C. (2003) Communicating with disabled children, *Adoption & Fostering*, 27(1): 26–35.

Stalker, K., Carpenter, J., Phillips, R., Connors, C., MacDonald, C. and Eyre, J. (2003) *Care and Treatment? Supporting Children with Complex Needs in Health Care Settings*. Brighton: Pavilion.

Tozer, R. (1996) My brother's keeper? sustaining sibling support, *Health and Social Care in the Community*, 4(3): 177–81.

Thomas, C. (1999) *Female Forms: Experiencing and Understanding Disability*. Buckingham: Open University Press.

Watson, N., Shakespeare, T., Cunningham-Burley, S., Barnes, C., Corker, M., Davis, J. and Priestley, M. (2000) *Life as a Disabled Child: a Qualitative Study of Young People's Experiences and Perspectives*. Final report to the ESRC Research Programme '5–16: growing into the twenty-first century'. http://www.regard.ac.uk.

Widdows, J. (1997) *A Special Need for Inclusion: Children with Disabilities, their Families and Everyday Life*. London: the Children's Society.

10

Breaking bad news

Jane Bloom

Introduction

Disclosure of bad news is probably one of the most difficult tasks health professionals face. Given that death and disability are part and parcel of clinical work, breaking bad news is very much a part of everyday practice. However, patients express dissatisfaction with this area of care and we, as professionals, are reputedly bad at it (Perkins *et al.* 1998; Barnett 2002).

There is a mix of standpoints here which this chapter attempts to explore in relation to the following:

- disclosure;
- bereavement;
- the social model of disability;
- emergence of guidelines;
- professional support;
- disclosing bad news;
- support for professionals;
- defences against anxiety;
- logical inconsistencies.

Disclosure

Bad news is defined as 'any news that drastically and negatively alters the patient's view of her or his future' (Buckman 1992: 11). For the learning disabled person, Read (1998) suggests that any change that creates feelings of anxiety, apprehension or fear can be perceived as 'bad' news. This can vary from moving house and leaving familiar staff to the death of a relative.

The varieties of clinical situations that trigger a need to break bad news are as many and varied as there are people. They can begin even before a child is born, and occur across traditional professional boundaries, from the cradle to the grave. There is a paucity of literature available on supporting loss generally, and particularly bereavement in people with a learning disability (Cathcart 1994a, 1994b, 1994c).

Bereavement theory

If the professional has some understanding of the process of grief, and how people relate socially, this may help them to understand people's responses in the clinical situation when they have to break bad news. Kubler-Ross (1970) describes five stages of grieving: denial, anger, bargaining, depression and acceptance. Feelings of unbearable sadness or anger come in waves and can be triggered by something related or apparently totally unrelated. People do not move through these stages logically and it can take up to two years for some resolution to occur.

Harper and Wadsworth (1993: 313) report that: 'People with learning disabilities display grief responses similar to those of other adults, a mixture of sadness, anger, anxiety, confusion, and pain and their ability to feel or display emotional behaviour during grief is not contingent on a conceptual level'. People with a learning disability are thought to have an understanding of the concept of death, like any other non-disabled person (McEvoy 1989), and they experience grief and loss profoundly (Emerson 1977; Conboy-Hill 1992; Hollins and Esterhuyzen 1997).

Bowlby (1944, 1951) wrote of the effects of the social context of deprivation and neglect on patterns of attachment and loss in relationships. Patterns of attachment were later researched and described by Ainsworth *et al.* (1971) and are now reliably identified, together with the family conditions that promote them. Attachment patterns are thought to develop differently in response to either secure or persistently unstable environments. For example, Bowlby thought that repeated parental threats of abandonment or punishment (normally made to the child to impose discipline) can create insecurity of attachment (see also Marrone 1998).

It is possible to foretell with some accuracy the persistence of patterns of attachment from as early as 12 months (Bowlby 1988: 124). According to Marrone (1998), the patterns identified in adult attachment interviews are as follows:

- secure;
- dismissing;
- preoccupied;
- unresolved.

Given that these patterns are identified in child and adult relating it would not take a great leap of the imagination to understand that they can find their way into other areas of care, including the way in which individuals break bad news or respond to hearing bad news.

Bowlby (1988: 32) suggests that healthy mourning includes: 'anger, directed at third parties, the self, and sometimes at the person lost, disbelief that the loss has occurred (misleadingly termed denial), and a tendency, often though not always unconscious, to search for the lost person in the hope of reunion'. The responses are similar in adults and children. That children are unable to mourn is untrue and that they should be protected from death is clearly not so. Bowlby suggests that inability to mourn in children is caused by not being given adequate information about what happened, or else having no one to sympathize with them and understand their feelings of loss, anger and sorrow or their yearning for a parent.

Psychotherapists believe that a large part of our mind is out of our conscious awareness. This is called the unconscious. We develop unconscious templates or fixed patterns of how we see the world and how we think it sees us and this may make us unhappy and lead to repeated patterns of difficulty. Childhood experiences are important in this (Specialist Psychotherapy Directorate 1995). Learning to move on and let go of patterns of thinking and relating is difficult and can only be done when there is hope. In this deep despair, anger and rejection in adults with learning disabilities can occur, as Hollins and Tuffrey-Wijne (see Chapter 32) demonstrate. Often the necessary emotional work to assist people in moving on can be done in a particular setting such as psychotherapy, where the treatment involves the repetition of negative thought patterns in relation to the therapist, called transference. When these patterns are experienced and understood in the therapy situation, they can trouble the person less (Specialist Psychotherapy Directorate 1995).

Sometimes, when there has been an associated emotional trauma that links in some way with the grief, such as when grief occurs as a result of a traumatic event like suicide or because of an unexpected medical event that might have been prevented, individuals may not follow a normal bereavement pattern. In such situations, should a person not be able to find ordinary comfort, expert professional help can be invaluable.

Exercise 10.1

How do you usually manage goodbyes?

How might this influence how you help your patient to say goodbye to their loved ones?

How might you improve the way you end your relationship with patients?

The social model of disability

Some people think that over-protective parents may smother a child's development and sense of identity, and that parents may later deny developing sexuality (Pantlin 1985). The difficulty of generalizing cause and effect here is that parents, like staff, can become easy targets and their relationships pathologized as failures (see Chapter 11). Curtis and Thomas (1997) describe many moving, painful and sad examples of how professionals' practice can disempower disabled women, undermining their confidence in their abilities as mothers. Though the women in this study were not learning disabled, the research attitude adopted to investigating a culture of neglect is relevant. Curtis and Thomas draw a clear distinction between the conventional view that revolves around issues of individual coping and risk, leading to questions such as whether a disabled woman can 'cope' with pregnancy and child care as opposed to a 'social model' approach where disability can be perceived and experienced in the context of social and environmental barriers that prevent people with impairments from experiencing full social inclusion.

(p. 203)

Empathizing with the situations people experience and are powerless to change, along with the deep disappointments they must bear, can be difficult. Quite often people in such vulnerable situations find themselves on the receiving end of attack and blame, or pity and prejudice. What is happening here? A culture of bullying, harassment and blame is beginning to emerge in the NHS (Kirkham 2000) and a picture of stereotyping (Kirkham *et al.* 2002). Analysis of the group dynamics involved in scapegoating can be found in Rose (2003).

Laing (1927), in thinking about the individual's mental health and its relationship to their family, moved from a medical to a social model, seeing the location of disturbance not in the individual but in the family. He argued that particular family dynamics gave rise to schizophrenia. Having met relatives who had read Laing, I noticed they felt a great burden of responsibility, guilt and suffering: that they had in some way 'caused' the problem. I wonder if their response to Laing's work mirrored something about the repercussions of naming and shaming, about secrets brought out into the open that are often difficult to bear, and also something about the problem of scapegoating.

It seems that what we need here is what Le Roy (1994: 207) calls 'outsight' as distinct from 'insight': 'Outsight relates to insights in the way that outside and inside relate . . . whereas insight refers to inwardly orientated expansion of awareness, outsight refers to the outward expansion of social consciousness and thoughtfulness'. An example of this is where so-called primitive tribes in Africa have a very different attitude to illness compared to western culture. When a member of the family is ill, they do not say 'My sister is ill', but 'I am ill in my sister'. This way of thinking does seem to have a social consciousness and thoughtfulness built into it, in that we are thought to be intimately connected in ways that must be recognized for healing to occur, and that healing is reciprocal, mutual and social.

Emergence of guidelines on breaking bad news

The importance of breaking bad news to the vulnerable in the right way is not underestimated in the literature (Buckman 1992; Faulkner and Maguire 1994; Kaye 1994). The approach is mostly described in behavioural steps that on the surface appear easy enough to follow.

Girgis and Sanson-Fisher (1998) suggest consensus-based guidelines as follows:

- give bad news in a quiet, private place;
- allow enough uninterrupted time in the initial meeting;
- assess the patient's understanding and emotional status;
- provide information simply and honestly;
- encourage the patient to express their feelings;
- respond to the patient's feelings with empathy;
- give a broad time frame for the prognosis;
- avoid conveying that 'nothing more can be done';
- arrange a time to review the situation;
- discuss treatment options;
- offer assistance in telling others;
- provide information about support services;
- document the information given.

The above guidelines can be considered in the context of breaking bad news to families as follows:

- It is usually best to break bad news to both parents at the same time, so that they can offer mutual support to one another.
- Subsequent to this, help families to make contact with other families and self-help groups who are often better at supporting/listening than professionals.

Another approach (Baile *et al.* 1997) involves the mnemonic SPIKES, referring to the following stages: Setting up, Perception, Invitation, Knowledge, Emotions, Strategy and summary. Buckman's (1992: 81) six-step protocol for breaking bad news and Read's (1998) adaptation of it involve variations on the theme. Read develops the approach for people with a learning disability, making further recommendations regarding multi-agency working. Read suggests that for people with learning disabilities, it is important to avoid any confusion in information-giving about the news, as this can complicate the grieving process, particularly if individuals have not been prepared for the impending death or have not been told why their life is changing so much. Particular attention needs to be paid to timing and pacing, checking understanding and repeating information to aid understanding, along with allowing sufficient silence to enable the expression of feelings.

There is disagreement over techniques for breaking bad news (Draper 2000–2002), and criticism that guidelines tend to be constructed from a professional standpoint and hence lack patient-centred reference (Arber and Gallagher 2003). All protocols tend to act as a guide to clinicians for helping to ease, as much as possible, situations that most patients experience as distressing and upsetting. Some identify the importance of breaking bad news as relevant to 'educating patients about their diagnosis and treatment, and increasing the likelihood that they will remember what they have been told' (Girgis *et al.* 1997). In general the principles can however help to remind doctors and nurses of the importance of attending to the patient's emotional state, in addition to providing information about their medical condition (Girgis and Sanson-Fisher 1998: 55).

It seems that guidelines can work towards enabling both helpful and defensive practice. Depending on how one looks at the process, guidelines can provide a channel for encouraging the natural intimacy necessary for good interpersonal relationships by enabling patients to express their feelings, but they can also defend against this with more focus on education. The balance could go either way and it might or might not be tailored to the patient.

Exercise 10.2

Look at the following website for information on the SPIKES approach to breaking bad news:

www.postgradmed.com/issues/2002/09_02/editorial_sep.htm

(Mueller 2002)

Think about a situation where you have had to break bad news. Identify which aspects of the approach you attended to, and which ones you omitted.

Identify the strengths and limitations of the approach as applied to your care.

Discuss with your colleagues how these guidelines might need to be adapted for people with learning disabilities.

Exercise 10.3

'Talking makes things worse!'

What do you think of this statement? What does 'worse' mean?

How would you know when to encourage patients to talk? What difficulties have you encountered when encouraging patients to talk?

Have you got a framework for thinking about these difficulties? Where might you go for help to think further about them?

Sensitive and effective professional support for families facing bad news

Pregnancy

Parents tend to assume their baby will be perfect, and antenatal screening tests can sometimes only give an indication of risk. Prenatal diagnosis of foetal malformation can feel like a bombshell. The mother may already have felt her baby moving and begun to form an attachment. In our tendency to idealize maternity, we can forget the ethical, moral and psychosocial dilemmas parents face.

Parents may respond differently to worrying results of screening tests, with some wanting to keep the baby and others wanting to terminate. The mother and father can also differ radically in their personal feelings about whether to go ahead with the pregnancy. The father can feel as if things have been taken out of his hands if the mother decides to go ahead against his wishes. At this uncertain stage in the pregnancy, if parents' views radically differ, their relationship can be seriously tested. Can they survive their own anxieties and negotiate their personal views and needs, while managing the love and hate stirred up in their relationship? I have known parents show great courage, and though they felt enormous distress they also looked forward to seeing their infant, showing concern, not avoidance of the developmental problems ahead. Those who choose to terminate may experience feelings of despair, misery, grief or relief (Raphael Leff 1993: 105–6).

There is another difficulty when conveying bad news. This is when there is a possible developmental delay that is a direct result of parental behaviour – for example, in the case of foetal alcohol syndrome. This is an extremely difficult situation, where guilt and blame can become overinflated. Parents can easily feel persecuted, and this feeling can be fuelled if they suffer paranoia or if others are judgemental.

Sometimes there is a link in pregnancy with an existing child having a particular abnormality. This can make hearing news about a similar abnormality in a subsequent pregnancy more accessible or more difficult.

The value of good psychological care is beginning to permeate the literature. Raphael Leff (1991: 466) suggests that 'what parents need most of all at this early point is the knowledge that it is safe to express all their feelings of disappointment, shame and grief without being accused of reject-ing the baby or failing as parents'. She goes on to discuss differing parental responses and cautions professionals on the importance of their non-verbal communication towards parents, making clear the link between parents' 'first contact' with others' responses to an abnormal baby, a mother's nor-mal vulnerability around the time of birth, and her sensitivity to 'subtle nuances of distaste or pity in the attitude of health professionals'. Tone of voice can be crucial here. One mother recalled that, 'The midwife handled the situation well, telling me about it in a gentle but direct manner' (Twelve-tree 1995: 23). To provide opportunity for adequate discussion, Raphael Leff (1991: 467) says that most specialists suggest that a multi-disciplinary meeting should be held three or four days after the birth, inviting the parents and all health care professionals involved.

It is important not to forget culture and spirituality in these situations. Sometimes this is not a clear-cut situation and practitioners may need to get to know parents while also following any hunches or intuition they have. Parents may not profess to a particular faith, and do not always require help or support from a spiritual leader. However, they might still benefit from some mention of whether spirituality is important to them, and in what ways the observance of cultural practices may help them to feel supported. This may turn on simple things like being accessible to members of the extended family, something with which many hospitals still struggle. Parents can take great comfort from knowing someone is interested in what they feel and think. Practitioners who can support their endeavours, for example in praying, lighting candles or visiting a place of worship, can be invaluable. Just enabling parents to have time to think quietly or letting them know they are remembered by those who do pray can be important.

At birth

When a child is born with a possible learning disability, the loss of the imagined perfect baby must be mourned before attachment to the living infant can take place (Raphael Leff 1991). Parents can experience great uncertainty and also inadequacy and loss of self-esteem at this time (Leon 1990). They have to cope with the emotions of grieving and may also feel shame (Leick and Davidson-Nielsen 1991). All the information profes-sionals can give may not always be enough to break through disbelief. And, of course, professionals also have feelings in these situations.

Sometimes when women are given bad news about their child they refuse to believe it. One woman was told by the paediatrician that her baby had a congenital heart abnormality, and needed further investigation. She repeat-edly responded, 'My baby will be alright, won't it?' The thought that it was not was understandably too difficult for her to process immediately. Another mother repeatedly begged the midwife to say her baby was breathing, when it was stillborn.

In one family the news of a genetic chromosomal abnormality with implications for normal development, inherited from the father, left the parents estranged from each other. The father felt unbearable guilt, blamed himself and initially rejected the child, while the mother continued to care for it. It took some weeks, lots of information about the condition, caring and supportive staff and a loving wife, before the father felt able to begin to accept the situation. In the meantime, staff were concerned about the mother, but she seemed to have a stronger sense of herself and possibly felt less responsible for the outcome, which helped her.

One group of students explored their experience of a woman who knew her infant had a chromosomal abnormality that carried developmental implications, discovered in the postnatal period. This mother had refused antenatal screening and continued to refuse further information about the disorder postnatally. She wanted to give her child the benefit of the doubt and to let it develop without her imagination and encouragement being hindered. The group wondered whether this woman was in denial of the implications, that she could not accept the loss of her 'imagined' perfect baby and wanted to believe it would be alright. The thought that she would be robbed of the precious moments of early motherhood and that all would be spoilt was perceived as unbearable for the mother.

Ordinarily mothers, and fathers, can feel great pressure, and it is a terrible burden for them, thinking they have to make their child's life perfect. Parents who feel they are in some way to blame for a child's developmental delay can be very hard on themselves, feeling terrible guilt. When parents experience feelings of shame it can get in the way of their seeking outside support, leaving them very isolated. It is important to remember that 'searching' and 'blaming' are part of the normal process of grief and that these things are not rational. In the BBC documentary, *The Talking Cure*, Caroline Garland, a psychoanalyst at the Tavistock Clinic, talks about the process of grief Mr Green experiences in coming to terms with the sudden death of his son in a road traffic accident: 'What Mr Green does is what every human being does, faced with a terrible event, which is to say I cannot accept that this was an accident. There is no such thing as an accident in the unconscious. We always attribute what happens to a somebody or something' (Garland 1999).

The wider context

I have known women who suspected a friend's child was showing developmental delay but felt that they could not mention it. The fear was that they would at best be ignored and at worst would lose their friendship. There is also a difficulty with timing. Paediatricians can experience different parental responses. Having seen a doctor for a year and then been told of a developmental delay, parents can respond angrily, wanting to know why they were not told earlier. And parents become similarly upset if progress turns out to be unduly optimistic.

There are other cases where parents have been told, for example, that the child will never walk, and then it does. In such circumstances parents may feel anger and resentment or else a sense of elation and strengthened self-belief that they have proved the doctors wrong.

The cycle of individual emotional neglect mirrored in the clinical team

Many have observed a neglect of emotional care of people with a learning disability. Read (2001: 27) notes 'an inherited legacy of practical, emotional and attitudinal difficulties', seeing their grief as being traditionally invisible and their emotional care overlooked (Kitching 1987; Oswin 1991; Conboy-Hill 1992). The psyche and the social are deeply connected. This is illustrated by the situation of a young learning disabled teenage mother whose child, prior to its birth, was placed under a court protection order. This young woman went on to experience a stillbirth. There was some evidence that this mother had herself been emotionally unsupported. Her parents showed no interest in her, she had been sexually abused and there was concern about this for the unborn child. When the child was stillborn, and the news was broken to her, she was unable to talk with staff. She was then left isolated. Members of staff felt unable to talk to her. A rumour went around the ward that it was better for her and for her child that it was stillborn. What does this little case study tell us? Read (1998) suggests that supporting a person with a learning disability may also involve supporting those around them, much as it would for non-disabled individuals in similar circumstances. The difficulty, however, is when *everyone* needs emotional support. The culture can easily become a depriving, neglectful and emotionally harrowing one for all.

It is difficult to define what full social inclusion would mean for a learning disabled mother who withdraws, wishes just to watch TV, talks to staff in a very limited way, does not seem to understand what has happened, and as yet has no emotional language to share her feelings. Social inclusion in this sense involves a whole range of social, sensory, cognitive, abstract intelligence, communication and behavioural challenges, both individual and group.

The literature often tends to focus on the social as opposed to the psychological. The idea of separating the individual's psychological world from the social group they live in is contested by group analysts. Separation of the individual from the group is thought to be an artificial division, as the social and psychological are intimately connected. S.H. Foulkes, the originator of group analysis, believed that the individual could not be abstracted from their social situation: 'What is inside is outside, the "social" is not external but very much internal too and penetrates the innermost being of the individual personality' (Foulkes 1971: 227). In the case example above, a cycle of deprivation was re-enacted, where the mother's emotional needs, and the staff's anxieties about meeting these needs, were neglected. Is it possible that the mother repeated a pattern of relating she had learned earlier? Certainly her parents had withdrawn and avoided her. Staff also appeared to have repeated the parental pattern. What was going on here? Thinking about the one-to-one relationships (e.g. mother and midwife, mother and own mother,

mother and baby), is of course important. Equally important is to go beyond this, to think about everyone involved: their psychosocial functions, social role and the meaning of what happened. The emotional challenges learning disabled people and their carers face intimately affect those individuals and their caring groups. As Hollins and Evered (1990) and Hollins and Tuffrey-Wijne (see Chapter 32) demonstrate, the whole is profoundly more than the sum of its parts.

A culture of cold, rejecting families with unwanted, bothersome children could be interpreted from this case example. But, whose family of origin is being mirrored here? What aspects of the individual, family and cultural group are now being re-enacted, waiting in hope for recognition and understanding? What are the implications of talking or not talking about this for the individuals, groups and organizations concerned and how are these issues thought about, and with whom?

Is this group at a stage in its development where it has the psychological capacity to bear to look at its interactions? If the staff could not face the young woman, was it that they just did not know how to engage with her? Did they not have the appropriate support themselves? Did they not have the skills? Did they feel hopeless and disappointed without feedback from her, or were they just being realistic about what could be achieved? Alternatively, were they merely re-enacting an unsympathetic management structure? And was this structure merely reflecting a wider social and cultural denial of feelings? How would one know? Should the individual be given priority over the group, or vice versa?

It is important to think about how to retain a multiplicity of perspectives, whilst being mindful of positions that might obscure, prejudice, privilege or disable particular points of view. There are important issues here for clinical staff, with enormous implications for clinical care. Furthermore, these issues do not sit neatly with behaviourally-driven practice guidelines.

The concept of resilience discussed by Grant *et al.* (2003: 143) is relevant here. They suggest that 'resilience should be viewed within a relational matrix'. They identify the view of Hawley and DeHaan (1996) of 'resilience as a process requiring constant adaptation and negotiation between the individual or family and the environment' (Grant *et al.* 2003: 163) and point to 'evidence suggesting the strengths of kinship as the basis of attachment' (p. 164). The word 'negotiation' is important here as is the concept of kinship, conjuring up images of dialogue and the importance of being able to talk with others and get support.

Exercise 10.4

What does support mean to you? Do you know of any support in your area that you could make use of, or introduce people to?

Who do you most identify with in the above case example? Who do you least identify with?

What do you make of this woman's case?

Disclosing bad news: tensions and possibilities

The word 'disclosure' conjures up ideas of hearing something previously unknown, perhaps a secret. Hollins and Grimer (1988) found that the three 'secrets' of death, sexuality and dependence were of particular importance to people with learning difficulties. Discussion on traditionally 'taboo' areas runs the risk of running into problems of naming, shaming and blame, leaving some individuals and groups subsequently isolated. So how can we continue to work together to think about difficulties that may be hidden, shameful, unbearable and unarticulated? Read (1998: 90) advises: 'Do not be surprised if the person with a learning disability does not react at all initially (sometimes it takes a while for information to be understood and acknowledged – days, months or even years) or reacts inappropriately'. Often this is related to impairment or environmental factors, but either way communication aids and assistive technologies may help (see Chapters 12 and 13).

In my experience with very able students I notice similar dynamics: they worry about laughing inappropriately, and quite often do. They sometimes need help to work through their embarrassment and shame. Furthermore, adults in therapy can experience grief, previously denied for many years and triggered unexpectedly in discussion. Similarly in education groups, people may struggle with sudden unexpected strong feelings they find threatening. While some group members might personally resonate with an individual's upset and share this, others might try to help, while others look on, feeling helpless and powerless. Some individuals might wish they were not there, while others might want to get on with something more practical.

There is good evidence that training professionals about how to break bad news has a positive impact on clinicians' communication skills (Kern *et al.* 1989) and that training works well in multi-professional settings. Benefits emerging from workshops include:

- 'the development of practice, the value of sharing, the benefit of feedback and team work' (Farrell *et al.* 2001: 765);

- increased confidence in professionals' ability to break bad news (Baile *et al.* 1997);

- students are 'rated as more effective' (Colletti *et al.* 2001).

The way in which bad news is broken is also linked with the subsequent emotional reaction of the receiver: 'When information given is perceived by the patient as too much or too little, and resultant concerns remain undisclosed and unresolved, there is a high risk that the patient will develop clinical anxiety and/or depression' (Maguire 1998: 188). Reports suggest that although disclosure may have a negative emotional impact in the short term, most patients will adjust well in the longer term (Gergis and Sanson-Fisher 1998). Girgis and Sanson-Fisher (1998: 55) suggest that the professional role is seen as helping to ease as much as possible a situation that most patients experience as distressing and upsetting. What does this helping mean and what is hoped for?

It is clear that professionals can feel quite a burden of responsibility and confusion here. In the effort to ease suffering as much as possible clinicians must ensure they neither silence nor encourage distressing and emotional feelings. But how far should they go with silencing or encouraging? Clinicians are guided here in the requirement to use empathy and open questions. These are both powerful tools, coming under the term 'probing' described by Egan (1990). Empathy can enable clients to access feelings they would normally not tune into, feelings they usually deny and defend against, and clinicians are further guided to confront patients' defences (e.g. 'denial' – see Buckman 1992). Professionals and patients need help here, but what does 'help' mean? Buckman (1992) makes some attempt to explore this, demonstrating how to use open and closed questions. He also discusses the difference between hostile and empathic responses, and how to remain patient-centred while continuing to be one's professional self. In the end, the underlying educational message aims to equip practitioners to manage the patient. But what is it that clinicians are hoping to manage?

Faulkner and Maguire (1994) give helpful and practical conversational examples of how a professional can help patients with difficult news. They demonstrate the requirements of sensitive timing and pacing, how one can acknowledge the patient's distress, check their understanding and gauge their level of awareness, denial and desire for knowledge. Implicit in all the examples provided is the notion that eventually a good psychological outcome with adequate acceptance and adjustment can occur, even though it might only begin the day before a patient dies. But even here, things go apparently unnoticed, as demonstrated in the following example from Faulkner and Maguire (1994):

Nurse Spry: As I understand it your main concern is not so much the cancer, because they are going to be able to remove all of it, but the fact you are going to need a colostomy. You are worried about it leaking and affecting your social life and personal relationships.

Mrs Bond: Yes that's correct.

Nurse Spry: Do you have any other worries at the moment?

Mrs Bond: Isn't that enough?

Nurse Spry: Well, it's important to check I haven't missed anything before we discuss what we might be able to do.

Mrs Bond: All right.

Nurse Spry: Which of these concerns is bothering you most?

Mrs Bond: Having to try and cope with the colostomy.

Nurse Spry: So shall we begin, then, by talking about what we might be able to do to try and help you with that?

Mrs Bond: Yes I would be grateful if you would.

I suspect a sensitive Mrs Bond would pick up fairly quickly whether her nurse could really empathize and would just accept that the best she could hope for was help with physical care. The angry acceptance of one's condition, which seems to be an entirely healthy response, goes unnoticed in this example. Additionally, the fact that the nurse holds the privileged position of having information about the patient, which the patient does not have, must surely be difficult for the patient but is not explored. What would informed consent mean here? Furthermore, what does this sort of response reveal about the nature of professional difficulties or the neglect in emotional care previously mentioned that people with learning disabilities face?

Exercise 10.5

Think of several clichés you have heard people use and discuss what you think these achieve.

Think of several statements, each not a cliché but an attempt at saying something that would encourage a person to bring the discussion back to what is being skipped over. Find words to talk about it in an acceptable way.

Support for professionals

Phipps and Cuthill (2002: 287) suggest that clinicians are faced with many personal difficulties in breaking bad news. These include: 'harbouring fears of the patient's unpredictable emotional reactions, feeling ineffectual and unable to deal with patient's expectations for a cure, fearing display of their own emotions, or that a revival of bad news personally received may be triggered'. In addition, Phipps and Cuthill point out that the clinician 'may use distancing tactics in discussing emotionally charged topics'. The word 'use' is interesting here, suggesting that clinicians have conscious control over their emotional responses, in ways unexpected of patients.

It seems that health care professionals are destined to re-enact the Greek myth of Cassandra – they, like her, are to be the ones who accurately foretell disastrous events, but the awful emotional impact and personal consequences for them cannot be really believed, felt or experienced, because they are to be packaged, serviced, managed and improved by teaching them how to behave in given situations. The steps towards breaking bad news overall seem to be disappointingly behaviour-driven with the purpose of getting the professional to move through the correct steps to help the patient to face up to 'reality' and understand their situation.

Ptacek and Ellison (2000) report on the difficulties of intimacy that 115 health care providers faced in bad news transactions, where there was a failure to explore emotional reactions. Ramirez *et al.* (1995) found that 28 per cent of doctors in their study reported they suffered from clinical levels of anxiety and depression and clinicians viewed communication difficulties as being a significant contribution to their stress and lack of fulfilment. Cohen *et al.* (2003: 459) found that in healthy medical students, the task of breaking bad news as compared to breaking good news produced 'significant increases in self-reported distress, and in measured cardio-vascular responses. There was also a significant increase in natural killer cell function 10 minutes into the task'.

Read (1998) develops Buckman's (1992: 11–31) list on the difficulties professionals face, as follows:

- fear of causing pain (against the caring role);
- sympathetic pain (you feel their discomfort/distress);
- fear of being blamed (as the messenger of bad news);
- fear of the untaught (many nurses are not taught to break bad news);
- fear of eliciting a response or reaction (for a person with a learning disability such a response may be wholly inappropriate, delayed, or indeed challenging);
- fear of admitting that they do not know (against both nursing and medical culture);
- fear of expressing emotions (goes against the professional image);
- ambiguity surrounding the phrase 'I'm sorry' (as a form of apology or sympathy);
- one's own fears (do you feel comfortable talking about death?);
- fear of hierarchical structures or individuals (e.g. you may support the person with a learning disability who wishes to see the body of his/her late father, but your colleagues may not);
- fear of saying the 'wrong' things (yet we know that saying nothing at all is often the worst thing to do).

The medical and nursing literature is full of examples and protocols aimed at helping teams to work together towards breaking bad news sensitively and compassionately. Practitioners are expected to help patients at this difficult time. Within this, there is some explanation of professionals' difficulties, but naming the feelings seems to be mostly as far as it goes. Curiously, there is little meaningful exploration of the feelings professionals experience in relation to their emotional work. Professionals and carers appear to be expected to regularly offer help of the sort they may never have received themselves. But can they give what they have never had?

Hollins (1993) notes that therapists working with learning-disabled patients need ongoing support and supervision from colleagues to enable them to contain the feelings of despair and anger projected by their patients. Failing to understand the meaning of strong feelings stirred up in the professional can lead to complications. There is nearly always a projection of difficult feelings, normally associated with grieving, but easily displaced onto professionals, for example, when a patient is angry with a professional. Anger is a normal part of the grieving process and is particularly evident when bad news is disclosed. If misunderstood, there is a channel here for displacement, where anger is not talked through. If it is acted on, a complaint may ensue. Talking about grief with a bereaved person requires professionals to make a judgement in an effort not to deny or misinterpret feelings. Grief, as an interpretation, should not be used routinely to explain away feelings of anger. Nor should the reality of the risk of litigation be used as a defence against getting close to the patient's painful feelings of anger. A delicate balance of dialogue is required. In the event of an actual complaint, it is probably necessary to rethink these boundaries as action has overtaken dialogue, which might make subsequent dialogue impossible, particularly for the clinician who has been blamed.

Problematizing, psychologizing, or ignoring professionals' feelings that normally occur in response to their patients places the buck straight back in their lap. Le Roy (1994) reminds us that silence about the suffering of any particular individual, family or group can serve a particular function: to keep certain thoughts outside our awareness. By keeping silent about the trauma of professional experience, secrets such as shame about attitudes, love, hatred, collusions, and abuse of power can remain in the cellar, so to speak. Professional secrecy keeps the fragile balance of the status quo safe and fails to differentiate between the suffering of the cultural group to which one belongs and the suffering of the individual or family one is trying to help. As Burman (2001: 191) observes: 'It is precisely those areas that are passed over as obvious, or are assumed, that call for investigation. For, at the point of convergence between what might be regarded as the individual and cultural unconscious (or perhaps what Dalal (1998) calls the social unconscious), they are where the roots of compliance and coercion live'.

Defences against anxiety and emotional pain

As far back as the 1950s, Menzies Lyth wrote in detail of the difficulties nurses face and how organizations defend themselves against their anxiety: 'By the nature of her profession, the nurse is at considerable risk of being flooded by intense and unmanageable anxiety' (Menzies Lyth 1988: 50). Menzies Lyth wrote about how the organization and bureaucracy of the nursing profession had failed to contain the high levels of anxiety and stress that nurses experienced.

Main (1989: 208–11) also wrote about professional anxiety regarding a clinical case of 'hopeless troubles' in a GP practice. The patient was the elderly sister of an elderly man. She was totally deaf (at least to the GP) and blind, confined to a chair, with little quality of life. Her brother looked after her. It was a hopeless, tragic, sad and painful case for the helpless doctor and his distressed patient. Main suspects that helplessness nearly overwhelmed the professional ego of the doctor and his private self nearly got involved in the tragedy, 'but he risked it and could get deeply involved'. Main suggests that 'love in professional work is largely unstudied and decidedly much less than hatred, which seems to be more respectable and less shamefaced'. Main suggests that all of us have weak spots in terms of intolerably painful encounters and that we inevitably erect defences such as laughter, forgetfulness, aloofness, denial, evasive professional cheerfulness, concentration on somatic troubles or the environment, and reassurance. He presents a case where the doctor's attempts to reassure the patient fail and he subsequently loses his temper, suggesting that all reassurance can be roughly translated as follows:

> Please stop being the way you are. I don't understand you and I don't know what to do and I can't stand being useless. I do not want to observe any more facts that disturb me. Therefore they do not exist. So please stop complaining. Now look, I really mean it! So watch it! For God's sake keep quiet! Never heard of baby battering? Shut up! Go to hell! My dear!
>
> (Main 1989: 208)

Main suggests that health professionals need to be strong enough to withstand and not be overwhelmed by major tensions such as dealing with a sense of helplessness. In other words, a strong ego is needed. He understands that this is an ideal state and we know it is achieved only intermittently when the health professional is in good shape. None of us dares be superior about this but it is important for furthering our care that we freely recognize that failures are common. We need to study their nature, the circumstances in which they arise, the defences used against anxiety and the clinical consequences.

Professionals experience many difficulties in containing grief and can be likened to parents in this sense. Parents can find it difficult emotionally to 'contain' a baby when it has been fed, winded, cuddled and so on, yet still it continues to cry and no physical problem can be found. Mothers can feel their maternal self threatened, and question whether they are 'good enough'. Likewise it is difficult for professionals to tolerate a patient who might make them feel powerless, useless or distressed. Balint (1963: 230) writes about the 'apostolic function' of the doctor: 'An especially important aspect of the apostolic function is the doctor's urge to prove to the patient, to the whole world, and above all himself, that he is good, kind, knowledgeable, and helpful. We doctors are only too painfully aware that this is a highly idealized picture'. There are important issues here, not least the protection of the patient's interest in ensuring a safe space for them to hear bad news and express their feelings, but also for clinicians who are also human and have to cope with their own difficult feelings.

Understanding relationships requires careful consideration and exploration to ensure sensitive and appropriate care. Such exploration has traditionally been neglected in the caring professions. The danger of this is that there will continue to be a great poverty of dialogue and practical know-how about how to personally and socially manage relationships for the best. Fraiberg *et al.* (1980) write movingly of how a young mother cannot give her child the emotional care it requires because she has not had emotional care herself when younger. The child is at risk of physical and emotional neglect. Advice and guidance on how to be a good parent fails and only with psychotherapeutic help can she move forward, increasing her confidence and resilience.

Given that there are similar parallels and difficulties between parental care and professional care, it is curious that a psychoanalytic or group analytic approach has been neglected by professionals. Most approaches seem to be behaviourally driven, working on the premise that if professionals know what is acceptable behaviour they can improve adequately with coaching.

Regular time structured into health care clinical work for the purpose of thinking about the meaning of professionals' behaviour and the intense feelings they experience in response to their patients has long been neglected in National Health Service practice (Savage 2004). Psychoanalytic practice has offered help in the assessment, preparation and facilitation of psychological work in the service of the patient by helping professionals to think psychologically about their patients and talk more openly with them (Balint 1963) (see Savage 2004: 28–32 for a moving account of the process of psychoanalytic clinical supervision during a Balint seminar programme for psychosexual nurses).

Exercise 10.6

What organizational function is served by superficially passing over professionals' feelings?

What unspoken cultural rules, beliefs and messages are expressed?

What ways of relating are expected? How do you comply with these ways of relating? How are you coerced into these ways of relating?

What choices do you have? What would be the implications of stepping out of the usual cultural pattern?

Logical inconsistencies with gaining consent to explore feelings

As the UK Learning Disability website demonstrates (UKLD 2003), consenting to decisions about care, emotional or physical, places particular demands on professionals. Whether guidelines on informed consent aid professionals in the ethical field of emotional distress evoked in the disclosure of bad news, and subsequent grieving, is hard to say. After all, how can clinicians help someone, learning disabled or not, give consent in advance to express their emotions when their feelings are not yet in their conscious awareness?

There seems to be a logical inconsistency, and perhaps some ambivalence, in a requirement that attempts to take account of an individual's rights, yet does not acknowledge the inherent paradoxes of this. Working with developing and emerging patterns of interaction may include unimagined shifts in defences towards growth and personal exploration. Proper training and clinical supervision in individual and group dynamics is required to understand and work with defence mechanisms. There is always the danger that individuals, professional or patient, can defensively blame the other for making them feel something that they had not consented to, or that one party takes advantage or is perceived to be taking advantage of the other. Acknowledging the difficult emotions stirred up in this process requires careful preparation and particular ethical and management structures.

Conclusion

Breaking bad news is not easy. From the cradle to the grave professionals and their patients face extraordinary dilemmas concerning what to do for the best. We live in a society that is moving towards the ever-increasing illusion of perfection, where disability is seen as something to be prevented. With the availability of prenatal testing, there may be social pressures to terminate pregnancies. Disapproval of disability may occur and there may be greater prejudice and discrimination. It is obviously important to listen to our patients and to have dialogue with them about their feelings. What is disappointing in the medical and nursing literature is the lack of genuine material that regularly demonstrates the personal struggles clinicians and patients must face together when there are interpersonal difficulties. When breaking bad news, professionals can sometimes find themselves at sea, required to personally negotiate uncharted territory with their patients. Psychological theories and guidelines, like maps and compasses, can be useful, but they can also be difficult to understand and apply, and emotional responses, like the weather, can be variable and unpredictable. Individuals and groups are complex, no single theory explains them and there is still much to study and understand.

When breaking bad news, professionals may find themselves doubting their judgements:

- Have we got all the information?
- Have we missed something?
- Is there something we should say?
- Is there something we shouldn't say?
- Are there regrets about things left unsaid?
- How can we know when we adopt positions of silence or of expertise whether we are acting in facilitation or constraint towards our own and others' development?
- How can we make sure that in an effort to provide psychological care or communicate bad news we are not tempted to use ready made words, taken-for-granted platitudes or clichés?

Professionals are not perfect: they make mistakes, but if they can try to understand these rather than bury them they can try not to repeat them.

Lack of emotional support, neglect and deprivation are probably the most significant factors that affect the emotional health of everyone, learning disabled or not, professional or patient. It is important for professionals to have a framework, like a map and compass, with which to think about how to talk with patients about emotional issues, and a place to regularly think about and get support with this. And we need to be mindful that our perceptions are coloured by our particular models. Psychotherapy, like nursing and midwifery, has held on to a non-medical model and an awareness that good relationships are crucial to caring. The broad variety of schools within psychotherapy offer a fertile arena for health care professionals to get support and help to develop new and different ways of thinking, understanding and talking with patients.

Raphael Leff (1993: 204) explains that psychotherapy works 'to release resources which have been occupied in defensive manoeuvres of dispersal, hiving off, deflection or silencing internal voices'. Working personally and professionally with difficult and repeated patterns of relating is not without its risks. It requires grit, determination, curiosity and motivation as psychic pain is re-experienced in the service of resolving repetitive conflicts and difficulties in patterns of thinking and relating.

Paulo Freire (1972) reminds us that the true focus of revolutionary change is not escape from oppressive situations but from the internalized oppressor within us, which is structured according to dominant myths, relationships and politics. The best method for liberation lies not in thinking it can be given as a gift. 'The correct method lies in dialogue' and 'Dialogue cannot exist without hope' (Freire 1972: 42, 64).

For professionals, patients and families who have suffered repeated patterns of neglect and deprivation, or are facing difficult dilemmas in hearing bad news, the experience of proper emotional care may be their first encounter with someone who talks kindly with them. It is a great privilege, and immensely rewarding, to be accepted and allowed to accompany professionals, individuals and families on their varied, uncertain and sometimes difficult journey.

Exercise 10.7

How are you going to improve how you talk with your patients? Where might you get help with this?

Resources

Group analysis
The Journal of Group Analytic Psychotherapy
www.sagepub.co.uk

The Group Analytic Society
258 Belsize Road
London
NW6 4BT
Tel: +44 (0)20 7316 1824
Fax: +44 (0)20 7316 1880
www.groupanalyticsociety.org

The Institute of Group Analysis
I Daleham Gardens
London NW3 5BY
Tel: +44 (0)20 7431 2693
email: iga@igalondon.org.uk
www.igalondon.org.uk

United Kingdom Council for Psychotherapists
167–169 Great Portland Street
London WIW 5PF
Tel: +44 (0)20 7436 3002
Fax: +44 (0)20 7436 3013
email: ukcp@psychotherapy.org.uk
www.psychotherapy.org.uk
Look under the psychoanalytic and psychodynamic section.

References

Ainsworth, J.D.S., Bell, S.M. and Stayton, D.J. (1971) Individual differences in strange situation behaviour of one-year olds, in H.R. Schaffer (ed.) *The Origins of Human and Social Relations*, 17–57. London: Academic Press.

Arber, A. and Gallagher, A. (2003) Breaking bad news revisited: the push for negotiated disclosure and changing practice implications, *International Journal of Palliative Nursing*, 9(4): 166–72.

Baile, W.F., Bast, R.C. Jr, Goldstein, M., Kudelka, A.P., Lenzi, R., Maguire, P., Myers, E.G. and Novack, D. (1997) Improving physician-patient communication in cancer care: outcome of a workshop for oncologists, *Journal of Cancer Education*, 12(3): 166–73.

Balint, M. (1963). *The Doctor, His Patient and the Illness*. Edinburgh: Churchill Livingstone.

Barnett, M.M. (2002) Effect of breaking bad news on patients' perceptions of doctors, *Journal of the Royal Society of Medicine*, 95(7): 343–7.

Bowlby, J. (1944) Forty-four juvenile thieves: their characters and home life, *International Journal of Psycho-Analysis*, 25: 19–52, 107–27.

Bowlby, J. (1951) *Maternal Care and Mental Health*. Geneva: World Health Organization.

Bowlby, J. (1988) *A Secure Base*. London: Routledge/Tavistock Books.

Buckman, R. (1992) *How to Break Bad News: A Guide for Health Professionals*. London: Macmillan.

Burman, E. (2001) Fictioning authority writing experience in feminist teaching and learning, *Psychodynamic Counselling*, 7(2): 187–205.

Cathcart, F. (1994a). *Understanding Death and Dying – Your Feelings*. Kidderminster: British Institute of Learning Disabilities.

Cathcart, F. (1994b). *Understanding Death and Dying – A Guide for Carers and Other Professionals*. Kidderminster: British Institute of Learning Disabilities.

Cathcart, F. (1994c) *Understanding Death and Dying – A Guide for Families and Friends*. Kidderminster: British Institute of Learning Disabilities.

Cohen, L., Agarwal, S.K., Baile, W.F., Henninger, E., Kudelka, A.P., Lenzi, R., Marshall, G.D. and Sterner, J. (2003) Physiological and psychological effects of delivering medical news using a simulated physician-patient scenario, *Journal of Behavioural Medicine*, 26(5): 459–71.

Colletti, L., Barclay, M., Gruppen, L. and Stern, D. (2001) Teaching students to break bad news, *American Journal of Surgery*, 182(1): 20–3.

Conboy-Hill, S. (1992) Grief, loss and people with learning disabilities, in S. Conboy-Hill and A. Waitman (eds) *Psychotherapy and Mental Handicap*. London: Sage.

Curtis, P. and Thomas, C. (1997) Having a baby: some disabled women's reproductive experiences, *Midwifery*, 13: 202–9.

Dalal, F. (1998) *Taking the Group Seriously*. London: Jessica Kingsley.

Draper, J. (2000–2002) *SkillsCascade.com*. www.skillscascade.com/badnews.htm (accessed 12 November 2003).

Egan, G. (1990) *The Skilled Helper: A Systematic Approach to Effective Helping*. Pacific Grove, CA: Brooks/Cole.

Emerson, P. (1977) Covert grief reactions in mentally retarded clients, *Mental Retardation*, 15(6): 27–9.

Farrell, M., Langrick, B. and Ryan, S. (2001) Breaking bad news within a paediatric setting; an evaluation report of a collaborative education workshop to support health professionals, *Journal of Advanced Nursing*, 36(6): 765–75.

Faulkner, A. and Maguire, P. (1994) *Talking to Cancer Patients and their Relatives*. Oxford: Oxford University Press.

Foulkes, S.H. (1971) *Selected Papers Psychoanalysis and Group Analysis*. London: Karnac Books.

Fraiberg, S., Adelson, E. and Shapiro, V. (1980) Chapter VII. Ghosts in the Nursery: A Psychoanalytic Approach to the Problems of Impaired Infant–Mother Relationships, in *Clinical Studies in Infant Mental Health: The First Year of Life*. London: Tavistock. 164–221.

Freire, P. (1972) *Pedagogy of the Oppressed*. Harmondsworth: Penguin.

Garland, C. (1999) *The Talking Cure*. London: BBC, 6 December.

Girgis, A. and Sanson-Fisher, R.W. (1998) Breaking bad news 1: current best advice for clinicians, *Behavioural Medicine*, 24(2): 53–9.

Girgis, A., McCarthy, W.H. and Sanson-Fisher, R.W. (1997) Communicating with patients: surgeons' perceptions of their skills and need for training, *Australian & New Zealand Journal of Surgery*, 67(11): 775–80.

Grant, G., Goward, P. and Ramcharan, P. (2003) Resilience, family care, and people with intellectual disabilities, *International Review of Research in Mental Retardation*, 26: 135–73.

Harper, D.C. and Wadsworth, J.S. (1993) Grief in adults with mental retardation: preliminary finding, *Research in Developmental Disabilities*, 14(4): 313–30.

Hawley, D.R. and DeHaan, L. (1996) Toward a definition of family resilience: integrating life span and family perspectives, *Family Process*, 35: 283–98.

Hollins, S. (1993) Group analytic therapy for people with a mental handicap, in S. Conboy-Hill and A. Waitman (eds) *Psychotherapy and Mental Handicap*. London: Sage.

Hollins, S. and Esterhuyzen, A. (1997). Bereavement and grief in adults with learning disabilities. *British Journal of Psychiatry* 17, 497–501.

Hollins, S. and Evered, C. (1990) Group process and content: the challenge of mental handicap, *Group Analysis*, 23: 55–67.

Hollins, S. and Grimer, M. (1988) *Pastoral Care and People with Mental Handicap*. London: SPCK.

Kaye, P. (1994) *A–Z Pocketbook of Symptom Control*. Northampton: EPL Publications.

Kirkham, M. (2000) *Developments in the supervision of midwives*. 2nd Edition. Previous ed: published as supervision of midwives 1996. Manchester: Book for Midwives.

Kirkham, M., Stapleton, H., Curtis, P., *et al.* (2002) Stereotyping as a professional defence mechanism. *British Journal of Midwifery*. **10**(9): 549–552.

Kitching, N. (1987) Helping people with mental handicap cope with bereavement, *Mental Handicap*, 15: 60–3.

Kubler-Ross, E. (1970) *On Death and Dying*. London: Tavistock.

Kern, D.E., Grayson, L.R., Barker, L.R. and Grayson, M. (1989) Residency training in interviewing skills and the psychosocial domain of medical practice, *Journal of General Internal Medicine*, 4: 422–31.

Laing, R.D. (1927) *Sanity, Madness and the Family: Families of Schizophrenics*. Harmondsworth: Penguin.

Le Roy, J. (1994) Group analysis and culture, in D. Brown and L. Zinkin (eds) *The Psyche and the Social World: Developments in Group-Analytic Theory*. London: Routledge.

Leick, N. and Davidson-Nielsen, M. (1991) *Healing Pain: Attachment, Loss and Grief*. London: Routledge.

Leon, E.G. (1990) *When a Baby Dies: Psychotherapy for Pregnancy and Newborn Loss*. New Haven, CT: Yale University Press.

Maguire, P. (1998) Breaking bad news, *European Journal of Surgical Oncology*, 24(3): 188–91.

Main, T. (1989) *The Ailment And Other Psychoanalytic Essays*. London: Karnac/ Free Association Books.

Marrone, M. (1998) *Attachment and Interaction*. London: Jessica Kingsley.

McEvoy, J. (1989) Investigating the concept of death in the mentally handicapped, *British Journal of Mental Subnormality*, 35(2): 115–21.

Menzies Lyth, I. (1988) The functioning of social systems as a defence against anxiety, in *Containing Anxiety in Institutions: Selected Essays*, vol. 1. Oxford: Free Association Books.

Mueller, P.S. (2002) Breaking bad news to patients: the SPIKES approach can make this difficult task easier, *Postgraduate Medicine Online*. 112(3). www.postgradmed.com/issues/2002/09_02/editorial_sep.htm (accessed 28 November 2003).

Oswin, M. (1991) *Am I Allowed To Cry?* London: Souvenir.

Pantlin, A.W. (1985) Group-analytic psychotherapy with mentally handicapped patients, *Group Analysis*, xviii(i): 44–53.

Perkins, J.J., Anseline, P., Gillespie, W.J., Lowe, A. and Sanson-Fisher, R.W. (1998) A preliminary exploration of the interactional skills of trainee surgeons, *Australian & New Zealand Journal of Surgery*, 68(9): 670–4.

Phipps, L.L. and Cuthill, J.D. (2002) Breaking bad news: a clinician's view of the literature, *Annals of the Royal College of Physicians & Surgeons of Canada*, 35(5): 287–93.

Ptacek, J.T. and Ellison, N.M. (2000) Health care providers' perspectives on breaking bad news to patients, *Critical Care Nursing Quarterly*, 23(2): 51–9.

Ramirez, A.J., Cull, A., Graham, J., Gregory, W.M., Leaning, M.S., Richards, M.A., Snashall, D.C. and Timothy, A.R. (1995) Burnout and psychiatric disorder among cancer clinicians, *British Journal of Cancer*, 71(6): 1132–3.

Raphael Leff, J. (1991) *Psychological Processes of Childbearing*. London: Chapman & Hall.

Raphael Leff, J. (1993) *Pregnancy: The Inside Story*. London: Karnac Books.

Read, S. (1998) Breaking bad news to people with a learning disability, *British Journal of Nursing*, 7(2): 86–91.

Read, S. (2001) A year in the life of a bereavement counselling and support service for people with learning disabilities, *Journal of Learning Disabilities*, 5(1): 19–33.

Rose, C. (2003) Scapegoating, *Counselling and Psychotherapy Journal*, July: 10–12.

Savage, J. (2004) Researching emotion: the need for coherence between focus, theory and methodology, *Nursing Inquiry*, 11(1): 25–34.

Specialist Psychotherapy Directorate (1995) *Psychoanalytic Psychotherapy Patient Information*. Sheffield: Sheffield Care Trust.

Twelvetree, S. (1995) Something's wrong, *Modern Midwife*, August: 22–4.

UKLD (2003) *A Guide to the Draft Mental Incapacity Bill – What does it mean for me?* www.uklearningdisabilities.co.uk (accessed 15 December 2003).

11

Experiences of family care

Bridging discontinuities over the life course

Gordon Grant

Introduction

For families with children or adults with learning disabilities, caregiving typically begins at an early stage in the lifecourse, continuing for many years, sometimes until the death of the caregiver. Over such a protracted period of time, parents and other family members face many challenges to their identities, to the structure and functioning of their support networks, to their capacity to maintain resilience in the face of daily stresses, and to their efforts to lead enriched lives outside the compass of their caregiving. Drawing from theoretical and empirical literature, and supported by case illustrations from the writer's own research, this chapter considers lifecourse experiences and discontinuities in family caregiving, and their implications for professional practice in relation to the support of families. To begin, it is necessary to ask the question 'who is the family?' and to challenge some popular stereotypes about family care of children and adults with learning disabilities.

Who is the family?

Posing the question 'who is the family?' may at first sight appear a little naïve, but since policy and professional practice is increasingly aligned to the idea of working in partnership with families (Department of Health 2001a, 2001b; Carers and Disabled Children Act 2000) it seems reasonable to say something about this.

Despite major economic, political and social changes, the family as an institution has still endured but family structures, family forms and the boundaries of families continue to be reshaped. In post-industrial societies people are marrying later, having fewer children, and becoming parents later in life. Women are realizing improved educational opportunities, greater control over their fertility, and increased participation in paid employment. People are also living longer so intergenerational ties may have greater significance, especially to those family members in caregiving roles. More significant than these developments perhaps is a growing acceptance of the diverse patterns of family life. In post-industrial societies the family can be represented in terms of the subjective meanings of intimate connections as well as formal, objective blood or marriage ties. As a result, no particular family form has a monopoly in terms of producing moral, autonomous, caring citizens (Silva and Smart 1999).

This applies equally to bringing up family members who happen to have disabilities. However, the influence of different family structures on the continuity and quality of care of disabled children at home remains a matter still meriting close and continuing research. In the context of changing definitions of 'family' for example, it is necessary to recognize the emergence, in recent decades, of families of choice, parenting across households, as well as parenting by people with learning disabilities (Booth and Booth 1999) (see also Chapter 22). The new genetics and sperm donorship will likely give rise to even newer family structures that have profound implications for forms of attachment, the enactment of reciprocity, and patterns of caregiving within families.

It is self-evident that 'the family' is more than the sum of those individuals who live in the same home. Improvements in health and survival together with social and geographic mobility lead to the dispersal of families, though not necessarily to their fragmentation. Technologies like the internet, email, cell phones and video links are contemporary means by which physical barriers to communication between family members can easily be accommodated, and responses to demands and crises dealt with. Such technologies represent one means by which care and support 'from a distance' can be brought into play. However, they cannot replace requirements for 'hands-on' support and care where direct contact, intimacy or constancy are necessary.

If families are to be supported to provide environments in which their disabled children can grow into contributing citizens, it will be important for health and social care professionals to take account of how families continue to define themselves in the face of changing technologies and cultural expectations.

Caregiving families

Stereotypes and half-truths?

Stereotypes about families with children and adults with learning disabilities abound within professional and academic discourses, though some of these appear to be more like myths and half-truths than positions substantiated by evidence.

Perhaps most common of all is a perception that some parents 'overprotect' their child, understate the child's true potential and reject help from services whenever it is offered. This leads to perceptions of such parents as being aloof, 'difficult to deal with' or even as perpetrators of the difficulties faced by their disabled children. Such perceptions ignore the fact that over the lifecourse parents may have had hopes raised and dashed many times by services and that they may well have good reasons to be sceptical, to withdraw from cooperating with services and to fall back on help from within the family circle. In this scenario, with parents acting as gatekeepers, it can be very difficult for professionals to gain access to the disabled child or adult at home, giving rise to professional anxieties about the child's 'best interests' (see also Chapter 5). The Andrews family typifies this view.

The Andrews family

Brenda and Stuart Andrews, wife and husband, are respectively sister and brother-in-law to Alan. Born with Down's syndrome, Alan had been living with Brenda and Stuart for 15 years since the death of Alan's father. Now aged 51 years, Alan had been showing symptoms of early onset Alzheimer's disease (AD), as evidenced by a major shift in his behaviour towards being withdrawn, uncommunicative and difficult to motivate. Stuart in particular found this difficult to cope with. For example, when Alan wandered off, pulled out his tongue or made facial grimaces, Stuart's typical response was to get angry even though he knew it may be a product of Alan's AD rather than malicious intent. Brenda's response was rather more measured and accommodative, but though she tried not to show her upset she still felt stressed by the situation. Brenda and Stuart described services as 'never having really shown any interest in them', and it was only a visit from a trainee social worker on a placement visit to the Andrews that triggered renewed interest in the situation. Despite this, recent professional attention focused on getting a clearer diagnosis of Alan's condition with a view to longer-term planning for him, rather than on identifying ways of helping Brenda and Stuart to manage Alan in a more agreed and consistent way.

For many years Brenda and Stuart had harboured scepticism about what services could do to help them – they resented paying charges for services and so made only minimal use of respite; they felt that services had not been very helpful in the recent past, and in any case took the view that Alan's problems were theirs, leading to a reluctance to engage services. Brenda and Stuart were perceived by the key worker as having dissimilar yet entrenched ways of coping with Alan at home, and this was believed to be contributing to Alan's behaviour problems.

A linked set of stereotypes concerns families as having agendas and needs that contrast with those of their children, rather than having mutual interests that are the natural product of interdependencies and reciprocities within the family. In this view, families are represented as being competitors against their disabled child for scarce professional resources. For instance, there is some evidence suggesting that professionals in key worker roles have a tendency to overstate differences in the needs and interests of parents and their disabled children (Williams and Robinson 2001a).

A further stereotype concerns presumptions about the widespread existence of stress and burden in families (Olsson and Hwang 2003), linked to a pathological view of families as passive, unresourceful and lacking in agency. Reinforcing this view therefore we still see services that prioritize stress reduction in families or providing them with a break from the 'daily grind' of caring. This position has been legitimized by a huge international literature obsessed by the stresses of bringing up disabled children at home.

Then there are families who are depicted as being paralysed by time, or frozen, as a result either of wanting to remember earlier times before they were engulfed by the pile up of caregiving demands, or being trapped by time and therefore unable to free themselves to do other things. In some defence of those suggesting a 'families as frozen' stance, the vast majority of the empirical literature about families of disabled children fails to consider temporal factors in family life due to the short-term nature of most research projects and their cross-sectional rather than longitudinal designs.

Exercise 11.1

Think of two or three families you know within your own social circle or other families with disabled children you have encountered from work or placement experiences. Ask yourself:

Which of the above stereotypes offers a way of characterizing each family?

What aspects of family life do these stereotypes capture well?

What aspects of family life do they fail to capture?

There is some truth in all of these stereotypes, but as such they only tell half the story. Before attempting to offer a fuller representation of the family caregiving experience, it is necessary to comment on theoretical perspectives that have informed family care studies.

Theoretical perspectives

Most prevalent within studies of families supporting children with disabilities are transactional stress-coping models (e.g. Lazarus and Folkman 1984; Orr *et al.* 1991). In these models people are seen as constantly appraising transactions with their environments; those seen as stressful (threatening or challenging) require coping to regulate distress or to manage the problem causing distress. The emphasis is very much on understanding the cognitive appraisals brought to situations, and the secondary and consequent appraisals of coping resources they can access to deal with these. Coping resources may be internal (e.g. skills, analytic ability) or external (e.g. finances, support networks). The huge body of literature based on these models has latterly come to realize that stresses are not unilaterally experienced and that coping has its rewards that can maintain people in potentially stressful situations for lengthy periods of time (Folkman 1997; Grant *et al.* 1998). Hence the coexistence of rewards and stresses in family care is quite common. Moreover there is mounting evidence about family strengths and resilience, the ability of families to embrace paradoxes in their everyday lives, and what disabled children and their families say about their everyday lives (Helff and Glidden 1998; Larson 1998; Connors and Stalker 2003; Grant *et al.* 2003b).

Commenting on the literature about adults in general, Aldwin (1994) has suggested that there are at least four ways that stress can result in positive effects:

- *the inoculation effect* – created by the expansion of people's coping repertoires through experience;
- *the increase in mastery effect* – which has more to do with improved self-confidence, skill and sense of control in dealing with situations;
- *changes in perspectives and values emerging from threatening circumstances* – leading to a reordering of a person's value hierarchy and improved coping;
- *the strengthening of social ties* under certain circumstances.

Through such means it is claimed that individuals develop improved self-understanding since it is thought that this leads to an explanatory or organizing framework for individuals that evolves over time. If true this might suggest that individuals and families become better able to cope with things over the lifecourse, even if they continue to live their lives under considerable pressures. However, evidence shows that services struggle both to understand how parents experience 'time' (Todd and Shearn 1996), how supportive services can best be tailored to fit family routines, and how they should be addressing the multiplicity of demands and obligations families face within and outside of their caring (Stalker 2003).

The search for explanations as to why some people appear to cope better than others under conditions of threat or adversity has led to an interest in resilience in individuals and families (see also Chapter 15). Prompting much of this interest was the work of Antonovsky (1987). His theoretical and main empirical claim was that maintaining a sense of coherence (SOC) in a challenging or apparently disordered world makes the difference between staying psychologically healthy or succumbing to life's vicissitudes. SOC was defined by Antonovsky as a:

> global orientation that expresses the extent to which one has a pervasive, enduring though dynamic feeling of confidence that (1) the stimuli derived from one's internal and external environments in the course of living are structured, predictable and explicable; (2) the resources are available to meet the demands posed by these stimuli; and (3) these demands are challenges, worthy of investment and engagement.
>
> (Antonovsky 1987: 19)

Antonovsky equated these parameters respectively as comprehensibility, manageability and meaningfulness, though he viewed the motivational component of meaningfulness as most crucial. There have been rigorous empirical tests of this model in the dementia care field though not yet, as far as is known, among families with children with learning disabilities.

Linked to the above, Hawley and DeHaan (1996) have attempted to integrate thinking about individual resilience to resilience as a family level construct. They suggest that: 'Family resilience describes the path a family follows as it adapts and prospers in the face of stress, both in the present and over time. Resilient families respond positively to these conditions in unique ways, depending on the context, developmental level, the interactive nature of risk and protective factors, and the family's shared outlook' (p. 293). Recognizing resilience thus seems to require us to investigate the following:

- individual dispositions, beliefs and values;
- familial, social and cultural resources that mould dispositions and opportunities;
- an ability to discern meaningfulness in what are often non-normative situations;
- capacity, linked perhaps to an understanding of individual and family history.

A further perspective worth mentioning here is the notion of 'boundary maintenance' and 'boundary ambiguity' within families. Due largely to the work of Pauline Boss (1988), this is an attempt to understand situations where there is some uncertainty about whether a person is 'inside' or 'outside' the family system. The boundary issue arises in circumstances where there is either psychological presence in the face of physical absence, or psychological absence in the face of physical presence, the latter being of particular relevance in families supporting people with cognitive disabilities where there are accompanying behavioural difficulties. Uncertainty as to the person's absence or presence is considered to hinder the family's ability to adapt to changes brought on by cognitive decline and shifts in behaviour patterns. In such conditions family caregivers can become immobilized, and fail to reorganize to meet new demands. Boss's work has concentrated largely on families with relatives with dementia.

Finally there is an argument to be made that families of disabled people are disabled by basically the same social barriers, prejudices and poorly conceived services as disabled people themselves (Dowling and Dolan 2001). In other words, the social model of disability (Oliver 1990) is just as relevant to an understanding of the everyday lives of families as it is to disabled people. This would stand in opposition to those adopting a families-as-competitors position, as described earlier. This being the case, it would therefore be logical to adopt a more systemic view of the family, where the ties that bind all family members together, as well as the rules and norms that underpin them, become important factors in understanding individual member and family-level needs and wants.

At the time of writing these appear to be the dominant theories and models informing family care research relevant to the lives of people with learning disabilities. However, there is still a considerable amount of largely atheoretical work being published that, in the writer's view, adds little to knowledge or to professional practice in working with families. Nevertheless, the perspectives briefly described above should be regarded merely as provisional or testable templates that may be helpful as guides to practice. There will be further cross-references to them in the following section.

Exercise 11.2

Revisit the families you thought of in Exercise 11.1. Now ask yourself:

What are the typical everyday challenges each family faces?

How do they deal with these challenges?

What theoretical perspectives best explain how each family deals with the situation?

Discontinuities and the lifecourse

Trajectories and clocks

For any family the lifecourse is always filled with ambiguities as well as with things that are more patterned and predictable. Individuals and families have only partial control over the environments in which they live, work and spend their leisure time so there are inevitably tensions and uncertainties about the interactions involved.

According to Heinz and Kruger (2001: 29), the lifecourse is 'a major institution of integration and tension between individual and society that provides the social and temporal contexts for biographical planning and stock-taking as well as for ways of adapting to changes in public and private time and space'. Using similar language, Clausen (1998: 196) suggests that the lifecourse can be likened to a developmental process in which the individual moves from being a helpless organism to a more or less autonomous person that: '(a) takes place in a changing cultural, social structural and historical setting; (b) increasingly involves individual choices as to the action taken; and (c) almost always entails both continuities and discontinuities'. In these definitions we therefore get the idea of individuals following pathways full of twists and turns where key transition points may be reached that can be life-changing. The birth of a child with lifelong disabilities in the family is perhaps a good example of a transition that may represent a major discontinuity for parents, or what has been called 'biographical disruption' (Bury 1982), yet in time it can also become transformative in more positive ways (Scorgie and Sobsey 2000).

Two metaphors are useful in helping to understand the processes involved – as clocks, and as journeys along trajectories.

Families face the ticking of different clocks and calendars that affect their choice-making and control over the entire lifecourse. Most obvious are the biological, physical and human development clocks of the disabled person and individual family members. Then there are social clocks representing the norms, values and rules about times when life events are expected to occur (Mills 2000). Finally there are calendars based on religious, family, employment or public service institutions. Families therefore may not always find their own expectations, 'schedules' and arrangements fitting neatly with demands and expectations set by other clocks or calendars. There may be culture and value clashes between families and services (see also Chapter 25). Families may find themselves carrying on caring for a long time and therefore 'out of synch' with other families. In addition they may find it hard to balance their use of private and public time.

The lifecourse can also be viewed as a journey along different time trajectories, each with their own routes and time demands. Journeying implies elements of agency, choice and control over the directions taken, though experiences and outcomes depend very much on perceptions of and responses to environmental demands encountered along the way. Four trajectories are considered below as a way of mapping family experiences of supporting disabled children over the lifecourse, and of spotting discontinuities. These are in turn: the caregiving trajectory, the development/disability trajectory, the family life cycle, and finally the service trajectory. Components of these are summarized in Table 11.1 which should be viewed as a heuristic device, rather than a definitive account of all the issues that will arise over the lifecourse.

The caregiving trajectory

Journeying along the caregiving trajectory can be likened to moving from a position as relative novice to ultimate expert. 'Stages' in the caregiving journey have been highlighted (Nolan *et al.* 1996; Grant *et al.* 2003a) that appear to signal important transitions. These have been described respectively as: 'building on the past' (before caregiving begins); 'recognizing the need'; 'taking it on'; 'working through it'; 'reaching the end'; and 'a new beginning'. Rather than describing these in detail here, some central points about continuities and discontinuities will be highlighted.

As Table 11.1 suggests, some families may find themselves having to contemplate bringing up a disabled child before the child is born, either because of genetic testing or because of prior knowledge of family risk factors for disabling conditions. Either way, moral and ethical questions are raised. Family members may feel uncomfortable about sharing details of possible hereditary factors within a close network of family and friends though genetic counselling may help with this (Pilnick *et al.* 2000). Although this 'building on the past' stage is really antecedent to 'hands-on' caregiving, it involves family members in information-seeking, planning and problem-solving, the

Table 11.1 Lifecourse trajectories

Caregiving trajectory	Development/disability trajectory	Life cycle	Service trajectory
Focus – effects of the 'stage' family carers have reached in moving from 'novice' to 'expert' carers	Focus – effects of construing disability as an ongoing process with landmarks, transition points and changing demands	Focus – effects of shifts in support network membership and intergenerational ties on values and adaptation	Focus – effects of transitions on development and adaptation as individuals move between health, education, social care and independent sector services
'Building on the past' – exposure to genetic counselling; caregiving ethics and values; acting on known risk factors for disability; 'caring about' invoked; pre 'caring for' stage	'Onset' – immediate or gradual; expected or unexpected	Family support network as: vehicle for transmitting values; opportunity structure for support; vehicle for substitute and complementary support; means of sustaining reciprocity	Is there a 'cradle to grave' commitment to family support agreed between services?
'Recognizing the need' – exposure to disclosure of disability; diagnostic limbo; biographical disruption; attachment formation; development of sense of coherence	'Course' – progressive, constant, relapsing/episodic; these being precursors of predictability	Support network dynamics affected by: death, incapacity or migration of family members; supportiveness of services	Compatibility of values and philosophy between services
'Taking it on' – novice and improvised caregiving; capacity to set limits on care; structures and routines for managing care; development of predictive competence	'Outcome' – impairment; disability and social-environmental barriers; shortened life expectancy; death dislocating	Potential for transfer of caregiving responsibility between family members to be dislocating	Continuity and reliability of support to families over the lifecourse

'Working through it' – managing 'invisible' care; realizing own identity needs; realizing caregiving rewards; achieving reciprocities	'Incapacity' – cognitive, sensory, mobility, energy and stigma; mediated by values, expectations and coping resources	Anticipation of future family support needs and care planning arrangements
'Reaching the end' – maintaining caregiving reciprocities; negotiation of future care plans; freedom to relinquish instrumental care; making ethical end-of-life decisions	Work-life balance important during working-age years	Commitment to tackling barriers that disable or marginalize families
'A new beginning' – freedom to commit to 'caring about' after relinquishing instrumental care; acting as an arbiter of care standards; maintaining meaningful involvement	Intergenerational ties, culture and ethnicity may be important in sustaining a commitment to family care	Ensuring families have a 'voice' alongside that of their disabled child
		Are family resources and expertise being incorporated into 'best practice'?
(Based on Grant et al. 2003a)	(Based on Rolland 1988)	

results of which have obvious life-changing potential. Engaging in such activity can be viewed as one of the manifestations of 'caring about' an unborn and possibly disabled child. Many parents in this position are likely to be dealing with probabilities and uncertainties about the outcomes, and even where disabled children are born the prognoses parents are offered by experts are not always reliable.

Because learning disability can be the product of a huge range of aetiologies, and indeed in many cases there is still no known cause, determination of developmental delay may be neither immediate nor accurate. Accordingly, parents can be left in a state of 'diagnostic limbo' for quite some time, which can itself be very disabling. Edelson's (2000) autobiography as a parent of a disabled son offers riveting descriptions of this phase of the family experience when the world seemed for a long time devoid of anyone who could 'make sense' of her son's condition. Such 'meaning-making' is remarkably difficult when, according to some commentators, 'parents must eventually focus attention on the present and future, maintain an accurate, undistorted view of the child's skills and abilities, hold a balanced view of the impact of this experience on themselves, and regulate their affective experience' (Pianta *et al.* 1996: 253). Even at such an early stage then, parents are thrust into having to rethink and make sense of present and future scenarios when they are probably still not in possession of all the facts, and may never be. In short, they are immediately catapulted into a time warp.

The conditions under which disclosure of disability is eventually made are especially important to parental and family adjustment, but there are still too many stories from families about negative experiences. Edelson's account is particularly evocative:

> I am somewhat alarmed to see that the doctor is flanked by five eager medical students. Their white coats belie the innocence of their fresh, young faces. The doctor practically rounds them up with his clipboard and prepares, it seems, to hold forth. My heart lurches into my throat.
>
> 'Your son has a rare brain condition called lissencephaly,' says the doctor. He is curt. It is clear that he is addressing his entourage as much as Jim and me. We still don't even know his name . . . 'I have the results of your son's MRI scan right here, I'm afraid,' says the doctor. 'Your own neurologist will discuss it with you further.'
>
> It is the Friday before the Labour Day long weekend. We are unlikely to track down 'our own' neurologist for several days. This unknown physician has just delivered tragic news in the middle of the crowded public hallway of an emergency department.
>
> (Edelson 2000: 41–2)

It is little wonder that families at this stage struggle to establish a sense of coherence (SOC) (Antonovsky 1987) where their capacity to make sense of the situation is under such severe threat.

In his review of earlier studies on the subject Cunningham (1994) describes parental dissatisfaction with disclosure as falling into three categories: the manner in which information was disclosed; problems with the information itself; and organizational arrangements. Although there are useful guidelines about good disclosure (see Chapter 10), there are still no guarantees that the practice of disclosure will be any better. It seems that professionals have special difficulties when 'bad news' has to be conveyed to individuals and families.

As families begin to 'take on' direct caregiving they are reported to improvise, and to discover the best ways of handling things very much by trial and error (Grant and Whittell 2000), for there are no books or 'handy recipes' for bringing up babies and young children, let alone those with disabilities. The Trevor family is a typical example. In this brief extract from an interview narrative, Mel Trevor is explaining the hit and miss nature of communicating with her 4-year-old daughter, Fiona:

Mel: The other hard thing is getting her to understand things. You have to repeat them over and over again. She picks up on most things quite easily but a lot of things she plays on it, and gets you quite frustrated and you don't know whether she is playing up or that she genuinely doesn't understand. That's the worst when you are sitting there and you are shouting at her and you're thinking, does she just not understand me, but when I questioned quite a few different people about it, they said to me to just treat her as if she did understand and would pick it up; even if she didn't, to just treat her normally anyway, to shout at her for doing something wrong.

Interviewer: So that is how you dealt with that?

Mel: Yes but I did get quite upset as to whether I was doing the right thing, should I shout at her or not? If I don't shout at her she'll get away with it, which she is very good at, playing the innocent . . . and [with Fiona] being the first [child] it was quite hard because you don't know what is normal.

Communicating meaningfully with a young child is basic to good care but the physical and psychological toll of doing so can be very taxing. During this phase it is common for families to spend lots of time information-seeking, yet setting limits on their caregiving to avoid burnout, and establishing structures and routines for managing things. It is something that helps to bring a degree of order and predictability into everyday life. It leads therefore to an 'increase in mastery effect', as previously described by Aldwin (1994).

'Working through it' connotes a proactive stance by families to maintain a sense of coherence (SOC) (Antonovsky 1987) in managing their affairs. It often coincides with a period during which families face a series of challenges to social and cultural norms, emphasizing the importance of social time (Mills 2000) – they may notice increasing differences in the emotional and intellectual development between their disabled child, siblings and other children. They will be reminded that theirs is likely to be a protracted period of caregiving – their disabled child continues to grow physically but as adulthood looms, rather ambiguous-looking issues of their child's adult citizenship status arise, for example about their autonomy, capacity and legal rights (Zetlin and Turner 1985; Simpson 2001). Furthermore, family members, parents in particular, have their own identity needs to think about – as wage earners, as people with vocational interests, as parents to other children, as people with obligations to the extended family, and so on. An unbridled commitment to caring for their disabled child may leave these other identity needs neglected. Mothers especially are reported to find combining employment with child care very difficult, a complex array of structural problems leading to mothers feeling marginalized and unfulfilled (Shearn and Todd 2000). At the same time, families typically report caregiving as being uplifting and rewarding as well as stressful, supporting Aldwin's (1994) assertions about the positive effects of challenges, and Larson's (1998) account of how parents manage paradoxes in their lives.

In 'reaching the end' of their caregiving careers, parents have reported increased reciprocities and interdependencies with their now adult children (Heller *et al.* 1997; Williams and Robinson 2001b), supporting Aldwin's (1994) assertions about how, under certain circumstances, social ties can be strengthened and changes in values and perspectives arise that help to sustain coping. However, it is still not clear whether such parents are effectively captives and dependent, for economic, physical and psychological reasons, upon keeping their disabled adult child at home.

In letting go to enable their adult child to live a more independent life in a home of their own, parents can find it very difficult to plan ahead with this in mind. Plans can be fragile and prone to change, with financial and legal matters far from clarified (Prosser 1997). During this stage of caregiving there is likely to be an accumulation of concerns and anxieties about what will happen after the death of the parents. Underlying this, parents can feel that others (statutory or not-for-profit agencies) will be unable to provide the standard of personalized support that they have given over a lifetime. Alternatively there can also be strong feelings from parents about the preference of predeceasing their sons or daughters.

The Crosby family

The Crosby family are fairly typical of others in this respect. David Crosby, 22 years of age, still lived at home with his parents, Margaret, 60, and Tom, 68. David, Margaret and Tom had for some time been discussing alternative permanent accommodation for David. Reflecting on the resolution of end-of-life issues, Margaret summed things up as follows:

> But I've always said, and a lot of parents say the same, I would rather grieve for David than have David grieving for me. I know then that David is safe. We've looked after him and he's safe and nobody can harm him; and he's not going to go into care where he's going to be

ill-treated and perhaps be abused, because they're very vulnerable, so trusting and can easily be hurt. They're very feeling and understanding, and that's what really worries me.

This can lead to even very well informed parents like Margaret and Tom again feeling trapped by time, aware of the balance of risks and benefits for David, yet paralysed all the same by indecision about future living options. However, some older parents never complete 'launching' their offspring towards a more independent life because they do not wish to, for reasons to do with the feelings of intimacy, assertiveness and sense of control they experience (Tobin 1997). The question still has to be asked – in whose interests is this?

Even after relinquishing responsibility for direct hands-on caregiving, families typically continue to 'care about' their adult relative, and express a desire to maintain some involvement in their lives. Where care and support is shared with agencies, families may have important roles to play as arbiters of care standards since they will still retain more particularistic knowledge about their relative, and know what works best for them. It is therefore important that families are not abandoned by services the minute that agencies take charge of things.

The development/disability trajectory

As suggested in Table 11.1, disability can be construed as an ongoing process with landmarks, transition points and changing demands. Categorizations of the 'disability trajectory' put forward by Rolland (1988) are helpful here. Though at first sight this has the appearance of being a medical view of disability, this is not really the case as it intersects with biological and psychosocial worlds.

The 'onset' of a disability may be immediate or gradual, and expected or unexpected, the particular circumstances of the onset creating potentially life-changing adjustments in families, as already described.

The 'course' of a disability may be progressive, constant or relapsing and episodic. For people with multiple disabilities and those with accompanying chronic illnesses there may be 'courses' running in parallel which complicate the everyday management of caregiving as well as the development of a predictive capacity in families. Where the 'course' of a disability is fairly constant and predictable then management and coping is likely to be easier. In progressive conditions, for example early onset dementia in people with Down's syndrome, families have to deal with symptoms that manifest in a stepwise or progressive fashion. Even though the course may to some degree be predictable, never knowing what challenges are just around the corner, and whether these are going to be comprehensible or manageable (Antonovsky 1987) is extremely taxing, as was seen in the case of the Andrews family described earlier.

The 'outcome' of a disability relates primarily to the expectation of death, and shortened life expectancy. Although the life expectancy of people with learning disabilities is steadily improving there are syndromes like the San Felipo sydrome and lissencephaly, among others, that lead to premature death. In circumstances like these, the compressing of time horizons can lead parents to act as if every day was the last for their son or daughter, resulting in an over-indulgent approach to caregiving that undermines the person's autonomy and self-image as a contributing citizen. Expressed another way, it represents a major discontinuity between the biographical or developmental clock of the person with a disability and the family's construct of social time (Mills 2000), as the typical timing of life events and family routines are thrown out of kilter.

'Incapacity' is the final dimension outlined by Rolland, comprising five areas: cognitive, sensory, mobility, energy and stigma. Different types of incapacity are seen to require different responses from families, mediated by their values, expectations and coping resources. Families who are more inclined to fostering autonomy generally limit incapacity while those that 'take over' increase incapacity. This highlights the importance of understanding the degree of congruence in the expectations and views of disabled people and their families about autonomy and interdependence. Shifts in incapacity will often trigger the need for a realignment of caregiving intensity and organization.

The family life cycle

Family life cycle considerations are concerned here with the effects on adaptation and everyday coping of shifts in support network membership and intergenerational ties. From studies of assessment practices with family carers, key areas of their lives are reported to be overlooked, including their health, housing, work, ability to continue caring, and their rights and entitlements (Williams and Robinson 2001a). Assessments, and continuing dialogue, tend to focus on mothers, to the exclusion of other family members, uncannily reflecting much of the research literature on family care which is based largely on maternal accounts. If this orientation is allowed to prevail, the support needs of the family unit are at risk of being neglected, as well as its helping resources and expertise.

In looking at the family support network as a whole, it is important to recognize the significance of the values, world views and cultural practices of family members since it is these that define and cement intra-family relationships. They will also alert practitioners to ways of helping that are culturally acceptable and therefore meaningful to families, thereby helping to sustain a resilient outlook as described by Antonovsky (1987). The family network can be looked upon as an opportunity structure for providing support and care, though it should be borne in mind that not all family members provide support, and not all support is received as supportive (Ell 1996). Indeed families are also a context in which abuse and neglect of people with relatives with learning disabilities occurs, though not as frequently as appears to be the case in services (O'Callaghan *et al.* 2003).

Family support networks undergo transformation and change as a result of death, incapacity or migration of family members, though to a degree these can be anticipated over the lifecourse. As parents age their health and capacity may decline; siblings can be expected to leave home at an age-appropriate time in order to set up their own home, or to pursue college or employment opportunities; and older family members who have been providing some help, support and advice may die at some point. Family support networks can undergo quite major transitions like these in relatively short periods of time, but the repercussions of these for a realignment of family support are not always picked up by front-line health and social care practitioners (Grant 1993).

The role of grandparents in supporting families of children with learning disabilities has until lately received little attention. There is no denying that grandparents can be a valuable resource in providing a wide range of instrumental and emotional support, but recent research indicates that relationships between parents and grandparents are not benign, and that conflict or disagreement with grandparents can affect the experience of stress in parents, mothers more than fathers (Hastings *et al.* 2002). This once again points towards the need for a better understanding of the basis of reciprocities within the family, in this case across the generations. In Hastings *et al.*'s (2002) study and in other research (Grant and Whittell 2000; Salovita *et al.* 2003) mothers and fathers appear to have different stress reactions and coping styles. The implications of these gender-related differences for consistent support to young and adult disabled children in the family requires closer investigation.

The service trajectory

The focus of the service trajectory is on the effects of transitions on family adaptation and development, as individuals move through different services. Over the lifecourse this is likely to involve serial encounters by people with disabilities and their families with health, education, housing, social care and independent-sector services. With each service sector being driven by its own values, philosophy, working methods and rules, families face a major challenge in obtaining and making sense of information about relevant services and supports, before they can begin to feel comfortable about using them. Despite considerable investment by policy-makers in promoting seamless services, there has been little empirical investigation of how transitions between services are experienced and evaluated by families right across the lifecourse. Investigations seem to concentrate on the early childhood years with experiences about disclosure of disability and early counselling (see earlier this chapter) or else transitions from child to adult services (e.g. Thorin *et al.* 1996; Simpson 2001). More integrated perspectives are required that take a longer-term view of the lifecourse, as in Bigby's (2004) recent work on ageing with a lifelong disability.

At the moment, there does not seem to be an agreed view, nationally, about what would be regarded as successful outcomes of service interventions for families supporting others with disabilities (Nicholas 2003), and this applies to families at all stages of the lifecourse. There are a whole series of questions to be asked here:

- Is there a 'cradle to grave' commitment to the support of families agreed between services?
- Is there compatibility of service values and philosophy between the different services?
- Is there continuity and reliability of support to families over the lifecourse?
- Are family resources and expertise being incorporated into best practice?
- Are the anticipatory needs and hopes of families being accommodated alongside those of the disabled person?
- Is there an agreed plan to tackle the barriers that disable or marginalize families?
- And who, on behalf of the family, is responsible for making sure that all this will happen?

Conclusion

The focus of this chapter has been family experiences of supporting children and adult members with learning disabilities, and discontinuities that can arise over the lifecourse. Discontinuities within individual lifecourse trajectories have been identified. It has been noted that these are often far from predictable and quite often not within the control of families. However, it is also necessary to scan across these trajectories to get a more complete picture of the range of challenges faced by families over the lifecourse. From the evidence available it seems that not all these discontinuities are yet within the field of view of services. One way of mapping these has been outlined in this chapter, together with a description of theories that may help to guide practice.

Perhaps the central message here is that families want more certainty in their lives, and an ability to be able to influence the present and future conditions under which good quality support and care for their child is provided. Greater recognition by professionals of the ways different 'clocks' and 'journeys' along lifecourse trajectories are experienced by families seems to be one means by which this could be achieved. This requires from professionals a shift towards empowering the family as a whole (Grant 2003), implying a need to understand how families:

- define themselves, and the importance of their social and cultural resources;
- describe their 'journeys' along different lifecourse trajectories;
- describe the basis of reciprocity and exchange within the family;

- demonstrate what family strengths, expertise and coping strategies are relevant to good care;
- manage their identity needs, and the competing demands upon their time and resources;
- frame concerns and preferences about their continuing involvement in future care and support arrangements;
- define disabling barriers, including services, that prevent hopes from being realized.

It seems appropriate to leave the last word to one of the families whose lives have been glimpsed in this chapter. In this short interview extract Margaret Crosby sums up past and present discontinuities, very much aware of comparisons with her peers:

> My husband and I, we've got a very strong marriage . . . In the beginning [following diagnosis of David's disability] you're all hurting and you're not really talking about the problem because you're protecting everybody. You don't want to hurt them. Do you know what I mean? I recall a holiday when we went away on our own. We booked with Shearings and went to Ireland. I didn't want David to know we were going because I didn't want him to be upset . . . I felt we really needed this holiday by ourselves. But you go away for a holiday and what happens? I enjoyed it but you're stricken with guilt because you've left him behind. You can never shut off. Whereas when I hear my friends talking, I'm not envious of them, don't get me wrong, but when they say, 'Oh we're going to so and so', they can go without any problem. If David was a 'normal' 22-year-old he would probably have a life of his own, a girlfriend, he could easily be married and living in a flat. I could say to my husband, 'Come on let's go', but we can't do that. Most people with disabled children or who are caring for them, you can't just do that because you've got to make arrangements . . .

Exercise 11.3

Consider the Crosby family:

First, identify the discontinuities that Margaret Crosby mentions in her experiences of family care.

Then consider what 'trajectories' are relevant in understanding the stance Margaret takes about going away on a holiday.

Based on your existing knowledge, what advice and help would you give to the Crosby family about their holiday plan?

References

Aldwin, C.M. (1994) *Stress, Coping and Development: An Integrative Perspective*. New York: The Guilford Press.

Antonovsky, A. (1987) *Unraveling the Mystery of Health*. San Francisco, CA: Jossey Bass.

Bigby, C. (2004) *Ageing with a Lifelong Disability: A Guide to Practice, Program and Policy Issues for Human Services Professionals*. London: Jessica Kingsley.

Booth, T. and Booth, W. (1999) Parents together: action research and advocacy support for parents with learning difficulties, *Health and Social Care in the Community*, 7(6): 464–74.

Boss, P. (1988) *Family Stress Management*. Thousand Oaks, CA: Sage.

Bury, M. (1982) Chronic illness as biographical disruption, *Sociology of Health and Illness*, 4: 167–82.

Clausen, J.A. (1998) Life reviews and life stories, in J.Z. Giele and G.H. Elder (eds) *Methods of Life Course Research: Qualitative and Quantitative Approaches*. Thousand Oaks, CA: Sage.

Connors, C. and Stalker, K. (2003) *The Views and Experiences of Disabled Children and their Siblings: A Positive Outlook*. London: Jessica Kingsley.

Cunningham, C. (1994) Telling parents their child has a disability, in P. Mittler and H. Mittler (eds) *Innovations in Family Support for People with Learning Disabilities*, Chorley: Lisieux Hall.

Department of Health (2001a) *Valuing People: A New Strategy for Learning Disability for the 21st Century*. London: Department of Health.

Department of Health (2001b) *Family Matters: Counting Families In*. London: Department of Health.

Dowling, M. and Dolan, L. (2001) Families with children with disabilities – inequalities and the social model, *Disability and Society*, 16(1): 21–35.

Edelson, M. (2000) *My Journey with Jake: A Memoir of Parenting and Disability*. Toronto: Between the Lines.

Ell, K. (1996) Social networks, social support and coping with serious illness: the family connection, *Social Science and Medicine*, 42(2): 173–83.

Folkman, S. (1997) Positive psychological states and coping with severe stress, *Social Science and Medicine*, 45(8): 1207–21.

Grant, G. (1993) Support networks and transitions over two years among adults with a mental handicap, *Mental Handicap Research*, 6(1): 36–55.

Grant, G. (2003) Caring families: their support or empowerment? in K. Stalker (ed.) *Reconceptualising Work with Carers: New Directions for Policy and Practice*. London: Jessica Kingsley.

Grant, G. and Whittell, B. (2000) Differentiated coping strategies in families with children or adults with intellectual disabilities: the influence of gender, family composition and the life span, *Journal of Applied Research in Intellectual Disabilities*, 13(4): 256–75.

Grant, G., Ramcharan, P., McGrath, M., Nolan, M. and Keady, J. (1998) Rewards and gratifications among family caregivers: towards a refined model of caring and coping, *Journal of Intellectual Disability Research*. 42(1): 58–71.

Grant, G., Nolan, M. and Keady, J. (2003a) Supporting families over the life course: mapping temporality, *Journal of Intellectual Disability Research*, 47(4/5): 342–51.

Grant, G., Ramcharan, P. and Goward, P. (2003b) Resilience, family care and people with intellectual disabilities, *International Review of Research in Mental Retardation*, 26: 135–73.

Hastings, R.P., Thomas, H. and Delwiche, N. (2002) Grandparent support for families of children with Down's syndrome, *Journal of Applied Research in Intellectual Disabilities*, 15: 97–104.

Hawley, D.R. and DeHaan, L. (1996) Toward a definition of family resilience: integrating life span and family perspectives, *Family Process*, 35: 283–98.

Heinz, W.R. and Kruger, H. (2001) Lifecourse: innovations and challenges for social research, *Current Sociology*, 49: 29–45.

Helff, C.M. and Glidden, L.M. (1998) More positive or less negative? Trends in research on adjustment of families having children with developmental disabilities, *Mental Retardation*, 36(6): 457–64.

Heller, T., Miller, A.B. and Factor, A. (1997) Adults with mental retardation as supports to their parents: effects on parental caregiving appraisal, *Mental Retardation*, 35: 338–46.

Larson, E. (1998) Reframing the meaning of disability to families: the embrace of paradox, *Social Science and Medicine*, 47(7): 865–75.

Lazarus, R.S. and Folkman, S. (1984) *Stress, Appraisal and Coping*. New York: Springer.

Mills, M. (2000) Providing space for time: the impact of temporality on life course research, *Time and Society*, 9: 91–127.

Nicholas, E. (2003) An outcomes focus in carer assessment and review: value and challenge, *British Journal of Social Work*, 33: 31–47.

Nolan, M., Grant, G. and Keady, J. (1996) *Understanding Family Care: A Multi-dimensional Model of Caring and Coping*. Buckingham: Open University Press.

O'Callaghan, A., Murphy, G. and Sinclair, N. (2003) The impact of abuse on men and women with severe learning disabilities and their families, *British Journal of Learning Disabilities*, 31(4): 175–80.

Oliver, M. (1990) *The Politics of Disablement*. London: Macmillan.

Olsson, M.B. and Hwang, P.C. (2003) Influence of macrostructure of society on the life situation of families with a child with intellectual disability: Sweden as an example, *Journal of Intellectual Disability Research*, 47(4/5): 328–41.

Orr, R.R., Cameron, S.J. and Day, D.M. (1991) Coping with stress in children who have mental retardation: an evaluation of the double ABCX model, *American Journal on Mental Retardation*, 95: 444–50.

Pianta, R.C., Marvin, R.S., Britner, P.A. and Borowitz, K.C. (1996) Mothers' resolution of their children's diagnosis: organised patterns of caregiving representations, *Infant Mental Health Journal*, 17: 239–56.

Pilnick, A., Dingwall, R., Spencer, E. and Finn, E. (2000) *Genetic Counselling: A Review of the Literature*, discussion paper 00/01. Sheffield: Trent Institute for Health Services Research.

Prosser, H. (1997) The future care plans of older adults with intellectual disabilities living at home with family carers, *Journal of Applied Research in Intellectual Disabilities*, 10: 15–32.

Rolland, J.S. (1988) *Families, Illness and Disability*. New York: Basic Books.

Salovita, T., Italinna, M. and Leinonen, E. (2003) Explaining the parental stress of fathers and mothers caring for a child with intellectual disability: a double ABCX model, *Journal of Intellectual Disability Research*, 47(4/5): 300–12.

Scorgie, K. and Sobsey, D. (2000) Transformational outcomes associated with parenting children who have disabilities, *Mental Retardation*, 38: 195–206.

Shearn, J. and Todd, S. (2000) Maternal employment and family responsibilities: the perspectives of mothers of children with intellectual disabilities, *Journal of Applied Research in Intellectual Disabilities*, 13: 109–31.

Silva, E.B. and Smart, C. (eds) (1999) *The New Family?* London: Sage.

Simpson, M. (2001) Programming adulthood: intellectual disability services and adult services, in D. May (ed.) *Transition and Change in the Lives of People with Intellectual Disabilities*. London: Jessica Kingsley.

Stalker, K. (2003) *Reconceptualising Work with Carers: New Directions for Policy and Practice*. London: Jessica Kingsley.

Thorin, E., Yovanoff, P. and Irvin, L. (1996) Dilemmas faced by families during their young adults' transitions to adulthood: a brief report, *Mental Retardation*, 34(2): 117–20.

Tobin, S.S. (1997) A non-normative age contrast: elderly parents caring for offspring with mental retardation, in V.L. Bengston (ed.) *Adulthood and Aging: Research on Continuities and Discontinuities*. Berlin: Springer-Verlag.

Todd, S. and Shearn, J. (1996) Struggles with time: the careers of parents with adult sons and daughters with learning disabilities, *Disability and Society*, 11(3): 379–401.

Williams, V. and Robinson, C. (2001a) More than one wavelength: identifying, understanding and resolving conflicts of interest between people with intellectual disabilities and their family carers, *Journal of Applied Research in Intellectual Disabilities*, 14: 30–46.

Williams, V. and Robinson, C. (2001b) 'He will finish up caring for me': people with learning disabilities and mutual care, *British Journal of Learning Disabilities*, 29: 56–62.

Zetlin, A.G. and Turner, J.L. (1985) Transition from adolescence to adulthood: perspectives of mentally retarded individuals and their families, *American Journal of Mental Deficiency*, 89: 570–9.

12

Promoting healthy lifestyles

Physical and sensory needs

Bronwyn Roberts

Introduction

As will be seen in this chapter, people with profound and multiple learning disabilities (PMLD) face enormous challenges in maintaining good physical health and well-being. Drawing upon both medical and social constructions of disability, this chapter examines conditions that affect many people with PMLD – cerebral palsy, visual impairment, hearing impairment – and the communication challenges they pose for practitioners. Based on the evidence, suggestions are made about how these challenges can be addressed.

Background

There is no universally accepted definition of PMLD. However, it is commonly associated with pronounced developmental delay with significant physical and sensory impairments and epilepsy (Ware 2003). Communication difficulties are also common (Kelly 2000), and some 80 per cent of affected individuals will have physical impairments that affect mobility. Some definitions have looked at functional skills to help classify individuals' abilities (Hogg and Sebba 1986), while Ware (2003) recognizes that people with PMLD need maximum assistance and 24-hour support, in all aspects of daily living. For this chapter the definition of PMLD will include people with a profound learning disability, people with sensory impairments and people with a physical impairment. Coordination of muscles, cerebral palsy and asymmetrical body shapes will also be considered as many people with PMLD experience some or all these conditions. In essence it is recognized that PMLD sufferers are people with high health and social support needs.

It has been estimated that there are about 210,000 people with PMLD and that around 65,000 of this number are children and young people (Department of Health 2001). The Department of Health also suggest that the number of people with severe learning disabilities may increase by around 1 per cent per annum for the next 15 years as a result of the growing numbers of children and young people with complex and multiple disabilities who are now surviving into adulthood (Department of Health 2001). These figures highlight the need for appropriate services to be developed for people with high support needs.

The care and nurturing of a child is a complex and multi-dimensional process, involving emotional, cognitive, physical and psychological aspects. This complexity of care increases when the child concerned has profound learning and physical impairments. Care can often appear to revolve around the daily living activities of eating, drinking, intimate personal care and getting dressed and undressed, which are essential activities if fundamental needs are going to be met. Roberts and Lawton (2001) showed that the majority of children with PMLD in their study required extra assistance or supervision with multiple areas of daily life. They looked at five activities (washing, dressing, meal times, during the night and keeping occupied) and found that more than 70 per cent of the children needed extra help to complete these activities. These findings further highlight the fact that children with severe disabilities have considerable extra care needs in many areas of daily life.

It is easy to think of people with PMLD as having a multitude of needs by concentrating on the impairments and the care needed, often utilizing a medical model of care – i.e. a predominant focus on medical conditions as defining the person. However, it is well documented (Department of Health 1995, 1998, 1999a, 1999b, 2001; Kerr 1998; Barr 1999) that the health care experience of people with a learning disability is far from adequate. Kerr (1998) suggests that the British health care system appears to be failing in meeting even the ordinary health care needs of this group, particularly in regard to health promotion and the identification of ill health. He recognizes a 'health divide' between people with learning difficulties and the rest of the population. Morris (1999) has a differing slant to these problems when she identifies that it is not the individual's needs that are complex, but the trials they have to endure to find appropriate help. The labels of 'profound', 'complex needs', 'multiple needs' and 'severe learning disability' also highlight obvious needs and impairments, often reflected in lists of what someone cannot, rather than what they can, do. In developing services to promote a positive and healthy lifestyle it is essential that we recognize the individual: a person unique in what they can achieve with their skill base enhanced by appropriate support services. The medical model of care highlights the deficiencies the person has, while other models highlight social barriers (Richardson 1997; Race 2002). Barriers to good health care cited by the Scottish Executive (2002) include:

- *physical barriers* – poor wheelchair access to health care facilities;
- *administrative barriers* – appointment times too short for people who

are non-verbal; waiting times to see GPs and consultants too long for people with poor concentration and for people who are hyper-active;

- *communication barriers* – inability of doctors to understand different communication styles, the difficulties of a person with PMLD to describe symptoms;
- *attitudinal barriers* – negative assumptions and attitudes about people with learning disabilities, for example not offering pain relief to people with a learning disability;
- *knowledge barriers* – limited theory and practice experience of the health needs of people with learning disabilities.

For children with cerebral palsy and associated impairments the task of maintaining basic physical activities of life can appear to be very simplistic. However to achieve a positive and healthy lifestyle and see the child from a positive perspective can be an enormous challenge.

Clare, a first-year student nurse, had her first placement with people who have complex care needs. She felt hopeless, useless and completely overwhelmed by the people she met: 'I felt really nervous, I didn't realise really what complex needs had meant, I didn't realise what people would look like. I didn't want to hurt anyone and I certainly didn't know how to approach someone. I didn't know what to say. Lunchtime was a nightmare. It sounds a simple task helping someone with a meal but it was really difficult'.

These challenges include enhancing life opportunities, building choices into everyday living (Ware 2003) and learning to communicate rather than teaching communication (Nind and Hewett 2001). We need to recognize that the health of any group is about positive lifestyles based on abilities and strengths that guide and enable interventions. Due to the nature of having PMLD some children miss out on essential learning opportunities that impact on how they know themselves and their environment. These missed opportunities are made worse if their environment is not manipulated to enhance their abilities. A visually stimulating room will not reward the child with a vision impairment, just as a room that utilizes sounds well will not reward a person with a hearing impairment. There are many different views regarding quality of life and how we perceive and measure it (see Chapter 7). However, in assessing quality, we must take into account all facets of the person including their physical, social, emotional and spiritual abilities and interests (British Medical Association 1999). Quality services must also control everyday environments, so that they stimulate and reward the person with PMLD. This chapter aims to identify practical strategies to help meet these challenges.

It has already been highlighted that a person with PMLD will have a variety of health care needs. It is essential that the person is supported to maximize their health state and in doing so it is possible to maximize their chance of having an active and fulfilling life. For example, a person with untreated chronic constipation will not be in the best state of health and will probably be lethargic and in pain. Understanding some of the main impairments faced by people with PMLD, and the barriers experienced in everyday life, helps to highlight what can be done to improve health, personal well-being and social inclusion.

Cerebral palsy

Cerebral palsy (CP) is a condition that affects both movement and sensation. It is caused by damage to different parts of the brain. The damage may occur before birth, at birth or in early childhood. As a result of this damage the child might have poor coordination, difficulties in balancing and unusual patterns of movement. Some children's movement may only be slightly affected and they can learn strategies to manage their condition, while others may be more severely affected requiring long-term support. At birth it is not always possible to identify which type of CP the child will have. Movement and coordination difficulties will be easier to identify as the child grows and develops (Rennie 2001). Depending on where the damage has occurred and the extent of the damage to the brain, the child may have other associated impairments. These include epilepsy, visual impairment, hearing impairment, communication, eating and drinking difficulties, emotional and/or behavioural difficulties and varying degrees of learning disability (Cogher *et al.* 1992; Miller and Bachrach 1995; Lacey and Ouvry 2000).

There are four main types of CP which describe the difficulties with movement and coordination that the child might have:

- *Hypertonic (spastic) CP*. Children with this type of CP have increased muscle tone. They may find their muscles becoming very stiff, especially when they try and move (e.g. when they reach out to a toy). This can reduce the amount of movement they have due to the hypertension in their muscles. It can also make the child fearful to move as they may have difficulties in balancing.

- *Hypotonic (flaccid or floppy) CP*. Children with this type of CP have a decrease in muscle tone. The muscles are soft and floppy with little strength in them. Having hypotonic muscles means that the muscles do not support the joints, resulting in the joints having an increased range of movement.

- *Athetoid CP*. Children with this type of CP have continuous and unwanted movements that they cannot control. Their limbs move in a slow writhing motion often described as snake-like movements. These movements increase when the child wants to complete an action. If the child wants to pick up a toy the arm and hand will writhe in all directions before landing on the toy.

- *Ataxic CP*. Children with this type of CP have lack of balance and demonstrate sharp and jerky movements. These movements describe all of their motion including the way they move their body or arm (e.g. when reaching out to touch an object), as well as movement of their whole body when they attempt to move around (e.g. start to crawl).

Exercise 12.1

Sitting in an easy chair, bend your arms up to rest on your chest. Clench your fists and tense your arm and shoulder muscles. Without releasing the muscle tension attempt to move your arms away from your body. It is very difficult if not impossible to do so. Maintain the muscle tension for several minutes and then relax. Be conscious of how your muscles ache and the strain placed upon them in the few minutes you have been doing this exercise. Take some time and reflect upon your feelings. How might hypertonia affect someone's voluntary movement?

Having CP will affect how a child moves, movement being an essential basic ability to react to surroundings and explore and learn about the environment. Movement is also a way of expressing our personality, emotions and moods. Movement for a child with CP can cause pain, discomfort and distress and this can discourage the child from moving. Alternatively, lax and weak muscle tone can make movement extremely difficult and often the reward is not worth the effort. Assessment of the child's ability to move is essential to all plans for learning and care. A few simple questions can help identify difficulties in movement:

- How does the child move when placed on the floor?
- Are there any abnormal patterns of movement?
- What does the muscle tone feel like?
- Does the child use one side more than the other?

Unfortunately the more severe types of CP can result in the development of unusual body shapes. This is due to the tightness of the muscles changing the shape of the spine, limb alignments and body symmetry. Primitive reflexes that disappear as the child develops normal movement patterns can be retained in children with CP and these also affect the shape and posture of the child. Long-term effects of gravity can pull the body into asymmetry and can 'flatten' the trunk and limbs. If the child uses one side of the body more than the other (e.g. always rolling to one side and not the other), the body will not develop symmetrically. This will make the development of balance, eye-to-hand coordination, perceptual skills and movements more difficult. It can also contribute to the development of muscle contractures, body and limb shape changes and hip dislocation (Stolk *et al.* 2000).

Exercise 12.2

Think about your body and the shapes it takes on when sitting, standing and lying down. How often is your position symmetrical? Symmetrical positions are often the most comfortable as our bodies are arranged equally and are balanced. How long can you sit in a position that is not symmetrical before you make slight adjustments to your position? We are constantly moving, if only slightly, so as to allow blood to flow, ease aching muscles and take weight off joints that are under strain. This constant movement also helps our digestion and elimination processes, lung performance and circulation. Reflect upon someone with CP and assess how much voluntary movement they have. Consider how their movements might affect their body systems and the impact this may have on their health state.

There are many methods of assessing posture and body shape (Pountey *et al.* 1990; Goldsmith and Goldsmith 1996), but there are four simple questions that can be asked to aid identification of body asymmetry (Lacey and Ouvry 2000: 18):

- Does the body tend to stay in a limited number of positions?
- Do the knees seem to be drawn to one side, or outwards, or inwards?
- Does the head seem to turn mainly to one side?
- Is the body shape already asymmetrical?

If the answer is yes to any of these questions, postural management is essential to support the body and to protect body symmetry. Maintaining symmetry is important for the body systems to work to their optimum capacity. An asymmetrical body can reduce the space for body organs and even compress them. In the worst scenario, organs and systems can even be pushed out of their usual position. A compressed stomach will affect the process of digestion, reduce the space available for food and may cause reflux. Compression on the lower bowel will affect the normal muscle contractions (peristalsis), slow down food passing through the digestive system and cause constipation. A chair that supports the child in symmetry and alignment is needed to ensure that food eaten can be processed effectively without causing the child digestive problems.

For a child with CP having their body supported in symmetry becomes a 24-hour necessity. We spend approximately a third of our lives sleeping so even sleeping positions need to be considered in promoting postural management. Whatever activities are occurring, symmetry of position must be central to the activity. Our first challenge is to identify appropriate positions to support body symmetry that can be utilized as part of the daily activities for the child. Posture management becomes integral to the activity and is not carried out as specific therapy.

Exercise 12.3

Think about a variety of play situations a child will enjoy. Identify two play activities that could be undertaken while the child is posturally aided in sitting up, lying on one side, lying on their back and standing.

Helping strategies

The following are some useful helping strategies:

- An asymmetrical body shape can affect the internal body systems. If the stomach and digestive tract are compromised, this may be managed by providing small nutritional meals more often, rather than attempting to provide a third of the daily requirements in three large meals. This strategy may help reduce reflux and aspiration.

- Treat a person's wheelchair with respect – people can spend long periods of time in their wheelchair, so that it almost becomes part of them. Avoid leaning on wheelchairs and 'kicking off' brakes.

- Be aware of the floor surfaces you are going over – some can be painful to people in a wheelchair. Think about how the sensations of different floor surfaces can become part of the way the person can identify where they are and where they are going.

- Ensure that all activities are planned around the person being in as straight and aligned a position as possible. Remember the internal body systems and how they function.

- As the person will spend a large portion of their day in different positions, on the floor, on their side, sitting or standing, change the environment around them so that they can use their eyes and ears as much as possible. What are they able to see while on the floor apart from other people's feet?

Visual impairment

The Royal National Institute for the Blind (RNIB) has identified that every year 27.5 million people need to have regular eye tests. However, only 15 million people do so. This means that 12.5 million people do not have a regular eye test (Department of Health 2003). People with intellectual disability have higher levels of impaired vision compared to the general population (Welsh Health Survey 1995). For children with complex care needs it is essential that they have regular eye tests to ensure that as practitioners we know exactly what they can see. Even people who are registered as blind can have some useful vision. It is also necessary to monitor any changes as people grow older so that treatments can be accessed that may enhance vision or use of vision. Optometrists and carers need to be aware of the high prevalence of vision defects and the importance of regular eye examinations in people with a learning disability (Woodhouse *et al.* 2003). Research has shown that up to three-quarters of all children with learning disabilities may have some kind of visual impairment (Sonsken *et al.* 1991).

Lack of clarity surrounding these exact numbers is due to the wide variety and types of visual impairment among children with learning disabilities. As damage to the brain is usually the cause of visual impairment in children with learning disabilities, there are many more kinds of visual difficulties that may develop. Children with learning disabilities may have:

- reduced visual acuity (clarity or sharpness of vision);
- visual field loss (may not be able to see above or below or to the sides);
- difficulty in hand-to-eye coordination;
- difficulty recognizing and matching objects;
- short- or long-sightedness;
- problems making accurate fast eye movements (scanning an object);
- problems keeping fixation on an object (they may might have uncontrollable eye motions);
- each eye may have a different impairment.

Exercise 12.4

Sit in a busy room for ten minutes with your eyes closed. How do you know who is in the room with you? Who is coming and going? What activities are going on? How do you feel? Are you relying on your hearing more? This exercise offers a very small insight into what it is like without visual input. Without visual cues it is also difficult to keep track of time, and many people will think the ten-minute exercise takes a lot longer.

It is important to observe how the child uses their vision and/or if they have *any* useful vision. We need to observe what distance they can see, what colours they react to, and what size of objects they can see and at what distance. The following questions will help you gain knowledge of how a child is utilizing their vision. They are designed as support information to take to an optician; they are *not* intended to replace a formal visual assessment.

- What colours does the child respond to?
- When do they appear to focus on your face as you approach them?
- Do they react to toys held in front of them at 6 inches, 12 inches, 24 inches, 48 inches etc.?
- In what position do they hold their head? Is it tilted or turned to one side? Do they appear to be looking upwards/downwards at an object?

- What lighting do they respond to best? Light directed on the object? Daylight? Soft lighting? Do they respond to light stimulation in a sensory room?

- Does the child respond better when the object is placed on a contrasting background (i.e. a yellow teddy against a black jumper, a red plate on a white placemat)? Visually busy patterns can hamper rather than enhance someone's vision.

- Are there times of the day when they respond better (i.e. first thing in the morning or after a bath when they are relaxed)? Try not to assess the child if they are tired or after a strenuous physiotherapy session.

This type of assessment will take time and require the child to be carefully observed in a variety of situations. A sensory room where light and colour can be controlled is a very useful resource during a visual assessment. If the child has low vision and experiences life in a blurred visual haze, the visual rewards and stimulation that encourage children to learn will not be present. Hence, many children with low vision 'switch off' and stop responding. Once the initial assessment is completed the sensory room can be utilized in many different ways to stimulate useful vision alongside the tactile and auditory skills that will be needed to supplement visual loss (Pagliano 1999). Non-visual ways of learning through touch, smell and hearing are essential to any child with low vision.

Helping strategies

- Use a sensory room to help identify when the person reacts to visual stimulation. Utilize all your knowledge about the person to maximize any vision assessment.

- Be aware of how differing eye conditions affect the person. Most people will have some useful vision, and changing the environment can help. Think about light and how this can be used; a simple strategy is to use an extra lamp to shine on a meal so that the person can see their food. Shadows can appear as dark holes, and will make walking across shadows cast on the floor very frightening. Harsh bright light can also cause problems for a person who has cataracts, causing them to squint and reduce their vision further.

- Colour and contrasting colours are often under-utilized when considering creating a pleasant homely environment which is useful to a person with low vision. Finding your way around can be very difficult when all the rooms and colour schemes blend in. Doorways can be made clear by having a contrasting door colour to the wall or door surround. Walls can have a contrasting border along them to facilitate movement from area to area. Plates can be placed on a contrasting placemat so that the edge of the plate becomes clear. Edges to steps can also be highlighted in a contrasting colour.

- Think about the sensations and noises differing floor coverings make and how could you use this to help identify rooms. Lounge areas could be wool carpets, while kitchens could be vinyl floor covering and toilet areas could be tiled.

- Noises will also be used to orientate and identify areas. Sounds of the fish tank, the toilet flushing and cutlery being placed on the table, noises outside, a ticking clock, the fridge motor and the washing machine, can all help a visually impaired person to identify where they are. Beaded curtains and wind chimes can be used on outside doors to identify that they *are* outside doors. Alternatively, constant noise such as the radio or television on all day can mask noises that act as auditory clues.
- Different shaped door handles can be used to identify different rooms.

Hearing impairment

There are an estimated 9 million deaf and hard of hearing people in the UK. There are about 20,000 children aged 0–15 years who are moderately to profoundly deaf. There are about 23,000 deaf-blind people. Some will be totally deaf and others will have some useful hearing (RNID 2003). People with learning disability have higher levels of impaired hearing compared to the general population (Welsh Health Survey 1995). Yeates (1991) identifies that the incidence of hearing loss is *much* higher in people with a learning disability: 37 per cent compared to 14 per cent of the general population, highlighting that hearing impairment in people with a learning disability is a significant issue. It is also recognized that children with CP are more likely to have a hearing impairment. For example, hypertonic quadriplegia and athetoid patterns of movement in all four limbs are associated with severe sensori-neural hearing impairment (Cogher *et al.* 1992). Inability to hear can have a major impact on independence and confidence, interaction and communication, so it is essential to minimize the impact of any hearing loss.

People with a learning disability may not be able to communicate a problem with their hearing. Changes in behaviour that may indicate a hearing loss can often be missed or misinterpreted. This is further complicated by the difficulties in recognizing the need for medical attention (Rogers *et al.* 1999). Mencap (1998) highlight that GPs find it difficult to identify when a hearing assessment is needed and are often dismissive of carers' concerns. Yeates (1991) notes that people with learning disabilities and hearing loss are a group that have experienced many problems accessing ordinary services, and that many consultants feel that people with learning disabilities cannot undergo hearing tests – the implication being that nothing can be done for them and that it will not make any difference if hearing loss is present in the individual. Questions to consider here include:

- Is the person not hearing?
- What are they not hearing?
- Are they unresponsive?

- Do they have a short concentration span?
- Do they have difficulties in coordinating their physical movements?
- Are they not responding to any auditory input?

To maximize hearing, audiologists recommend that people with learning disabilities, especially children, should receive a regular hearing assessment every two years, especially for those judged to be at higher risk. The examination is also the opportunity to look for any problems in ear health and to ensure that even a little hearing can be used beneficially. The answers to the following questions will help the audiologist in assessing the person more effectively. These may indicate that they might need help with hearing:

- How long is their concentration span?
- Do they respond differently to male and female voices?
- Do they respond better when eye contact is gained?
- When the television is on or music is playing do they sit close to the speaker?
- Do they respond to vocalizations?
- Do they respond to gestures such as pointing?
- Do they respond better in a quiet environment?
- Have they developed any unusual behaviours (i.e. bending of the outer ear, making noises to themselves, slapping the ear, poking the ear or banging the head)?

These questions are designed to help you gain knowledge of how a person is utilizing their hearing. They are to support information taken to an audiologist; they are *not* intended to replace a formal hearing assessment.

Exercise 12.5

Listen to a piece of music that you enjoy. Now turn off the treble and listen: the music will sound very different. This is similar to what people with a hearing impairment might hear when they have high frequency (Hz) hearing loss. Now listen to the piece again with the bass turned off. This is what a person might hear with low frequency (Hz) hearing loss. Music sounds different and may not be comfortable for the person with hearing loss to listen to. In fact some music can be quite painful depending on the hearing loss.

In helping a person utilize their hearing we need to concentrate on their being aware of sound, identification of the sound, where the sound is coming from, what they like to hear and what volume is needed for them to hear. A sensory room is an ideal place to help assess hearing skills as noise volume and location can be controlled and changed to assist the assessment and to stimulate residual hearing.

Exercise 12.6

Think of two activities that would help you understand how well a child can hear.

Helping strategies

- Always approach a hearing impaired person from the front, as they will not hear you approaching.
- Encourage them to utilize their hearing ability. A sensory room is a useful area to control sound for assessment and stimulation purposes.
- Remember that some frequency hearing loss can cause pain when hearing certain frequencies. Ensure you understand any hearing assessment and the implications it may have. Identify sounds that cause alertness and pleasure so that these can be used appropriately.
- Control everyday sounds so that any residual hearing can be utilized. Turning the television off or moving away from background noise may help.
- Hearing alarms should be supplemented by vibration and/or lights.
- Skill development needs to utilize touch and vision, showing and feeling rather than telling.

Communication

As professional carers we talk about normalization, person-centred planning, partnership working, multi-agency and multi-disciplinary teams and methods of working, planning and reviewing care. However thoughtfully prepared, care can often be about physical care based 'around' the child with PMLD. This type of care can be very time-consuming and physically tiring to the carer, becoming a routine of postural positioning and movement. It can lack the positive interactions that makes caring for someone else rewarding. Rewards for carers of people with PMLD are often of a long-term nature: skill development can take a long time, and carers can miss out on immediate feedback, which we all need to maintain positive interactions. Interactions can be judged as beneficial because we have made the person laugh or smile, but being told that I can make the person laugh or smile has further frustrated me due to the limited nature of the interaction, the child or person reacting to me rather than a two-way communication. Caldwell (1998) suggests that we need to 'get in touch' with people who appear locked in their own world. It is time we learnt 'new languages' based on the abilities and communication skills of the person with PMLD. Not all formal methods of communicating will be appropriate, so first we need to observe how the person communicates. How do they communicate that they are thirsty? Want to move? Ask what is happening next? We need to learn each individual's 'language' and so become adept at learning to communicate rather than teaching communication (see Chapter 13).

It is well known that there are barriers to communication. Some children with learning disabilities, especially if they have additional needs, may have experienced limited learning and life opportunities. This, in addition to other people's low expectations of someone with high support needs, creates additional communication difficulties. Practitioners may also feel they do not have the time or they may interpret communications to help meet their own needs, or be preoccupied and fail to focus on the individual (Bradley 2001). The person with PMLD will have all the needs of any person and additional needs dependent on how their physical, sensory and cognitive impairments affect their status. Each person is different and it is the difference that we need to concentrate on rather than the similarities. Each person will experience and perceive the world in a different fashion, a world that is very different to the visually- and sound-orientated world that other people experience.

Bradley (1994) identifies several challenges facing people with PMLD who want to be effective communicators:

- they may have visual impairments ranging from no useful sight to some useful vision;
- they may have a range of hearing impairments;
- they may not have reached a development level where speech is processed and has meaning;
- they may have physical impairments which affect speech or the physical coordination needed for gesturing or formal signing;
- they may be sensitive to touch or be wary of touch;
- they may communicate in idiosyncratic ways.

To interact meaningfully with a person who has PMLD it is important to learn about their world and how they communicate. It is the 'idiosyncratic' ways they communicate that are vehicles for effective two-way communication. It is extremely difficult for someone with PMLD to learn and utilize 'our' communication methods, whether these be oral, visual or tactile. It is far more effective for practitioners to learn how the person they care for communicates, 'tuning in' (Nind and Hewett 2001) to the person's unique face and body movements or pre-verbal communications, allowing us to recognize intentional communication signals. Without this 'tuning in' we fail to notice, recognize and interpret these signals. If these signals are not responded to, the person may give up trying to communicate, leaving us with only one-way communication. This 'tuning in' will mean, for professional carers, that they become multi-communicators, learning as many methods of communicating as the number of people they care for.

'Tuning in'

We need to observe closely, assess and interact by:

- use of eye contact, blinking – voluntary and non-voluntary – and eye gaze;
- reading facial expressions and small facial movements;
- recognizing intentional movements of the body which can be difficult when someone has CP;
- turn-taking in making noises, copying behaviours and responding to pulling faces;
- use of appropriate touch and physical contact;
- reading the person's body language, understanding what is intentional movement and what is not;
- utilizing personal space – this may mean recognizing that for a person in a wheelchair this includes their chair;
- making time and enjoying 'tuning in', this is fun time;
- focusing on the individual and not the activity.

Make a note of all your interventions and identify patterns of behaviour, facial expressions and noises. Remember the person with PMLD may have very little purposeful self-controlled movements. They may rely on a subtle movement of the eyelid or a jerk of a toe. We must not miss these. A person with CP can function differently from day to day and sometimes hour to hour. We need to be able to recognize this and change strategies to accommodate these changes.

Children with PMLD will only communicate when they have a reason to do so. They may have had many experiences of their attempts at communicating being ignored or misunderstood. This leads to the child giving up trying and relying on family members or support workers to meet their needs. As professional carers we need to learn not to anticipate and meet every need as part of our daily caregiving. We need to think about what the person *can* communicate and create opportunities for them to do so. For example, instead of offering drinks on a regular basis so that the child is never thirsty, think about how we can use this situation to create an opportunity to communicate.

Case study: *Seema*

Seema would sit in her wheelchair apparently unaware of her surroundings. She spent a lot of time sleeping. Her only enjoyment was eating and drinking and due to her CP she was totally dependent on her carer and the speed that the carer helped her with her meal. It was noted over time that if food was offered too soon Seema would lower her head slightly, as she had limited control of her head. If the food was given too slowly then Seema would grunt and lift her head. To communicate to Seema that it was mealtime her carer would take her to the table and then lift her head and make Seema's grunting noise, offering her some food. Food was delayed several seconds to encourage Seema to ask for her next spoonful. Within weeks Seema was controlling the speed she ate her meal and was developing a two-way conversation with her carers.

Helping strategies

- Learn and practise 'tuning in'.
- Monitor and record all actions and behaviours so that any intentional communications can be identified.
- Produce a communication tool that identifies how the person communicates. This may take the form of photographs capturing the person communicating, line drawings showing limited movements that indicate communications or a written description of the activity. Individuals will have their own unique tool. These tools should be portable and replaceable so that they can go with the person wherever they go.
- Do not give up. Pre-verbal intentional communications can be very difficult to recognize.
- Practise turn-taking. This is one of the basic elements of communication. Pat-a-cake and peek-a-boo are useful activities in encouraging turn-taking.
- Acknowledge and validate communication no matter how basic.

Conclusion

Knowing the individual, their skills and abilities, communication methods and how they interact with and perceive their environment is essential if practitioners are to be effective in helping people with PMLD. This will mean taking time, using keen observations, monitoring and recording all behaviours and working in partnership with all significant individuals and teams. We must be mindful that regardless of the application of 'social' and 'medical' models we are always dealing with a unique individual. A multi-dimensional assessment that takes account of medical and social constructions of disability is obviously important in understanding how people with PMLD perceive and adapt to everything life.

References

Barr, O. (1999) Care of people with learning disabilities in hospital, *Learning Disability Practice*, 2: 29–35.

Bradley, A. (2001) *Understanding Positive Communications*. Kidderminster: BILD Publications.

Bradley, H. (1994) *Encouraging and Developing Early Communication Skills in Adults with Multiple Disabilities*. Focus fact sheet. London: RNIB Publications.

British Medical Association (1999) *Withholding and Withdrawing Life-prolonging Medical Treatment*. London: BMA.

Caldwell, P. (1998) *Person to Person – Establishing Contact and Communication with People with Profound Learning Disability and Extra Special Needs*. Brighton: Pavilion.

Cogher, L., Savage, E. and Smith, M.F. (1992) *Cerebral Palsy: The Child and Young Person*. London: Chapman and Hall Medical.

Department of Health (1995) *The Health of the Nation: A Strategy for People with Learning Disabilities*. London: Department of Health.

Department of Health (1998) *Signposts for Success in Commissioning and Providing Health Services for People with Learning Disabilities*. Wetherby: Department of Health.

Department of Health (1999a) *Saving Lives: Our Healthier Nation*. London: HMSO.

Department of Health (1999b) *Once a Day*. Wetherby: Department of Health.

Department of Health (2001) *Valuing People: A New Strategy for Learning Disability for the 21st Century*. London: Department of Health.

Department of Health (2003) *Registered Blind and Partially Sighted People Year Ending 31 March 2003, England*. London: Department of Health.

Goldsmith, J. and Goldsmith, L. (1996) *A Carers' Guide to the Management of Posture*. Ledbury: The Helping Hand Company.

Hogg, J. and Sebba, J. (1986) *Profound Retardation and Multiple Impairment Development and Learning*. Vol. 1. London: Croom Helm.

Kelly, A. (2000) *Working with Adults with a Learning Disability*. Oxon: Speechmark Publishing.

Kerr, M. (1998) Primary health care and health gain for people with a learning disability, *Tizard Learning Disability Review*, 3(4): 6–14.

Lacey, P. and Ouvry, C. (eds) (2000) *People with Profound and Multiple Learning Disabilities: A Collaborative Approach to Meeting Complex Needs*. London: David Fulton.

Mencap (1998) *The NHS – Health for All?* London: Mencap.

Miller, F. and Bachrach, S.J. (1995) *Cerebral Palsy: A Complete Guide for Care Giving*. Baltimore, MD: Johns Hopkins University Press.

Morris, J. (1999) *Hurtling into the Void: Transition to Adulthood for Young Disabled People with Complex Health and Support Needs*. Brighton: Pavilion Publishing/Joseph Rowntree Foundation.

Nind, M. and Hewett, D. (2001) *A Practical Guide to Intensive Interaction*. Kidderminster: BILD Publications.

Pagliano, P. (1999) *Multisensory Environments*. London: David Fulton.

Pountey, T.E., Mulchahy, C. and Green, E. (1990) Early development of postural control, *Physiotherapy*, 76(12): 799–802.

Race, D.G. (ed.) (2002) *Learning Disability: A Social Approach*. London: Routledge.

Rennie, J. (ed.) (2001) *Learning Disability, Physical Therapy, Treatment and Management: A Collaborative Approach*. London: Whurr.

Richardson, M. (1997) Addressing barriers: disabled rights – the implications for nursing of the social construct of disability, *Journal of Advanced Nursing*, 25(6): 1269–75.

RNID (2003) *Facts and Figures on Deafness and Tinnitus*. London: RNID.

Roberts, K. and Lawton, D. (2001) Acknowledging the extra care parents give their disabled child, *Child: Care, Health and Development*, 27(4): 307.

Rogers, R., Mills, L. and Buckle, J. (1999) Providing equal access to primary care services, *Learning Disability Practice*, 2(1): 24–5.

Scottish Executive (2002) *Promoting Health, Supporting Inclusion: The National Review of the Contribution of all Nurses and Midwives to the Care and Support of People with Learning Disabilities*. Edinburgh: Scottish Executive.

Sonksen, P., Petrie, A. and Drew, K. (1991) Promotion of visual development of severely visually impaired babies: evaluation of a developmentally based programme, *Developmental Medicine and Child Neurology*, 33: 320–35.

Stolk, J., Boer, T.A. and Seldenrijk, R. (eds) (2000) *Meaningful Care: A Multidisciplinary Approach to the Meaning of Care for People with Mental Retardation*. London: Kluwer.

Ware, J. (2003) *Creating a Responsive Environment for People with Profound and Multiple Learning Difficulties*. London: David Fulton.

Welsh Health Survey (1995) *Health Evidence Bulletins: Medical Conditions in People with Intellectual Disability*. Cardiff: HMSO.

Woodhouse, J.M., Adler, P.M. and Duignan, A. (2003) Ocular and visual defects amongst people with intellectual disabilities participating in Special Olympics, *Ophthalmic and Physiological Optics*, 23(3): 221–32.

Yeates, S. (1991) Hearing loss in adults with learning difficulties, *British Journal of Medicine*, 303(6800): 427–8.

13

Communication and people with learning disabilities

Lesley Cogher

Introduction

In trying to understand how people with a range of learning disabilities experience communication, it is useful to define the characteristics of communication. The following working definition is suggested: 'Communication occurs when two or more people correctly interpret each other's language and/or behaviour'.

There are many possible definitions of communication but the following characterization has been developed from a number of writers on language and communication such as Grice (1975), Chomsky (1976) and Miller (1981). Critical features of communication are that:

- *it is at least two-way* (two or more people are always involved in a communicative act, sometimes directly, sometimes indirectly, over the telephone or through the written word);

- *it may be verbal or non-verbal* (behaviour that may have a meaning for someone is common; for example, yawning may indicate that someone is bored; however, to be communicative, a behaviour has to be intentional);

- *it may not always be successful* (either party to the communication might need to work hard to repair misunderstandings or misinterpretations);

- *interpretation is needed* (successful communication involves a shared code or culture; the code need not be spoken language, it can be mimes, signs or gestures, pictures or writing).

The above list highlights the social and cultural context in which communication occurs. Each of us brings knowledge of our world and our experience in social situations to bear on our understanding of other people and what they might mean by what they say. Our knowledge of the world may be similar to a degree if we have been raised in a similar way, for example attended the same school, lived in the same area or watched the same programmes on television. It will never be *exactly* the same because of our own unique experiences in our family groups. So, if a person with learning disabilities went to a special school and lived in sheltered housing, their knowledge of the world would differ from that of their communication partners who may have gone to mainstream schools or even university, and each of these would differ from those who had travelled on a gap year. How would these differences affect the content and quality of the communication interactions that might occur between these groups of people?

In this chapter I will describe the underlying skills required for communication to develop, the overall sequence of communication development, what can go wrong with communication, the effect that communication breakdown can have on potential interactions and the role of communication partners.

Communication skills

By the time we reach adulthood, our communication skills have largely been acquired. Infancy and childhood are therefore critical periods in which to acquire, practise and develop the skills of communicating.

The skills required for communication to develop, for the purposes of explanation, can be split into individual skills, although all skills work in interaction with each other during communication. This can be seen in the language skills model (see Figure 13.1). The left-hand side of the figure

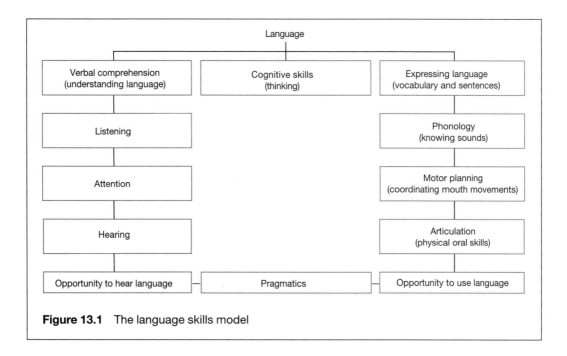

Figure 13.1 The language skills model

shows the skills and opportunities that are required for communication to develop.

Input

Opportunity to hear language

It is possible to gain much language experience from listening to the conversations of others, if meanings are made clear by the context (e.g. at the dinner table or when dressing). Background language forms a large part of a young child's experience and is as important to them as direct conversation.

However, some language learners may not have the opportunity to hear good-quality language from which they can learn. If students have limited mobility and cannot move towards the source of their interest or if their fellow students or those with whom they have most interaction do not use language, their opportunities may be severely reduced.

Hearing

Clearly the language learner also needs the ability to hear and it is quite clear what limitations hearing impairment puts on the development of speech and language (see Chapter 12).

Attention and listening

It is not enough just to hear sounds and language. There has to be an intention to interpret what is said, and we call this listening. Listening can be defined as hearing with the purpose of understanding. Language development can be vulnerable where the person has difficulty in giving attention to the language in their environment, such as people with concentration problems as part of their learning difficulties.

Language processing

The next stages of language ability include both input (understanding of language) and output (expression of language) as well as a central processing component. In order to understand what is being said it is necessary to:

- extract the meaning from words and the sentences used (language comprehension);
- process what is understood by comparing with experience and developing a response (thinking);
- generate the appropriate vocabulary and sentence structures to convey this meaning back to the communication partner (expressive language).

Language output

There are several stages to language output. Having decided which words and sentence structures will best represent what the speaker wants to say, further planning is required, involving:

- linguistic rules which refer to style of pronunciation, intonation and stress patterns;
- motor planning, the organization and sequencing of appropriate mouth movements;
- the ability to move the mouth in a coordinated way in order to produce speech sounds;
- the opportunity to use the speech and language in an interactive way.

It should be noted that output can be via oral speech, signs, pointing to pictures, use of objects of reference, writing, the use of a talking book, or even a high-tech communication aid, but all of these require some sort of motor planning and output ability from the complex physical act of writing to pressing a switch to activate a synthesized or digitized speech machine.

Exercise 13.1

Imagine a person was unable to speak. In what ways might they make themselves understood?

Pragmatic competence

The final central box in Figure 13.1 is labelled 'pragmatics' which refers to the use of language in social situations. In order to do this successfully the communicator needs to understand which of a range of social styles to use in a given situation. For example, it would not be appropriate for a child to refer to his teacher as 'mate' or for a football supporter to be formal in interaction with others on the terraces. Most adults know when swearing is inappropriate and in which circumstances it can be tolerated, but this is learned behaviour and relies on subtle interpretation of social clues and rules, memory and awareness of social timing.

Pragmatics, then, is knowledge about linguistic communication and includes recognition of the social uses of language and the importance of context in making speaking and listening choices. As children become skilled language users they interact with a variety of speakers and gain access to differing patterns of input. They engage in disputes with their peers, report on their activities, ask questions and generally experiment with language acquisition.

For a person with learning difficulties, the complex interaction of all the above communication skills may make effective communication one of the more vulnerable areas of their lives.

Development of communication

It was argued above that infancy and childhood are critical to developing communication skills. Below I outline key ideas to development during this period. The support provided during this time is critical, and a principal reason why the work of speech and language therapists begins as early as possible.

The detailed developmental sequence of speech and language in babies and children is well documented (e.g. Sheridan 1973). In typically developing people, the bulk of language competence is learned by age 6, with further refinement of vocabulary and sophistication of sentence structure continuing to develop throughout their lives. For people with learning difficulties, the pace of language and communication development may sometimes be significantly slower, such that there appears to be very little intentional communication. It will be useful therefore to outline some of the key developmental stages of communication.

This chapter is about people of all ages with learning difficulties but, in discussing language development, there needs to be a strong reference to the childhood years. People with learning disabilities are vulnerable to delay in learning skills in general, and this may particularly be the case with a complex set of skills like communication. Some people may, for example, have achieved the communication skills that might be expected of a young child. This is not to say that they will behave like a young child but that their processing is at a much reduced level from what is expected for their age.

Infants usually start to say their first words around 1 year old and put two words together at 18 months old. If a child has not started to talk by the time he or she is 2 there is usually concern on the part of parents and health visitors. However, other stages of language development may be less well understood. When, for example, do children understand the prepositions 'in', 'on' and 'under'? When can they use pronouns like 'he' and 'she' correctly? When do they learn the difference between 'ask' and 'tell'?

In a sense, these milestones are quite unimportant. When we meet a new person, particularly a person who may have learning difficulties, we are not assessing whether or not they understand pronouns, we are engaged in the business of communication with them and the most important question that we ask is, 'What is the person intending to communicate?', and when we interpret their intention this gives us clues towards their meaning. So it is important to look at the development of language, speech and communication skills in the context of the main task of the communicator, which is to 'learn how to mean'.

The infant and young child – learning to talk

Early meaning

Children must develop basic communication skills before they can be expected to use language for the purpose of communicating. This pre-linguistic development starts at birth.

The baby's first task is to ensure continuing care. Daniel Stern (1977) maintains that a strong tendency exists in the vast majority of us to respond in a fairly stereotypical and predictable way to the sight of a baby. The newborn baby has facial characteristics which are designed to encourage people to care for it and, just when this instinctive reaction on the part of the parents might be wearing a bit thin, the smile appears and is a very powerful social motivator for the parents. The baby's cry is an alerting factor which ensures a response from the parents in terms of comfort, presentation of food and general physical care. The parents' responses to the cry and the smile help the child to develop knowledge about the communicative power that they have, such that from approximately 3 months the child will vocalize, coo or cry with the express intention of getting attention or of obtaining food, comfort or physical care.

Early experience of the human voice in pleasurable situations helps the baby to attune to language. Baby games and songs help the infant to learn rhythm and anticipation of events that become associated with language. Understanding develops in close reciprocity with expression.

Joint attention

For communication to take place, the participants must be able to share a 'frame of reference'. In the early stages of language development babies and children establish reference by looking and/or pointing and/or sound-making.

In babies and very young children the communication partner tends to follow the child's attentional lead and interpret meaning in their behaviour accordingly. This ability of people to share attention on an object or activity is central to successful communication and is known as 'joint attention'. As the baby becomes older, the communication partner can increasingly draw the child's attention to something instead of just following the child's attentional lead, and the balance gradually shifts so that subsequently attention can be shared on more equal terms. At around 9 months, the baby can look at an object, towards his or her mother and back to the object to indicate interest.

Children of around 4 to 5 years of age can cooperate for short periods of time in attending entirely to an adult-directed task.

Evidence that the communicator is trying to get a specific message across is gained from eye contact, eye direction and body language, as well as speech. For a person with learning disabilities it may be necessary to increase the parent's or carer's awareness of where the communicator's interest is directed. They also develop the ability to recognize reference by watching eye direction or by pointing.

Participation

Early language is learnt through verbal routines in familiar situations. The baby comes to anticipate and expect events to follow the build-up (e.g. dinner arrives after clattering of plates, cooking smells and preparation of the table).

In contexts such as these, a person with learning difficulties begins to expect certain language strings (e.g. 'dinner's ready', 'wash your hands' or 'sit down'). Having learnt this framework he or she can begin to recognize word boundaries when other situations arise (e.g. 'it's bedtime', 'wash your face' and 'lie down') (Bruner 1975). This sort of social and environmental scaffolding for language development is vital but should not preclude choice-making on the communicator's part.

Intention

Perhaps the most powerful factor in the development of communication is the interpretation of intent even if, as in the very young baby, the intent does not exist. Interpretation allows the interaction to be spontaneous and child-led and teaches turn-taking, contingency (i.e. the consequences of behaviour – children learning communication skills learn that their vocalizations have an effect on their environment, e.g. the child says 'more' and gets more food), timing and joint attention, as well as specific verbal and non-verbal representations of the world. Understanding and expressive language can develop in a social context as the baby learns that certain behaviours lead to a predictable outcome. This helps to bring the behaviour under voluntary control.

A very young baby behaves in an instinctive way. As previously noted, all behaviour can communicate and the parent or carer tends to interpret richly the child's behaviour as having meaning. There is no sense of reciprocity at this stage, but the child learns about the communicative power of his or her behaviour. Interaction with a baby often involves exaggerated facial expression and seemingly bizarre vocal pitch changes which hold the baby's attention and maximize learning. Stern (1977) called these adult behaviours 'infant-elicited social behaviours'. With the development of the smile and its potent effect on adult behaviour, opportunities arise for the baby to learn such communicative prerequisites as turn-taking and cause and effect. The baby also learns about initiating, responding to and maintaining social interaction in that, with the smile, he or she signals a readiness to interact, then that the interaction is going well and, in the event of a breakdown, a desire to re-engage in the interaction.

Early characteristics contributing to communication

Most babies are predisposed to look at faces (Fantz 1966), their principal interest being in the eyes and mouth. This predisposition helps the baby to learn that important messages are sent by the face and not just by using eye contact. Also, the infant can attract and hold the attention of adults. Joint attention and reference have their roots in the early months when parents watch the direction of the baby's eyes and reinforce the interest by moving the object closer and/or talking about it. Eye contact and eye pointing become meaningful and communicative.

Language learning

The young infant does not cooperate with any of his or her carers' requests or demands at this stage. However, from 3 months up to 4–5 years, there is a gradual shift towards a more equal balance of turn-taking and cooperation, listening and talking. Many parents intuitively provide the child, during daily activities, with language he or she can for the most part understand, with new elements introduced gradually, basing their language on knowledge of the child's current vocabulary. The child therefore receives understandable language input in an environment where he or she is able to make more sense of new vocabulary.

Much of the child's language is learnt actively through play and daily activities. The child learns not only the names of objects but also actions (e.g. run, clap, eat); positions (e.g. in, on, under); and qualities (e.g. big, red, long). In facilitating language it is important to include all types of words and resist the temptation to restrict language to labels. The child's language acquisition will be helped if he or she has experience of as many activities as possible and these activities are discussed in terms of past, present and future, positive and negative. Understanding is an active process usually learnt in the context of expressive physical interaction with the environment – talking, showing, looking and so on. A person with learning disabilities may have limited opportunities in this regard.

Communication in the school-age child

The school-age child is expected to be able to communicate fully and to use language to interact with family, peers, teachers and others. As well as verbal development, the school-age child should have grasped many of the rules of social interaction, for example acceptable strategies for initiating, maintaining and terminating conversations. Language and communication skills are also used in a child's social life outside school, in play sessions with other children and in organized activities such as Cubs or Brownies.

A child with learning disabilities may have a limited range of social opportunities and may also have to rely on alternative methods of communication such as Makaton signing or a symbol system to augment their communication. They may only participate to a small extent in the rough and tumble of primary-age children communicating. This is exacerbated in situations of segregation where, for example, the child attends a special school.

Communication in young people and adults

Raffaelli and Duckett (1989) suggest that, in adolescence, conversation becomes the major medium of social interaction rather than the shared activities typical of the younger child. Moreover in adolescence and adulthood friendship is often negotiated by just talking. Adolescents are able to think more abstractly and this is reflected in the language that they use.

In young people there is continuing development of vocabulary and language structure skills towards those of an adult, but there will be a significant use of slang and the dialect of the adolescent. This is also the time when the younger person tends to move away from the intensity of family relationships and seek out an identity within his or her peer group. Attendance at a special school can be isolating because school friends are unlikely to live nearby. However, adolescents with learning difficulties at mainstream school may find themselves unable to keep pace with their physically and mentally more agile peers. Some children may have the opportunity to attend clubs provided for both able-bodied and disabled youngsters. However, this broadening of relationships does not necessarily mean that relationships are benign or fulfilling. Bullying and abuse can of course occur (see Chapters 9 and 16).

By adolescence, children have mastered the basic skills of language learning and have started to achieve goals in producing and understanding narratives and complex sentences. They are able to make inferences and do some critical thinking. Their sentences are longer, with more subordinate clauses, and show an increase in technical terms. They learn to manipulate meanings through understanding the multiple meanings of words, and they start to understand language that has a figurative rather than literal function. They are much more able to make coherent jokes and use metaphors, proverbs and idioms correctly. They pick up and use slang as part of their social group, and this is important for peer acceptance.

As an adult the development of language and communication skills seems to be inextricably bound up with achieving personal autonomy and independence. From 18 years we expect people to vote, be able to drink in pubs and make most major life decisions. However, young people with learning disabilities have often not been able to achieve such independence, and it may therefore be hard for them to establish an adult role in the community and access adult decision-making. Work opportunities often depend on an ability to communicate effectively in a number of settings, from requesting more work materials to commenting on the food in the cafeteria, and an environmental analysis may be necessary to develop a comprehensive list of possible communication situations and partners. By environmental analysis I mean a review of all the possible communication partners in a person's life and a breakdown of their opportunities for communication. The importance of this point is illustrated by recent findings from a study of supported employment that shows that people with learning disabilities can often find themselves working by themselves, and that social inclusion in the workplace is yet to be claimed (Wistow and Schneider 2003).

In order to consider this further the next section will focus on the tasks of the communicator and the tasks of the communication partners in communication.

Exercise 13.2

Think of a person with learning disabilities that you know. How would they communicate: in a work setting; in a social situation with friends; at home? What are the issues for this person?

Communication tasks

In any communication there are parties whose roles vary throughout the interaction.

The tasks of the communicator

In order to be effective the communicator must show intention to communicate. So what are the indicators of intentional communication? Evidence that:

- the communicator is trying to get a partner's attention;
- the communicator is trying to get a specific message across;
- the communicator is clearly waiting for a response; and
- if no response is forthcoming, further attempts will be made through repetition or showing displeasure.

The communicator must also intend to make sense of the communication attempts of their communication partners.

The tasks of the communication partner

The range of a person's potential communication partners will vary during the course of their life, and the main task of the communication partner is to intend to make sense of the interaction.

The baby and young child tend to communicate primarily with their parents, then extended family are included. The child then goes on to communicate with teachers and care staff and, to varying degrees, friends. As an older child and young adult, as well as the people already mentioned, there will be a need to extend the circle of friends and acquaintances, and the communicator may be expected to interact with service staff such as shop assistants, bus drivers and postmen as potential communication partners. With adulthood comes the opportunity to interact with work colleagues and others related to their community and leisure activities. It will be seen later (Chapters 23 and 28) that maintaining these relationships beyond a superficial level can be very difficult for people with learning disabilities. Language development is inevitably implicated in this.

Communication partners need not be just one person. Communicators could be having a conversation with one other person, taking regular turns, interrupting or being interrupted, or could be having a night out in a small group with people chatting freely and simultaneously with someone occasionally holding the floor. Alternatively, the communicator could be at a lecture or gathering of a larger group, either as part of the audience or indeed the speaker. These, and many more possible scenarios, need to be taken into consideration when evaluating what a person's communication needs might be in any given situation. Consideration of the type and number of communication partners will determine the type of communication that needs to take place if it is to be successful. What does the communication partner need to do which helps the communication?

- expect the communicator to want to communicate and look for active signals;
- apply active understanding (i.e. rich interpretation of what the communicator may be trying to convey);
- reframe the communication in his or her own words to show understanding, requesting clarification or physical clues such as pointing if the message is not understood;
- be aware that the communicator may need time to get their message across, and be receptive to potential communication;
- respond in a timely and appropriate manner;
- be consistent in responding to the same behaviour or sound in the same way.

Activities that do not help the success of interactions include the following:

- distracting the communicator to a new activity or issue;
- ignoring;
- making an unrelated response;
- interrupting;
- not giving time to complete the utterance;
- breaking off to talk to another;
- being too helpful in talking for the communicator.

What can go wrong with communication?

Age-related difficulties

In this section I consider developmental stages once again, drawing attention to some of the more specific communication challenges facing people with learning disabilities.

Across the age range many difficulties can occur, and it is also important to note that early experience of communication failure can influence future development into adulthood.

Babyhood

The baby's sounds and gestures encourage interaction from adults, and evidence that the baby can understand, such as waving 'bye bye' or clapping along to a song, leads adults to expect and try to elicit yet more. The baby with learning difficulties may be slow to respond to these initiatives and this may result in extinction of the adults' positive communication behaviour.

Speech output skills may be affected as babies with learning difficulties may have low muscle tone. This can result in a difficulty in producing babble sounds which contain consonants, and they may lack experience in producing sounds, thus affecting their acquisition of a phonological system. Disordered oral sensation may also occur and be compounded by the lack of experience of mouthing toys if the baby has been late to do so. Using speech in a communicative act requires accuracy and timing, skills usually learnt in the baby stage through babble, imitation and interactive games.

Babies also use body posture, gaze and facial expression to augment their speech attempts. A baby with learning disabilities whose intention to communicate is hampered by physical or cognitive impairment may experience frustration.

Illness in the early months can disrupt the balance of early interactions with parents, as described in the section on communication development in young children. The sick baby may not be available for social interaction; the anxiety of the parents may jeopardize the interaction; and the disclosure of a diagnosis which suggests learning disabilities in the future may also throw the development of interaction off-balance (see Chapter 10).

Preschool

It is central for the preschool experience of all children to learn to interact with a variety of other children. Communication skills provide the primary means of controlling the social environment – friends, siblings, classmates, parents, caregivers, relatives and teachers – but simply placing children with disabilities in the same educational environment as preschool children without disabilities does not automatically facilitate high-quality social interactions.

Children need early socialization experiences in order to build up a variety of language functions. Breakdowns occur when one participant in the communicative interaction fails to respond to a partner's utterance requiring a response. For example, if a child says, 'Do you want to play ball?' to a friend and the friend fails to say anything, a breakdown has occurred. Similarly, if the friend appears to respond with irrelevant information, for example, 'Red one', breakdown will occur. Communicative breakdowns may be attributable to sensory impairment, memory deficit, or delayed or disordered aspects of language. Repairs of communicative behaviour tend to rest with the more sophisticated communication partner but research has shown that children with specific difficulties with language tend not to request clarification if they do not understand (Donahue *et al.* 1982).

Children with expressive speech problems who find it difficult to be understood may become aware of their failure to communicate and may become reticent to speak or may rely on simple predictable context-based language structures.

Primary school

Research suggests that children between the ages of 2 and 7 engage in verbal interaction between one-third and two-thirds of the time spent in free play (Goldstein and Kaczmarek 1992). Mueller (1972) reported an average of 3.3 utterances per minute per child, with a suggestion that children adapt the frequency of their contribution to that of their partners (Kohn 1966). However, Beckman (1983) found that children without disabilities interact more frequently with other children without disabilities than they do with children with disabilities in integrated settings.

Guralnick and Paul-Brown (1986) have shown that children without disabilities reduce the level of their language in accordance with the developmental sophistication of their playmates with disabilities. This works to the advantage of children with disabilities but may overall give them fewer communicative experiences (Goldstein and Katczmarek 1992). Nuccio and Abbeduto (1993) found that school-age children with mild-to-moderate learning difficulties tended to use what would be regarded as impolite non-interrogative (demanding) forms when requesting an object, whereas their learning-age peers without disabilities tended to use polite forms (e.g. 'Can I have another toy?').

Secondary school

Bliss (1985) found that adolescents with learning disabilities were less good at selecting socially acceptable forms for their request than would be expected from the evidence of their cognitive functioning. There is also evidence that understanding social motivation during interactions can pose a problem to people with learning difficulties, particularly if the speaker is not familiar to them, or if the interaction is not embedded in their highly familiar routine.

Case study: *Pauline*

Pauline is a very articulate person with Asperger syndrome. She has good spoken language and is very interested in No Smoking signs. However, she doesn't understand other people's language well. People overestimate her skills because she can talk well and, when she does not understand or respond to what they say directly, they think she is being difficult or ignorant. As she has Asperger syndrome, Pauline finds it difficult to make reciprocal relationships on equal terms with other people, but her good expressive language skills in the context of poor understanding make her seem aggressive and uncaring and make it even harder for her to develop relationships.

Exercise 13.3

Discuss how you might support Pauline to express her views in work, social or familial situations.

Adulthood

Research has shown that people with learning difficulties reveal delays in all aspects of their speech, language and communication performance (Abudarham and Hurd 2002). As well as limited language use and problems with speech intelligibility, they also show delays in their use of social information to make decisions about the appropriate social style to adopt, and may be delayed in understanding social motivations. However, in adulthood they do tend to show some ability in understanding language when it is embedded in highly familiar interaction routines (Abbeduto and Rosenberg 1992).

It is not uncommon for people with learning disabilities to appear socially gauche or inappropriate in interactions. Abbeduto and Rosenberg (1992: 347) attempt to account for this in terms of difficulty with skills at a pragmatic level:

> When making a request such a speaker may select a linguistic form at random because they are unable to retrieve information about their addressee, e.g. his or her status because, as part of their cognitive problems, they have poor organisation of retrieval from long-term memory, poorly developed interpersonal goals and motive, a lack of knowledge about other people's intentions and beliefs, and other limitations in social competence or knowledge of and reasoning about the social world which can limit the effectiveness of linguistic communication. For example, people may have difficulty making polite requests because their poor perspective-taking skills prevent them from anticipating the reaction of their addressee to an impolite request.

It may be that the person with learning difficulty lives in a supported environment where there is a high turnover of care staff, and the concomitant difficulties in establishing rapport and relationships can result in communication breakdown. Where there are a number of carers on shifts it may be that nobody fully understands the extent of the person's understanding and may pitch the language too high or too low for the language learner. It has also been shown that staff can sometimes overestimate a person's understanding of verbal language, or fail to identify non-verbal behaviour as a means of communication (Purcell *et al.* 1999).

Case study: *Nigel*

Nigel has autism and lives in a very caring home with quite a strict routine because of shift patterns and care routines. Meals are always provided on time. Staff are concerned that Nigel sometimes becomes angry around supper time and when he does it tends to be on a Saturday. Supper is always at 5.00 p.m. on a Saturday, when Nigel enjoys watching the football results. Because of the rather strict routine he does not have the opportunity to watch the football results and then eat his supper or say that he wants to eat earlier. Nigel does not have the skills to refuse his supper or negotiate postponing it. Living in a routine has meant that Nigel does not need to ask for food, nor does he have the opportunity to reject it. He does not have the opportunity to hear anyone else negotiating or making choices about food. As well as his primary difficulty of autism, therefore, Nigel lacks experience in managing choices and negotiating. He does not know that he can ask for change and therefore doesn't or hasn't the motivation to learn the language he needs to do so. When there is a conflict between his routine meal times and his focused interest, Nigel finds it difficult to cope and tends to have a tantrum which requires help to calm him down.

In spite of and perhaps as a result of the staff in Nigel's home making every effort to make residents comfortable, Nigel has lacked the opportunity and experience for developing skills of negotiation and he has only aggression to resort to when he is frustrated.

Exercise 13.4

Think of one person with learning disabilities with whom you have worked. Can you think of ways you might facilitate his or her ability to communicate?

A person with learning disability has to communicate with a range of people on a personal level and, indeed, on a service level, and here further risk can arise. Depending on the degree of support required, a person with learning disability will have to react to life events with appropriate actions (e.g. illness should lead them to consult a doctor, but they may be required to communicate their symptoms to a precise degree, which might lead to misunderstanding or misdiagnosis in a busy consultation).

A recent report by the National Patient Safety Agency (NPSA) (2004) highlights that patients with learning disabilities may have difficulty communicating and may in fact not be listened to as carefully in matters of health, which can result in severe risk for them. The NPSA report quotes a survey entitled 'Speaking up' which found that people with a learning disability rarely feel that they have enough time to communicate their needs to their GP.

Similarly, housing issues or respite arrangements may need to be negotiated and the person with a learning disability will need support with this – as long as, of course, the support person takes the time to listen accurately and check that they have correctly interpreted the wishes of the communicator.

Above all, on the issue of communication, services must, while respecting confidentiality and dignity, communicate with each other in the best interests of the person with a learning difficulty. Vulnerable people need services to work sensitively in tandem with each other with the person with a learning disability at the centre. To this end person-centred planning (see Chapter 24) using MAP and PATH (Pearpoint *et al.* 1993) techniques can be a major communication resource. These are techniques involving drawing or other visual representation that actively involve the person with a learning disability in planning their environment, activity and life aims.

Looking back to the input/output communication model (Figure 13.1), difficulties or vulnerabilities in any of these areas can cause speech, language or communication problems. Communication breakdown can occur if communication partners have expectations that cannot be met.

Communication breakdown in learning disability

A person with a hearing impairment will be vulnerable in the vital part of the chain for building up listening skills, verbal comprehension and thinking with language. The expression of language will obviously be affected by this difficulty with input, and the ability to produce accurate speech sounds may also be affected. In contrast, others may have difficulties more associated with processing, understanding or verbalizing. Studies indicate that these may be impairment-specific, but even when distinctive aetiologies are evident there can be huge variation in communication and language development (Tager-Flusberg 1999; Chapman and Hesketh 2000).

A person with cerebral palsy is likely to be vulnerable in all areas, as their opportunity to hear and use speech and language will be severely reduced by a lack of mobility. Although hearing may be intact, it will be difficult for the person with cerebral palsy to have learnt how to localize sound and to listen, as a result of not being able to turn their head at will as a young child (see Chapter 12). Although many people with cerebral palsy have preserved intelligence, some may not, and their exposure to a range of language will be limited, because of fewer opportunities and their reliance on others to move them to stimulating situations. This can also result in an impoverished vocabulary. In addition, people with cerebral palsy, particularly those with the more severe types, will have significant difficulty in producing mouth movements which can be coordinated to make intelligible speech (Cogher *et al.* 1992). Many people with cerebral palsy rely on alternative methods of communication, such as communication books or digitized speech aids.

Franklin and Beukelman (1991) found that augmentative communicators primarily respond to rather than initiate communication interactions. They tend to produce a limited number of turns and a limited number of communicative functions, and often fail to repair, that is they often fail to bring the communication back on track if there has been a breakdown. Franklin and Beukelman found that the speaking partners tended to dominate conversations and structure interactions to require minimal responses from users of augmentative communication systems. People who use augmentative and alternative communication (AAC) systems act on as few as 50 per cent of the available conversational opportunities during the course of an interaction (Light *et al.* 1985). AAC supports oral speech. For example, we all tend to use natural gesture when speaking and this 'augments' our meaning by giving extra clues. AAC is required when a person is unable to use speech at all and needs to communicate in other ways. AAC systems can involve signing and/or visual systems (e.g. pictures, symbols, letters).

Signing

There are a number of signing methods mainly developed by the hearing impaired community: e.g. British Sign Language, the Paget Gorman sign system. These languages vary in how the signs are made with hand shape and position and also in terms of how many grammatical markers such as tense and plurality that they convey.

The Makaton Vocabulary Development Project used signs from British sign language to develop a vocabulary of signs which are relevant to the experiences and needs of people with learning disability. 'Signalong' works on similar principles.

Visual systems

Depending on the person's cognitive ability to process visual information, objects, photos, drawings, symbols or letters can be used within AAC. Objects of reference have already been mentioned above. It is also possible to use photos, pictures or symbols to point to by hand, fist, head or eye, to indicate meaning. These can be on a board, tray or in the form of a 'talking book' or 'talking mat'. The child can also hand over these pictures to convey meaning as in PECS (Picture Exchange Communication System) (Bondy and Frost 1992). Symbols systems such as Rebus and Mayer-Johnson can be generated using computer programs such as Widgit and allow more condensed meaning, giving more options for communication providing the person has cognitive skills to that level.

Another form of AAC used in combination with visual systems is battery-operated or electronic communication aids which the child activates to produce spoken words, phrases or sentences. These aids vary in complexity from one-hit, single message aids (e.g. Big Mack made by Prentke Romich) through to 4, 8 or 32 message aids and more. The more complex the aid, the more intellectual ability is required to use it.

Case study: *George*

George is a young man with cerebral palsy. He has preserved intelligence and understands the language of others very well, but has no intelligible speech. Through support workers and the internet, he is working for a degree in computer science and he has a number of 'buddies' who help him take part in a number of social activities. However, George uses a wheelchair and has to use a communication aid as he does not have adequate oral movement for speech. Programming what he wants to say into his communication aid takes slightly longer than spontaneous speech, and he therefore finds it hard to interact in group conversation in the pub. He is always two or three sentences behind, and the group dynamic means that it is hard for people to wait for him to speak. People who don't know George imagine that, because he can't speak, he has difficulty in understanding, and when they talk, they may talk to his carers rather than directly to him.

Exercise 13.5

How do you think George feels when people don't hear what he has to say? What would make it easier for George to communicate in this environment?

Fostering communication

Communication occurs all day and every day, and the fostering of communication in children and adults with learning disabilities should reflect this by recognizing that the families, teachers and other communication partners are the best resource. Written programmes may cause stress as they have to be read and assimilated into child rearing and interactional practices. Also, the programme writer's style of interaction with children may not correspond with that of the parents, and their interaction may become stilted and unnatural. If, as a result, they then abandon the programme, they may feel guilt and their relationship with the child and therapist may suffer as a result. As experts on their child (see Chapter 11), parents and carers can be equal partners in the facilitation process with the therapist, and it is important to develop the team for the person with learning difficulties, who can make joint decisions about appropriate strategies for improving communication.

All potential communication partners of the person with learning disabilities can be responsible for enhancing and facilitating the communication partnership. MacDonald (1985) outlines some natural teaching principles, the understanding of which can contribute to a positive communicative environment, for example:

1　*The ubiquity principle* – all behaviours communicate. Every behaviour potentially carries a communicative message and the communication partner can richly interpret behaviours to facilitate the communication, except possibly in the case of self-stimulatory stereotypical behaviours where it might be best to distract the communicator.

2　*The systems principle* – this is the principle that there are multiple members of the team or system for any one person and each needs to be a target for training. The child or person with learning difficulties is not the only receiver of therapy or training. Communication partners should also receive training.

3　*The joint attention principle* – communication is more likely to occur if the communication partners can focus on the interest and activity of the communicator.

4　*The expectancy principle* – communication partners need to behave as if they expect the child or person with learning difficulties to communicate; they need to wait and listen.

5　*The trade-off principle* – if the person has an effective but non-desirable method of communication there must be a significant and immediate result if they are to be encouraged to replace this effective behaviour with a new one that has no proven benefit, as in the following case study.

Case study: *Robert*

Robert is a young man with severe learning difficulties and visual impairment. As a young child he regularly put his hand down his nappy and smeared faeces. When he did this he would be attended by a carer who would change and clean him. In time Robert became aware that smearing could be an alerting tool. He began to reach for his nappy to get attention or to avoid an activity. If Robert were successfully to use a single-message communication aid or an object of reference the 'payoff' for him would have to be immediate, clear and effective enough to prevent the undesirable behaviour.

There are a number of facilitation strategies which aim to enhance the communication skills of a person with learning disabilities, for example intensive interaction (Nind and Hewett 2001) in which the communication partner pays close attention to and responds adaptively to behaviours which may be communicative. Speech and language therapists may develop, in conjunction with users and carers, strategies that are designed to build vocabulary, grammatical or speech or social skills. However, in an inter-action it is most important that the intention behind the communication is recognized and acknowledged so that it can be 'functional' even if not age-appropriate in terms of language or clear in speech production.

Roland and Schweigert (1993) suggest that functional communication:

- occurs in everyday real life and natural situations;
- results in real consequences, the act affecting the environment, with changes in accordance with the intent of the communication;
- includes but is not limited to spontaneous communication – communi-cation skills are not fully functional if the communicator is incapable of using them except when prompted to do so.

Some people may not be able to use speech at all as their main method of communication and may need to use alternatives. As recognizing and responding to alternatives to oral communication is not currently a common experience for most people, it may be necessary for supporting organizations to arrange regular training for groups of carers and people working within the learning disability community.

In the future, the increase in children with special needs being educated with their peers in mainstream schools may bring greater understanding of a range of communication styles on the part of the wider community.

Alternative methods of communication

Use of sign

Signing should be considered as a positive alternative or augmentative method of communication. Makaton signing, British sign language and Signalong are signing systems that have been used positively with popula-tions of children and adults with learning disabilities as they provide a multi-sensory approach to communication (Paul 1995) and can help with understanding as well as expression. Makaton is a sign vocabulary devised for use with people with learning disabilities, and the vocabulary items, which are presented in stages, reflect the common experiences and needs of people who have limited cognitive ability.

Use of symbols

Objects of reference are miniature objects or parts of objects which represent very closely an activity or an idea. For example, a key may be used to indicate going out as it refers to the key of the door, car keys etc., or a piece of coat fabric or shoelace may indicate going out. A cup, or a bottle, or a straw, whatever is relevant to the person, may indicate drink. When the planned activity is about to take place, the person is given the object of reference to hold and then the activity continues. They come to associate the object with the activity and are passed the object every time the activity is imminent. In time, some people learn to select an object and hold it or hand it to someone to indicate that they want the activity to take place. Each person has their own customized vocabulary and set of objects that are easily understood by them. Objects can have written labels on them to enable carers who might be unfamiliar with this system to understand the person's communication. It is also possible to use textured material as symbols, particularly if the person has a visual impairment.

Some people with learning difficulties will benefit from using *pictures* as an aid to communication. There are a number of different types of pictures from photographs which represent as close to real objects as possible, through to lined drawings which represent the idea in some detail, to symbols which are abstract representations of the idea. The pictures can be used in a number of ways: the person can be encouraged to pick a picture and hand it to their communication partner to get an idea across. A structured programme to enable this is called the Picture Exchange Communication System (Bondy and Frost 1992); alternatively, the pictures can be assembled into a sequence to give the users information and allow them to continue to look at the sequence over time to remind themselves of the information. Picture sequences may be used in, for example, dressing or work tasks.

Use of communication aids

A Big Mack, a single message switch, can help a person with very limited communication skills to signal that they need attention or request that an activity is repeated. Clearly just one message significantly limits communication options but there are communication aids which can convey longer and more complex messages, the level of aid being influenced by the person's general learning capacity

Because communication and language play a central role in human development and behaviour throughout a person's life, the facilitation of communication and any therapeutic intervention that needs to take place must work across disciplines. It should not be exclusively the province of the speech and language therapist to manage communication. While they have analytical and facilitation skills in the area of communication, they cannot be with the person in crucial communication settings. The communication plan for the individual must therefore be agreed across the team for that individual and implemented by everyone in typical everyday settings. The presence of a speech and language therapist may mean that other members of the team abdicate responsibilities for communication to the speech and language therapist, but this can be counterproductive for the person trying to communicate.

Conclusion

Good communication lies at the heart of enabling people with learning disabilities to be heard, understood and respected. It requires that we pay attention both to the foundations of how people with limited verbal articulacy seek to communicate and to the skills and communicative competencies of families and health and social care practitioners.

People with learning disabilities may not understand as much language as you would expect of a person of their age, so:

- use short sentences;
- use gestures/pointing to support what you say;
- don't talk too fast, but there is no need to talk loudly.

People with learning disabilities may take longer to process language, so:

- give them a little more time to make a response;
- wait and listen.

People with learning disabilities may find it hard to express themselves, so:

- give them time and listen;
- try hard to understand what they are trying to express;
- help out if you can, but don't put words in their mouth or rush them;
- if you don't understand, say so and see if the person can tell you another way.

People with learning disabilities may have been limited in their life experiences, so:

- offer communication opportunities (i.e. give choices, try not to assume).

You might use a number of augmentative or alternative communication approaches to enable the systems of input, processing and output to be successfully achieved.

A sensitivity to features of the language skills model described in this chapter may be helpful in reminding us of how to take account of these matters in an integrated way. Rolling out arrangements for advocacy, person-centred planning and the inclusion of people with learning disabilities in decision-making forums will heighten the importance of the contributions they can make in shaping their own lives and influencing others. Allied to these important changes, helping staff to communicate more effectively will have a centrally important part to play in promoting the well-being and social inclusion of people who are too easily marginalized because of a 'poverty of speech and language'.

Resources

Big Mack
Prentke Romich Company
1022 Heyl Road, Wooster, OH 44691, USA
Tel: +1 (330) 262 1984
www.prentrom.com

BLISS
Blissymbol Communication (UK)
c/o ACE Centre, 92 Windmill Road, Oxford, OX3 7DR
Tel: 01608 676 445
www.blissymbols.co.uk

British sign language
British Deaf Association
1–3 Worship Street, London, EC2A 2AB
Tel: 0800 6522 965
www.britishdeafassociation.org.uk/bsl/

Makaton
Makaton Vocabulary Development Project
31 Firwood Drive, Camberley, Surrey, GU15 3QD
Tel: 01276 61390
www.makaton.org

Mayer Johnson Symbols
Mayer-Johnson LLC
PO Box 1579, Solana Beach, CA 92075-7579, USA
Tel: +1 (800) 588 4548
www.mayer-johnson.com

Paget Gorman
Paget Gorman Society
2 Downlands Bungalows, Downloads Lane, Smallfield, Surrey, RH6 9SD
Tel: 0134 284 2308
www.pgss.org

PECS
Pyramid Educational Consultants UK Ltd
Pavilion House, 6 Old Steine, Brighton, BN1 1EJ
Tel: 01273 609555
www.pecs.org.uk

Rebus
Widgit Software Ltd
124 Cambridge Science Park, Milton Road, Cambridge, CB4 0ZS
Tel: 01223 425 558
www.widgit.com

Signalong
The Signalong Group
Stratford House, Waterside Court, Neptune Close, Rochester, Kent, ME4 4NZ
Tel: 0870 7743752
www.signalong.org.uk

Talking Mats
AAC Research Unit
University of Stirling, Stirling, FK9 4LA, Scotland
Tel: 01786 467645
www.psychology.stir.ac.uk/AAC/infosheet.htm

References

Abbeduto, L. and Rosenberg, S. (1992) Linguistic communication in persons with mental retardation, in S.F. Warren and J. Reichle (eds) *Causes and Effects in Communication and Language*. Baltimore, MD: Paul H. Brookes.

Abudarham, S. and Hurd, A. (2002) *Management of Communication Needs in People with Learning Disability*. London: Whurr.

Beckman, P.J. (1983) The relationship between behavioural characteristics of children and social interaction in an integrated setting, *Journal of Early Intervention*, 7: 69–77.

Bliss, L.S. (1985) The development of persuasive strategies by mentally retarded children, *Applied Research in Mental Retardation*, 6(4): 437–47.

Bondy, A.S. and Frost, L.A. (1992) *The Picture Exchange Communication System (PECS)*. Newark, DE: Pyramid Educational Consultants, Inc.

Bruner, J.S. (1975) The ontogenesis of speech acts, *Journal of Child Language*, 2: 1–40.

Chapman, R.S. and Hesketh, L.J. (2000) Behavioral phenotype of individuals with Down syndrome, *Mental Retardation and Developmental Disabilities Research Reviews*, 6: 84–95.

Chomsky, N. (1976) *Reflections on Language*. Glasgow: Fontana.

Cogher, L., Savage, E. and Smith, M.F. (1992) *Cerebral Palsy: The Child and Young Person (Management of Disability)*. London: Chapman & Hall.

Donahue, M., Pearl, R. and Bryan, T. (1982) Learning disabled children's syntactic: proficiency on a communicative task, *Journal of Speech and Hearing Disorders*, 47: 397–403.

Fantz, R.L. (1966) Pattern discrimination and selective attention as determinants of perceptual development from birth in A.H. Kidd and J.L. Rivoire (eds) *Perceptual Development in Children*. New York: International University Press.

Franklin, K. and Beukelman, D. (1991) Augmentative communication: directions for future research, in J. Miller (ed.) *Research on Child Language Disorders*. Austin, TX: Pro-Ed Inc.

Goldstein, H. and Kaczmarek, L. (1992) Promoting communicative interaction among children in integrated intervention settings, in S.F. Warren and J. Reichle (eds) *Causes and Effects in Communication and Language*. Baltimore, MD: Paul H. Brookes.

Grice, H.P. (1975) Logic and conversation, in P. Cole and J. Morgan (eds) *Syntax and Semantics, Volume 3, Speech Acts*. New York: Academic Press.

Guralnick, M.J. and Paul-Brown, D. (1986) Communicative interactions of mildly delayed and normally developing preschool children: effects of listener's developmental level, *Journal of Speech and Hearing Research*, 29(1): 2–10.

Kohn, M. (1966) The child as determinant of his peers' approach to him, *Journal of Genetic Psychology*, 109: 91–100.

Light, J., Collier, B.K. and Parnes, P. (1985) Communicative interaction between nonspeaking physically disabled children and their primary caregivers: Part II – communicative function, *Augmentative & Alternative Communication*, 1(3): 98–107.

MacDonald, J. (1985) Language through conversation: a model for intervention with language-delayed persons, in S. Warren and A. Rogers-Warren (eds) *Teaching Functional Language: Generalization and Maintenance of Language Skills*. Baltimore, MD: University Park Press.

Miller, G.A. (1981) *Language and Speech*. San Francisco: W.H. Freeman.

Mueller, E. (1972) The maintenance of verbal exchanges between young children, *Child Development*, 43: 930–8.

National Patient Safety Agency (2004) *Understanding the Patient Safety Issues for People with Learning Disabilities*. London: NPSA.

Nind, M. and Hewett, D. (2001) *A Practical Guide to Intensive Interaction*. Kidderminster: BILD Publications.

Nuccio, J.B. and Abbeduto, L. (1993) Dynamic contextual variables and the directives of persons with mental retardation, *American Journal of Mental Retardation*, 5: 547–55.

Paul, R. (1995) *Language Disorders from Infancy through Adolescence: Assessment and Intervention*. St Louis, MI: Mosby.

Pearpoint, J., O'Brien, J. and Forest, M. (1993) *PATH: A Workbook for Planning Positive Possible Futures*, 2nd edn. Toronto: Inclusion Press.

Purcell, M., Morris, I. and McConkey, R. (1999) Staff perceptions of the communicative competence of adult persons with intellectual disabilities, *British Journal of Developmental Disabilities*, 45(1, 88): 16–25.

Raffaelli, M. and Duckett, E. (1989) 'We were just talking . . .': conversations in early adolescence, *Journal of Youth and Adolescence*, 18: 567–81.

Roland, C. and Schweigert, P. (1993) Analyzing the communication environment to increase functional communication, *Journal of the Association for Persons with Severe Handicaps*, 18: 161–76.

Sheridan, M.D. (1973) *Children's Developmental Progress: From Birth to Five Years*. Windsor: NFER.

Stern, D.N. (1977) *The First Relationship: Infant and Mother*. Cambridge, MA: Harvard University Press.

Tager-Flusberg, H. (ed.) (1999) *Neurodevelopmental Disorders*. Cambridge, MA: MIT Press.

Wistow, R. and Schneider, J. (2003) Users' views on supported employment and social inclusion: a qualitative study of 30 people in work, *British Journal of Learning Disabilities*, 31(4): 166–74.

PART THREE

Independence

Adolescents and the younger adult

Part Three of this book considers independence in relation to adolescence and younger adulthood in the lives of people with learning disabilities. This is an especially important period for young people with learning disabilities and their families, for it heralds key transitions in their lives. Most obvious are the transitions from adolescence to adulthood, and from child to adult services. It may also be a period when familiar figures like siblings and friends are moving away to pursue careers or set up home. Accompanying these transitions for those involved are growing sensitivities about typical and normative behaviours and the fulfilment of adult roles and identities. Steps towards a more independent life also bring with them challenges, risks and adult protection issues that can be life-changing for both individuals and families. Chapters in this section provide the reader with an appreciation of how these issues are experienced in the everyday lives of people with learning disabilities, what services are doing to address them, and how health and social care practitioners can provide important help.

Beginning with some narrative accounts from adolescents and young people, Chapter 14 by Margaret Flynn and Philippa Russell points to many of the disabling barriers that young people face. It draws the reader into a critical appreciation of a range of important elements, including:

- socially constructed barriers that young people with learning disabilities report and which impinge upon their development of self-concept;

- young people's aspirations for schooling and employment and barriers between school and taking up employment;

- barriers to the development of role models and the implications and actualities for young people's self-definitions;

- aspirations and barriers to developing friendships, relationships and a social life;

- growing up in a culture of assessment, examinations and reviews.

Chapter 15 continues to draw from some narrative accounts by people with learning disabilities. Peter Goward and Linda Gething focus the reader's attention on the identification of factors that support both younger individuals and groups of people with learning disabilities in developing resilience, despite their encountering adversity. In particular the reader is invited to consider:

- the construction of scientific certainty and its limitations;
- the concept of resilience;
- the growing awareness of protective factors in relation to the individual, their support networks and the environment;
- factors that undermine resilience;
- the social construction of difference and the potential for reconstruction and renegotiation of social identities;
- the concepts of reciprocity and distributive competence;
- resilience through shared action and the disabled rights movement.

In Chapter 16 Margaret Flynn and Hilary Brown encourage the reader to consider the wider contexts in which abuse takes place, critically appraising the more typical methods of prevention and pointing to examples of best practice. With the help of case examples, the reader is enabled to reflect upon a range of issues surrounding independence, autonomy, national policy and the primary prevention of abuse. In particular the chapter supports a critical appreciation of the following factors:

- the nature of independence, autonomy, power, empowerment and protection;
- the policy context in which community living occurs;
- manifestations of abuse;
- making sense of incomplete information surrounding incidences of abuse;
- proactive approaches to abuse prevention and detection;
- building primary and tertiary systems of prevention into service delivery;
- staff training implications;
- external professional scrutiny of practitioners and governmental scrutiny of services.

Chapter 17 reviews the nature and causes of behaviour that challenges services, together with the main strategies employed in support of people who exhibit such behaviour. To assist the reader to develop a broad appreciation of the nature and causes of challenging behaviours, Sally Twist and Ada Montgomery outline the mainstream approaches that may assist the person with a challenging behaviour to lead a fulfilling and healthy lifestyle. The reader is assisted to understand:

- definitions of challenging behaviour, its nature, functions, modes of expression and prevalence;
- additional contributory factors;
- mental health and challenging behaviour;
- blocks to understanding challenging behaviour;
- assessment of challenging behaviour;
- support and intervention;
- staff training and support;
- safety factors.

In Chapter 18 Alex McClimens and Helen Combes explore sexuality and young people with learning disabilities. Views of people with learning disabilities in relation to sexual needs and identity are discussed. Additionally the reader is invited to adopt a self-reflexive approach and ask themselves how they might think, feel or act in similar situations to those faced by people with learning disabilities, with a view to understanding:

- the historical context in which the sexual needs and sexual identity of people with learning disabilities are set;
- the meanings of sexuality to young people and those assisting them;
- the issues concerning behaviour, risk factors, gender, contraception, parenting, relationships and consent;
- factors that determine the marginalization of individuals/groups;
- implications for social and health support service providers/carers.

In Chapter 19 Nigel Beail offers the reader some detailed examples of what happens to people with learning disabilities when they encounter the criminal justice system as either complainants, witnesses, accused or offenders. Drawing from the most recent research, the chapter introduces the reader to a series of case examples, enabling a critical appreciation of the support needs of people with learning disabilities at each stage of the process. In particular the following are critically examined:

- the historical view of criminality and learning disability;
- vulnerability of people to crimes committed against them;
- why people with learning disabilities come into contact with the criminal justice system;
- what happens to people with learning disabilities at different points in the criminal justice system and the difficulties they encounter;
- how people may be supported at each stage of the criminal justice system;
- mitigation factors;
- victim support;
- guidance for 'appropriate adults' and police officers.

Chapter 20 draws the reader into the world of day services and the prospects of employment in the lives of young people with learning disabilities. Mark Powell and Margaret Flynn examine the tenacious grip of the day services model, a model that remains irrespective of current policy and the promising opportunities emerging within the social economy that places people before profit and social benefit before return on investment. This chapter therefore points to 'work' initiatives that are developing as alternatives to day services. Using accounts from people with learning disabilities the reader is drawn into a critical examination of the following:

- the importance and meanings of work;
- the tenacity of day service provision;
- the development of a social economy and work alternatives to day services;
- supported employment and social firms;
- holistic approaches to tackling social, economic and environmental matters;
- policy and practice initiatives that have led to the promotion of independence through work.

Counselling services are increasingly regarded as an important therapy in helping people cope with major life events, transitions in the life cycle and traumas. As several chapters within this book illustrate, people with learning disabilities are likely to face more than their fair share of adversity, yet they are also likely to have fewer friendships and relationships that can support them during and after such events (see e.g. Chapters 15, 16 and 23). Access to counselling services can, therefore, offer a valuable means of helping people with learning disabilities to understand such major life events, transitions in their life cycle and traumatic experiences. Ultimately, therefore, such access has a potential to assist those who have suffered adversity to cope, thereby fostering resilience and perhaps recovery. In the final chapter of Part Three, Jill Jesper and Jayne Stapleton draw from case examples in order to outline the therapeutic potential of counselling in relation to people with learning disabilities. In particular the following aspects are addressed:

- the purposes of counselling;
- counselling processes;
- the skills of counselling;
- types of counselling.

14

Adolescents and younger adults

Narrative accounts

Margaret Flynn and Philippa Russell

I was always being asked difficult questions, personal questions. Some of them were frightening. What was I going to do in adult life? I needed preparation for some of those questions. It seemed easier just not to answer. But really I had important things to say. I needed someone to break the questions down so that I could answer them. I felt quite frightened when someone asked me about my future. But I needed to talk about it, if only someone would understand. I think they went away saying he's got a learning difficulty, there's no point in talking to him.

(John, looking back on his teenage years when a severe speech impediment and cerebral palsy made communication difficult except through the use of Makaton, in Russell 1998a: 24)

Introduction

The material on which this chapter is based is drawn from a variety of work – a recent anthology (Murray and Penman 2000) along with studies and focus groups which explore selected domains of young people's life experiences (e.g. Flynn 1998; Russell 1998a, forthcoming). It is not proposed that these narratives and extracts from interviews promise authentic information about the experience of adolescence. More accurately, they are glimpses of young people's self-selected chronologies in which some experiences of adolescence are featured. The adolescence described may have been subject to the change arising from the young people's interaction with new experiences as they 'look back'. The first section summarizes what is known about the experience of adolescence. It presents two women's experience of school and their challenges to educational structures. The next section explores young people's concerns about the existence of a parallel special school system and the absence of role models as they prepare to leave school. The enduring aspiration of employment against the pull of day services and the socially constructed shadows and silences surrounding medical realities and other matters of importance bring this section to a close. The next section considers the layered subject of people's friendships and relationships, bearing in mind that most of us recognize that a lack of friends is undesirable, regardless of the time spent with families. Finally, we look at identity matters – young people's self-definitions and the groups to which they assign themselves – which serve to affirm adolescents as somebodies. The aim is to consider how young people talk about and make sense of their adolescence, their experiences as children and young disabled people and the implications of these for their adulthood.

Context

Broadly, this chapter is concerned with the times in young people's lives which predate their being viewed as legally and ethically equal to make decisions for themselves. This life phase challenges beliefs about the appropriateness and scope of parental authority which links with an underlying uncertainty about the moral status of young people (e.g. Purdy 1992). Adolescence marks the end of childhood and the beginning of adulthood as physical growth is completed and the skills required for adult roles and responsibilities are acquired. It is a period of enormous change as young people begin to have adult capacity, although their behaviour may occasionally be more childlike than adult. Not surprisingly, the age range defining adolescence varies according to the setting, the purpose of the definition and the individuals involved (Cotterell 1996; Blustein *et al.* 1999). It is noteworthy that research has consistently assembled evidence which demonstrates that the better we know people with learning disabilities, the more we discover that their aspirations, wants, values and pleasures fall within the range of desires common to most of us and that most young people aspire to what we recognize as an ordinary life (e.g. Kuh *et al.* 1986; Le Touze and Pahl 1990; Flynn and Hirst 1992).

The subject of being with peers who do not have disabilities, and in turn inclusion in mainstream education opportunities or segregated special schools, exercises many young people and their families. While some positive aspects of segregated residential schools and colleges are acknowledged (e.g. Thomas *et al.* 1996), there are some remarkable barriers to be lowered and removed before local schools are assisted to become inclusive:

> I believe that we shouldn't be in special schools. Everyone should be together so we can mix and make new friends with all kinds of people. All people are different. We should not be sent far away and educated in places we don't want because of our differences. I have been to two special schools. In one, one of the teachers made a stuffed fish for us and

two bunny rabbits. I took them home and I destroyed them because I didn't make them for myself. How do we learn to do things for ourselves if teachers do it for you? Why do we need schools if we don't learn anything for ourselves? I also went to a mainstream school and I had been there for five years when the Headmistress turned around and said 'What is this "mongol" person doing in my school?' My mother took her to High Court and we won and she lost. I was bullied at special school . . . Sending us to special school is not the best for us. We are still called names and bullied. We don't want special schools. We don't need special treatment. We want our human rights . . . I went on to college and work. Now I work on my stained glass. I am independent. I do my own things. I was brought up to be independent and disciplined. From my mother.

(Anya Souza in Murray and Penman 2000: 78–9)

I didn't like being kept apart from the other children when I went to my primary school. I had to eat downstairs and everyone else ate upstairs. No one asked me what I thought about it or how I could have eaten with the other children . . . children know about the people who work with them better than the adults. I had a helper who wouldn't let me go in the playground. Now I write my helper's job description and we have got it sorted . . . I wanted to go to my local mainstream school. I am a part time pupil there but only because the toilets are inaccessible. The leisure centre next door is fully accessible and they were happy for me to use their toilets – but that wasn't acceptable! So I go to mainstream part time but have to be driven 12 miles to a special school to use their toilet. By the time I have got there it is too late to come back . . . I go to and from school in a taxi. But I'd like to spend time after school with my friends like everyone else, to go to the library, to do homework together. I asked if I could bring a friend home with me but was told the insurance wouldn't allow it. I tried to argue there was plenty of room and the taxi must be insured for passengers anyway. The next thing I knew was that someone I didn't know was sharing the taxi with me and there wasn't room for my friends! I wasn't asking for much, only to use the taxi service better.

(Lucy Mason and Maresa Mackeith quoted in Russell 1998b: 42–3)

Clearly there is more to inclusive education than opening doors and having the names of young people with disabilities on the registers. The challenge to the whole school system is to prepare all young people to participate fully in the lives of their communities.

Exercise 14.1

Think of the parents you know, who have young children with a learning disability.

How would you make sure that they understood all the options for the education of their child?

What information and advice would you offer, if they expressed strong preferences for a mainstream or for a special school?

What sources of independent advice might be available in their communities?

Most importantly, how would you convey a positive picture of the children's future and the importance of high-quality educational experiences in achieving good outcomes?

Some horizons of experience

Schools have unavoidable impacts on young people, not merely on their learning, but on their ways of behaving and their attitudes towards further education, work and adulthood. The organizational conclusion of adolescence may be attenuated by extending the ages at which young people leave school (typically at 19 years) and colleges (at ages up to 25 years) if they go directly from school. The preceding and following narratives illuminate the perplexing eligibility criteria and obstacles that prevailed as parents sought to identify the right kind of education for their children and challenge the perceptions of difference which impacted on their daughters' lives:

> I am 24 years old . . . have problems with communication and coordination. I also have mild learning difficulties. I live at home with my parents and younger brother . . . In 1997 I went to Portland College, Mansfield for two short assessment visits . . . It was a bit strange at first because it was my first time away from home. Fortunately that didn't last long because we were looked after by Care Tutors who were nice and friendly. I tried out different subjects such as Computers, English, Maths and Horticulture. They had a full programme of activities at weekends and evenings . . . There was also a lot of independence training which was very useful . . . I was delighted when they offered me a place on their Further Education Course for two or three years. That was the good bit. I then had to try and get funding to pay for the course. I applied to the Further Education Funding Council. I had to fill in a lot of forms and provide details of everything I had done since I left school. It seemed to take ages before I got a reply and unfortunately they turned me down. That, of course, was the bad bit. I was very disappointed. I appealed against the decision but they wouldn't change their minds. I am pleased that I have now been employed as a messenger in the postroom at Porterbrook House. I really enjoy the work and I have the same terms and conditions as all the other workers . . . I hope that I will have more good things than bad in the future.
>
> (Sally Mason in Murray and Penman 2000: 213–14)

By the time I was 13 I was well into my secondary school. It was the Sheffield's Maud Maxfield School for the Deaf. I am not deaf, and to this day I do not know why I was sent there. My looks had been very much improved, but the earlier name calling had left its mark. I was very insecure until I was about 15 years old. From the deaf school I was transferred to an open air school and it was here that I decided to change my name . . . I was a good dancer. This was achieved by going into Working Men's Clubs . . . My father in his mistaken wisdom tried to bribe young boys to dance with me by buying them drinks, but when my father disappeared, so did my partners. But I had a fighter's spirit and I danced on with my girlfriends as partners . . . In my young adult years there were still the knocks and bangs such as the man who admitted he'd only gone out with me for a bet . . . I met my future husband in a pub. He was not a dancer but he was a wonderful man. We got married . . . I was 24 years old. We had four very handsome boys . . . the experiences, good and bad, have made me who I am today. I am an ordinary woman who just happened to be born with a double hare lip and cleft palate.

(Anne Hunt in Murray and Penman 2000: 32–3)

These narratives touch on many topics: the tenacity of a parallel, special education system and an enduring reluctance to educate children and young people with disabilities – or even with a hare lip and cleft palate – in local, mainstream schools; the arbitrariness of the ways in which classifications are made and the implications of this for children's education; the critical arena of self-expression in shaping young women's lives; and parental efforts to enable young people to sample ordinary experiences and preclude potential isolation.

In the late 1980s, a large, nationally representative sample of children and adults with disabilities was interviewed to assess the financial and social consequences of disability, including effects on employment and mobility, and to provide information about the use and need for health and social services (Martin and White 1988; Martin *et al.* 1988, 1989; Bone and Meltzer 1989; Smyth and Robus 1989). Seventy-nine young people with learning disabilities were interviewed to complement the main OPCS surveys (Flynn and Hirst 1992). This study confirmed that young people had not been emancipated from the 'day care' assumption which special school leavers often encounter; and that local adult and further education agencies addressed the need for scarcity of day services for adults with learning disabilities by providing courses for people with special needs. It also confirmed the widespread underemployment and unemployment of young people with learning disabilities. It indicated also young women's generally impoverished employment status, when considered alongside that of young men, and arguably the absence of encouragement for them to be economically active (and resonated with such earlier research findings as Asch and Sacks 1983 and Hahn 1983).

I'd like to meet an adult disabled person, I mean, someone who is like me. I don't know any disabled people. I'm Black and everyone talks about my culture – but I have a disabled culture too, don't I? I'd like a few role models. Most of all I want a job.

(Russell 1998a: 3)

It would be really great to meet grown ups who are disabled like me and getting on with their lives. They could really tell me what I need to do to get a job, get a home of my own. I can't see myself as a grown up if I don't meet anyone like me.

(Russell 1998b: 32)

Such observations attest to the significance of wanting to learn from the insights, perspectives and experiences of older people who have had similar life experiences, and to construct self-images that are influenced by people whose lives appear enviable. They also attest to the importance of experienced mentors who may describe their situational influences and their ways of perceiving, explaining and understanding the preoccupations of adolescence.

The subject of employment as an enduring aspiration unifies the findings of many studies, focus groups and workshops examining the post-school opportunities and aspirations of school leavers with disabilities (e.g. Anderson *et al.* 1982; Flynn and Hirst 1992; Flynn 1998). This aspiration cannot easily be set aside as the effects of not having a job reach far beyond unemployment, as these extracts from Flynn (1998: 2, 2, 3, 5, 7) demonstrate:

It's not very easy on Income Support because if you get employment you're only allowed £15.00 a week.

[You can't] retire [from a day centre] because you lose your place.

We work in environments where we're not paid . . . We don't want to be taken advantage of.

Mum wakes me at 8.30. I have breakfast with my mum. I get washed, clean my teeth and put the radio on. A big ambulance thing comes. It picks up three wheelchairs and a walker. I get to the centre at about 10.00. I sometimes go to [another centre] and go to the light room as well. At 10.30 we have coffee and a tea break. Then it's the light room until dinner time [mid-day until 1.30pm]. After, I watch TV, play games on the computer . . . after tea break I get ready to go home. I wait for transport. People get dropped off then home at last.

Social services said we should have our education classes at the Technical College like everyone else. Now hardly anyone has education classes . . . you can't stay on a course at college for a very long time but some of us learn slowly. This does not mean we are not progressing . . . If you have a lot of disabilities you do not get to go to college . . . Members would like to do courses that would help them to get a job . . .

other Members would like to do courses for leisure . . . in other words, our Members would like the same opportunities as everyone else.

Such reflections, routines and experiences capture the terrains yet to be negotiated if young people with learning disabilities are to envisage themselves as employees. The insistent question, 'What do you want to do when you grow up?' is familiar to most young people whose prospective autonomy is taken for granted. Answers may refer to living and working circumstances, travel, adventure, intimate relationships, marriage and parenthood. Such aspirations are known to have sustaining qualities. Although life in uncertain times may render us unwilling to think ahead, most of us anticipate that we will be instrumental in shaping our own futures. What the preceding quotations confirm are the starkly finite options available to young people with disabilities. Entering paid employment, leaving the parental home, having intimate relationships, getting married and perhaps having children are widely regarded as markers of adulthood. By 'silencing' such topics (e.g. Fine 1995) the experiential conditions of young people's lives are effectively ignored:

> When I was 14 I suddenly realised how little I knew about my disability. My parents did not want to discuss it and my teachers and friends were silent if I raised the issue. I wanted to know what the options were. How can you have a 'transition plan' if you don't know what jobs you could do? I began to watch things on TV, to read bits in the newspaper. I imagined dreadful things, I would get worse, I was really ill, I might die. I couldn't sleep at night and my schoolwork got worse. I felt really depressed. Then the school nurse talked to me and asked what I was worrying about. She was really helpful and practical. She told me about a group of young people in my town. She gave me information to read and told me about a national organisation for my disability. She also said I could ask to see the doctor on my own if I wanted – but I should tell my parents how I felt. In the end we wrote them a letter. I didn't want secrets. They were really upset to find I had been so worried. I went to see my paediatrician and he was wonderful, very helpful. I wish people would realise that we do want information about ourselves. We do want to meet other disabled people. We don't want to be seen as problems. I have my own health plan now and that's good.
>
> (Peter in Russell 1998b: 52)

> Realising that my disability may get worse. Nobody at home would talk about it. I never met any disabled people at my school. When I was 14 they started saying, 'You can't' and I heard things. Now I know I might die young. That's awful. There are a lot of places for parents to get information, but no one seems to want to do that for me.

> I want to know if I can have children. My parents don't want to know. They just say 'Look after yourself first.' But it matters doesn't it? Could I? And if not, why not?

> I don't know much about sex education. They do it at school but lots of

parents withdraw their children so it isn't much use. I may be disabled but I'm human like everyone else. And I can't just disappear down town to buy something to read.

I'd like to talk about incontinence. It's an awful subject isn't it? But it stops me going on school trips. I think it will stop me getting a job. What about girlfriends? Could I ring up the GP and get him to send me somewhere? I don't want my parents around.

(Young people in Russell 1998b: 92)

Yes, I really worry about the future. I know some people [with cystic fibrosis] do really well now. But some die. Some of the kids I've seen at my hospital have died. It's scary really.

(Young person in Russell 1998a: 3)

Such fundamental concerns bring to the foreground what is not being said to young people. It can be perceived as protective not to discuss the implications of people's medical conditions and disability. Yet such a hide and control stance can be endorsed by the wider context and wander into other topics of enormous significance to young people:

- 'The most important thing is loving each other, helping each other, emotional health.'
- 'You need to know every part of the body to help you explain.'
- 'No, I don't get embarrassed. Men and women are all the same in a way. Just different.'
- 'Parents tell you about having babies.'
- 'And that you don't just come out with things like that!'

Parents in some localities questioned whether sex education was necessary for their child's development, perhaps confirming the sense of censorship which appeared to characterize the sexuality of young adults. A local project found that the majority of parents interviewed did not know whether or how sex education was taught in the schools or how to teach some of the issues at home. Neither did they know whether menstrual cycle care featured in the curriculum for young women (Pearson *et al.* 1997):

Difficulties arose in one special school where they undertook no special health education, sex education or more neutrally, training in first aid. The families of some young people with learning disabilities wanted assistance with preparing their relatives for adulthood and the possibility of sexual relationships. Primary health care teams were anxious not to take a lead on this subject in order not to 'medicalise' sexuality. The local authority questioned why this and associated subjects should be seen as the unique responsibility of social care providers.

(Pearson *et al.* 1997: 68)

Sexuality has a central place in negotiating the transition to adulthood. The tasks of integrating sexual feelings and desires into a positive self-identity, which includes a positive sexual self, are complex. Values and norms about masculinity and femininity interact with family expectations about what constitutes acceptable behaviour, and yet, examination of these structured silences and shadows speaks of disproportionate exclusion, and more partitions to be dismantled. Pearson *et al.* (1997) identified superficially neutral boundaries to controlling what it is that young people with learning disabilities may be taught, in school, by health care professionals and social care professionals. However, these have far-reaching consequences for young people and expose the dynamic of exclusion.

Improvements in the level and quality of personal, health and sex education for young people with learning disabilities (crucial as these are) will not in themselves guarantee social inclusion and positive personal relationships for young disabled people. A survey of the views of young disabled people between 16 and 24 (Disability Rights Commission and MORI 2002) found that over 35 per cent (regardless of their disability) expected to have more difficulties in making relationships in adult life and finding a partner than their non-disabled peers. Thirty-two per cent noted their difficulties in accessing a social life (which might be reasonably expected to generate the friendships and connections from which most people form closer individual relationships as adults). They commented on their over-dependence on parents and family members to facilitate social and leisure activities and the lack of freedom to just 'hang out' with their peers.

However, the survey clearly showed that the aspirations of young disabled people mirrored those for young people without a disability. The survey covered young people with a range of disabilities (including learning disability), and there was no difference in views expressed between the different disability groups represented. Key aspirations included:

- a well-paid job by the time the young people reached 30;
- the opportunity to travel;
- a home of their own;
- a partner and a family;
- to have attended university or to have continued education and training for a career.

Relationships mattered to those participating in the survey. Perhaps most worryingly, respondents in the 21–24 age range were twice as likely as those aged 16–20 to say they felt lonely a lot or all of the time. In effect, school and college had produced a range of friends and social activities which reduced or disappeared when young people dispersed to find work or to continue education or training outside their home areas. There was also a marked drop in confidence about the future as young people grew older. The survey found that one in three of the participants believed that they would be earning less than other people of their age by the time they were 30. Sixty-six per cent had problems with public transport (essential for a social life as well as potential employment).

The importance of access to a social life and employment in order to develop friendships was a key theme within the Disability Rights

Commission survey (2002). A young woman (Russell 2003: 13) similarly observed with some sadness that:

> . . . they talk about sex all the time at school, don't get pregnant, all that stuff. But they talk about it like learning to ride a bike. There's no point in learning to ride a bike if you don't understand the rules of the road and if there are no roads to ride on! It's a trick, nothing more. Me, of course I'd like a boyfriend. But I'd like some friends first – good mates teach you things, they look out for you. I'd feel safer if I got out more, learnt to hang out with the others. Otherwise all this stuff about condoms and HIV, it's stupid, isn't it? What I want is someone to help me get a life! No point in learning about sex and stuff, if you can't go anywhere without your mum tagging along behind you. Clubs, pubs, cinemas, just hanging out with your mates – I can't do it. Mum's there at 12.00pm with the car and I'm Cinderella – but I never get to the ball!

Exercise 14.2

Recalling your own experience of adolescence, what were your preoccupations as a teenager and which, if any, were 'silenced'? What did being 'grown up' mean to you?

Aspirations and realities

Our lives are not interesting. A fantastic life would be moving into a hostel on my own and staying there and having lots of money so I can retire into the country and not come back. I really want a girlfriend who is thinking about me now. I don't want people who help me. I like friends. I like an independent life. Now I just sit up and watch TV and listen until 5.00 in the morning. I go to sleep at 5.00 in the morning and 5.00 in the afternoon to make up my sleep. I like watching things about getting jobs . . . I've tried to get one before but things have stepped in my way . . . I like working with people . . . I'd love to go to sleep really tired after a hard days work.

My life would be fantastic if I was happy, engaged and married; I could do sports when I wanted; read books; do crosswords and play snooker.

I'd like a conversation with me and my girlfriend. They can't tell me what to do with my life. I get picked on at the [day] centre and I haven't done anything. They get me mad sometimes. In the centre they think I talk too much. I would be really happy if people didn't get at me all the time. I like making coffee for people. I'd like lots of money to be able to buy my girlfriend an engagement ring. I'd like a job and I'd like to be boss.

I like training to move into a group home or flat with Adam. I like Adam's company. I would be really happy if we could get married and settle down . . . I think Adam would like a job. I'd like to go out with Adam for a meal. I'd like to see different countries because I read loads of travel books. I'd like to work in a coffee bar serving people. I like visiting places with Adam. I'd like a lot of money so I can go into an expensive shop like C&A and get lots of things from there.

(Flynn 1993: 3–4)

It's about hopes and dreams, isn't it? School is really important. It's children's work, isn't it? Grown-ups go to work every day to earn their money. If you want to get a job, you have to go to work at school first, to learn lots of things. I want a good job, I want to get on in life. So I want a good school, then I've got a better chance, haven't I? I want to go to college, all that stuff, I'm tired of people saying 'can't'. But my school says 'you can', that's good. I feel they're fighting for me.

(Quotations from young people's focus groups in Russell 2003: 15–16)

Enduring friendships, and close and enjoyable relationships are recurring themes in the literature about adolescence. Concerns with belonging, being included, making and keeping friends and group affiliation are important sources of status and reputation (Cotterell 1996). Milardo (1992) proposed that friendship networks can be regarded as concentric circles, with very few in the centre (close friends or best friends) and friends and acquaintances in the outer circles. While school is a key location for meeting and making friends, out of school settings also play a part in developing closer friendships. Young people's confiding relationships were explored by Flynn and Hirst (1992). One in ten of the study sample claimed not to confide in anyone and over half confirmed that they confided in their mothers. The importance of families was similarly endorsed by young people in a focus group (Russell forthcoming), who stressed their (often reluctant) reliance on parents to act as supporters, advocates and, of course, as chauffeurs.

When contrasted with young people who did not have disabilities, this signalled more reliance on their parents for emotional support than young people generally. This was particularly the case for young women. We concluded that confiding in parents, especially mothers, as opposed to other adults or special friends, was widespread and that this was clearly linked to being in the parental home. It also crucially linked with opportunity. Two parent focus groups (Russell forthcoming: 28) identified the lack of accessible and safe transport for after-school and weekend activities as a major barrier to independence for their children. The parents regretted what one family saw as:

an old fashioned and interfering constant presence in our daughter's life. We are committed to giving her maximum independence, but that often means my husband or I picking her up from a club at 2.00am. If we have to get up for work at 6.30am the next morning, that's a real burden for us. We do it for Lily's sake. But she worries about us and we know she sometimes won't go out when she wants to, because she thinks we are too tired.

And yes, we've tried to book independent transport. But Lily didn't feel safe with the driver who turned up. So that idea came to a full stop and we're back as the taxi drivers. My husband even got pulled over by the police one evening – they thought he was a kerb crawler! He explained about Lily and how he had to hang around waiting for her. They were very nice about it. But it did not feel nice at the time. And of course it's not nice for Lily, she deserves a young person's life – but most of her time she's stuck with two sixty pluses who'd really just like an early night, but who have to act as her 'best friends'!

The importance of young people's weekday activities in terms of offering possibilities for non-family relationships was confirmed with just over two-thirds of the study sample referring to people who lived in their neighbourhoods. A few young people described adult figures such as teachers as their friends. Although many young women said that they saw their friends in their spare time, they were less likely to do so than their male peers. We expected the incidence of contact with friends to increase with age, reflecting greater freedom of movement as the young people got older. However, more of those in their early twenties were found to have limited social contact with their peers. The incidence of seeing friends also pointed to the particular isolation of young people with extensive support needs. The study suggested that it is more difficult to make new friends after leaving special school and to keep in touch with friends made at school (Flynn and Hirst 1992). However, the Disability Rights Commission and MORI's national opinion poll survey (2002) also found extensive problems in retaining old friends and making new friends in a cohort of young people aged 16–24, regardless of whether they had attended mainstream or special schools. One young woman of 23 who had attended a mainstream school and a local college commented in a personal communication that:

Round here, most young people go away to work or college. They move on. I'd like to move on too. But where do I go? Yes, I'd like some new friends. But I can't afford taxis. My support worker doesn't work evenings. There aren't any safe buses and things to travel on. I thought it would get better when I left school. Actually it's worse. And I don't feel safe where I live . . . there are some nasty kids, I don't go out after dark any more. Really, I feel like an old lady. And I'm 20 years young.

Other young people have made similar comments:

The name calling was painful. I got called 'spastic' and 'mongol'. They shouted at me 'cos I got learning difficulties and I don't read and write well. They said I was a dummy because I didn't get any homework. Well I went to my teacher and said I've got to learn to read and write, 'Help me!' She did and I've got a briefcase like the other kids for my papers now. I do homework just like them. If they call me spastic I just laugh.

I hear people talking about me to mum. They're sorry for her, having me. She says, 'Don't worry – she's great!' She helped me to speak up for myself. She said, 'It's your life and you've got to say what you want.' I'm on the Student Council at school now, the first Disabled Student.

The word respite care. Actually I love my link family and I know mum and dad need a break. To be honest I need a break from them too! But the word respite I looked it up in a dictionary and it said, 'Relief from burden'. It worries me. Am I a burden? I don't want to be but I expect I am, and I needn't be. I said to mum, 'If we had a wish list for the new bathroom, a better wheelchair, a wider front door, accessible shops, then I wouldn't be a burden to anyone.'

Being cared for! No one else is cared for when they are 13. I'd prefer to talk to someone about support and not care. I'm not the family dog! I want to be in charge.

(Russell 1998b: 91–3)

Identity matters

A key challenge for many young disabled people is that of developing an independent and confident identity amidst an ongoing procession of assessments, examinations and reviews. Russell (2003) found that many young people with disabilities or special educational needs were acutely aware of the constant assessments, reviews and target-setting which set them apart from their non-disabled peers.

In a series of focus groups with young disabled people (Russell 2003: 18), many participants described their anxieties about constant assessment. One pupil commented that: 'I'm sick of assessments all the time. The other kids, they do tests and SATS and things, and I get assessments. Why? One of the lads, he said I was like a second-hand car. I must always be breaking down, to have all these people fussing over me. I felt really bad, sort of singled out.' Another noted that: 'It'd be OK if they assessed you, like, for things you could do. But all they want to do is find out what you're bad at! I'm sick of being a problem, I want them to help me find out what I'm good at.' A third talked angrily about assessment for the Disability Living Allowance:

They sent someone to the house, like, and my mum and me, we had to go through all the things I couldn't do. My mum said, mind you don't look too good when he comes, we need the money. I think the money should be to help me move on, not to keep me stuck here. We do need the money, I can't use the bus and mum hasn't got a car. So we just sat there and made a list of what I couldn't do.

But sometimes assessment is seen as having a positive purpose. One young person described how:

> the school really helped me make a video of my day, when I wanted help and what help I needed to learn. The good thing was that the video showed what I could do on my own. It made me feel in control. They were asking me what do you want to do, what job do you want, let's work together. That felt really good, like I really mattered. I felt I had something to show all those people at the review, like 'this is me and this is where I'm going'.

For many young people, getting the right support is crucial. One young man (Russell forthcoming) described angrily how, when he first attended a mainstream school, the learning support assistants decided it would be easier to group all those needing some support at lunchtime round one table. He was angry and upset that he and other pupils with disabilities or special educational needs were, as he put it,

> . . . sat around like little kids, when all we needed was some help in standing in the queue and carrying our trays back. We didn't want the staff to go and load the food up for us. Half the time, we didn't want what they had chosen and then we got told off like little kids for not eating it up. And they kept mopping the table all the time – as if the other kids weren't spilling things too. The other kids, they took the micky and called us the 'rabbit table'. That's because our helpers made us eat salad all the time – no chips, no pudding. Talk about the Nazis! We're fifteen, for heaven's sake!
>
> (Russell forthcoming: 30)

This boy, Paul, finally plucked up courage to tell a teacher about his humiliation. The response was positive – a round-table discussion, some very embarrassed learning support assistants and the end of segregated eating. Very importantly, Paul and his friends are now involved in recruiting their own personal assistants and in training them and other staff in the school to avoid a repeat of the 'rabbit table'. Paul, reflecting on the experience, commented that:

> . . . the staff, they did mean well but they saw us as babies! They made us feel like babies too. Funny thing is, when I went to a special school, they were the other way round – pushing us to do more for ourselves. But I guess we were pioneers at 'X' school. We were their first disabled students and they learnt on the job. What I've learnt is that you have to speak up – and if you do, people listen. That's inclusion but it's hard work.
>
> (Russell forthcoming: 31)

Thus at a time when self-conceptions are emerging, some young people are highly attuned to being perceived as different and their daily interactions, and exposure to the views of others, yield opportunities for affirming these perceptions. Name-calling which hinges on young people's disabilities is harrowing at a time when self-conceptions and group identification are developing. Being acutely attuned to the verbal bullying and harassment others provides unsought information about the attitudes and values of others. At a time when young people spend time in public places with their peers, being part of a group which nurtures belonging and endorsement, and a sense of place, some young people experience being devalued. Further, their bullying may be a means of affirming the identity of the peer group which is so exclusive.

Witnessing the sympathies extended to a parent and understanding why a father buys young men drinks so that his daughter will not be a wallflower speaks of a significant parental role in making the experience of connectedness possible for their children. It would be inaccurate to cast this role as cotton-wool protectiveness. It reveals a reassurance to their offspring that they are accepted in their families and that inclusion and membership are important. In being overtly supportive and pre-empting the possibility of rejection, they act as best they can to give their offspring the confidence to meet these new challenges.

The mother who asserted of her daughter, 'She's great!' declined to focus on her daughter's disabled identity and simultaneously reassured her acquaintance, and as significantly her daughter, that her sympathy was unmerited. This is a role that is also performed by teachers, as the teacher of the young woman with Down's syndrome demonstrates. She responded to her pupil's desire to be as her peers: a reader and a writer and to have homework as they did. While the name-calling persisted, this young woman had new resources to draw from in dealing with it.

Politicization arrives early for some young people with disabilities:

> What do we want from life? Like everyone else we want to have our own homes, our partners, we want to be healthy, we want to see our families and friends. Disability isn't an end, it's a beginning. We like to think 'can do' not 'this is a problem'. If you talked to us more, you would know that disabled people are real people with things to say. Please hear us!

> It's not just us who are disabled and make the problems. It's the big world out there. Just think, if we made it better out there, then all sorts of people would be better too – mums with pushchairs, old people, dogs and things like that. I play sport, I go to school, I'm a scout and I help in a club for older people. We did citizenship in the National Curriculum the other day. That's me. I'm a citizen, not a problem!
>
> (Young people in Russell 1998b: 93)

Exercise 14.3

You are the headteacher of a mainstream school. How do you deal with the peer ridicule described in this chapter?

You are a teacher. How do you explore the subject of group identification with adolescents?

Conclusion

Listening to, and learning with, young people with learning disabilities breaks important ground. There are no shortcuts to realizing the practical, pragmatic and humane benefits of engaging children and young people in decision-making and in discussion about their identities and their lives.

References

Anderson, E.M. and Clarke, L. in collaboration with Spain, B. (1982) *Disability in Adolescence*. London: Methuen.

Asch, A. and Sacks, L. (1983) Lives without, lives within: the autobiographies of blind women and men, *Journal of Visual Impairment and Blindness*, 77(6): 242–7.

Blustein, J., Levine, C. and Neveloff-Dubler, N. (eds) (1999) *The Adolescent Alone: Decision Making in Health Care in the United States*. Cambridge: Cambridge University Press.

Bone, M. and Meltzer, H. (1989) *The Prevalence of Disability among Children*, OPCS Surveys of Disability in Great Britain, Report No. 3. London: HMSO.

Cotterell, J. (1996) *Social Networks and Social Influences in Adolescence*, Adolescence and Society Series. London: Routledge.

Disability Rights Commission and MORI (2002) *Survey of Young Disabled People Aged 16–24*. Disability Rights Commission, Research and Evaluation Unit (available via the Disability Rights Website at www.drc-gb.org).

Fine, M. (1995) Silencing and nurturing voice in an improbable context: urban adolescents in public school, in M. Fine (ed.) *Disruptive Voices: The Possibilities of Feminist Research*. Ann Arbor, MI: University of Michigan Press.

Flynn, M. (1993) *Consultation with People with Learning Disabilities*. North Yorkshire Community Care Plan 1994–1995. Manchester: National Development Team.

Flynn, M. (1998) *Customer Research with People with Learning Disabilities*. York: City of York.

Flynn, M. and Hirst, M. (1992) *This Year, Next Year, Sometime . . .? Learning Disability and Adulthood*. Manchester: National Development Team.

Hahn, H. (1983) *'The Good Parts': Interpersonal Relationships in the Autobiographies of Physically Disabled Persons*. Wenner-Gren Foundation: Working Papers in Anthropology, December, pp. 1–38.

Kuh, D., Lawrence, C. and Tripp, J. (1986) Disabled young people: making choices and future living options, *Social Service Research*, 15(4&5): 1–30.

Le Touze, S. and Pahl, J. (1990) *A Consumer Survey Among People with Learning Disabilities*. Canterbury: Centre for Health Services Studies, University of Kent.

Martin, M. and White, A. (1988) *Financial Circumstances of Disabled Adults Living in Private Households*, OPCS Surveys of Disability in Great Britain, Report No. 4. London: HMSO.

Martin, M., Meltzer, H. and Elliot, D. (1988) *The Prevalence of Disability Among Adults*, OPCS Surveys of Disability in Great Britain, Report No. 1. London: HMSO.

Martin, M., Meltzer, H. and Elliot, D. (1989) *The Prevalence of Disability Among Adults*, OPCS Surveys of Disability in Great Britain, Report No. 2. London: HMSO.

Milardo, R.M. (1992) Comparative methods for delineating social networks, *Journal of Social and Personal Relationships*, 9: 447–61.

Murray, P. and Penman, J. (eds) (2000) *Telling our own Stories: Reflections on Family Life in a Disabling World*. Sheffield: Parents with Attitude.

Pearson, M., Flynn, M., Maughan, J. and Russell, P. (1997) *Positive Health in Transition: A Guide to Effective and Reflective Transition Planning for Young People with Learning Disabilities*. Manchester: National Development Team.

Purdy, L.M. (1992) *In Their Best Interest? The Case Against Equal Rights for Children*. Ithaca, NY: Cornell University Press.

Russell, P. (1998a) *Making Connections: Challenges and Opportunities in Transition Planning*. London: Council for Disabled Children.

Russell, P. (1998b) *Having a Say! Disabled Children and Effective Partnership in Decision Making*. London: Council for Disabled Children.

Russell, P. (2003) Reports of consultation focus groups with parents and young people, in *Report of the Ministerial Working Party on the Future Role of Special Schools*. London: Department for Education and Skills Publications Unit.

Russell, P. (forthcoming) *'Families In': Report of a European Union Study of the Lives of Families with a Child with a Learning Disability in Five Member Nations*.

Smyth, M. and Robus, N. (1989) *Financial Circumstances of Families with Disabled Children Living in Private Households*, OPCS Surveys of Disability in Great Britain, Report No. 5. London: HMSO.

Thomas, A., Legard, R. and Chetwynd, M. (1996) *Student Voices: The Views of Further Education Students with Learning Difficulties and/or Disabilities*. London: Social and Community Planning Research, Skill, National Bureau for Students with Disabilities, The Further Education Funding Council.

Independence, reciprocity and resilience

Peter Goward and Linda Gething

Introduction

This chapter argues that the modern era's emphasis on scientific knowledge
has inadvertently disadvantaged certain sections of society, most notably
those people with a learning disability. Within this context people are seen as
vulnerable and at risk, thus overlooking their capacities, talents and ability
to survive adversity. Using examples from the lived experiences of Sophie, a
young woman with a learning disability, the different types of protection
that accrue from daily living and contribute to a sense of resilience are
explored. Importantly, a link is made between putative differences, positive
experiences, self-esteem and resilience. Using examples of 'parenting'
the chapter closes by identifying reciprocity, the ability to 'give' as well as
'take', as a means through which such positive experiences can be socially
generated.

One of the key features of the modern era is a collective faith in science
and certainty. Modernity's central quest is to find out the true and indisput-
able facts about things. If science cannot immediately discern the meaning
then the answer is to look harder, with increasingly complex instruments. In
many cases this stance has proved immensely successful and rendered enormous benefits. We, and I suspect you, are very grateful that biologists took
the time to painstakingly dissect the human body to better understand how
it functions, that medical scientists began to understand disease and provide
inoculations and treatments, that public health pioneers mapped out the
pattern of illness around the 'Broad Street' pump that led to better public
health, and that finally the mysteries of DNA and the genetic code are being
broken. As students in the health and social care arena you will have first-
hand experience of the effects of the modernist allegiance to science and
quantification in such things as quality assurance mechanisms, wherein
the assumption is that benchmarks and standards inevitably lead to quality
care.

Exercise 15.1

Identify five ways in which science has had a beneficial effect on your health and well-being.

Identify five ways in which you think science has negatively affected how you live your life.

The theories and notions that have underpinned illness and vulnerability were, and to some extent still are, hugely consequential to our capacity to conceptualize and deliver treatment, care and support. For example, Darwin's theories on natural selection contributed to the idea that some people, and indeed some cultures, were superior to others and therefore that some people and collectives were naturally inferior socially, physically or intellectually. The works of Bowlby, Harlow, Freud, Piaget and others generated ideas that appeared to suggest that if a child was not brought up in a certain way, if things did not occur in a prescribed order or if adversity intervened at a crucial phase, then dire consequences would inevitably ensue. Arguably, scientific interventions such as medication and surgery were found to be ineffective for people with intractable, chronic or psychologically/ intellectually based 'illness'. When this challenged medical and scientific superiority the 'evidence' was metaphorically 'brushed under the carpet' of sanatoriums, colonies and asylums and the people therein labelled 'at risk' and 'vulnerable'.

The past experience of people with learning disability is clearly illustrated by Ryan and Thomas (1987). They describe the dominant influence of medicine over the lives of many people with learning disability perceived to be far in excess of any medical problems that they may have presented. This contributed to an ideology of people with learning disability as being sick, helpless and needing to be taken care of.

Perceiving people as sick, incurable and dependent has led to behaviour that confirms these perceptions. Hence an expectation of underachievement is likely to compound the problems of people with a learning disability. Changing attitudes is never easy at the best of times and even when it does occur it often moves so slowly that the pace is barely perceptible. Perceptions of people with a learning disability in the past still prevail in whole or in part in contemporary society.

Increasingly, feminist and postmodernist challenges have been posed to the all-pervasive centrality of scientific truth and many of the stances that were previously seen as immutable, unchallengeable and 'taken for granted' are now being reappraised. Thus the notion that everyone who has suffered from maternal deprivation, been late with potty training or in any way deviates from the norm will throughout their life suffer the consequences in terms of risk and deficiencies is being increasingly, albeit slowly, replaced by an emphasis on competency and resilience.

The notion of resilience

Resilience is not the polar opposite of risk and therefore a resilient person is not one who has never experienced any difficulty. Rather, a resilient person can be conceptualized as someone who has experienced adversity and not only survived but become more hardy in the process; what Radke-Yarrow *et al.* (1990) refer to in their title as 'hard growing' children. If a person has never been faced with a problem or has never been exposed to any sort of risk then they could not claim to be resilient, for how would they know? This is similar to me not being able to claim that I do not suffer from altitude sickness because I have never been up a mountain.

Facing and overcoming some sort of a problem is therefore an inherent component of resilience and led early theorists to label resilient children as 'invulnerable' and 'invincible' because of their ability to thrive in the face of adversity. While an attractive notion, such children are not, like the frying pan, Teflon-coated. Nor are they like the cartoon coyote who tries to capture the roadrunner and in the process gets pulverized by a falling rock but gets back up and is miraculously intact.

Being resilient does not mean that people do not feel pain or that they are inured to suffering but that there are factors that, in a way not yet fully understood, appear to act as buffers that protect a person against 'going under'. This metaphor is apposite as the buoyancy that not going under suggests is evident in the title of Wolin and Wolin's book, *The Resilient Self: How Survivors of Troubled Families Rise Above Adversity* (1993). Similarly, Jacelon (1997: 123) notes that 'resilience is the ability of people to spring back in the face of adversity' and Dyer and McGuiness (1996: 276) define resilience as 'a global term describing a process whereby people bounce back from adversity and go on with their lives'.

Exercise 15.2

If you can, try and recall a situation that was difficult for you at the time but subsequently you felt helped you develop and grow stronger. What were the things that helped you get through that difficult period? What were your feelings afterwards?

Throughout this chapter we will use the experiences of a person with learning disabilities to inform and illustrate various points. Sophie is 23 and a very active member of her self-advocacy group. Her story as told to her group will be used to illustrate sections of this chapter. While her experience is unique to her it may also mirror that of some other people with a learning disability.

Sophie has experienced more than her fair share of adversity. She remembers children making fun and laughing at her in the street. She also remembers children pushing her around and on one occasion she had to go to hospital because a boy had thrown a stone at her and it had cut her eye. However, what she recalls with the most passion is her sadness at not being allowed to play with other children. She spent many hours watching them play through her bedroom window. After the stone-throwing incident her father refused to let her join in their games.

Sophie has thrived in the face of adversity, she has faced her frustration and her experience of loneliness and now has a social network that is not significantly different from her peers. She has a gregarious nature and an infectious laugh that draws people to her like a magnet. However, Sinason (1992) warns us that the smile is often a guise. There are potential dangers of overestimating people's powers of recovery. We should therefore be cautious in allowing the promotion of resilience to lead to overlooking the importance and impact of people's suffering.

The nature of protection

Dyer and McGuiness (1996: 277) observe that the pathway towards becoming resilient is a dynamic and iterative one that 'is highly influenced by protective factors'. Rutter (1985) in discussing the nature of protection suggests that there may be some difference in the way that differing factors generate protection and thus resilience. The distinction he makes is between prophylactic factors that serve to prevent untoward impact, a little like body armour protects people from bullets, and palliative factors which attempt to minimize and limit the damage following adverse impact. Garmezy (1985), in noting the buffering effect of protective factors, categorizes them under three broad headings: personality or dispositional factors, family-related factors and social or environmental factors. While the categorical systems proposed by Rutter and Garmezy at first sight seem very different they are compatible once the factors themselves are unpackaged.

Dispositional factors

These are the most extensively researched and therefore numerically the greatest category and include such diverse elements as sociability, autonomy, intellectual capacity, creativity, internal locus of control, high energy levels, gender, ordinal position among siblings or being an only child. As all of these factors are to a greater or lesser degree present from birth, or at least from a very early age, they can be equated with the prophylactic qualities described above. They are the factors that help construct a shield, perhaps even before the child is able to purposively affect his or her environment, and as such there is an inbuilt element of chance. I had no control or ability to affect which gender I was born to, how many brothers and sisters came before me, or how outgoing, intelligent or placid I appeared to others. Cederblad *et al.* (1995), who studied nearly 600 people over a 40-year period, place particular emphasis on a placid, 'easy going' temperament and intelligence as being important as children develop into resilient adults. She concludes that this is because they 'increase the coping capacity of an individual . . . If a person is high on sociability . . . he/she can also get a little help from his friends' (p. 18). This would seem to place people who have learning difficulties at a disadvantage.

Exercise 15.3

Try and remember what you were like as a small child or, if you are able, talk to your parents and get their views. How many of the dispositional protective factors did you appear to possess? In what ways, if at all, do you think they helped you in later life?

While Sophie has a learning disability that for many would be sufficient to view her as vulnerable, she also has a range of dispositional protective factors on which to draw. These include that she is female, is sociable and outgoing, has no physical markers of difference and is active and physically robust. However, the potential these have for offering protection is negated by the absence of other, more socially-related issues such as prejudice, discrimination and the resultant exclusion and lack of opportunity to make meaningful contributions.

For a person with a learning disability life's losses may be profound. From birth, issues of loss may affect the person because of the very nature of their difference. Many of the difficulties that people experience are because they are treated differently from the norm and perhaps partly because of their being sheltered from challenging opportunities.

Sophie recounts that when she was 6 her mum died from cancer. She has only known this fact for the past three years. She remembers being sent away on holiday as a treat for her birthday. When she arrived home her mother was gone. When she asked where her mother was she was often told 'she has gone to a better place'. Her family, although loving and caring, had assumed that she was incapable of understanding her mother's death. This is not an uncommon experience for people with a learning disability, as noted by Hollins (1995). She suggests that families comfort themselves with the hope that the person with the learning disability has not noticed. An additional problem created by this conspiracy of silence is that the person with the learning disability has no one to confide in. Sophie says that she did not feel able to talk about her mother's whereabouts or share her feelings of sadness.

The very nature of the learning disability experience exposes individuals to what could be perceived as adverse life events. They experience oppression similar to that experienced by other oppressed groups. This is located in barriers that deny opportunities in family, work, leisure, education and so on (Oliver 1990). Oppression also takes the form of negative labelling, stereotyping, sexual abuse and violence.

Family-related factors

In these factors there is the possibility of interactions that are supportive and helpful in times of adversity and so the protection is of the buffering, palliative kind. Writers such as Beardslee and Podorefsky (1988), Baldwin *et al.* (1993) and Egeland *et al.* (1993) note that being required to help and take on responsibility, clear rules and sanctions, shared values and celebrating family events are all significant contributors to the development of resilience in the face of adversity. McCubbin *et al.* (1998) and also Antonovsky and Sourani (1988) observe that family factors are most effective when they work collaboratively rather than in isolation and thus form a unified 'family schema' or 'a sense of coherence'. This coherent approach can be seen in the following example.

John Finn was a Gypsy Traveller who had learning difficulties and exhibited challenging, impulsive behaviour. Because of some bad experiences with health and social care services his family, like many other Traveller families, avoided contact with the wider community and 'looked after our own [family schema] in a way that fits in with what we does [sense of coherence]'. John had his chores to do and was expected to contribute to the family economy by helping his dad collect scrap. While doing this he functioned as part of the family work unit and because Traveller communities generally shun waged labour and place less value on literacy and numeracy he was an accepted and valuable part of the team. Gypsy and Traveller communities are usually closely-knit, kin-based collectives but are frequently dispersed across a wide geographical area. So when John 'lost it' as his mum described it and became overly boisterous or when his family needed some respite he was taken, along with his own trailer (caravan), to one of his relatives and their family several miles away where he helped them and contributed to their income. Over time this pattern was repeated until eventually John circled back to his 'Ma' who was by now rested and refreshed. At no time during such periods of community respite care was John ever out of contact with his family. He was always within his culture and not exposed to ridicule or culturally insensitive practices and, as with any other family member, when it was his birthday the whole extended community celebrated with John wherever his 'home' was at the time.

Similarly, Sophie's experiences support the notion that taking on responsibilities and early exposure to helping are all protective and help generate a degree of resilience. After the death of her mother, Sophie lived with her father and two older brothers. They have a very close and loving relationship and have a great influence over her decisions. She will often punctuate her conversations with, 'Well Dad says . . .' or 'Russell doesn't think . . .' or 'David thinks that I should . . .' In many ways she appears to have taken on the traditional female role of housekeeper within the family.

She takes great pride in this role and appears to have gained confidence and self-esteem from the skills that she has developed. She will say, 'I make a great cup of tea' and 'Dad says that I can iron a shirt just as good as Mum'. Whenever a conversation involves household duties, Sophie takes the opportunity to boast about her adeptness.

Exercise 15.4

How does your family, however you determine it require family members to be helpful; set and maintain rules and standards; celebrate significant family milestones such as birthdays?

Try and think of how these things have influenced the way that you are now and imagine how different you would have been if they had not occurred.

Social factors

Of all the protective factors this is the least well described. Although Wamboldt and Wamboldt (1989) discuss the possible impact of myths, stories and customs, this appears to be from a position in which the myths and stories are told by the powerful and successful. The heroism of living a life filled with the potential for ridicule, discrimination, oppression and putative failure, as experienced by many minority groups including those based on ethnicity, religiosity, sexual orientation or physical and intellectual difficulties, has yet to find its way into modern myths and stories. Possibly the only social factor to be given any serious consideration in the bulk of the literature is the presence of alternative caregivers including individuals of significance from outside the family (Luthar and Zigler 1991). Those old enough to remember the film *To Sir with Love* will recall the resilience that Sydney Poitier, as a respected teacher, helped his pupils attain. Younger readers may relate more easily to the similar storylines of films such as *Dangerous Minds*.

Exercise 15.5

Did you ever have someone outside of your family who, in some way, helped shape your life? In what ways do you imagine things would be different if they hadn't been there?

Perhaps because the main epistemological thrust for studies into risk and vulnerability has been rooted in medical and developmental psychology, understandably, the psychological gaze falls first on the individual and their intrapsychic and interpersonal processes. This may partly account for the lack of overt attention on social protective factors. Also, in the study of children and their development, the salient collective is the family unit and it is not until later that a wider social vista becomes influential and therefore visible in research findings.

However, as the role of health as opposed to illness, and competencies instead of deficiencies, has become more central, then issues concerning social inclusion and connectedness have grown in importance. Arguably, within the fields of sociology and anthropology, there has been a much richer discussion relating to social influences on health and resilience, including the damaging effects of social exclusion. One of the richest sources of debate is located within the literature on ethnicity and the social construction of difference.

Miri Song (2003), in describing how minority ethnic identities can be constructed, reconstructed and negotiated, identifies that a minority status does not inevitably lead to risk and vulnerability. Protection and resilience are thought to be achieved through recognizing that power and control are distributed unequally and that by celebrating difference the resultant increase in esteem leads to resilience.

People with learning disabilities have many things in common with people from ethnic minority groups in that both collectives can experience discrimination, disempowerment and yet can also show remarkable resilience in the face of the adversity caused by perceptions of what being different means.

Them and us

Miri Song (2003: 45) writes that 'A distinct ethnic identity is central to a group's efforts to differentiate themselves from other groups'. This idea echoes the work of the Norwegian anthropologist Frederick Barth who in 1969 highlighted the importance of 'the ethnic boundary that defines the group, not the cultural stuff that it encloses' (p. 15). The notion of a boundary presupposes that there are those who are within the boundary and those who are without. As the boundary is not a physical thing but a socially constructed one it therefore requires regular reiteration of the differences between those inside or outside in order to maintain it. Both Barth and Song focus on race and ethnicity to describe how it is possible for minority groups to gain esteem and cultural kudos through showing resilience in the face of discrimination and oppression. For example, in some young ethnic collectives being 'bad' is seen as 'good' and therefore offers protection through enhancing feelings of belonging to the group, by accentuating the difference between the 'cool' us and them – the prosaic white majority (Song 2003).

Jenkins (1998) draws a parallel between ethnicity and incompetence (learning difficulties) through the shared sense of exclusion by a hegemonic society in that 'Categorisations of incompetence and "racial" categorisations are often dimensions of hierarchical schema of human adequacy and acceptability: as sexual partners, mates, affines, colleagues, neighbours and so on' (p. 2). Having mates, colleagues and partners is not only something that people usually take for granted but is a means whereby we gain social support in times of trouble. Other chapters in this book describe in more detail some of the positive and negative effects that personal and social networks, culture, leisure and employment have on the lives of people with learning disabilities. Therefore here it is enough to identify that this applies equally to people with learning disabilities. However, this does not mean that if people choose to adopt different ways of associating and different ways of choosing and forming friendships and relationships then this is in some ways inferior or less meaningful than patterns constructed by the social majority.

It is therefore possible for people with learning difficulties to gain the self- and minority group esteem that Song's subjects have by recognizing and reframing difference in a positive way. However, to do this there needs to be a recognition of the power imbalance inherent in Jenkins' notion of a categorization of human adequacy. If higher levels of esteem contribute to a felt sense of resilience then people need the opportunity to gain esteem through positive life experiences.

In Chapter 22 of this book, Llewellyn and McConnell draw our attention to the fact that support is not always supportive as it depends on how it is perceived by the recipient. They describe how 'competence inhibiting' support takes over, thereby undermining confidence and recreating dependence.

To the observer, the interdependency that exists between Sophie and her family is evident. However, this is rarely acknowledged by any of the parties concerned. They exercise control over Sophie while at the same time relying on her contribution to the household. This of course could be, as reflected in the findings of Oakley (1974), the result of a lack of value placed on housework by society in general. But Mitchell (1997) claims that families often find difficulty with the concept of adulthood in their sons and daughters with learning disability.

Giving and receiving care is something that most individuals experience at various stages in their life. Many individuals with learning disability like Sophie find that their experience is unique as many of their relationships throughout their lives can be defined as caring. They are extensively defined by others as dependents, vulnerable, people in need of care and protection. The notion of care can be disabling as the person in receipt of care is often assumed to be passive and dependent (Morris 1993).

Care and protection can present themselves in many guises but on a day-to-day level can often result in things being done for the person, preventing their autonomy and independence. This may arise from negative attitudes and low expectations but it can also arise from benevolence and wanting to be helpful. The consequences are that people are often deterred from taking risks and making mistakes and are also denied the opportunity to achieve success.

Sophie tells us about her schooldays:

I used to go to Nana's for tea after school 'cause Dad was at work. I was really naughty at Nana's, I threw my tea on the floor. She'd get cross and shout at me that made me more upset. You see I used to see Granddad behind Mr Khan's shop, he was watching me. I knew how to cross the road, I pressed the button and waited for the green man, and then I'd see Granddad and feel really mad.

Any sense of achievement and independence that Sophie felt due to this accomplishment was shattered by seeing her grandfather watching her. Other examples where the sense of achievement is negated are when tasks are 'finished off' by the well-meaning individual. The fastening of the missed button, straightening the slightly crooked tie, putting the last hair in place, and so on . . .

Opportunities to take control and make decisions can also be limited for the person with a learning disability: 'The freedom to exercise choice is seen as a motivating force that assists learning and is vital to the concept of self' (Jackson and Jackson 1998: 22). The disabling effects of limited choice are illustrated in the following personal (L.G.) experience.

I don't usually arrive early for work, I park my car on a plot of waste land that serves as a car park and is well managed by the very helpful car park attendant who directs us into our spaces so that every square inch of the waste land can be utilized effectively. Last week I arrived uncharacteristically early, the car park was empty; there was no helpful attendant to direct me to my space. Where should I park? The decision was overwhelming and I was left feeling incompetent. This would also have been the conclusion of any bystanders who had the time to watch me shunting backwards and forwards across the car park before I eventually chose a space and left my car – still with the slight doubt that I was not in the right place.

The above examples show that all people including those with 'special needs' need to feel special and gain esteem by doing the very ordinary everyday things others take for granted but which are often placed out of their reach. However, this does not always happen and there are many reasons given for why people with learning disabilities may feel socially excluded and not very special. One that is particularly relevant to the notion of protection and resilience is that relating to 'tragedies'.

Learning disability is often portrayed as a family 'tragedy' (Hill and Hill 1994). People comment on the negative picture given to them as prospective parents of a child with Down's syndrome. All parents develop expectations of their child's future based on their own experience. Therefore, at the time of diagnosis of their child's disability parents can find their cosy expectations of becoming mothers and fathers shattered. This can lead them to perceive a child with a learning disability as a 'tragedy' in the family which can contribute to the child being perceived and treated as different. This difference is not necessarily the positive sense of difference that Miri Song discusses, but a negative one that focuses on passivity, helplessness and incompetence.

Oliver (1990) makes the claim that policies and practices that are concerned with doing things for people, rather than enabling them to do things for themselves, are maintained by the ideology of personal tragedy theory. The language of dependency, impairment, burden and multiple needs represents those who are dependent as less than complete individuals. Disability becomes the sole or major identifier of the person, thus erasing individual traits and abilities and negating the possibility of individual growth, development and change.

Viewing people as useless and unable to take care of themselves decreases the power of individuals to take control over their lives and essentially increase dependency. Morris (2001) observes that those who cannot take care of themselves are not allowed to take their place in society; this inevitably leads to social exclusion. Segregated schools, leisure facilities and further education opportunities are still commonplace and the majority of people with learning disabilities are unemployed and live in relative poverty.

For many people with learning disabilities the findings of Morris (1993: 164) are a mirror of their experience. She found that the lived experiences of, and the meanings they attach to, social exclusion for young people with learning disabilities was:

- not being listened to;
- having no friends;
- finding it difficult to do the kinds of things that non-disabled young people do, such as go shopping, go to the cinema, go clubbing, etc.;
- being made to feel that they have no contribution to make, that they are a burden;
- feeling unsafe, being harassed and bullied;
- not having control over spending money, not having enough money.

Sophie can certainly identify with the young people in Morris's study. She will begin many sentences with, 'I am not allowed to . . .' Her family, although loving and supportive, have found it difficult to move from protecting her as a child to allowing her to have the independence of an adult. They have struggled to protect and keep her safe while denying her the opportunities to take risks. Families can be crucial in enabling the achievement of independent lives and developing confidence and self-esteem. Although Sophie has a well-defined and valued role within her family this has not been extended beyond the family. The close relationship that she is experiencing appears to be hindering her from becoming a self-reliant individual. She will also make the comment that 'they will miss me if I left home'. Williams and Robinson (2001) demonstrate that many people with learning disabilities take responsibilities within the family and help to support their parents. However, no one appeared to recognize this situation as *mutual* care. An acknowledgement of mutual care would not only bolster self-esteem but begin to redress any power imbalance through the enactment of reciprocity.

The notion of reciprocity

The essence of reciprocity is captured by Finch and Mason (1993) who state that 'Reciprocity provides the glue that holds the community together. I help you, you help me, and everyone is happy'. The mutuality that is central to reciprocity is echoed by Jordan (1996: 165) who defines it as 'the notion that meaningful communication and economic exchange require respect for the social value of each member, and willingness to obey very basic principles, such as taking turns . . .'. Tones (1997: 40) links reciprocity to health promotion through its ability to generate empowerment: 'In short, empowerment has to do with the relationship between individuals and their [social as well as physical] environment; the relationship is reciprocal'.

From the above it can be seen that for reciprocity to make people 'happy' it is dependent on 'taking turns'. Therefore, by inference, not 'taking turns' would make people sad and disempowered.

Exercise 15.6

Have you ever found yourself in a situation in which you are passive and somebody else is doing everything for you, being extremely nice to you and accepting nothing back in return?

How did you feel 'early on' in this period?

Did your feelings change over the course of the event?

How did you think the other person felt?

Sophie describes a situation where she experiences a degree of reciprocity through having a defined role and the feeling that her family would miss her presence. This clearly bolsters her self-esteem by making her feel valued and thus helping her face adversity (i.e. to be resilient). She has the responsibility for most of the household tasks and provides support to her father and brothers. Yet they see themselves as the carers of Sophie. Because she is identified as a victim or burden the emphasis appears to be on her incapacity and not her capabilities. She does not appear to contribute to the decision-making within the household and will constantly defer to her father's and brothers' opinion. This could be seen as a carefully orchestrated attempt by her family to maintain the boundary between 'us' (the family) and 'them' (everyone else) in a laudable but ultimately unhelpful desire to protect Sophie. However, Margalit (2003) stresses the importance of reciprocity in fostering a wider range of interpersonal relationships and its close relationship with the experience of resilience. The notion of dependency associated with learning disability can create a power imbalance in relationships where reciprocity exists but is not acknowledged or allowed to extend beyond family members. Hudson (2003) notes that overly controlling parental autonomy where the person is not allowed to make decisions, take responsibility and develop a degree of independence and control are factors that can impede the transition to adulthood. Part of being an adult usually includes relationships with people outside of the family, accessing their help and support but also being open, helpful and supportive to them. Thus, for Sophie, the lack of contact with a broader range of people outside the family could be seen as limiting her ability to meet others and form the sorts of friendship and personal relationship that most other young women take for granted, including having a family of their own (see Chapter 22).

The evidence from parenting

As noted earlier, resilience can only exist in the presence of adversity. Feldman (1986) is clear that being born to parents at least one of whom has a learning difficulty is an adverse condition. This finding was the result of studying the interactions of 12 mothers with learning difficulties and their 2-year-old children.

Despite the significant lack of consensus on what behaviours are consistent with a successful meeting of the above criteria, the assumption is that it is the parents' learning difficulties, rather than their socioeconomic status and social exclusion, or a whole range of other factors, that generate such putative dangers. Feldman concludes that such children run the '. . . risk of developmental delay, cultural-familial retardation, maltreatment and neglect . . .' (p. 777).

Similarly, McGraw and Sturmey (1993) in their study of the difficulties clinicians face in the early detection of parents who have learning difficulties noted that 'Half of the learning-disabled parents known to services are being reported for abuse and neglect and a quarter are having a child removed from their home' (p. 113). However, more encouragingly they also found that the 'pregnancies appeared to give them [the parents] a sense of pride and increased self-esteem' (p. 107). They also observed that while some parents were likely to be more restrictive and punishing 'some children appear to have resilience to damaging, negative environments and manage to thrive despite their exposure to such poor care' (p. 110). This they attributed to 'interactions with other people from inside and outside of the home environment' which prompted McGraw and Sturmey to highlight the 'importance of long-term social support for such children and their families' (p. 110).

This more positive outlook is replicated and enhanced by Tim and Wendy Booth (1998). In recognizing that resilience is generated by (usually iterative) exposure to adversity, they recognized that it is likely to take time to manifest itself, unlike vulnerability which is more immediately evident. The Booths focused their attention on adults who had been brought up by parents, at least one of whom had a learning disability. This enabled them to obtain a more balanced picture as the angst generated immediately after adversity had been tempered by time and the opportunity for reflection. Their findings supported the notion that external support was a key factor in developing individual and family resilience and highlighted two aspects in particular. The first was a network of supportive relationships which, in their study, included school friends, helpful neighbours, support workers and people from agencies such as school, church or health care services. The second was a sense of participation and involvement such as working, being part of the local community, belonging to clubs and joining in with ceremonies and celebrations. The key feature in this was that the person felt able to draw support from the community but also that they could contribute something.

Booth and Booth (1998: 98) refer to the combination of the two aspects identified above as 'distributive competence' which 'attests to the fact that parenting is mostly a shared activity and acknowledges the interdependencies that comprise the parenting task'. The notion that a shared approach to managing life's vicissitudes through a network of external support in which those supported are active contributors is an important one. Its importance is not to be measured only by externally judged indicators of success such as whether health visitors think that parents are 'good enough' or that the child is thriving. It must also be gauged more subjectively by the parents and their offspring on the basis of their happiness, their felt sense of success and the effects on their levels of esteem. This resonates with findings about the quality of life and healthy ageing in people with learning disabilities (see Chapter 33). As discussed earlier, esteem is a crucial mediator between protective factors and resilience and therefore anything that lowers self-esteem is unlikely to be maximally protective and therefore would fail to act as an effective buffer between the person, risk and vulnerability.

Many parents reading this will be familiar with the importance of sharing responsibilities and of having support from a range of people in the process of bringing up children. How refreshing it is when a neighbour offers to help do the shopping, how glad we are when a niece babysits, and how comforting when the health visitor assures us that it's normal for a baby to cry. However, in all of this we, as parents, know that we will assume a central role in the child's upbringing and will be able to influence the intensity, volume and nature of the support offered. In this way we can gain a great deal of pleasure and self-esteem when we see our efforts rewarded in the first smile, the first word and the first teetering attempt at walking, and know that we were central to it happening. However, this is not always the case for some parents.

Learning disability is often the sole reason why children are removed from their parents (O'Hara 2003). Parents with a learning disability constantly live with this fear and therefore have additional pressures to those of family life and bringing up children. There can be a complexity of services involved and the possibility of encounters with people who have negative preconceived ideas about people with learning disability being parents is a reality. Guinea (2001) found that the pressure that these parents experienced was primarily environmental and not associated with any lack of competence in parental skills. In her study most parents lived close to their extended families, and they provided much of the external support. Such social support may be positive but, as identified by Llewellyn and McConnell (2002), it can also prevent mothers from creating social networks. Llewellyn and McConnell found that many mothers did not have friends or support from their neighbours and were in reality socially isolated.

Conclusion

The White Paper *Valuing People* (Department of Health 2001) reinforces the importance of social inclusion, choice, advocacy, rights and independence. For Bates and Davis (2004) social inclusion means ensuring that people with learning disabilities have access to the same range of social roles and activities as their non-disabled peers.

With today's increasing awareness of human rights, people with a learning disability are challenging the history of exclusion and are establishing their rights as citizens. People First of Canada has found a new way to build a national and international organization in which education is the key strategy (McColl and Bickenbach 1998). Most major towns and cities in the UK have an established People First group. Such groups are speaking to university students, professionals, employers, government officials and families about their experience of discrimination and the changes that need to occur. They are also participating in research and speaking at conferences. A key to their struggle is to replace the old patterns of exclusion and segregation with the right to social inclusion and participation.

Goodley (2000) states that this movement of self-advocacy captures resilience in the face of adversity. People with a learning disability are speaking for themselves and are challenging the labels that define them as incapable. As Goodley confirms, 'they are not passive recipients of oppression, they are active resilient social members'.

Sophie has all the hopes and dreams of many young women. These include being able to have a job, somewhere nice to live, to get married and have children. Through the telling of her story she has demonstrated resilience, particularly as much of the power and control in her life is not within her command. Negative attitudes and values are as much a barrier for people with learning disability today as they were 20 years ago, so Sophie still has many challenges to face. Hopefully, the resilience that she has demonstrated will continue to flourish and help her to realize her hopes and dreams.

References

Antonovsky, A. and Sourani, T. (1988) Family sense of coherence and family adaptation, *Journal of Marriage and the Family*, 50: 79–92.

Baldwin, A., Baldwin, C. *et al.* (1993) Contextual risk and resiliency during late adolescence, *Development and Psychopathology*, 5: 741–61.

Barth, F. (1969) *Ethnic Groups and Boundaries: The Social Organisation of Cultural Difference*. London: George Allen & Unwin.

Bates, P. and Davis, F.A. (2004) Social capital, social inclusion and services for people with learning disabilities, *Disability and Society*, 19(3).

Beardslee, B. and Podorefsky, D. (1988) Resilient adolescents whose parents have serious affective and other psychiatric disorders: importance of self-understanding and relationships, *American Journal of Psychiatry*, 145(1): 63–9.

Booth, T. and Booth, W. (1998) Risk, resilience and competence: parents with learning difficulties and their children, in R. Jenkins (ed.) *Questions of Competence*. Cambridge: Cambridge University Press.

Cederblad, M., Dahlin, L., Hagnell, O. and Hansson, K. (1995) Intelligence and temperament as protective factors for mental health: a cross-sectional and prospective epidemiological study, *European Archives of Psychiatry and Clinical Neuroscience*, 245: 11–19.

Department of Health (2001) *Valuing People: A New Strategy for Learning Disability for the 21st Century*. London: Department of Health.

Dyer, J. and McGuiness, T. (1996) Resilience: analysis of the concept, *Archives of Psychiatric Nursing*, X(5): 276–82.

Egeland, B., Carlson, E. and Sroufe, L. (1993) Resilience as process, *Development and Psychopathology*, 5: 517–28.

Feldman, M. (1986) Research on parenting by mentally retarded persons, *Psychiatric Clinics of North America*, 9(4): 777–96.

Finch, J. and Mason, J. (1993) *Negotiating Family Responsibilities*. London: Routledge.

Garmezy, N. (1985) Stress resistant children: the search for protective factors, *Journal of Child Psychology and Psychiatry*, book supplement No.4. Oxford: Pergamon.

Goodley, D. (2000) *Self-advocacy in the Lives of People with Learning Difficulties*. Buckingham: Open University Press.

Guinea, S.M. (2001) Parents with a learning disability and their views on the support received: a preliminary study, *Journal of Learning Disabilities*, 5(1): 43–56.

Hill, G. and Hill, D. (1994) article in *Woman*, 11 July.

Hollins, S. (1995) Managing grief better: people with developmental disabilities, *The Habilitative Mental Healthcare Newsletter*, 14(3).

Hudson, B. (2003) From adolescence to young adulthood: the partnership challenge for learning disability services in England, *Disability and Society*, 18(3): 259–76.

Jacelon, C. (1997) The trait and process of resilience, *Journal of Advanced Nursing*, 25(1): 123–9.

Jackson, N. and Jackson, E. (1998) Choice-making for people with a learning disability, *Learning Disability Practice*, 1(3): 22–5.

Jenkins, R. (1998) Culture, classification and (in)competence, in R. Jenkins (ed.) *Questions of Competence*. Cambridge: Cambridge University Press.

Jordan, B. (1996) *A Theory of Poverty & Social Exclusion*. Cambridge: Polity Press.

Llewellyn, G. and McConnell, D. (2002) Mothers with learning difficulties and their support networks, *Journal of Intellectual Disability Research*, 46(1): 17–34.

Luthar, S. and Zigler, E. (1991) Vulnerability and competence, *American Journal of Orthopsychiatry*, 61(1): 6–22.

McColl, M.A. and Bickenbach, J.E. (1998) *Introduction to Disability*. London: Saunders.

McCubbin, H., Futrell, J., Thompson, E. and Thompson, A. (1998) Resilient families in an ethnic and cultural context in H. McCubbin, E. Thompson, A. Thompson and J. Futrell (eds) *Resiliency in African-American Families*. Thousand Oaks, CA: Sage.

McGraw, S. and Sturmey, P. (1993) Identifying the needs of parents with learning disabilities: a review, *Child Abuse Review*, 2: 101–17.

Margalit, M. (2003) Resilience model among individuals with learning disabilities: proximal and distal influences, *Learning Disability Research and Practice*, 18(2): 82–6.

Mitchell, P. (1997) The impact of self-advocacy on families, *Disability and Society*, 12(1): 43–56.

Morris, J. (1993) *Independent Lives*. London: Macmillan.

Morris, J. (2001) Social exclusion and young disabled people with high levels of support needs, *Critical Social Policy*, 21(2): 161–83.

O'Hara, J. (2003) Parents with learning disabilities: a study of gender and cultural perspectives in East London, *British Journal of Learning Disabilities*, 31: 18–24.

Oakley, A. (1974) *Sociology of Housework*. Oxford: Blackwell.

Oliver, M. (1990) *The Politics of Disablement*. London: Macmillan Press.

Radke-Yarrow, M., Sherman, T. *et al.* (1990) Hard growing: children who survive, in J. Rolf *et al.* (eds) *Risk and Protective Factors in the Development of Psychopathology*. Cambridge: Cambridge University Press.

Rutter, M. (1985) Resilience in the face of adversity, *British Journal of Psychiatry*, 147: 598–611.

Ryan, J. and Thomas, F. (1987) *The Politics of Mental Handicap*. London: Free Press.

Sinason, V. (1992) *Mental Handicap and the Human Condition*. London: Free Association Books.

Song, M. (2003) *Choosing Ethnic Identity*. Cambridge: Polity Press.

Tones, K. (1997) Health education as empowerment, in M. Sidell *et al.* (eds) *Promoting Health*. Buckingham: Open University Press.

Wamboldt, F. and Wamboldt, S. (1989) *Family Myths: Psychotherapy Implications*. New York: Haworth Press.

Williams, V. and Robinson, C. (2001) 'He will finish up caring for me': people with learning disability and mutual care, *British Journal of Learning Disabilities*, 29: 56–62.

Wolin, S.J. and Wolin, S. (1993) *The Resilient Self: How Survivors of Troubled Families Rise above Adversity*. New York: Villard Books.

16

Managing independent living

Safeguarding adults with learning disabilities
against abuse

Margaret Flynn and Hilary Brown

Introduction

This chapter addresses issues of empowerment and protection: twin aspirations which are usually set up as opposite ends of a continuum to be
somehow weighed up and offset against each other. This is not our view, as
we consider them to be inextricably intertwined. Experiencing abuse or neglect is to experience in the raw what it is like to be disempowered: it follows
that you cannot exercise power in your life if you are not being appropriately
protected from abuse or neglect. Independence is sometimes represented as a
state of insularity within which one has no needs and is presented with no
risks, but independent people *manage* rather than *avoid* relationships and
risks. Adults in our society are rarely independent: they get their needs met
by a mixture of sustaining relationships, paying for assistance and negotiating with helping agencies. People with learning disabilities will also draw on
these sources of support to varying degrees. People protect themselves in a
range of ways, by living in secure premises, insuring their property, checking
out new friends, being careful in their sexual lives, listening to the advice of
their families and friends, getting input from their doctor, accessing the
police or domestic violence agencies if they have need of them, and seeking
help from a range of agencies in a crisis.

It helps to think critically about how the elements of our title, Managing
independent living . . . safeguarding adults . . . learning disabilities . . . abuse
are defined, as this is not self-evident. Is independence a function of the
capabilities of an individual or of the relationship between individuals and
their environment? Moreover, if adults are believed to be self-reliant and
equal to attending to their self-maintenance, why and in what manner can
their independence be protected and fostered? What are the necessary or
sufficient conditions for conferring the status of 'independence' on adults
with learning disabilities, given the constancy of their support needs – albeit
to different degrees and levels of intensity – according to life events and

stages? 'Abuse' can be seen as a vague, all-encompassing term, embracing crimes against property, as well as the violence, neglect, discrimination, humiliation, sexual assaults and mistreatment visited upon disabled children, young people and adults (Brown *et al.* 2000; Brown 2002). The chapter aims to encourage consideration of the wider context in which abuse occurs and an appreciation of the means of prevention.

A metaphor

To address the imprecision of, and the relationships between, independence, management and abuse, we have decided to use the metaphor of a river from its source to a delta. The river represents independence – it is sometimes fast-moving, it is subject to seasonal flooding, it has shallows, low waters, muddy waters, and it is charged with undercurrents of self-determinism. The river has a couple of major tributaries, both of which shape it. They are abuse, and separately, management or oversight. The former brings dangerous undertows and pollutants and the latter reinforcing, nurturing strength and occasional lifeboats as, towards the end of its course, the river makes hesitant progress to the delta.

What makes us 'independent' has early 'upstream' origins in which our parents are expected to play critical and nurturing roles. Our ability to manage what goes into and comes out of the body is an early potent symbol of being independent that is strongly associated with the parental role. The role of nurturing and advancing our skills may persist throughout the lives of our birth, foster, adopted or chosen parents, or it may be brought to a premature end. A growing and complex constellation of capacities and competencies, sufficient to comprehend, analyse and make choices and decisions about a host of preoccupations that make up human experience and ultimately determine how we decide to live our lives, characterizes the maturing river. Such currents control us, our decisions and our actions.

While there are no adults whose job it is specifically to guide and nurture our independence, the roles of peers, teachers, health and social care professionals, friends, partners and work colleagues, for example, can be instrumental in each of us becoming more or less self-governing and they may become part of the oversight tributary. For those of us whose independence appears likely to be compromised, throughout childhood, adolescence and beyond, parents and family caregivers may elect to provide support for very extended periods and/or seek assistance to do so. We are not describing a discrete and linear process as our river metaphor perhaps implies. Many families experience discontinuities and biographical disruptions, and lone individuals, as well as lone family caregivers, may be especially exercised (Blustein *et al.* 1999; Grant and Whittell 2003).

The abuse tributary is unobtrusive. It can modify its flow as its need determines and is capable of invoking admiration, trust and unbelievable horrors, including exploitation, alienation and drowning. The true and profound nature of its flow is captured by the ease and stealth with which it steals and poisons the lives and resilience of its victims, and their loved ones, and assures would-be rescuers that they are misguided or even way off course. But vulnerability to abuse is commonly assumed to be a function of the person in isolation rather than an expression of complex interactions between the person and their carers or environment. Analysis shows that far from being 'over-protected', people with learning disabilities are often chronically 'under-protected', being exposed to more dangerous situations than others, with less chance that abuses will be noticed and fewer opportunities to be rescued or supported than are offered to other citizens. It is as if the river flows between more hazardous banks and when it hits danger it creates stagnant pools and goes underground.

Visionary policy expectations

How does policy characterize independence? There is a great deal of evidence suggesting that policy champions independence but it does so in ways that barely acknowledge the interdependence of our lives. If we scroll back over the last 30-plus years, we see that independence is an enduring policy cornerstone and arguably easier to envisage for someone whose support needs are not extensive:

> Most mildly handicapped school-leavers are able to go directly into open or sheltered employment, possibly with special help from the Youth Employment Service. Some need a period of training in an Adult Training Centre first . . . The object of this special training and work or occupation is to develop work habits and to increase self reliance generally, so as to help each handicapped person to live a more independent life . . .
>
> (DHSS/Welsh Office 1971: paras 154–5)

> Helping people to lead, as far as is possible, full and independent lives is at the heart of the Government's approach to community care. Improving the services that enable them to do that is a continuing commitment shared by all concerned.
>
> (DHSS/Welsh Office 1989)

> Promoting independence is a key aim for the Government's modernisation agenda. Nowhere is it of greater importance than for people with learning disabilities. While people's individual needs will differ, the starting presumption should be one of independence, rather than dependence, with public services providing the support needed to maximise this. Independence in this context does not mean doing everything unaided.
>
> Like other people, people with learning disabilities want a real say in where they live, what work they should do and who looks after them.

But for too many people with learning disabilities, these are currently unattainable goals. We believe that everyone should be able to make choices. This includes people with severe and profound disabilities who, with the right help and support, can make important choices and express preferences about their day to day lives.

(DoH 2001: para. 2.2)

So although policy asserts the importance of independence and, latterly, choice in respect of people with learning disabilities, endemic ambiguity haunts their margins. Policy suggests that excessive control and paternalistic services have had their day, and in their stead we wield 'independence' and 'choice'. However, if the worlds of those living independently strain or come apart, policy offers neither answers nor safe harbours. It persists in paying homage to pioneer images of self-reliance. How viable is a life of maximized independence? Would we recognize it? Most people with learning disabilities live with their birth families and have always done so. Is this the independence successive governments have so willingly endorsed? If it is not, then should we be cutting the ties to this tenacious policy theme or embarking on its neglected analysis and, as importantly, setting out what it means for adults with learning disabilities and their families?

Exercise 16.1

What rites and events do you associate with being 'independent'?

There is something more solid in a consideration of 'abuse'. While we may not know about the sum of its manifestations, and different definitions may challenge our efforts to record it and measure it over time, we know that it should be warded off if people's lives are not to be derailed:

There can be no secrets and no hiding place when it comes to exposing the abuse of vulnerable adults . . .

In recent years several serious incidents have demonstrated the need for immediate action to ensure that vulnerable adults, who are at risk of abuse, receive protection and support. The Government gives a high priority to such action . . . The circumstances in which harm and exploitation occur are known to be extremely diverse, as is the membership of the at risk group . . .

Abuse is a violation of an individual's human and civil rights by any other person or persons . . . [it] may consist of a single act or repeated acts. It may be physical, verbal or psychological, it may be an act of neglect or an omission to act or it may occur when a vulnerable person is persuaded to enter into a financial or sexual transaction to which he or she has not consented, or cannot consent . . . can occur in any relationship and may result in significant harm to, or exploitation of, the person subjected to it . . . main different forms of abuse: physical . . . sexual . . . psychological . . . financial or material . . . neglect or acts of omission . . . discriminatory abuse . . .

(DoH/Home Office 2000: Foreword, paras 1.1 & 1.2, paras 2.5–2.7)

While public inquiries and undercover TV programmes have intermittently illuminated the nature and reach of abuse in the lives of vulnerable populations, we are attuned to our culture's ambient climate of minimizing and outright denial of abuse (e.g. MacIntyre 2003). As O'Connell Higgins (1994: 10) observed of the 'Holocaust deniers': 'If such uncertainty exists in the face of organised, abundantly documented evil, no wonder less centralised abuses are overlooked. Most of the traumatised bear no remaining physical manifestations of their abuse and have no witnesses'. Thus it is not surprising that abuse and safeguarding vulnerable populations are insistent, if recent, themes in government policy, not least as the consequences transcend individual suffering.

Exercise 16.2

What makes you feel safe?

Four illustrative case studies

The following case studies exemplify and amplify the phenomenon of abuse in an array of locations. They describe the circumstances of people we have met (Flynn and Brown 1997; Brown 2002) and people whose circumstances have been described to us by their relatives and support staff (Flynn and Whitehead in press). Necessarily, people's names and identifying details have been changed.

Case study: *Michael*

Michael lives in a long-stay hospital. He does not speak. He uses a wheelchair and he rarely leaves his 'high dependency' ward. Michael requires help with his personal care, including shaving, washing, feeding and drinking. He wears pads as he is doubly incontinent. A recurring phrase in Michael's casenotes is, 'Michael bruises easily'. Although he lives in a 'hospital' the assumption that Michael's bruising is due to some unnamed medical condition is not verified by health professionals and no investigations are sought.

The arrival of a new, unqualified assistant is a watershed in Michael's life. She witnesses a colleague thumping Michael.

Some contextual details

Neither the ward manager nor the hospital's chief executive regard themselves as managing Michael's independence; Michael is not registered with a GP and has no other contact with primary care professionals. He has no visitors and little is known of his family; none of the ward staff are qualified; none have received any training about creating and sustaining safe services; and the hospital has minimal experience of investigating the abuse of patients.

Managing Michael's safety

Michael requires a more proactive approach to his safety than that which the ward and hospital adopted. He has relied on, and will continue to rely on, public services for his day-to-day support. He is known as a man who is unequal to protecting himself or seeking help to challenge the 'bruises easily' smokescreen. Given that this myth has been transformed to the status of a fact, Michael's ordinary health needs require attention and being registered with a GP is an important safeguard on two counts: that he or she would be independent of the hospital and also that he or she would be in a position to offer screening and other interventions available to other men of the same age as Michael. People's relatives and friends also have legitimate interests in safety. Occasionally, some are labelled as 'overprotective' by professionals as a means of accounting for their attentiveness to the safety of their loved ones. Michael's life would be enhanced in many ways if people could be identified to be involved and 'look out' for him, becoming attuned to his likes, dislikes and his ways of communicating, sounding alarms when he appears distressed or unwell and exploring the scope for sharing activities with him inside and outside the hospital environment.

Case study: *Doreen*

Doreen lives with her sister and large family in a depressed part of a large city. She attends a day centre and a residential respite service every three months. Staff from the respite service and the day service collaborate in working with Doreen. They are concerned that she is her sister's unpaid cleaner, cook and child minder and that she has very little money for 'spends', irrespective of her welfare benefits. Over time, staff encourage Doreen to be interested in her personal hygiene and help her to save from her modest income for deodorants, bath gel and shampoo. While puzzled that Doreen opts to leave her purchases in the day centre, and shower when she arrives each morning, they are so animated by the results and by Doreen's pleasure in her 'smellies' they turn their attention to her appearance. It takes many months for Doreen to save enough money to buy a new outfit and she goes shopping with two women staff with whom she gets on well. She is excited by her purchases and returns home animated. The following day Doreen is not wearing her new clothes and is evasive when staff ask her about them. It takes several days for Doreen to disclose that her sister returned them to the store 'to get the money back'.

Some contextual details

Doreen is grateful that her younger sister, who is a single parent, has 'taken me in – otherwise I'd be in a home'. Doreen's sister does not welcome contact with staff from the day service or the respite service and has on occasion been verbally abusive to them. She views Doreen's welfare benefits as *her* money, not least as she describes herself as her sister's carer. Doreen has told staff that she would like her own home but she cannot discuss this with her sister as she fears it would make her angry.

Managing Doreen's safety

Irrespective of Doreen's abilities, she is not well placed to disentangle her interests from those of her sister's or to challenge the purview of her sister's decision-making. The mantra of 'independence' is not helpful in this situation as it offers no framework for discussing interdependence, belonging, intimidation or compliance. Furthermore, there appear to be no limits to the amount of domestic work expected of Doreen.

It is only when someone proactively intervenes to assert appropriate boundaries for Doreen that a space can be made within which she is free to exercise choice. Care managers have important roles in safeguarding vulnerable people and identifying one for Doreen marks a turning point in her life. The new care manager is not intimidated by Doreen's sister and has challenged her for gaining financially and using Doreen's skills rather than supporting Doreen. Having spent time with Doreen and staff who know her well and like her, she outlines the plan that Doreen should have her own tenancy with the support that she needs (most particularly regarding money management and risk of exploitative relationships). In the short term, to address Doreen's stress at what this means for her relationship with her sister, Doreen is spending more time in the independence unit of her respite service. Staff are removing the labels from Doreen's newly-purchased clothes so that they cannot be exchanged and are supporting her to put an agreed sum every week into a Post Office savings account. They keep her savings book locked away in their care. They have a means of logging how she spends her money, tracking receipts and keeping a note of the staff who accompany her when she goes shopping 'for my bottom drawer!' Doreen benefits from being supported by women who are committed to changing her life for the better and helping her achieve her formerly unstated aspirations.

Case study: *Ben*

Ben lives in a residential service with five other people. He has a few words. He can name his favourite TV programmes and recognizes the actors and actresses. He indicates his wants by pointing and taking the hand of a member of staff. Ben is very overweight and has put on six stone since he moved into the service. He has a very affable nature and he laughs a great deal. What prompts his laughter is not always clear. A male member of staff calls Ben 'Fatso' and 'Hippo' and his mostly female colleagues do not challenge him. A member of staff in the day centre asked the unit manager why he thought that Ben was referring to himself as 'Fatso'. The manager said that it was 'just a joke'. A substantial change in Ben's demeanour is linked to the arrival of a new resident called Tim who begins to 'look after' Ben. Staff welcome Tim's help as Ben requires so much more of their time than other residents. There is insufficient continuity for them to ask why Ben has ceased to laugh and, as he is so large, his rapid weight increase goes unmonitored and unremarked. Several months after Tim's arrival a member of the waking night staff hears Ben screaming. She finds him naked and bleeding from his anus. Tim is in his bedroom, also naked and pleading with Ben to 'Shut up'.

Some contextual details

Ben's very elderly mother is in a nursing home and has Alzheimer's. He has no siblings but a cousin has always taken an interest in him and she assisted her aunt in negotiating long-term help for Ben. Ben's cousin visits every couple of months and on each visit has expressed dismay to staff about his weight gain. She is told that it is Ben's 'choice' to eat lots of what he likes. Although she has complained to the local authority the independent inspection report indicates that she is being 'unduly overprotective' and states that '. . . Ben should be allowed to develop now that he is in an independent setting'. Ben's service relies heavily on transitional, agency staff. In terms of his support needs, Ben requires more help than his co-residents; the residential service's mission statement asserts that it aspires to 'maximizing potential . . . maximizing independence'; the local day service cannot accommodate Ben for more than three mornings a week. When Ben was initially admitted to the residential service, 'he was such a handful we got some medication for him'. Little is known of Tim's history prior to his transfer to the residential unit.

Managing Ben's safety

Ben is disadvantaged by being in a service with no appreciation of the importance of his health and safety. Unqualified transitional staff have bought into the ideology of 'independence' and 'choice' and this acts to deflect them from paying proper attention to his weight gain, most particularly since Tim's arrival in the service. Ben's cousin is not regarded as a source of valuable information about Ben, or indeed as someone who is sufficiently committed to him to alert the service to her concerns. Nobody has asked her how the family sought to keep Ben safe in his previous life. Although Ben is registered with a local GP, support staff in the residential service are unaccustomed to collaborating with the GP or the practice nurse with and on behalf of residents.

Case study: *Michelle*

Michelle attended a day service with a poor reputation. A member of staff, who was feared by many of his colleagues, ensured that Michelle came to work in his section. Although Michelle became agitated and increasingly reluctant to attend the day service, this was variously attributed to: her menstrual cycle; stubbornness; challenging behaviour; possible early-onset menopause and/or (most shamefully) 'attention seeking'. When a member of staff and a friend of Michelle from another part of the day centre walked into this man's 'office' they were shocked to see him hurrying to adjust his trousers and Michelle crying and rocking on a chair before him. He was verbally abusive to his unexpected visitors and concluded by telling them to 'f***ing knock in future'.

Some contextual details

Michelle is a timid woman who has had many addresses since her parents signalled they could not manage her as a young teenager. Many years in a long-stay hospital were followed by several years in a large hostel, two family placements combined with respite, a group home with a couple of people she had known from the hostel, a few months of living 'independently' in a supported tenancy (during which time she is believed to have been raped by a man who claimed to have been interested only in 'helping her') and at least three co-tenancies since. Although Michelle speaks she can rarely be persuaded to talk and becomes distressed if staff are persistent.

Managing Michelle's safety

Michelle's abilities perplex the people who support her and those who manage the services she uses. Michelle can use local and national public transport; she can manage household routines; she can assist others in managing their household routines – and yet she is described as 'an innocent' when it comes to her own safety. She is supported by day centre staff with a very limited appreciation of what it takes to keep her and other people safe. Michelle has a loyal, if fairly new friend, Mona, who appears close to her and seeks her out in the day service. It has the promise of being a mutual friendship as Michelle has been observed to talk to Mona.

Disquieting conclusions

Events in Michael, Doreen, Ben and Michelle's lives point to several sets of conclusions:

- Abuse can happen anywhere, even in services that are regularly inspected.

- The perpetrators of criminal and abusive acts may be close relatives, people who are paid to have a duty of care, other people with disabilities and strangers.

- The people who know that a threshold has been crossed and subsequently alert authorities to criminal and abusive acts may be close relatives, people who are paid to have a duty of care, other people with disabilities or strangers (AIMS Project 1998a, 1998b).

- It may be necessary to challenge unscrupulous relatives for regarding people's welfare benefits as payment for their caring, especially if their care is erratic or neglectful (Brown 2003).

- People who do not know how to relate well to colleagues are unlikely to be appropriate 'support' staff to people with learning disabilities. If currents of bullying, cruel joking, sexism, racism and homophobia are allowed to become established and go unchallenged there is no holding back the tide of abuse as it bears down on people who use the service.

- Although consequences are assigned to having such labels as 'highly dependent' and 'independent' these are neither necessarily protective nor prescriptive of the nature of assistance required.

- Support staff may develop ways of talking about their work which provide an unhelpful 'cover' for poor practice and which can lead to inherently harmful interpretations of 'independence' and 'choice' as cues for non-intervention (e.g. Flynn *et al.* 2003).

- Access to independent primary care is not yet a 'given' for all adults with learning disabilities, even though they may have long-standing conditions which warrant scrutiny and their care staff may be operating on the basis of pervasive misinformation and diagnostic overshadowing so that a learning disability means that someone 'bruises easily'.

- Not everyone can alert others to their abuse, especially if it takes place within an ongoing relationship, service or family culture. Even if someone else is raising the alarm on their behalf, it can be extraordinarily difficult to challenge the views of professionals or the often superficial findings of regulators.

Taking a lead

It follows that to take a lead against abuse, service managers have to make sense of incomplete information, emerging policy and guidelines, and complicated experience. Their task is similar to that of those addressing the ills of secretive software companies. They write reams of code to protect the software, which in turn yield more flaws, and as more products are introduced to the market, more codes are required. They know too that the authors of software viruses, bugs and worms thrive on finding flaws in the security systems. Software companies are not assisted by their secrecy and it is frequently observed that they would benefit from an 'open source' approach which relies on many people collaborating on the software problems and fixing them as they arise. Similarly, it is tempting for service managers to identify 'the problem', take measures to ensure that it is unlikely to recur, and unwittingly deflect the attentions of would-be abusers to other weaknesses in the service system.

Most staff working with people with learning disabilities are without professional qualifications and training. They can be isolated in their work settings and from the larger communities of practitioners. It falls to managers to ensure that staff are supervised and have opportunities to work alongside experienced and competent practitioners if poor and idiosyncratic practices are not to take root and flourish. Moreover, long working hours and the non-involvement of unions render work settings/services vulnerable to abusive practices. Managers should be finding out what can be done to recruit and retain high-quality staff through structural routes such as by negotiating improved terms and conditions, offering customized training opportunities (most particularly if services are offered to people with complex support needs), and ensuring that policies in respect of people's safety and health are credible and known to staff. This is a much more robust strategy than one of bringing in poorly-qualified staff, exposing them to challenges that they cannot meet and then rooting out individuals without changing the infrastructure which has led to the breach in standards. An 'open source' approach would engage all staff with the subject of people's safety and health (e.g. Flynn and Whitehead in press).

A service's track record is revealing. Managers should take stock and be attuned to the histories and range of support needs of all service users. How have known incidents of abuse and criminal acts been addressed to date? Do all service users have contact with individuals who are independent of the service and what measures are taken to ensure that these people are safe? How is poor practice dealt with and challenged? Is attention paid to the safe groupings of service users? Does the service have a history of using medication and/or 'restraint' and 'punishment' to deal with difficult behaviours? Such questions should figure prominently in considerations of service management. Looking at a service's history is important, not merely as a means to glean an approximation of events, but also as a means to understand the attitudes and assumptions of the narrators, to justify exclusions or restrictions and to identify sources of, and triggers to, improvement and reform.

Working to achieve safer services

Strategies to prevent abuse are often predicated on unsophisticated and/or muddled models of causation. They confound abuses which are deeply embedded within the structure of services, with those which arise out of individual cruelty, exploitation or perversion on the part of an individual perpetrator. They advocate single 'one-size-fits-all' approaches to identification of abuse which lead to naïve 'scatter gun' approaches such as inspections and checklists while the river flows on underground.

A more differentiated understanding of abuse leads to a more complex model in which different stages of prevention and levels of intervention can be mapped out. Models borrowed from health promotion assist in this kind of analysis in that they are based on a separation of efforts designed to stop an illness occurring at all, from strategies designed to facilitate early identification, through to treatment and intervention to mitigate the effect of the illness and promote recovery (see Brown 2002). If applied to the prevention of abuse it can be seen that:

- primary prevention involves setting up a safe and well-ordered environment, screening unsuitable staff out of the workforce and paying attention to recruitment, induction and supervision;
- secondary prevention involves alertness to signs and symptoms of abuse so that any concerns are picked up quickly and any further abuse 'nipped in the bud'; it is at this stage that the policies and procedures set out in *No Secrets* (DoH/Home Office 2000) are most pertinent with their emphasis on early reporting and prompt investigation;
- tertiary prevention involves taking action to support and protect individuals who are known to have been abused and taking steps to return a service to a 'norm' of working within safe limits.

Not only is it important to act at all stages in this unhappy process, but it is also imperative to operate at all levels – to work with individual service users but also with staff teams and service policies. Commissioners and regulators of services need to be mindful of dangerous currents and undercurrents and take full responsibility for the perverse incentives they build into systems which are often more skilled at protecting business interests than the interests of vulnerable service users. Legal changes have proved necessary and helpful to address anachronisms and gaps in law and inadequacies in applying it within the criminal justice system. Society needs to be challenged about the way that the needs of marginalized groups are distorted in public policy and political discourse: tax minimization or avoidance needs to be seen as a form of pin-striped abuse with the same stigma as any rape or bruise.

But while the primary prevention of abuse is the ideal, the foregoing case studies demonstrate how difficult this is to achieve, not least as we have to factor in people's individual histories alongside their service histories. What is clear is the importance of taking action at all levels and, minimally, highlighting the risks of inaction (ARC/NAPSAC 1993; Brown 1996, 1999; Brown *et al.* 1996a, 1996b, 1998; Brown and Thompson 1997; Flynn and Brown 1997; Brown and Stein 2000, 2001).

Exercise 16.3

Why bother about the abuse described in this chapter? Why shouldn't we get on with our lives and let adults with learning disabilities get on with theirs?

At the individual level

An introduction to being and feeling safe can arise from (or be compromised by) being part of a family. This renders the contribution of schools, colleges, health and social care services critical. At an individual level, there is neither a step-by-step formula nor an off the shelf solution. Prevention should reflect a stance, a willingness to see beyond such descriptions as 'mild learning disability in mainstream school', or 'deaf and moderately learning disabled', by considering people's histories, including their exposure to unsafe services and people; asking families how they have kept their relatives safe and reflecting with them how continuity of efforts between the family and services might be practised; exploring with support staff how they keep themselves and their loved ones safe; and considering how 'assertiveness training', for example, may be customized and made relevant to this young man or woman, as from today. The concerns have to be:

- to help people recognize and resist abusive acts and, as importantly, to seek help if they are victimized;
- to ensure that service users, relatives, visitors and staff understand the importance of their roles as 'lookouts' or 'alerters' with and on behalf of people who do not communicate their distress in readily understandable ways;
- to examine the unstated assumptions, unspoken prejudices and constraints of labels and ideologies and, rather than take them for granted, evaluate them in the light of the larger purpose of people's health, well-being and safety.

It matters that people know there are remedies beyond a service when bad things happen to them. In turn, there are growing examples of the police contributing to people's learning about personal safety.

At the service level

Policies are key preventive tools in reducing the likelihood of abuse and assault. They should be shaped by research findings and outline the parameters within which decision-making takes place. Services are likely to have developed approaches and policies regarding: the recruitment and screening of potential staff; complaints; personal development planning; confidentiality; risk-taking; sexuality; challenging behaviour; control and restraint; handling money; and administering medication, for example.

Staff training is one process for articulating a reliable understanding of abuse and responsibility for preventing this resides with services. Staff should be attuned to signs of abuse and distress and, in hand with supervision, they should be orientated to listening to, and learning from, people with learning disabilities, and identifying the boundaries of effective and safe practice. They should be encouraged to revisit what is known of the struggle of adolescents as their competency and autonomy rise up forcefully – and put this alongside what is known of the person for whom they have lead responsibility.

Professional regulation is another tool in the abuse prevention kit. While it may appear remote from weak practice in an isolated service, it can be instrumental in ensuring that those responsible for abuse are prevented from working with vulnerable people. The overwhelmingly complicated experience of preventing abuse gives weight to: staff knowing what to do with their concerns and which referral routes to use; staff being attuned to the complementariness of their roles alongside those of other practitioners; making the complaints procedure known and accessible; knowing what information should be shared and what is confidential; anticipating and clarifying when intervention is justifiable; defining when, and in what circumstances, a police inquiry should be instigated; assisting people to identify the help and protection they require without jeopardizing action against perpetrators; and making sense of the lessons learned about enhancing the safety of vulnerable people (Brown 2002).

At the government level

The external scrutiny of services, setting targets for developing professional skills in specialist and mainstream provision, clarifying channels of communication and routes through which action should be taken, and developing means to strengthen legal protection are critical means of raising standards within services for vulnerable people. Maximizing resources and setting appropriate measures of success and 'performance indicators' are necessary as is the design of accountability structures that not only bring to justice those who abuse but confront those who have real power and responsibility for setting up and perpetuating unsafe services for people who, despite the rhetoric, depend on them.

> **Exercise 16.4**
>
> A rich relative has left many millions of pounds to a charity promoting the needs of vulnerable adults whose lives have been compromised by abuse with the proviso that it should be used 'to optimize the best outcomes'. How would you advise them to spend it?

Conclusion

One service summed up an approach to the prevention of abuse when they put forward, as a strapline for their adult protection policy, the ill-conceived slogan 'less intervention = more autonomy'. Fortunately, this was abandoned because, of course, it does not. Abuse actively undermines a person's autonomy, whether that is as a result of the deliberate grooming and targeting of a vulnerable person carried out in order to exploit them financially or sexually, or as the consequence of more pervasive neglect of their human rights, personal development, health or well-being. When abuse is at issue more, not less, intervention is needed to safeguard real autonomy and that will be as true in new direct payment schemes and supported living arrangements. Independence is something to be nurtured and safeguarded. It should not be seen as a rallying cry for abandonment or withdrawal: when people are left to sink or swim, many sink.

Returning to our metaphor of the river with benign and less than benign tributaries, our lives are continuous with those who have lived before us. There are more markers perhaps that assert the importance of warnings and safeguards if we are to be safe – lifebelts, warnings of the dangers of deep water or dangerous currents – which in their widest scope reflect the history of prevention. Beyond the delta there are further markers: safe harbours, trained lifeguards, lifeboats, lighthouses, warnings of the dangers of high tides and fast incoming tides – i.e. the future is similarly replete with safeguards, but the advancing and retreating waves may be experienced as merciful and joyfully fluid or as threatening further unsought experience.

People with learning disabilities do depend on others and when they are placed or left in situations like those of Michael, Doreen, Ben or Michelle they are often not able to raise the alarm or swim for safety. A 'choice' to stay in such impoverished circumstances is often no more than a 'choice' between a rock they know and a hard place they fear. They may be choosing independently but their choice has the same validity as that of a thirsty person 'choosing' to drink dirty water. The challenge is upriver and it involves cleaning up the water supply.

References

AIMS Project (1998a) *The Alerter's Guide and Training Pack*. Brighton: Pavilion Publishing.

AIMS Project (1998b) *The Investigator's Guide and Training Pack*. Brighton: Pavilion Publishing.

ARC/NAPSAC (1993) *'It Could Never Happen Here': The Prevention and Treatment of Sexual Abuse of Adults with Learning Disabilities in Residential Settings*. Derby: Association of Residential Care.

Blustein, J., Levine, C. and Neveloff Dubler, N. (eds) (1999) *The Adolescent Alone: Decision Making in Health Care in the United States*. Cambridge: Cambridge University Press.

Brown, H. (1996) *Towards Safer Commissioning: A Handbook for Purchasers and Commissioners on the Sexual Abuse of Adults with Learning Disabilities*, Need to Know series. Nottingham: NAPSAC. Available from Pavilion Publishing, Brighton.

Brown, H. (1999) Abuse of people with learning disabilities: layers of concern and analysis, in N. Stanley, B. Penhale and J. Manthorpe (eds) *Institutional Abuse: Perspectives Across the Life Course*. London: Routledge.

Brown, H. (2002) *Safeguarding Adults and Children with Disabilities Against Abuse: Integration of People with Disabilities*. Strasbourg: Council of Europe.

Brown, H. (2003) What is financial abuse? *Journal of Adult Protection*, 5(2): 3–10.

Brown, H. and Stein, J. (2000) Monitoring adult protection in ten English local authorities, *Journal of Adult Protection*, 2(3): 19–31.

Brown, H. and Stein, J. (2001) Crossing the divide: the role of inspection units in protecting vulnerable adults, *Journal of Adult Protection*, 3(1): 25–34.

Brown, H. and Thompson, D. (1997) Service responses to men with intellectual disabilities who have sexually abusive or unacceptable behaviours: the case against inaction, *Journal of Applied Research in Intellectual Disability*, 10(2): 176–97.

Brown, H. and Egan-Sage, E. with Barry, G. and McKay, C. (1996a) *Towards Better Interviewing: A Handbook for Police Officers and Social Workers on the Sexual Abuse of Adults with Learning Disabilities*, Need to Know series. Nottingham: NAPSAC. Available from Pavilion Publishing, Brighton.

Brown, H., Brammer, A., Craft, A. and McKay, C. (1996b) *Towards Better Safeguards: A Handbook for Inspectors and Registration Officers on the Sexual Abuse of Adults with Learning Disabilities*, Need to Know series. Nottingham: NAPSAC. Available from Pavilion Publishing, Brighton.

Brown, H., Flynn, M. and Maughan, J. (1998) *A Template for Reviewing Individual Cases Assessed Under Adult Protection Policies*. Tunbridge Wells: Salomons Centre.

Brown, H., Wilson, B. and Kingston, P. (2000) Comment: unpacking 'discriminatory abuse', *Journal of Adult Protection*, 2(3): 17–18.

DHSS (Department of Health and Social Security) and the Welsh Office (1971) *Better Services for the Mentally Handicapped*. London: HMSO.

DHSS (Department of Health and Social Security) and the Welsh Office (1989) *Caring for People: Community Care in the Next Decade and Beyond*. London: HMSO.

DoH (Department of Health) (2001) *Valuing People: A New Strategy for Learning Disability for the 21st Century*. London: Department of Health.

DoH (Department of Health) and the Home Office (2000) *No Secrets: Guidance on Developing and Implementing Multi-agency Policies and Procedures to Protect Vulnerable Adults from Abuse.* London: Department of Health.

Flynn, M. and Brown, H. (1997) The responsibilities of commissioners, purchasers and providers: lessons from recent National Development Team Inquiries, in J. Churchill, H. Brown, A. Craft and C. Horrocks (eds) *There are no Easy Answers – The Provision of Continuing Care and Treatment to Adults with Learning Disabilities who Sexually Abuse Others.* Chesterfield: Association of Residential Care and National Association for the Protection from Sexual Abuse of Adults and Children with Learning Disabilities, with the Social Services Inspectorate/Department of Health.

Flynn, M. and Whitehead, S. (eds) (in press) *Bruises Easily? Keeping People Safe.*

Flynn, M., Keywood, K. and Fovargue, S. (2003) Warning: health 'choices' can kill, *Journal of Adult Protection*, 5(1): 30–4.

Grant, G. and Whittell, B. (2003) Partnerships with families over the life course, in M. Nolan, U. Lundh, G. Grant and J. Keady (eds) *Partnerships in Family Care: Understanding the Caregiving Career.* Maidenhead: Open University Press.

MacIntyre, D. (2003) There should be a law against it, *Society Guardian*, 17 December.

O'Connell Higgins, G. (1994) *Resilient Adults: Overcoming a Cruel Past.* San Francisco: Jossey Bass.

17

Promoting healthy lifestyles – challenging behaviour

Sally Twist and Ada Montgomery

Introduction

It is estimated that approximately 10 per cent of young adults with learning disabilities accessing services exhibit challenging behaviour (Emerson *et al.* 2001). This chapter aims to provide a framework for identifying what challenging behaviour is and understanding why some young people with learning disabilities exhibit such behaviour, and suggest ways of responding to young people who present with challenging behaviour. It is anticipated that this information will increase the knowledge, skills and confidence of carers supporting young people with learning disabilities who exhibit challenging behaviour and, thereby, promote healthy and positive lifestyles for those individuals.

What is challenging behaviour?

A widely accepted definition of challenging behaviour is that described by Eric Emerson (2001: 3): 'culturally abnormal behaviour of such intensity, frequency or duration that the physical safety of the person or others is likely to be placed in serious jeopardy, or behaviour which is likely to seriously limit use of, or result in the person being denied access to, ordinary community facilities'. The essential elements of this definition are that the behaviour:

- is unacceptable by social standards, taking into consideration issues such as the person's age, social class, and ethnocultural background;
- imposes a significant cost to the person – for example, physical harm to self, social rejection, exclusion from recreational, educational or employment opportunities;

- imposes a significant cost to others – for example, physical harm, property damage, emotional distress.

This definition is the starting point in understanding challenging behaviour as it enables us to identify problematic behaviours that warrant further exploration.

Examples of challenging behaviour

Some examples of challenging behaviour include:

- Verbal aggression
- Shouting
- Stripping
- Stealing
- Anal poking
- Self-injury
- Withdrawal from others
- Physical aggression
- Persistent screaming
- Inappropriate sexual behaviour
- Property damage
- Smearing of faeces
- Disturbed sleep
- Non-compliance

Prevalence of challenging behaviour

Most studies investigating the epidemiology of challenging behaviour have researched the prevalence of different types of challenging behaviour, that is, the number of people in the population under study who at that time exhibit challenging behaviour. The results of a study (Emerson *et al.* 2001) indicated that between 10 and 15 per cent of people with learning disabilities in contact with services presented with challenging behaviour, and that most exhibited two or more different types of challenging behaviour. Correlational analyses of variables associated with different types of challenging behaviour indicate that an increased prevalence of such behaviour is seen in the following groups: men; people aged between 15 and 35 years; people with severe learning disability; people with additional disabilities (e.g. sensory impairment, communication difficulties); and people with specific syndromes and disorders, such as autism (Emerson 2001).

Understanding challenging behaviour

> **Exercise 17.1**
>
> Imagine the following scenario. You have a headache and would like some painkilling tablets. You find it difficult to talk to your carers. You have no direct access to painkilling tablets in your house, and you are unable to leave the house without support. How would you let other people know what is wrong? How would you get your needs met? You might try to communicate non-verbally that you have a headache by pointing at your head. Now imagine that your best efforts at communicating your needs are not being understood by your carers. What would you do next? How would you get the attention of your carers? If the pain was getting very bad you might start to hit your head. How would you feel if your carers then began to chide you, advise you to stop behaving in this way, ignore or isolate you? There are many ways you might behave or feel in this situation – for example, you might withdraw from everyone and hope the pain subsides; your behaviour might escalate until you significantly harmed yourself or someone else; and you might feel angry, upset or worried. Your reactions might vary depending on the situation – for example, whether this had happened before, your relationship with your carers, or how bad the pain was. Now try to imagine how you would feel if a carer spent some time trying to understand what was wrong, and after a period of time worked out what you were trying to communicate and gave you what you wanted.

The valuable learning points from Exercise 17.1 scenario are:

- Everyone has needs, many of which require the support of others to fulfil. These include the need for food, clothing, shelter, physical, emotional and social care, opportunities to learn and develop skills and relationships, and access to community facilities, to name but a few. Individuals with learning disabilities have the same needs as people without learning disabilities; however, the way they express those needs may be different.

- Behaviour is a way of communicating our needs. A young person with learning disabilities may use challenging behaviour to communicate something to others, and it may be that using challenging behaviour is the most effective way for the person to communicate their needs at that time. Emerson (2001) argues that the task of understanding challenging behaviour involves investigating what the purpose of the challenging behaviour is for the person in their life – what does it do for the individual? This is often described as developing an understanding of the 'function' of the challenging behaviour.

- Challenging behaviour is not unique to people with learning disabilities. The exercise above did not necessarily describe someone with a learning disability; it could equally apply to someone finding it difficult to talk after dental surgery. In some situations behaviours can escalate and become problematic, often when we need support and others fail to understand and meet our needs. Unfortunately, the consequences of exhibiting challenging behaviours are often different for people with learning disabilities, compared to people without learning disabilities. For example, they may be subject to negative labelling, physical abuse, inappropriate medical or psychological interventions, exclusion or neglect (Emerson 2001).

- Challenging behaviours often have multiple contributory factors. The same behaviour may be expressing several different needs – for example, the need to communicate 'I have a headache', 'I need some painkillers', and 'I would like some emotional support or some activity to take my mind off the pain'. Similarly, different behaviours may be used to communicate the same need – for example, pointing at the head and hitting the head to tell people 'I have a headache' – and this may vary depending on personal and environmental factors. It should also be noted that no two individuals are the same, and although two people may exhibit virtually identical challenging behaviour they may be communicating very different needs. Similarly, two people engaging in different challenging behaviour may be expressing similar needs.

- The task of understanding what the person is trying to communicate using challenging behaviour may be difficult and time-consuming, but it is also likely to be very rewarding. Blunden and Allen (1987) noted that the term 'challenging behaviour' conveys that the behaviour presents a challenge to the carers rather than the person exhibiting the behaviour.

Exercise 17.2

Reflecting on what you have just read, think about your own behaviours. What behaviours have you exhibited that could be thought of as challenging? For example, being short-tempered with a friend, banging a door, regularly getting up in the middle of the night because you cannot sleep. List the behaviours, then write a brief explanation of why you exhibited each one.

The task of understanding challenging behaviour – being a detective

There are a multitude of possible needs that an individual may wish to communicate to others, which can make the role of attempting to understand and meet those needs a somewhat daunting one. It is important to remember that in most situations you will be aware of many of the needs of the individuals for whom you are caring, and in many cases the individual will find an effective way of communicating their unmet needs. However, there may be some situations where the individual uses challenging behaviour as a means of communication. Here, the role of the carer supporting the individual is rather like that of being a detective; trying to find clues to understand why the person is behaving in the way they are (SETRHA and the Tizzard Centre 1994). Below are listed several areas for further investigation. It may be that several of these factors contribute to an understanding of why the individual exhibits challenging behaviour.

Personal characteristics

Knowledge of an individual's personal characteristics provides a better understanding of the person as a whole, and may help to determine the reasons why that person is exhibiting challenging behaviour. Obtaining information about the person's cognitive, sensory and physical impairments and how these impact on their skills and functioning can be helpful. For example, problems such as difficulties concentrating, understanding what people say or how they feel, finding it hard to cope with change, having to use a wheelchair or a hearing aid, or struggling to make friends may all contribute to situations that result in challenging behaviour. Information about the individual's personality characteristics can also help to assess challenging behaviour, and differentiate between behaviour that is 'normal' for that individual and behaviour that is 'challenging'.

Personal history

It is helpful to know about an individual's personal history – what life events they have experienced, where they have lived, where they have gone to school, whether they have experienced any trauma, what is their family background, who are their role models, what values, attitudes, prejudices have they been subjected to – as these factors may influence their personal functioning and their reactions to future events. For example, consider a young woman who over the last few years has exhibited uncharacteristic challenging behaviour during the Christmas period. Finding out that the young woman's mother died on 24 December 2001, and that she dislikes changes to her usual routine (a common experience over the Christmas period with parties and suchlike), suggests that she may be likely to experience some distress during the Christmas period. This might help to explain the increase in challenging behaviour and, thereby, point to ways to support the individual through a potentially difficult time.

Physical needs

A person may engage in challenging behaviour to communicate their physical needs. The scenario described in Exercise 17.1 illustrates that an individual may engage in challenging behaviour to communicate that they are in pain. There are many different reasons why someone may be experiencing pain – for example, toothache, ingrowing toenails, muscular pain, menstrual pain, constipation or an ear infection. Other physical problems people may be experiencing include poor sleep, physical illness or food allergy.

Relationship/emotional needs

A young person may exhibit challenging behaviour as a way of communicating their feelings. Individuals with learning disabilities experience a range of emotions. However, as a result of their disabilities or their experiences they may find it difficult to recognize and express those feelings. Gathering information about loss or bereavement, changes of staff, changes of residents/friends, house/family dynamics, changes in routine and family problems can help to identify whether the individual is using challenging behaviour to communicate their unmet relationship or emotional needs.

Mental health issues

While reviews of the literature demonstrate that prevalence rates of mental health problems in adults with learning disabilities vary considerably, with reported rates of between 10 per cent and 80 per cent depending on the study variables, there is evidence to suggest that the rate of psychiatric disorders is higher among people with learning disabilities compared to the general population (see Campbell and Malone 1991; Borthwick-Duffy 1994 for reviews). Young adults with a diagnosis of learning disabilities and mental health problems are described as having a 'dual diagnosis'. A study (Moss *et al.* 2000) investigating the prevalence of psychiatric symptoms in adults with learning disability and challenging behaviours found that an increase in the severity of challenging behaviour was associated with a higher rate of psychiatric symptoms, and that self-injurious behaviour seemed to be related to higher levels of anxiety symptoms. Adults with mental health problems often present with behavioural disturbances, such as aggression, withdrawal, mood disturbances, self-injury or antisocial behaviour (Fraser and Nolan 1994). Thus, if a young adult with learning disabilities exhibits challenging behaviour, another important factor to consider is the possibility of unrecognized mental health problems, such as anxiety disorders, depression, schizophrenic or psychotic illness, or acute confusion (O'Hara and Sperlinger 1997) (see also Chapter 27).

Experiencing abuse

An individual may exhibit challenging behaviour to communicate that they are being abused or exploited in some way. Until recently the abuse of adults with learning disabilities had not been acknowledged and addressed in any systematic way. However, it is now widely accepted that such adults may be the victims of physical abuse, sexual abuse, psychological/emotional abuse, financial abuse and neglect (Brown 1997). Indeed, many individuals with learning disabilities may be at increased risk of abuse as a result of their personal vulnerability due to lack of knowledge of abuse, poor understanding or limited communication skills, and also because of the settings in which they live, work and socialize (Brown 1997). It is important that those caring for individuals with learning disabilities recognize that abuse occurs and that challenging behaviour may be a means of an individual communicating that abuse. Carers should be aware of the appropriate steps to take to address the problem (see also Chapter 16).

Environmental influences

Another important variable to be considered when trying to understand why a person is exhibiting challenging behaviour is their environment. Environmental factors to investigate include: size and layout (too big, overcrowded, too small, too much too little furniture, too close to others?); access (access to other rooms, areas, outside, escape route, safe place, privacy?); noise levels (too loud, too quiet, source of noise, type of noise, continuous noise, sudden unexpected noise?); decoration (mirrors, ornaments, lighting, floor coverings, soft furnishings?); demands of the environment (too demanding or complex, over-stimulating, too much to understand or process, boring, does it require constant re-evaluation, too monotonous?); and activities (no outings, always at home, nothing to occupy self?). In addition, it may be important to investigate whether there has been a change in the environment.

Any of these factors could be experienced as stressful by an individual living, working or socializing in the environment, and could result in behaviours that are interpreted as challenging. For example, consider a situation where a young man with learning disabilities walked into his lounge, threw a chair through the window, then left and refused to return. When escorted back into the room by a staff member and encouraged to talk about what was wrong he became increasingly agitated and his behaviour escalated to screaming, verbal abuse, and attempting to throw an object towards the window. The young man was redirected to the kitchen for a cup of tea, where he was able to tell his carer why he became distressed. This was the first time the young man has been in the room since it was decorated. He became distressed when he saw the new orange curtains, as they reminded him of a residential establishment where he had lived as a child and where he had negative experiences.

This example illustrates how changes to the environment can cause distress for an individual, and how if that distress is not recognized the behaviour can quickly escalate to challenging behaviour presenting significant risk of harm. One advantage for the carers in this situation was that when he was removed from the environment and supported to reduce his anxiety the young man was able to communicate the reasons for his distress. Developing an understanding why someone exhibits certain behaviours can be even more challenging for staff when the person is unable to directly communicate their distress.

Lack of opportunities for development

Most young people relish the opportunity to attend social events, develop friendships, take part in sports, learn new skills at college or work, or pursue an interest. It is possible, therefore, that a young person with learning disabilities may present with challenging behaviours because of their frustration and distress relating to the lack of opportunities available to them.

Blocks to understanding challenging behaviour

Clements (1997: 84) cautions that 'making judgements and interpretations about other people and their needs is not a simple, scientific matter. It is a social process of construction and can be seriously flawed'. He identifies three potential blocks to effectively understanding challenging behaviour:

- lack of understanding of the complexity of human behaviour and the multiple contributing factors;
- making attribution errors about the function of the behaviour – one person's understanding of another person's behaviour will be influenced by a variety of factors, such as their relationship with the individual, their own emotional state, their past experiences and the power relationship between the two, and this may lead them to the wrong conclusions about the function of the challenging behaviour;
- the influence of personal attitudes and values, prejudices and stereotypes.

Therefore, it is important to take these factors into consideration when investigating what a person is trying to communicate by engaging in challenging behaviour.

Exercise 17.3

'Not waving but drowning': try and think of three examples of situations when you have misread the behaviour of friends or family members because of a snap decision or assumption you have made.

Responding to challenging behaviour

The first step in responding to an individual who is exhibiting challenging behaviour is to complete an assessment of the behaviour. Such an assessment is necessary as it enables the formulation of hypotheses about why the individual is exhibiting the challenging behaviour. The second step is to design and implement an intervention. This should be based on the hypotheses about why the challenging behaviour occurs. The third step is to evaluate the effectiveness of the intervention – i.e. does the intervention work to reduce the behaviour? If an intervention is not effective it may be necessary to conduct further assessment, modify the hypotheses and implement an alternative intervention. Thus, responding to challenging behaviour is often an ongoing and circular process of assessment, formulation of hypotheses, intervention and evaluation. These processes are described in more detail below.

Assessment of challenging behaviour

The purpose of an assessment is to try and answer the following questions:

- What does the person do that is challenging?
- How does the challenging behaviour get in the way of the person achieving a positive lifestyle?
- What is the function of the challenging behaviour (i.e. what needs is the person trying to communicate via their challenging behaviour)?

What does the person do that is challenging?

In order to answer this question the first piece of information needed is a detailed description of the behaviour. For example, a description of the behaviour of someone who throws objects might be 'the young lady picks up objects from the mantelpiece and throws them across the room. She aims the objects at people or objects in the room'. Information about the sequence of the challenging behaviour can also assist in planning effective interventions. Although at times it may seem that challenging behaviour occurs 'out of the blue' this is not often the case. It is more likely that there is a sequence of behaviour that leads up to the challenging behaviour. Returning to the example above, it might be observed that prior to throwing objects there is a sequence of build-up behaviours that begin with the young lady vocalizing loudly, followed by her holding her head in her hands, then by her moving to the mantelpiece and lifting up and replacing objects repeatedly.

Further useful information would include details about when the behaviour happens (date and time), where the behaviour happens (specific locations) and how often the behaviour happens. It may also be useful to know what the individual is doing when the behaviour occurs, who they are with and how they seem to be feeling.

This type of information can be gathered by people (staff, carers, relatives) who are in regular contact with the individual, simply by observing the person in their usual surroundings and making a note of what happens. If more detailed information is required it may be useful to design a recording form, covering the areas described above. Validated assessments of challenging behaviour – for example, the Aberrant Behaviour Checklist (Aman *et al.* 1985) – can also be used to assess challenging behaviour and monitor change.

How does the challenging behaviour get in the way?

The next stage of an assessment would be to determine how the challenging behaviour gets in the way of the young person achieving their full potential for a positive and healthy lifestyle. For example, this might include an assessment of whether the young person's challenging behaviour affects their opportunities for developing positive personal relationships, participating in social, recreational, educational and occupational activities, empowerment and choice, or access to appropriate services. In the past, many young adults with learning disabilities who exhibited challenging behaviour were excluded or had limited access to ordinary community settings and lived in segregated and restrictive environments. O'Brien's (1987) interpretation of the philosophy of normalization and social role valorization in terms of five fundamental accomplishments for service delivery for individuals with learning disabilities (competence, community presence, community participation, respect and choice) can be a useful framework in the assessment of challenging behaviour. For example, during an assessment of a young lady who exhibits self-injury, characterized by frequently hitting herself in the face, we might question whether she has the opportunity to learn new skills (competence), whether she is excluded from community facilities because of her behaviour (presence), whether she has the option of going to the local pub for a drink with friends (community participation, choice), and whether she is supported to present herself positively and perceived by carers in a positive light despite her challenging behaviour (respect).

In many cases a risk assessment of the challenging behaviour would also be valuable at this stage, to identify the level of risk of harm to the individual themselves, others involved in the individual's care, and/or damage to property. This information could then be used to design reactive strategies to manage the behaviour when it occurs in order to minimize risk.

What is the function of the challenging behaviour?

In some situations it may be a relatively straightforward task to identify the function of the challenging behaviour, by detailed description or closer observation of the behaviour. However, in cases of severe and enduring challenging behaviour the task of identifying the function can be complex, and require a detailed analysis of the behaviour in question. Under these circumstances a multi-disciplinary team approach to assessment is recommended. It was noted earlier that a young person with learning disabilities may exhibit challenging behaviour to express a range of needs. Therefore, assessment by a range of professionals with expert knowledge can be valuable. In some cases the involvement of workers with specialist knowledge of challenging behaviour, such as the challenging behaviour team, a specialist behavioural nurse or a clinical psychologist may be necessary. Emerson (2001) provides a comprehensive review of descriptive and experimental methods for the functional assessment of challenging behaviour. He tabulates the advantages and disadvantages of different approaches, including structured interviews, antecedent-behaviour-consequences (ABC) charts, scatter plots and various experimental analyses, and interested readers are directed to this text for further information.

Interventions for challenging behaviour

There are several texts providing detailed descriptions and evaluation of interventions for challenging behaviour (e.g. Donnellan *et al.* 1988; Carr *et al.* 1993; Zarkowska and Clements 1994; Emerson 2001). Here, a brief overview of the process of intervention and the range of approaches available is provided.

In theory, a comprehensive, multi-disciplinary assessment of a young person who exhibits challenging behaviour should provide a wealth of information, facilitate the development of hypotheses about the function of the behaviour, and support the development of an appropriate intervention. In practice, assessment is likely to show that the behaviour varies in frequency and intensity depending on different contextual factors, has different functions at different times and in different situations, and that there are several possible reasons why the individual might be exhibiting challenging behaviour. Thus, designing and implementing an effective intervention is rarely straightforward.

For example, analysis of a young man's challenging behaviour suggested that one reason he was hitting his head on the staff room door was that he was thirsty, as every time he engaged in this behaviour he was redirected by staff to the lounge and given a drink. The assessment raised concerns about the frequency with which the young man was requesting drinks, and prompted investigation of his physical health needs. It was also hypothesized that the young man might use the challenging behaviour to initiate social contact with members of staff, as the behaviour occurred less frequently when he was engaged with others. The assessment revealed that the young man had no effective, alternative ways of communicating these needs. This demonstrates that even in this simple example there are several areas for possible intervention, such as helping the young man to develop alternative means of communicating, exploring options for engagement in social relationships, and further medical investigation.

It is recommended that interventions for challenging behaviour are:

- *Individually-tailored* – an intervention based on a comprehensive assessment of the individual's challenging behaviour, personal characteristics and environmental factors. When planning interventions the key principles of rights, independence, choice and inclusion, outlined in the government White Paper *Valuing People* (DoH 2001) should be considered. Thus, it may be appropriate to involve the individual, perhaps with the support of an advocate, in decision-making about interventions.

- *Evidence-based* – there is a growing body of research investigating the effectiveness of different interventions for challenging behaviour (see Emerson 2001; Beail 2003), and it may be useful to consult relevant studies when selecting an intervention. It should be noted that effective monitoring of challenging behaviour before, during and after the implementation of an intervention also allows 'practice-based' evaluation of the effectiveness of a specific intervention for that individual.

- *Multi-faceted* – in most cases a 'multi-component intervention package' (Emerson 1998: 143) will be necessary, which involves different approaches and multi-disciplinary involvement. In cases of severe challenging behaviour a multi-faceted approach is likely to include both reactive and proactive/preventative strategies for managing the behaviour.

- *Graded* – in terms of the restrictive and invasive nature of the intervention. Research indicates that physical restraint is frequently used in the management of severe challenging behaviour for adults with learning disabilities living in residential settings (Emerson *et al.* 2000). Recently published guidelines for the use of physical intervention for people with learning disabilities (DoH/DfES 2002) recommend that physical interventions should, wherever possible, only be used in the management of challenging behaviour when other strategies have been tried and found to be unsuccessful, or in emergency situations where the risk of not intervening outweighs the use of minimum force. Hence, good practice in developing interventions for challenging behaviour would dictate that the package of interventions should include a graded hierarchy of strategies, starting with the least restrictive or invasive interventions and moving towards the use of physical restraint or emergency medication only as a 'last resort'.

- *Clearly documented and evaluated* – strategies for intervention should be clearly documented and accessible to individuals involved in the young person's care, preferably in the form of care plans approved at a multi-disciplinary level. Care plans are likely to include a rationale for the chosen intervention package, clear guidelines explaining how the intervention will be implemented and plans for evaluation of the effectiveness of the intervention. For example, evaluation might include ongoing monitoring of the challenging behaviour and assessment of changes in other variables, such as the young person's self-esteem, mood, physical health or engagement in activities.

Outlined below are various approaches to intervention that could be implemented.

Reactive strategies

There will be some emergency situations when it will be necessary for a carer supporting a young person exhibiting challenging behaviour to take immediate action to reduce the risk of harm to the individual or others, or damage to property (Murphy *et al.* 2003). This type of intervention, known as a 'reactive strategy', often takes the form of restrictive physical intervention or emergency administration of medication. The British Institute of Learning

Disabilities policy framework for physical interventions (Harris *et al.* 1996) describes three categories of physical intervention: direct physical contact between staff and client (e.g. holding); the use of barriers to limit freedom of movement (e.g. locked doors); and the use of material or equipment to restrict or prevent movement (e.g. arm splints). The Department of Health and Department for Education and Skills (DoH/DfES 2002) guidelines recommend that restrictive physical interventions should be used as infrequently as possible, that there should be clear policies and procedures for their use and that staff who may be required to intervene in this way should receive the appropriate training and support.

A distinction should be made between the use of reactive strategies to manage emergency situations and the planned use of these interventions as a 'last resort' to manage an individual's challenging behaviour. In this situation physical interventions should only be used when other less intrusive strategies have not worked.

Preventative strategies

The Department of Health and Department for Education and Skills (2002) outline primary and secondary prevention strategies for working with young people who exhibit challenging behaviour.

Primary prevention strategies include: ensuring that young people have suitable levels of support (i.e. that there are enough staff/carers and that those staff/carers have received appropriate training); ensuring that young people are supported to reduce conditions that may trigger incidents of challenging behaviour; care plans for challenging behaviour; and access to appropriate educational, occupational and recreational opportunities.

Secondary prevention strategies include:

- recognizing and knowing how to intervene at the first stages of a behavioural sequence that can develop into challenging behaviour (e.g. knowing that the first signs of anxiety include increased muscle tension, restlessness, signs of flushing and dilated pupils);
- skills in the use of de-escalation/diffusion and distraction techniques (e.g. de-escalation is a set of verbal and non-verbal skills that may help to reduce the level of arousal); verbal skills include speaking slowly, clearly and at low volume, being non-judgemental, listening carefully, clarifying the problem, answering truthfully and being supportive; non-verbal skills involve keeping your distance, making appropriate eye contact, showing that you are listening and being aware of your own body language – it should be relaxed, non-confrontational and open;
- developing multi-disciplinary care plans, use of medication and access to appropriate health care.

Behavioural interventions

In recent years, behavioural interventions have been perhaps the most widely used and most prolifically researched techniques in the treatment of challenging behaviour, particularly for adults with severe learning disabilities. This is an extensive area, and for further details readers are directed to Donnellan *et al.* (1988), Carr *et al.* (1993) and Emerson (2001). In a review of 103 outcome studies to establish best practice for interventions in challenging behaviour, Agar and O'May (2001) found evidence for the effectiveness of behavioural interventions for challenging behaviour, particularly when interventions were informed by functional assessment.

Emerson (1995) provides an excellent overview of the pros and cons of different behavioural approaches for challenging behaviour. Examples of behavioural approaches include: stimulus fading, non-contingent reinforcement, differential reinforcement of other behaviour (DRO), differential reinforcement of incompatible (DRI) or alternative (DRA) behaviour, extinction and punishment.

Medical interventions

Since physical and mental health problems can contribute to challenging behaviour it is essential that young people have access to appropriate health care services, in order that their heath needs are appropriately diagnosed and treated. One area of ongoing debate is the use of medication to treat challenging behaviour. Tyrer (1997: 205) noted that:

> psychotropic drugs are widely used in people with learning disabilities and often with poor indicators . . . these drugs are often used when there is no evidence of psychiatric or medical illness. They are widely employed in patients who are behaviourally disturbed in order to control aggression and self-injurious behaviour.

Medication can be an essential element of a multi-faceted intervention for challenging behaviour, and it is important we move towards providing a clear rationale and evidence base for the use of medication, and provide ongoing monitoring and evaluation of the effectiveness of medication on an individual basis.

Environmental interventions

Functional assessment may reveal certain environmental conditions (activities, people, approaches or situations) that trigger challenging behaviour, which if removed or avoided are likely to result in fewer incidences of the behaviour (Clements 1997). For example, if it is hypothesized that a young person exhibits challenging behaviour when the environment is too noisy, then an intervention might involve an overall aim to provide quiet living and working environments, alongside a series of strategies to manage situations when high noise levels are unavoidable, such as access to quiet areas and distraction via engagement in activities or social interaction.

Clements (1997) identified several potential changes to the social system of which the young person is a part that may be effective in reducing the incidence of challenging behaviour; for example, promoting positive attitudes towards the individual, resolving potential conflicts within the social system, ensuring the individual has the opportunity to make choices, structuring the young person's time and planning activity appropriately for that person, improving engagement levels and adapting communication systems to the young person's needs.

Psychotherapeutic interventions

In recent years there has been a growth of interest in the use of psychotherapy with adults with learning disabilities to improve emotional well-being, enhance self-esteem and develop skills (such as assertiveness, relaxation, anger management and relationship-building). However, research investigating the effectiveness of different therapeutic approaches is in its relative infancy. If it is determined that a young person is exhibiting challenging behaviour as a way of expressing emotional distress it may be appropriate that they are offered a psychotherapeutic intervention. Examples of therapeutic approaches include:

- *Cognitive-behavioural interventions* (e.g. Stenfert Kroese *et al.* 1997) – self-management interventions which assume that emotional and behavioural problems are related to the young person's cognitive impairments and lack of skills, teach self-monitoring, self-instruction, self-control, problem-solving and decision-making alongside relaxation therapy and social skills training. Cognitive-behavioural therapy is based on the premise that an individual's emotions and behaviour are influenced by their cognitions, and aims to effect change in the young person's distorted or negative thinking, beliefs and attributions, thereby resulting in positive changes to mood and behaviour.

- *Psychodynamic psychotherapy* – through the development of a relationship with the therapist, the individual develops an understanding of the defensive processes they use to manage psychological distress. Clients are encouraged to explore their early experiences and their emotional reactions to events.

- *Family therapy* – in contrast to cognitive-behavioural and psychodynamic approaches, family therapy intervenes at the level of the family. All family members are invited to sessions and encouraged to contribute to developing an understanding of problems in relation to difficulties experienced within family relationships. Fidell (2000) argues that systemic family therapy has obvious advantages for use with this client group, because of the stresses that the experience of having a learning disability place on the individual, the family and the organizations that support them.

In a recent commentary on the effectiveness of psychotherapy interventions for adults with learning disabilities, Beail (2003) argues that although the research is limited there is evidence that individuals make improvements in cognitive-behavioural and psychodynamic psychotherapy that are maintained at follow-up.

Exercise 17.4

Planning strategies for supporting a young person who exhibits challenging behaviour can seem complicated and difficult, and you may feel as if you do not know where to start. In order to plan interventions for challenging behaviour you may need to develop skills in assessing the range of interventions required, considering what information will be needed to plan and implement those interventions, and how to evaluate the effectiveness of them. To illustrate this process, try the following example.

Think of what information you would need to know, what you would have to plan and organize, and what interventions you might use, when taking a young person who exhibits challenging behaviours (in the form of physically aggressive outbursts and stealing) to a local pub for lunch. Now think of what information you would need to know, what you would have to plan and organize, and what interventions you might use to accompany the same individual on a two-week holiday in Blackpool.

Staff/carer support and training

People who support individuals with learning disabilities and challenging behaviour may experience a range of distressing events, for example physical assault, verbal abuse, emotional distress, property damage or theft. Staff, carers or family members may be the victims themselves, may witness such events, may have to live or regularly work in environments where challenging behaviours are exhibited, may have to conduct assessments and intervene to manage behaviours of this type and may be required to support others who have experienced such events. Therefore, the needs of carers supporting young people with learning disabilities who present with challenging behaviour cannot be overlooked. Below we address the issues of personal safety, staff support and training.

Personal safety

When working with young people who exhibit challenging behaviour staff/ carers may be at risk of physical assault and may need to take steps to ensure their personal safety. The law is clear on self-defence. Everyone has a right to defend themselves, particularly in cases of physical assault on one's person. However, carers/staff can find this difficult, as they may feel that taking steps to defend themselves is in conflict with what they see as their duty of care. The dilemma is that in many cases not responding can have serious consequences and carry a high risk of injury. So, if you are physically assaulted you are within your rights to defend yourself. The key legal issue is that your response must be in proportion to the risk presented to you. In other words, if a person were to nip you and you responded by hitting them, resulting in them falling to the floor, this would be considered excessive use of force and could result in assault charges being made against you. Thus, the law allows you to defend yourself but requires that your response is reasonable and in proportion to the threat/risk that you are in. The law also requires that you demonstrate a willingness to disengage, that you act with benevolence and in the other person's best interests, and that you act to maintain your own safety.

Challenging behaviour is by definition socially unacceptable, and in some severe cases can result in significant harm to others (e.g. physical or sexual assault), property damage or theft. In cases such as this it may be appropriate to involve the police and proceed with criminal investigation of the individual's actions. This type of intervention may be necessary to ensure the personal safety of people in contact with the individual.

Training

Wherever possible, carers/staff working with people with learning disabilities and challenging behaviour should have the opportunity to attend a recognized and approved training scheme for managing challenging behaviour/violence and aggression. Training courses usually include learning about risk assessment, reactive and preventive management strategies, physical intervention, personal safety, and how to support and maximize the safety of the individual exhibiting the challenging behaviour. Research demonstrates that training can be effective in increasing an individual's understanding, skills and confidence in dealing with incidents of challenging behaviour that impose a significant risk, can increase knowledge and confidence in the use of distraction, diffusion and non-aggressive physical intervention techniques, and can enable carers to read situations with greater clarity, manage their responses in a controlled and responsible manner and resolve situations without incident or injury – thereby reducing the risks to everyone involved (Allen *et al.* 1997; Allen and Tynan 2000).

An assessment of challenging behaviour may highlight issues where the knowledge or skills of the staff/carers is limited. In order to intervene effectively to reduce an individual's challenging behaviour staff/carers may benefit from support from professionals with expert knowledge of these issues. In addition to this, specific training on issues such as challenging behaviour, facilitating communication skills, specific physical or mental health problems, autism, dementia and the use of non-confrontational techniques is likely to be valuable for staff/carers who directly support the individual on a regular basis and who are largely responsible for implementation of care plans.

Staff support

Working with young people who exhibit challenging behaviour can be difficult, potentially dangerous and emotionally demanding for carers. Research findings indicate that staff working in residential settings supporting individuals with learning disabilities and challenging behaviour feel significantly more anxious, less supported and have lower job satisfaction than staff supporting individuals who do not present with challenging behaviour (Jenkins *et al.* 1997). We feel it is important that people caring for young people with learning disabilities and challenging behaviour also have access to appropriate support. Examples of different types of staff support include: team meetings where information about assessment, formulation, intervention, care planning and evaluation can be discussed; advice, recommendations and support from members of the multi-disciplinary care team; clinical supervision; access to appropriate training; critical incident debriefing; ongoing staff support groups; and psychological consultancy.

Conclusion

This chapter is an overview of ways of understanding and responding to young people who exhibit challenging behaviour. It provides information to enable carers to recognize behaviour that is challenging, develop hypotheses about why young people might behave in this way, and offer ideas for assessment and intervention. Overall, the chapter aims to support carers to feel more confident and knowledgeable when working with young people who communicate their distress through challenging behaviour.

Of course, how one evaluates the efficacy or otherwise of any form of behavioural intervention or therapy must be predicated upon a consideration of numerous factors. Not least among these are the ethics involved, the presumptions made about the behaviour in the light of the earlier assessment and the emerging results in terms of both actual and potential outcomes. Despite the professional's best efforts and intentions, sometimes interventions may not succeed in quite the way that was anticipated. For these reasons, evaluation is better understood not as an 'end stage' but rather as an integral and dynamic component that extends throughout the process of intervention. By such evaluative means, practitioners are better placed to respect not only the dynamic and holistic nature of human behaviour and understanding with which they are engaged, but also the person from whom it is derived.

Exercise 17.5

The aims of this exercise are to normalize challenging behaviour and give the reader the opportunity to work through the process of developing a strategy to change behaviour.

Readers are asked to think of something that they do that may be considered by others to be 'challenging' – that is, any behaviour that another person may find unacceptable, upsetting or difficult to understand. For example, swearing, nail biting, smoking, driving too fast. Once you have identified the behaviour that you do, apply the following process:

Define the problem (e.g. swearing, smoking).

Measure the frequency of occurrence (e.g. every second word, 20 per day).

Analyse when the behaviour occurs (e.g. throughout the day, evenings only).

Work out why the behaviour occurs (e.g. enjoyable, angry, worried, form of self-expression, habit).

Identify times when the frequency of the behaviour increases or decreases (e.g. increased swearing when angry, increased smoking when at the pub).

Generate positive objectives for reducing the behaviour (e.g. reduce swearing to get on better with people and present a more positive image of self, stop smoking to save money, improve health, live longer).

Devise an intervention which consistently reinforces behaviour change (e.g. make swear box and save money for a special treat, have a health check, get some nicotine patches, save up money usually spent on cigarettes).

Identify reasons why behaviour reoccurs, and change intervention (e.g. forget to put money in swearbox so no money saved – put in IOUs; identify times when it is most tempting to have a cigarette, such as after a meal or in the pub, and plan to do something to keep busy at those times, and get some support from others in the same situation).

References

Agar, A. and O'May, F. (2001) Issues in the definition and implementation of 'best practice' for staff delivery of interventions for challenging behaviour, *Journal of Intellectual and Developmental Disability*, 26(3): 243–56.

Allen, D. and Tynan, H. (2000) Responding to aggressive behaviour: impact of training on staff members' knowledge and confidence, *Mental Retardation*, 38(2): 97–104.

Allen, D., McDonald, L., Dunn, C. and Doyle, T. (1997) Changing care staff approaches to the prevention and management of aggressive behaviour in a residential treatment unit for persons with mental retardation and challenging behaviour, *Research in Developmental Disabilities*, 18(2): 101–12.

Aman, M.G., Singh, N.N., Stewart, A.W. and Field, C.J. (1985) The aberrant behaviour checklist: a behaviour rating scale for the assessment of treatment effects, *American Journal of Mental Deficiency*, 89: 485–91.

Beail, N. (2003) What works for people with mental retardation? Critical commentary on cognitive-behavioural and psychodynamic psychotherapy research, *Mental Retardation*, 41(6): 468–72.

Blunden, R. and Allen, D. (1987) *Facing the Challenge: An Ordinary Life for People with Learning Difficulties and Challenging Behaviour*. London: King's Fund.

Borthwick-Duffy, S.A. (1994) Prevalence of destructive behaviours: a study of aggression, self-injury and property destruction, in T. Thompson and D.B. Gray (eds) *Destructive Behaviour in Developmental Disabilities*. Thousand Oaks, CA: Sage.

Brown, H. (1997) Vulnerability issues, in J. O'Hara and A. Sperlinger (eds) *Adults with Learning Disabilities: A Practical Approach for Health Professionals*. Chichester: Wiley.

Cambell, M. and Malone, R.P. (1991) Mental retardation and psychiatric disorders, *Hospital and Community Psychiatry*, 42: 374–9.

Carr, E.G., Levin, L., McConnachie, G., Carlson, J.I., Kemp, D.C. and Smith, C.E. (1993) *Communication-Based Intervention for Problem Behaviour: A User's Guide for Producing Positive Change*. Baltimore, MD: Brookes.

Clements, J. (1997) Challenging needs and problematic behaviour, in J. O'Hara and A. Sperlinger (eds) *Adults with Learning Disabilities: A Practical Approach for Health Professionals*. Chichester: Wiley.

DoH (Department of Health) (2001) *Valuing People: A New Strategy for Learning Disability for the 21st Century*. London: Department of Health.

DoH/DfES (Department of Health and Department for Education and Skills) (2002) *Guidance for Restrictive Physical Interventions: How to Provide Safe Services for People with Learning Disabilities and Autistic Spectrum Disorder in Health, Education and Social Care Settings*. London: DoH/DfES.

Donnellan, A.M., LaVigna, G.W., Negri-Shoultz, N. and Fassbender, L.L. (1988) *Progress without Punishment: Effective Approaches for Learners with Behavioural Problems*. New York: Teachers College Press.

Emerson, E. (2001) *Challenging Behaviour: Analysis and Intervention in People with Learning Difficulties*. 2nd edn. Cambridge: Cambridge University Press.

Emerson, E. (1998) Working with people with challenging behaviour, in E. Emerson, C. Hatton, J. Bromley and A. Caine (eds) *Clinical Psychology and People with Intellectual Disabilities*. Chichester: Wiley.

Emerson, E., Robertson, J., Gregory, N., Hatton, C., Kessissoglou, S., Hallam, A. and Hilery, J. (2000) Treatment and management of challenging behaviours in residential settings, *Journal of Applied Research in Intellectual Disabilities*, 13(4): 197–215.

Emerson, E., Kiernan, C., Alborz, A., Reeves, D., Mason, H., Swarbrick, R., Mason, L. and Hatton, C. (2001) The prevalence of challenging behaviours: a total population study, *Research in Developmental Disabilities*, 22(1): 77–93.

Fidell, B. (2000) Exploring the use of family therapy with adults with a learning disability, *Journal of Family Therapy*, 22(3): 308–23.

Fraser, W. and Nolan, M. (1994) Psychiatric disorders in mental retardation, in N. Bouras (ed.) *Mental Health and Mental Retardation: Recent Advances in Practices*. Cambridge: Cambridge University Press.

Harris, J., Allen, D., Cornick, M., Jefferson, A. and Mills, R. (1996) *Physical Interventions: A Policy Framework*. Kidderminster: BILD Publications.

Jenkins, R., Rose, J. and Lovell, C. (1997) Psychological well-being of staff who work with people who have challenging behaviour, *Journal of Intellectual Disability Research*, 41(6): 502–11.

Moss, S., Emerson, E., Kiernan, C., Turner, S., Hatton, C. and Alborz, A. (2000) Psychiatric symptoms in adults with learning disability and challenging behaviour, *British Journal of Psychiatry*, 177: 452–6.

Murphy, G., Kelly, P.A. and McGill, P. (2003) Physical intervention with people with intellectual disabilities: staff training and policy frameworks, *Journal of Applied Research in Intellectual Disabilities*, 16(2): 115–25.

O'Brien, J. (1987) A guide to personal futures planning, in G.T. Bellamy and B. Wilcox (eds) *A Comprehensive Guide to the Activities Catalogue: An Alternative Curriculum for Youth and Adults with Severe Disabilities*. Baltimore, MD: Paul H. Brookes.

O'Hara, J. and Sperlinger, A. (1997) Mental health needs, in J. O'Hara and A.

Sperlinger (eds) *Adults with Learning Disabilities: A Practical Approach for Health Professionals*. Chichester: Wiley.

SETRHA (South East Thames Regional Health Authority) and the Tizzard Centre, University of Kent (1994) *Understanding and Responding to Difficult Behaviour*. Brighton: Pavillion.

Stenfert Kroese, B., Dagnan, D. and Loumidis, K. (eds) (1997) *Cognitive-Behaviour Therapy for People with Learning Disabilities*. London: Routledge.

Tyrer, S. (1997) The use of psychotropic drugs, in R. Oliver (ed.) *Seminars in the Psychiatry of Learning Disabilities*. Glasgow: Bell & Bain.

Zarkowska, E. and Clements, J. (1994) *Severe Problem Behaviour: The STAR Approach*. London: Chapman & Hall.

18

(Almost) everything you ever wanted to know about sexuality and learning disability but were always too afraid to ask

Alex McClimens and Helen Combes

On the subject of sex, silence became the rule.

Foucault (1990: 3)

Introduction

Here, we are breaking the silence. This chapter aims to inform people about the sexual needs and sexual identity of individuals with learning disabilities. As well as reviewing the literature when we began to write this chapter we decided to be honest with ourselves about the subject. We looked to our own lives and personal experiences – including our experience of working with individuals who have a learning disability. Since part of our argument is premised on the notion that sexuality is core to self-identity (Foucault 1990) it is inevitable that some degree of autobiography will have influenced our writing. This is not to suggest that we are promoting our own brand of white, middle-class professionalism about sexuality. Rather we are seeking to make a case for individuality, for difference and self-expression over conformity. To this end we have at all times encouraged the reader to position themselves in the narrative and ask themselves what they would do and how they would feel with the circumstances we describe. Only by adopting a self-reflexive stance can any of us hope to appreciate such a complex issue, which brings to the fore the ethical and moral dilemmas we have to face when working with people with learning disabilities. Our remit then is to examine sexuality and whether this term has any meaning for individuals with a learning disability and those involved in their care. This means that the discussion will have a broad focus on all of those elements that constitute sexuality and will include, but not be confined to, issues that revolve around the physicality of sex.

The research and background to this chapter has emerged through conversations we have had with people about sexuality, particularly with the people known to us through our research and clinical work. We have of course been influenced by the published literature on sexuality and learning disability. This chapter will look at the social and historical influences on how the sexuality of people with learning disabilities has been described and perceived. We see sexuality as covering a wide range of issues – sexual behaviour, representations of gender, knowledge of risks, contraception, parenting and the formation and maintenance of relationships. Sexuality is an integral part of our identity which includes how we present ourselves in the community. Our background work has helped us to see sexuality as a developmental process, which emerges and changes through our experiences and contact with other people and human services. We describe our construction of these developmental stages in accordance with the theme of this book, which emphasizes a life cycle approach.

We think that the fullest expression of sexuality emerges when people start to work and become financially and emotionally independent. When do you think people become sexually active? What contexts help this to happen? When do people cease to be sexually active? We feel that this full expression of sexuality may be different for people with learning difficulties for two main reasons. Firstly, people with learning disabilities may not be seen as mature enough to engage in intimate sexual relationships. Secondly, they do not usually have the opportunity for full-time work. Both of these reasons conspire to marginalize people and this leads to a contested adult status. Does this describe any individual you know or care for?

We have used quotes from people with learning disabilities to illustrate how they feel about their own sexuality and sexual identity. We have used real stories but different names throughout to protect the innocent. We will consider how human services might be able to help people with learning disabilities to overcome difficulties and to develop the kinds of relationship that they may wish to explore with others. Finally, just a few words on what not to expect from this chapter. This is not a 'how to' manual. As Tom Shakespeare has observed, it's mostly not a question of 'how to' but 'who to' do it with that bothers people (2000: 161). Besides, there are instruction manuals available (Stein and Brown 1996; Downs and Craft 1997). Neither is this a sexual health catalogue. We do not address directly the clinical aspects of reproduction and contraception. In effect, we ignore more areas than we explore but in considering sexuality and learning disability we invite the reader to take up the challenge and investigate those topics for themselves and with those they care for.

The chapter will advance by considering the legal and historical context that frames our current understanding. Then we will go on to explore some views we have canvassed from individuals who have learning disabilities before concluding with some thoughts on the implications for services.

The social and historical context

Historically, people's understanding of the sexuality of those with learning disabilities seems to have been based upon stereotypes (Bancroft 1989: 618). This often led to a 'safety first' attitude from carers and families who sought to protect people with learning disabilities from any sexual contact or knowledge. This ignorance in turn helped contribute to the high levels of abuse that exist within the field (McCarthy 1999). In the current climate of litigation it is difficult to balance the need for protection against the principle of risk. Given a choice between empowerment and protection, services will generally opt for protection over risk. Keywood puts the problem in context when she remarks that 'To choose between protection and empowerment is no choice at all' (2003: 31). It is when staff are placed in this situation that inertia sets in and the need to empower and enable gets lost in risk assessment.

In practice terms, the policy of segregation reinforced ignorance as men and women were cared for in separate environments. Partly due to the principles of normalization and the trend towards community care, such attitudes and practices have become less prevalent in the past 30 years (see Chapter 2). This does not mean that the sexuality of people with learning difficulties is now free from taboo. Despite the growing literature (Craft 1994; McCarthy 1999), which suggests that attitudes are changing, prejudice and ignorance remain. As will be shown in the following pages, some of these attitudes prevail in communities as well as in professional and family groups.

The legal context

Throughout our lives our behaviour is regulated by laws, codes and rules. This is evident in the way that relationships between carers and those they care for are subject to scrutiny. The focus of much discussion is in the area of sexuality and the rights and wrongs of sexually-oriented behaviour. This means that people are often confronted with their own personal prejudices and biases (both about sexuality and about what it means to have a learning disability) throughout their working lives. The ethical dilemma people working within services are most often faced with is whether or not someone is able to consent to a sexual relationship.

Consent

The Human Rights Act (1998) states that all people have the right to express their sexuality, to have a family life and intimate relationships, free from prejudice and victimization. These rights exist whether or not the person has the capacity to consent. If we consider again that legislation has come into existence to protect the rights of a vulnerable group then it is perhaps clear that it is our responsibility to ensure that these rights are upheld. In England and Wales, the law currently presumes that everyone has capacity (although this may change under the new Mental Health Act). However, regardless of the legal position, it is more likely that capacity will be questioned when the person has a learning disability. There is currently no clear legal position on learning disability and capacity to consent. There are clear guidelines for capacity to undergo medical treatment, but the position on whether someone has the capacity to choose to have a sexual relationship remains unclear. Case law to date seems to favour having a sexual relationship, even if it may seem to others to be abusive (see *R.* v. *Jenkins*, January 2000). The Sexual Offences Review Team reviewed the rights of people to have a private life free from exploitation, but as yet there is no formal legislation to help people to uphold these rights. However, at the time of going to press there is a draft Mental Capacity Bill going before Parliament, which may help to clarify the decision-making process. In the meantime we have developed a flow chart (see Figure 18.1) which we hope will help you to illustrate your decision-making process.

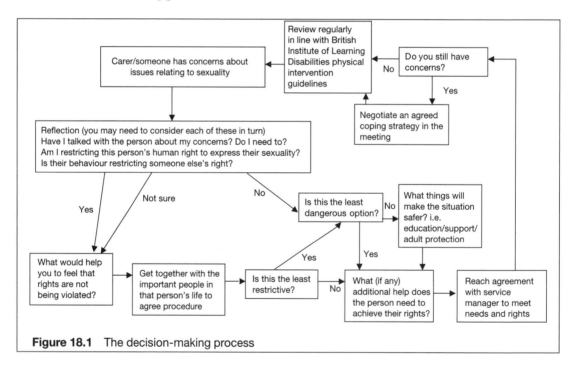

Figure 18.1   The decision-making process

Exercise 18.1

So how do we uphold the rights of an individual to express their sexuality, free from the potential risk of victimization? We feel that it is important to consider ourselves at this point. How would we want people to talk about our own sexuality? If we were at risk of being abused or exploited would we want it to be discussed at a multi-disciplinary meeting? If that team, because of its duty of care, felt that the issue needed to be talked about, what would make that discussion safe for you?

The situation is much clearer if abuse has taken place and the complaint has gone into the legal domain. Here again we can refer to case law. Although a professional opinion can be given and taken into account, the decision about whether or not the perpetrator has capacity comes down to the decision of the jury. As such the decision is not a unilateral one. If we consider the jury as a model of working, how can this be replicated within the care setting? Can this model be replicated without one professional opinion overriding the views of others involved in the decision-making process?

Exercise 18.2

Think about the first time you consented to a 'sexual' relationship. How did you make the decision to consent? How would we be able to use this scenario to help someone with a learning difficulty to make an informed decision about a sexual relationship?

Teaching versus learning about sexuality

When considering our duty of care, another important thing to bear in mind is whether it is possible to teach aspects of sexuality and sexual health or if they develop through personal relationships and a process of learning. If aspects of sexuality can be taught, then it is presumably our duty to teach people if we feel that they are either vulnerable or at risk. We would argue that aspects of our sexuality (as a process) are probably learnt through our relationships with others, whereas we can teach some issues – for example, to do with sexual health and well-being. People can be prompted and reminded about their sexual health. So, if our main concern is that someone is at risk of contracting chlamydia or AIDS then within our duty of care it is essential that we help the person to learn how to protect themselves against such risks. There is information available on the web about resources that have been specifically developed for people with learning disabilities (see www. sexualhealth.com; www.thpct.nhs.uk). Most sexual health clinics are able to offer a range of services to many diverse groups, and should not exclude on the grounds of disability.

However, the question of whether we can teach people about their own sexuality opens up a wealth of ethical dilemmas. This is perhaps because other aspects of sexuality may well change through the relationships and conversations we have with other people. It is important to consider therefore whether one individual can decide what is, and is not, appropriate behaviour. To help to clarify these issues the authors ran a series of workshops about sexuality. We felt that it was important to help people to express their own feelings about their sexuality and to find out from those people where their ideas about their own sexuality had come from.

Let's talk about sex . . .

Working forward from the premise that we have a duty of care towards the people we work with it then follows that this must include some recognition of their rights and needs in terms of their sexuality. The question remains though, how exactly do we address this? We now outline one attempt at engaging people in some open discussion about their experiences of sex and their attitudes to sexuality.

Both of us had worked for some time with a group of adults with learning disabilities who attended a local day service. We were introducing research methods to the group with a view to future empirical work. In another part of their curriculum, these people were exploring popular culture and it was via this medium that we tried to instigate some discussion on how people present themselves in public. From this discussion, we made the link to expressing sexuality.

This was a mixed gender group of 20 adults with an age range between early twenties and late fifties. We first made the group aware of our intention to write about the topic and gave assurances about confidentiality and anonymity. Included in this exercise was a written note to parents and carers informing them of the topic. Two parents wrote back outlining their concern and asking that their son or daughter should not participate in the group. One member of staff also opted out of this stage.

Exercise 18.3

Should paid staff be allowed to opt out of sessions they feel uncomfortable with if sexuality is an integral part of our sense of self? How can services enable people to opt in to this work?

After a few sessions of general discussion, we moved on to a more focused topic. We discussed representations of men and women in popular magazines. Each of us had picked out a picture from a popular magazine and talked about why we felt attracted to, or interested in, that person. Building on this we asked the group to think back to their first experience of being attracted to someone else. We asked them to think about how this felt. We chose to explore 'first time' experiences for three reasons. We felt these early experiences might be more memorable and so spark discussion. We also thought that these formative experiences might have influenced how the individual then developed their own ideas and sexual identity. Finally, we reasoned that such memories might also be 'safe' in the sense that any current relationships were less likely to be implicated.

As the session progressed we charted the talk on a flip chart and gave everyone the opportunity to write down their own experiences on a short questionnaire at the end. We did this to give people who contributed less to the verbal debate the chance to have their say (although everybody did say something). This device also focused responses on six topics under two headings. Looking at 'the first time' we asked people to recall their first kiss, first date, first boy/girlfriend. Then, to check understanding, we asked people to say what they felt three words meant to them. These words were, sex, love and friendship. During the course of these sessions various individuals asked to speak to us privately about their own sexuality. We have not been able to include their stories because these discussions took place beyond the scope of our public debates. However, one member of the main group wanted to write their story, knowing that it would be published. We are happy to include it here.

My first kiss!

It started one month after I started at senior school. Rebecca was the hottest girl at school at the time. She was going out with my friend Bill. Marge said, 'Why don't you Rebecca go out with S and I go out with Bill?'

One dinner time I was playing rounders and I hit a homer. At the end of dinner time me and Rebecca kissed each other on the lips and then the bell went to signal the end of dinner time. On the school bus home a couple of kids told me that she was a two-timing bitch. That night I couldn't stop thinking about her and that kiss. The next day she didn't turn up for school. Then I had all weekend to think about what had happened that Thursday. Monday came and she was at school. She told me it was over between us.

The discussion soon demonstrated that some preconceptions of people with learning disabilities as innocent, childlike or asexual were probably based on prejudice rather than any empirical observations. The group told us about a boyfriend who had 'a sexy arse' and of a girlfriend (described as a 'bird') who had 'big knockers'. Someone fancied their sister's husband, and two people, one of whom was in the group, were 'outed' as regularly having a snog behind the day centre equivalent of the bike shed.

The material generated by the questionnaire also revealed a range of awareness and experience. When asked to define 'sex', responses varied. Two individuals had this to say: 'I think it's rude. It means somebody touching you. I don't like to talk about it because it's vulgar' or similarly, 'Don't touch bodies. It would be rude. And I'd tell my mum and dad.' Another said, 'I've heard about it. So she can have a baby. It's cheeky and rude'. A different kind of answer emerged in 'Going out with girlfriend/boyfriend. Go to their house when no one there. Go to bed together.'

When asked to describe their thoughts on 'love' we got these varied replies: 'I don't know. I've got no clue.' Or, 'Lotsa long time. Happy heart, beat faster' or 'It's nice. I love my mum.' On the subject of 'friendship' there was more commonality. Of the 13 written responses, 4 specifically mentioned 'talking' as a component of friendship while 8 spoke of having a friend with whom they spent some time. This strong association of time spent talking underlines the value of relationships in general and highlights the need to engineer networks of relationships that can be used to support individuals with learning disabilities.

These activities were then linked to popular television as the discussion moved on to how couples are seen in public life. The links between marriage, being in a couple and having children were seen as accidental rather than strictly necessary as we debated the Simpsons, the Beckhams, and Madonna and Guy Ritchie.

Reference to goings on in a soap opera brought age difference under scrutiny. What the group showed here was an appreciation of how things are as well as how things ought to be. A ten-year age gap between a group member in their fifties and their partner was dismissed as irrelevant yet a unanimous verdict of 'No' accompanied the question 'Can a 20-year-old go out with a 10-year-old?' The follow-up question about at what age it was OK to kiss someone you fancy brought responses within the range from 14 to 18.

One member of the group had seen two men in bed on a TV soap. Two group members offered examples of friends who were in lesbian couples, one of whom had children. We checked what people understood by the terms lesbian and gay. Lesbians, according to our respondents, loved other women and gay men loved other men. The consensus was that as long as people were happy and agreed then this was OK. Again the group show that even when their immediate personal experience cannot accommodate some of these issues they can still refer to cultural resources to construct a position. On the evidence available from this small sample that position is always one of inclusion and understanding.

Playing mums and dads: Part 1

The work undertaken with the group is in no way definitive but it at least demonstrates that for these individuals sexuality and its expression was a live issue and that they were fully aware of themselves as sexual beings. Compare this group's construction of their sexuality with the experiences of other individuals with whom we have met and talked. The two case studies that follow demonstrate the gulf between innocence and experience. Whereas the group discussion had been based on genuine life lessons, none of these had transcended the emotional barrier that separates happy recollections from the harsh reality of loss, sorrow and regret. These emotions represent the flipside of adult sexuality. Both informants in the case studies are in their forties and the stories they relate bring into question the overall effect of the regulating agencies that exist to control our own access to our own bodies. Tricia begins by describing her feelings for an old flame. Harry then relates how a relationship went wrong.

Case study: *Tricia and John*

It were him I used to meet every night at half past eight. We used to stay in the house or go to the pub. His name was John and when I was at home and he used to come and pick me up some nights, can't remember if it was every night, I'll say some nights, at half past eight to go out . . . he'd come and sit and watch telly for a bit or we used to go to the pub, it were only a minute's walk from me mam's. He used to take me out Saturday and Sunday. Go to the pictures Saturday night. Sometimes Sunday too.

Yeah, we'd go to the pictures and then when he used to bring me back from the pub we used to have some lovin dovin in the passage, in the back passage, never in the house, always in the passage.

Me mam wanted me to marry him. She never said right out though. I had fits in them days but I got an idea when she died she wanted me to then. He were very nice, John. We never, y'know, like you shouldn't do. You know [mouthed silently] 's-e-x'. Even John wouldn't go right through everything. He were kind. If I'd stayed at home I'd have liked to settle down wi' John.

Now? Well, I'd love to get married. I've felt that way . . . Oh, for a long time. I don't know what I can do. I always wanted to marry John before I left home but there were my fits wi' epilepsy and I don't think I can have kids, wi' me women's problems. I'd have loved some. If I'd got married I'd have got some little children of my own who hadn't got homes. Adopt them. I'd like to see John again, though. He might be married now or have a girlfriend . . . there might be somebody else, I suppose.

Tricia relates her story with the benefit of 20 years' hindsight. Having read this passage it is worth thinking about whether Tricia is fully in control of her own sexual identity and destiny. There are clearly clinical considerations. Tricia is aware, for example, that her epilepsy might have conspired against her, though quite how she is not sure. She also mentions that she has 'women's problems'. The vagueness of the term suggests more than a reluctance to engage in specific talk: it suggests an ignorance of what exactly these problems are and how they might be resolved. But Tricia is clear about one thing and that is her wish to get married and have children. Many of us can sympathize and empathize with that wish.

Playing mums and dads: Part 2

'Narratives about identity are therefore significant sites of power struggles in refiguring what it means to be human. What people with an intellectual disability offer everyone in society are stories of how to live as unique individuals in relation to one another. These stories challenge any dominant notion of social homogeneity' (Fullagar and Owler 1998: 446).

One of the dilemmas that frequently recurs when discussing the whole concept of learning disability is the humanity of the individuals who comprise this social group. This is seldom more apparent than when discussing sexuality. Myths still pervade the topic with individuals regarded as occupying either end of a spectrum that stretches from predatory animal instinct to childlike innocence. Such ingrained prejudice is difficult to counter with any appeal to reason or research. To address this, the following account makes a direct appeal to the emotions. The man who tells us part of his story has a learning disability. He also has two children. This fact makes him a father. Under any other circumstances this would have been a sad story. The tragedy is that the regulation of this aspect of his sexuality by governing agencies conspires to make a failure of his fatherhood.

When discussing inarticulate subjects, Booth and Booth point to the differences between interview research and narrative research (1996: 56). They see this as founded on the individual who has a story to tell. Harry, who we will soon meet, is just such an individual. Booth and Booth also posed a question in their paper about how exactly to overcome some of the silences that inevitably occur in the one-to-one interview situation. In this case, the option was quite simple: keep the tape machine running. To have interrupted the flow of confession would have denied Harry his moment. The extract that appears here is a distillation of hours of transcript that Harry contributed for previous life history research. The episode that he relates reveals how in one the fullest expressions of sexuality available to modern western cultures, the parental couple bringing up children, any doubt over disability brings the normalizing machinery of the social services into action. Shotter (1993: 7), speaking about identity and belonging, describes a framework for 'becoming someone'. He suggests that:

> if one is to grow up and to qualify as a self-determining, autonomous person with one's own identity – to feel that one has grown up to be 'someone', someone who 'counts' in one's society – then, although one must grow up as a human being within that society, that in itself is not

enough. For even as a participating member of it, one can still remain either dependent on other members of it in some way or under their domination in some other way. To be a person and to qualify for certain rights as a free, autonomous individual, one must also be able to show in one's actions certain social competencies, that is, to fulfil certain duties and to be accountable to others in the sense of being able to justify one's actions to them, when challenged, in relation to the 'social reality' of the society of which one is a member.

If we believe this then we must believe that Harry 'counts' in this sense. What follows is just part of his story.

Case study: *Harry and Rebecca*

I met Rebecca at work. She came for an interview job and . . . it were about a month or a month and a half and I asked her out. Then, since, y'know, we started being friends and started taking her out n' that. When I asked her out she said, 'Yes, I would.' I asked her in a nice polite way and she said yes. That was when I was working on the forging.

I remember, once, taking her to catch the bus, outside the market, and she used to wave to me and she said, 'Don't wait for the bus, come back wi' me.' I used to say to her, 'I'll be alright.' This was when she was living wi' her mum and dad. Before she got caught, a long time before. I says, 'I can't', 'cos sometimes she never used to want me to go at night . . . I don't know . . . she's changed. I would have done but my mum and dad wanted me to come back. Things were different then.

Later she would stay at our house nearly every Friday. We used to go all o'er, everywhere. It were alright then. All things seem to change when you get . . . you're young, things pass on and you have to do different things in life, don't you? That's what it's all about. But when you have a date for the first time, you don't rush straight into things. You take one step at a time. That's what we did.

'Course it didn't stay that way for long. We just started going out like, as friends, and then, y'know, we shouldn't have rushed into it but . . . well, I may as well tell you; I've got a girl and a boy which I don't see. It upsets me that I don't see them but I think that in the long run they're better off where they are. They're getting looked after, getting clothes bought, and getting toys and presents at Xmas.

We'd never talked about it, never even occurred to us. These things happen; you make these mistakes and they just happen, don't they? But then you've got to do something about it, you can't blame the other person and say it's their fault; it takes two to tango. Both to blame. It just happened. No contraceptive. Should have done. We just never discussed it. Should have done.

We never lived together at all. I don't think we could live together . . . we'd always be arguing. I don't think Rebecca was bothered about living together. Because when people get married they always have so long then start having a divorce. I mean, everybody argues, no matter who it is. We all fall out in one way or the other. It's just a thing what goes off in life.

Things started to change then, after the kids arrived. We kept arguing. She wanted me to do something and I wouldn't do it. Like help. Most of the times I did but sometimes I didn't. I'd say something like, 'Oh, I'm tired.' That upset her a bit. That's why I only see her once a week now. She couldn't cope because the kids went into care. Well, Harry's in foster care and Sasha's been adopted. Everybody took to her straight away and they say what a nice girl she is but sometimes, if I talk about it, it upsets me and I just burst out crying sometimes. I know it isn't nice but that's the way it goes. The kids are looked after and that's all I can say.

I don't see the kids though, about eight years since I saw them last. I get photos, that's all. Rebecca sees them. What it is, the reason I don't get contact, is because they don't know who the father is of the kids. Social don't know. When they went into care they asked Rebecca about it but they didn't ask me. I felt hurt. When you see your kids it hurts you a bit, but when you don't see your kids it hurts you even more, deep down, than when you do see them. You understand? It's how it goes. It's hard. It's a shame when you don't see your kids. My lad's going away somewhere wi' the people who are looking after him, she told me. It's good that he gets a holiday.

But when they get older they'll come and look for me. Sasha might not 'cos it's too far, like. But Harry will. I don't know where they live though, do I? Rebecca knows.

Exercise 18.4

Ultimately we have to ask if things could have been any different for Tricia and Harry. Even without access to the autobiographical background we must conclude that information on contraception, on women's reproductive health issues, on parenting and nurturing skills would have benefited these people. What can we do as health care professionals to assist people in these very common circumstances? What other agencies might have usefully been involved? And crucially, how can we liaise successfully so that the outcomes are mutually satisfactory for all concerned?

In the next section we explore some of the issues that directly affect health care professionals when they try to plan care around the expression of sexuality by individuals with a learning disability. We approach this area from an oblique angle as we take in some of the relevant aspects of labels and labelling theory.

Labelling theory revisited

'Being sexual costs money. You need to buy clothes, to feel good about, and go places to feel good in' (Shakespeare 2000: 161). We asked our group to look through a variety of glossy magazines and to select images of people they felt attracted to. We found that the photographs selected were chosen on the basis of the clothes that the people featured were wearing – we were told that pictures were chosen because the people were glamorous or pretty. A quick glance in the mirror will be enough to reassure the reader that one of the main areas by which people express their sexuality is in the way they choose to present themselves to the world. The mere fact that we get dressed in the morning says as much about our sense of self as it does about the external environment. So we ask the reader to reflect: what governed your choice of clothing this morning?

There are many ways of dressing up or dressing down. The effect is the same. Some of the more obvious are hairstyling, make-up or accessories. These apply across the gender divide. Beyond this, there are semi-permanent adornments such as tattoos, body piercing, jewellery and eyewear. All of these were in evidence within the group. Fashion, lifestyle and, more specifically, brand awareness influence the acceptability of all of these adornments – none of them comes cheap. While neither of the authors are particularly label-conscious both find themselves drawn to brands and packaging – neither would be seen outside without their Converse All-Stars and to appear in public minus the iPod is of course a social taboo. In addition, if other people discuss our sexual orientation it is essential (to us at least) that the label is the right one – not one given through assumptions. Labels identify and can give us a sense of belonging to a particular group.

The serious point here is that many people with learning disabilities will possibly be equally as label conscious as their carers both in terms of what clothes they wear and how they are described as people. To be denied the opportunity to express one's sexual identity – either through dress or through behaviour may have a profound impact on our psychological and emotional well-being. And yet, given the structure of our society, many people with learning disabilities find themselves disenfranchised and unable to participate in shaping their sexuality as they might wish. For example, some members of the group found it difficult to travel independently and had to rely on other people to help them. This clearly compromises their ability to make and maintain relationships. In a society where to be is to be seen we can ask what price sexuality if you cannot afford the tram fare, with apologies to Hilary Brown (1993).

Exercise 18.6

Where does this leave the health care professional? If, as we have hinted, economics is important for maintaining sexual identity, what kind of interventions will be successful? Is it necessary to include these issues as part of a plan of care? Look in the mirror and consider a poster of a contemporary pop diva or a boyband; could you see yourself dressed that way? Could you see a client you have cared for dressed that way?

For some individuals who have motor impairments the sense of self can likewise be affected. Morgan (1999) offers numerous examples of women who feel that the way their bodies are prevents them from participating in the ideal of woman that they see in the media. The act of walking in stiletto heels, for example, while thought of as glamorous by some and practised by many, would be either dangerous or impossible for most individuals with some varieties of cerebral palsy.

Yet because certain images predominate in the media, many of our clients, and probably just as many of their families and carers, must look on from the side as youth and beauty parade what passes for the norm. However, in the UK the average dress size is a 16 while on the catwalk it is an 8. Many men will be more familiar with a six-pack of beer than toned abdominal muscles. Few of us can approximate the images portrayed in the pages of the glossy magazines. However, can we assist our clients to dress so that they strike a comfortable blend between fashion and function? What sort of conversations might help people to understand these disparities?

And if people with learning disabilities perceive that they do not resemble celebrities in looks or fashion, how closely do they match them in terms of their expressions of sexuality? The support that such individuals receive from those who care for them is crucial in achieving this level of personal satisfaction. For example, Christina *et al.* (2002) found in a survey of staff attitudes that there was a very high degree of consensus when staff groups were asked to reflect on issues concerning the expression of sexuality. Of the staff groups surveyed, 93 per cent agreed that women with developmental disabilities have the same sexual desires as others. Approximately 91 per cent felt that the sexuality of a woman with developmental disabilities is an important part of who she is, and 95 per cent felt that women with developmental disabilities should have the freedom and opportunity to express their sexuality.

Exercise 18.7

Do you think these statistics are reflected through care plans? How can you promote and enable the expression of sexuality through care planning? This is the focus of the next section.

Care planning: *reductio ad absurdum*?

One of the chief tasks for the health professional in providing care for individuals with a learning disability is to compile some plan of care. Whether this is done in collaboration with the individual or whether it is arrived at by professional consensus, any such plan must address certain core areas. To clarify our thoughts here we have referred to Maslow's hierarchy of needs. Maslow [1958] 1987 argued that psychological well-being and adjustment was contingent on various needs being met. He developed these into a hierarchy – with the basic biological and physiological needs being the most essential. If any of these needs were denied in early development then, Maslow argued, people would be continually seeking ways for these needs to be met. These biological and physiological needs included the need for air, food, drink, shelter, warmth, sleep and sex. He then argued that people needed to feel safe – this safety was provided through maternal protection (the protection by carers and significant others), security and the law. Then there is the need to belong and be loved, which occurs through family relationships, friendships and affection. Finally we strive to achieve all that we are able, to be given responsibility and to have status. Once these esteem needs are met then there is the potential for self-actualization through personal growth and fulfilment.

As well as the apparent social ramifications there remains a biological imperative here. All of us, for example, must eat and drink. To this end it is common practice for professional carers to discover the likes and dislikes of the person in their care and to incorporate such choices into a planned menu. Details such as the temperature and consistency of drinks will be noted. Allergies to wheat or nuts will be important. Does this individual feed themselves or do they require help with the act of eating? Do they need liquidized or puréed food; special adaptations in cutlery, or seating position; or do they require a special diet for health or cultural reasons? All of these considerations will form the basis of a plan of care that covers the physical and social aspects of eating and drinking. Nobody would dream of neglecting this aspect of care. And although we are not arguing that food and drink are of the same category as sex, how many of us are or have been guilty in the past of neglecting the sexuality of the individuals in our care?

If we consider for a moment that we also have a serious responsibility – a duty of care – towards the individuals we look after, then this must apply to all areas and aspects of that care and at all times. This must therefore include sexuality. Consider the need to make the environment safe for those who occupy the home, the clinic or the centre. It is now common practice to undertake risk assessments about almost any activity of daily living. This is in part a response to legislation and the culture of litigation but it is also a common-sense notion that derives from a basic instinct to avoid harm. Models of nursing, popular in the 1980s, made much of the so-called nursing process. Hence the cycle of assessment, planning, implementation and re-evaluation implied a final outcome. In a purely medical/clinical model this may have had some value where cure is seen as an end point to the process of caring. In translating this to a setting characterized by learning disability it seems to be of limited value. Notwithstanding this criticism the Roper *et al.* (1996) model, based on Virginia Henderson's thinking, capitalized on a reductionist approach by which being human is equated to participation in the 12 activities of daily living: the need for air, food, drink, shelter, warmth, sleep, sex, safety, love, achievement, responsibility and status.

Exercise 18.8

While we do not advocate this as a particularly beneficial approach to take with the people in our care it can still be a useful exercise to perform for our own instruction. In our experience of care planning we find two activities of daily living are frequently ignored or at least given scant attention. These are death and dying and expressing sexuality. Given that we will all die one day and that until then we will live as sexual beings, then ignoring these activities appears to be a flawed response. Concentrating on the latter topic we ask the reader to imagine that they must complete their own care plan to cover the issue of expressing sexuality. What topics might be included here? For example, would frequency and duration be part of the plan? Would the planning process reduce the element of spontaneity or limit the location? Who else might be involved and how would you go about making your preferences known? And would you be happy for these details to be written down, recorded and read by others?

Service responses

Many services provide living conditions for people with learning disabilities and it is in this context, perhaps, that our attention focuses on care planning. We feel that it is essential that services begin to see people with learning disabilities as sexual beings. We would challenge whether aspects of sexuality can be quantified in the same way as eating and drinking. Conversations about 'sexuality' and relationships should become part of the discourse. There is an increasing drive to provide person-centred care – which assumes change as part of the life cycle. This more accurately reflects the way people change and avoid stagnation (Duffy and Sanderson 2004) – with people having more choice and autonomy over their lives. These approaches challenge predominant models of how to plan care.

We have found that the groups we have worked with greatly valued having the time to talk about friendships, relationships and sex. These people have told us about the frustrations they have with maintaining relationships – particularly when they live in care homes, where it is difficult to meet people and to keep relationships private, which we would argue is an essential part of any early relationship. If talking about sex ceased to be a taboo, then it may provide people with an opportunity to ask for space or to explore concerns about sexual health. These conversations have to take place within a trusting relationship. Within the new models of supported living this should become feasible, with people being able to exercise more autonomy in determining the structure of their lives.

These new models of care are partly funded by new monies. For example, Direct Payments and Supporting People monies have the potential to increase personal choices. For some this may well mean a corresponding increase in socialization. Increased socialization means meeting people. Meeting people means forming relationships. Relationships are the basis for all community involvement. Community involvement is one of the principal goals of person-centred care.

In addition to these personal (or group) conversations you may also feel it is important to discuss sexuality within person-centred meetings. Any person-centred approach should consider the changing nature of the person – including their sexuality. It should take a life cycle approach by identifying the person's hopes and dreams for the future. These meetings should include people that the client wishes to invite: friends, family members and other key people. For those living in supported accommodation this will often involve professional carers. The meeting should consider whether the current context is the least restrictive – is it enabling the person to explore their sexuality (if they wish to)? If it is not, then you might consider how as a group you can help with this in a way that is not coercive. It is important to balance out individual rights with your own (and others') duty of care to the individual. Most family members are concerned that their son or daughter or their brother or sister could be at risk of being abused or of being exploited or rejected. You must listen to and respect these views. You may wish to challenge such views, but this should be in a safe and enquiring way.

There is much more of a dilemma, of course, when there are current concerns about risk or abuse. If one is concerned about health risks then one's duty of care would suggest that a carer should support someone in getting appropriate advice. If there are risks to sexual health (for anyone) then it is possible to seek advice from a sexual health clinic. You may need to support the person to attend the clinic. Advice on contraception is available from a GP or family planning service.

If as a carer you are concerned that someone has been raped, or that there is ongoing abuse, then the situation is more difficult. Most areas have adult protection procedures and guidance and these should be followed. If your concern is the victim/survivor of abuse then your duty is to help them to access appropriate help and advice. This may involve contacting Rape Crisis (www.rapecrisis.org.uk), helping them to give evidence to the police etc., or accessing counselling services. The police and courts will decide whether or not psychological assessment for capacity or sexual knowledge and understanding is necessary. The same applies for the perpetrator of abuse if they have a learning disability.

Conclusion

This chapter has tried to illustrate the importance of sexuality for human identity while maintaining a focus on the identity of people with learning disabilities. It has considered the historical context, which has led to denial of the sexuality of people with learning difficulties. Most of the chapter has been derived from the conversations we have had with people with learning disabilities about their identity – including sexuality and significant relationships. These conversations have highlighted how important it is to people that their sexuality is recognized. We have also tried to consider the ethical dilemmas that this may raise for staff working in human services. To this end we have tried to think about ways to raise these issues into people's conscious awareness. We feel that in the first instance it is important that these issues become part of the ordinary discourse. This enables questions to be asked and prejudices to be challenged. Otherwise, silence will be the rule once again.

We have deliberately talked in broad terms about sexuality so that we do not exclude people. We are all sexual beings, and no one view should dominate another, by suggesting that there are 'rules' that should be followed. The paradox of working with people with developmental disabilities, however, means that they may well wish to talk with us about 'the rules'. Not to enter into this conversation would be to risk denying people their sexuality.

We have tried to emphasize the importance of sexuality to people's lives. It is a mistake to focus solely on sexuality at one particular stage of the person's life – our own sexual identity changes throughout our lives and from person to person. Sexuality is a broad term which can be expressed in many different ways and should not be confined to one particular norm – i.e. it can encompass chromosomal and physiological differences as well as sexual preferences.

The administration of care often means that service systems try to categorize people in order to make sense of and understand them. However, to separate sexuality from the person is to deny a large part of the person's life and their potential for development and growth. Our duty of care means that we cannot ignore sexuality and should direct people to services that are available to help these people to understand and make sense of their sexuality. We do not wish to deny that sometimes there are risk issues related to sexuality. However, it is also important to remember that people have their own sexual identities which will develop *in spite of* service interventions. There remains, however, a role for carers in assisting people in how they present themselves to others.

Finally, we want to leave readers with a thought to take away. Sexuality as an area for discussion is rife with power relations, whether these are between men and women or between people with and without disabilities. This means that for health care professionals there is an urgent need to be aware that when we engage in any talk on the subject we are re-enacting these power relations. And whatever our gender or orientation, our professional alignment may lead people to see us as holding the power.

References

Bancroft, J. (1989) *Human Sexuality and its Problems*. Edinburgh: Churchill Livingstone.

Booth, T. and Booth, W. (1996) Sounds of silence: narrative research with inarticulate subjects, *Disability & Society*, 11(1): 55–69.

Brown, H. (1993) What price theory if you cannot afford the bus fare? Normalization and leisure services for people with learning disabilities, *Health and Social Care*, 2: 153–9.

Christina, L., Stinson, J. and Dotson, L.A. (2002) Staff values regarding the sexual expression of women with developmental disabilities, *Sexuality and Disability*, 19(4): 283–91.

Craft, A. (ed.) (1994) *Practice Issues in Sexuality and Learning Disabilities*. London: Routledge.

Downs, C. and Craft, A. (1997) *Sex in Context*. Brighton: Pavillion.

Duffy, S. and Sanderson, H. (2004) Person-centred planning and care management, *Learning Disability Practice*, 7(6): 12–16.

Foucault, M. (1990) *The History of Sexuality, Volume 3: The Care of the Self*. London: Penguin.

Fullagar, S. and Owler, K. (1998) Narratives of leisure: recreating the self, *Disability & Society*, 13(3): 441–50.

Keywood, K. (2003) Supported to be sexual? Developing sexual rights for people with learning disabilities, *Tizard Learning Disability Review*, 8(3): 30–6.

McCarthy, M. (1999) *Sexuality and Women with Learning Disabilities*. London: Jessica Kingsley.

Maslow, A.H. ([1958] 1987) *Motivation and Personality*. New York: Harper & Row.

Morgan, S. (1999) *Body Image*. London: Routledge.

Roper, N., Logan, A.J. and Tierney, W.W. (1996) *The Elements of Nursing: A Model for Nursing Based on a Model of Living*, 4th edn. Edinburgh: Churchill Livingstone.

Shakespeare, T. (2000) Disabled sexuality: towards rights and recognition, *Sexuality and Disability*, 18(3): 159–66.

Shotter, J. (1993) Becoming someone: identity and belonging, in N. Coupland and J.F. Nussbaum (eds) *Discourse and Lifespan Identity*. London: Sage.

Stein, J. and Brown, H. (1996) *Sexual Abuse of Adults with Learning Disabilities: The Quiz Pack*. Brighton: Pavillion.

19

Supporting people with learning disabilities within the criminal justice system

Nigel Beail

Introduction

People with learning disabilities may initially come into contact with the criminal justice system as a suspect or a complainant. If charged, the suspect becomes a defendant in court and then, if found guilty they continue as an offender, with disposal needs such as prison, special hospital or probation. Victims of crime become complainants and attend court as witnesses for the prosecution. People with learning disabilities may also witness a crime and be required to give statements and then appear in court for the prosecution or the defence. However, by whatever means they come into contact with the criminal justice system they may find the experience frightening, bewildering and stressful. In recent years research concerning offenders has increased considerably but interest in complainants or witnesses has only received modest attention. This chapter will look at the various stages of the criminal justice process and examine the support needs of people with learning disabilities who come into contact with it. The chapter will draw on the most recent research on offenders and witnesses with learning disabilities in relation to the criminal justice system, with accounts of some personal experiences.

The belief that there is a link between criminality and learning disability persisted throughout the first three-quarters of the twentieth century (Lindsay 2002). However, real evidence for such a link has never been proven. Indeed, Holland *et al.*'s (2002) review found little evidence to support the view that learning disability predisposes people to engage in criminal behaviour. There would appear to be very little in the way of reliable evidence concerning the prevalence of offending among people who have learning disabilities. McBrien (2003) identified 14 published studies conducted in the UK during the 1990s, which reported prevalence rates among offender populations. She identifies significant problems in interpreting these studies. They were carried out in a range of settings at different stages of the criminal justice process. For example, some studies were carried out in custody, some at the court stage, some in prisons and some with those on probation. The size of the populations studied also varied considerably. Interpretation was further hampered by the fact that there was no consistent approach to the identification of learning disability. The assessment approaches included self-report (whether the person feels they have reading problems, learning difficulties or attended special school), historical information (known user of learning disability services), the Quick Test (Ammons and Ammons 1966) and short forms of standardized intelligence tests. None of the studies carried out assessments that would be appropriate to make a formal diagnosis of learning disability. The prevalence rates ranged from 1 per cent using *IDC-10* criteria (WHO 1992) in a prison survey to 21 per cent using self-report from those entering a remand prison. However, further assessment of that group on a short form of a standardized intelligence test found no one with an IQ score below 70. Thus, it is questionable what these studies are actually telling us.

McBrien (2003) has also reviewed studies which have investigated the prevalence of offenders among populations of people with learning disabilities. She found only five surveys, of which only two had been published. These studies only concerned people with learning disabilities who were known to services. The problem with this approach is that many people with learning disabilities are not known to services. Also, no assessments were carried out of those known to services. McBrien excluded two studies, as their prevalence rates were unclear. Of the others the rates ranged from 2 to 9.7 per cent.

People with learning disabilities are at greater risk of having a range of crimes committed against them, compared to other sections of the population. Studies have found higher incidence of physical and sexual assault and robbery, theft and burglary (Wilson and Brewer 1992; Brown *et al.* 1995). There are also laws which have the aim of protecting people with learning disabilities from exploitation. For example, under the Sexual Offences Act 1956 it is an offence for a man to have unlawful sexual intercourse with a woman who is a 'defective'. Men with 'severe mental handicap' are given protection under the Sexual Offences Act 1967. The terms 'defective' and 'severe mental handicap' have been redefined to mean severe impairment of intelligence and social functioning by the Mental Health (Amendment) Act 1982. In fact, in legal proceedings in the UK, the term 'mental impairment' – as defined in the Mental Health Act 1983 – is often used instead of 'learning disability'. There are also laws which make it illegal for staff to allow adults with severe impairment of intelligence and social functioning to have sexual relations on any premises they are responsible for. These issues are discussed in detail in Gunn (1996).

Identifying those with learning disabilities when they come into contact with the criminal justice system

It is important that people with learning disabilities are identified when they come into contact with the criminal justice system. Due to their significant limitations in learning and social functioning they are disadvantaged and therefore vulnerable. They may have limited or no understanding of legal procedure, they are more likely to be acquiescent, suggestible and compliant in police interrogations or interviews and, as such, they are at risk of making false confessions or statements. Those convicted and given custodial sentences may cope poorly within the prison system and may be vulnerable to bullying and abuse by more able inmates. Also, in the UK, people with learning disabilities are officially seen as vulnerable and are entitled to certain legal protections under the Police and Criminal Evidence Act 1985. Further, for offenders, learning disability may be used in mitigation. Thus, it is important to support people with learning disabilities when they come into contact with the criminal justice system. However, we can only support them if we have procedures in place to ensure that their learning disability is identified.

When a person is arrested the police officer tells them, 'You are under arrest' and then tells them the caution: 'You do not have to say anything. But it may harm your defence if you do not mention, when questioned, something which you later rely on in court. Anything you do say may be given in evidence'. This is a long statement, which many people with learning disabilities may not understand. However, they may not tell the police officer that they do not understand. Once arrested the person has to be taken to a police station and presented to the custody officer. The custody officer's job is to look after people who are under arrest. In order to support persons who have learning disabilities who come into contact with the criminal justice system we need to identify them as soon as possible. What can be achieved will depend on the organization of inter-agency working. It is the custody officer who is most likely to observe that a person has learning limitations. Many areas now have nurses and social workers working in a liaising role between the police and health and social services. They are more familiar with the signs of learning disability and can help custody officers develop skills to detect the presence of such disability. They can provide a clinical opinion and advise the police whether further assessment is needed.

Mr A was arrested and taken to the police station. The custody officer had concerns about his understanding and asked the court liaison nurse to interview him. She shared the officer's concerns about his learning ability and also asked Mr A about his educational history. This revealed that he had attended a special school. However, further enquiries made through the local community learning disability service produced no reports or documents to state that he had a learning disability. Many people with learning disabilities are not in contact with or supported by specialist learning disability services and may not have an adequate assessment of their disability. This was the case for Mr A and so he was then referred to the local clinical psychology service for a full diagnostic assessment. As Mr A was over the age of 16 his consent to the assessment was sought. This is a legal requirement and no one can give consent for any assessment or treatment for a person over 16 years other than that person. Mr A consented to the assessment. The outcome was a formal diagnosis of learning disability. The psychological assessment also raised concerns about Mr A's mental health and vulnerability to abuse. A report was compiled and recommendations were made for treatment and management.

In some situations the alleged offender may not be capable of consenting. Here, the health care professional should consult with colleagues and others involved in the person's life and consider what is necessary for their health and well-being, and what will be in their best interests. In such circumstances the discussions concerning the decision-making process must be fully documented.

Victims of crime who have learning disabilities also need their disability to be identified. In a large-scale sexual abuse inquiry by several police forces, the police contacted former attendees of several residential schools by letter. The former pupils were all now adults in their twenties and the police were not aware that some of them had learning disabilities. Mr B received one of these letters. As he was unable to read, his care worker read the letter. The letter was asking Mr B if he was aware of any abuse taking place when he was at school. The care worker did not feel confident to deal with this matter on her own and so contacted a social worker at the local community team for adults with learning disabilities. The social worker contacted the clinical psychologist for learning disability services due to her experience in working with sexual abuse victims. The psychologist visited Mr B at his home and explained that he had been sent a letter by the police and what was being asked. Mr B said he had not been abused and did not know anything about it. However, the psychologist continued to visit Mr B at home as he may want to ask more questions about the letter, may have been disturbed by it or may have been denying past abuse. When the psychologist paid a second visit, Mr B said he wanted to see her in private and then disclosed a catalogue of abuse that had taken place over a number of years. With Mr B's consent the psychologist contacted the police who were keen to interview Mr B. His learning disability was explained so that the police were aware that they needed to make special provision for the interview.

Mr B was known to services and therefore information regarding his learning disability could be communicated to the police. Mr A, however, was not known. When he was taken to the police station the custody officer raised concerns and discussed these with the court liaison nurse. However, the method they used was similar to that employed in the studies reviewed by McBrien (2003). A criticism of these methods is that they have varying results and do not provide for an immediate formal diagnostic assessment. Thus some form of quick screening procedure is needed that is reliable and valid.

One screening tool that has been used is the Ammons Quick Test

(Ammons and Ammons 1966). This is a quick and easy test to apply and does provide an estimate of IQ. However, it is very dated and has not been re-standardized or updated. Thus IQ estimates may now be less reliable than desired. A more recently standardized screening tool is the Hayes Ability Screening Index (Hayes 2002). This was specifically developed for use by non-psychologists to identify offenders who may have a learning disability. It is a screening battery that consists of self-report questions, a spelling test, a join the dots test and a clock drawing test. The test takes between five and ten minutes to administer. The tool was developed in Australia and has not been standardized in the UK. However, it is likely that results in the UK will be similar to those in Australia. Thus, it is increasingly being used as a screening instrument for identifying offenders who may have learning disabilities and need to be referred for a full diagnostic assessment by a clinical psychologist. However, the test is only likely to be used if custody officers and interviewing officers have some skills in identifying the presence of learning disability in the first place. This involves checking that the person retains and understands information given and when interviewing does not rely on yes non-responses. Police officers need to be aware that people with learning disabilities have a tendency to answer yes/no questions in the affirmative and may also fail to disclose their disability.

When a person is placed under arrest, the custody officer tells them their rights. In addition to their right to remain silent, the person also has the right to consult a solicitor, the right to have somebody informed of their arrest and detention, and the right to consult a copy of the *Codes of Practice* (Home Office 1995) and to obtain a copy of the custody record. After advising detainees of their rights the Custody Officer gives them a leaflet explaining their rights. It is here that the police should check a detainee's understanding. The liaison nurse or social worker can play a significant supporting role here. If they are inexperienced in the field of learning disability they can contact the local community service for people with learning disabilities for further advice and support. This is important because people with learning disabilities may not understand the right to remain silent. The leaflet explaining their rights while being detained is complicated and cannot be understood by most detainees. People with learning disabilities are particularly disadvantaged as their reading skills are also limited or absent. Due to memory difficulties the information is not retained and therefore not comprehended. It is probably not encoded because it is too complicated (Gudjonsson 1992). Thus, it is only if the learning disability is identified that people with learning disabilities receive fair treatment.

Mr A was offered treatment as an alternative to continuing his journey through the criminal justice system. However, after attending four sessions with a clinical psychologist, where he did not engage, he refused further sessions and ended the treatment. This information was fed back to the court liaison service, but Mr A had broken contact with them. A few weeks later a solicitor in another jurisdiction contacted the psychologist who formally assessed and diagnosed Mr A's learning disability. Mr A had been arrested and charged for another offence but this time his learning disability had not been identified. Thus the police, without anyone else present, interviewed Mr A. It was the solicitor, who was not appointed until after the police interview, who identified possible learning disability and made further enquiries.

Being interviewed by the police

In the UK the Police and Criminal Evidence Act (PACE) *Codes of Practice* (Home Office 1995) has important provisions for interviewing special groups. It states: 'A juvenile or a person who is mentally disordered or handicapped, whether suspected or not, must not be interviewed or asked to provide or sign a written statement in the absence of the appropriate adult unless . . . delay will involve an immediate risk of harm to persons or serious loss of or damage to property'. Thus, it is important that the police are aware that the person has a learning disability so that PACE is not violated. When Mr A was arrested for the second time his learning disability was not identified and therefore PACE guidance was not followed. When this happens the defence lawyers may argue that the statement produced from the interview with the detainee is not admissible in evidence.

The person chosen to fulfil the appropriate adult role may be a relative or 'someone who has experience of dealing with mentally disordered or mentally handicapped persons but is not a police officer or employed by the police'. Thus professionals who work with people with learning disabilities may fulfil this role. The police should inform the appropriate adult that he or she is not simply acting as an observer but: 'first, to advise the person being questioned and to observe whether or not the interview is being conducted properly and fairly, and secondly, to facilitate communication with the person being interviewed'. In order to assist, the appropriate adult needs to be familiar with the detainee's expressive and receptive communication skills and be aware of their response style to open and progressively closed questions.

In the UK, detained suspects are told their rights again prior to being interviewed and the interview is audio-recorded. Mr C was interviewed by two police officers about allegations concerning sexual acts with underage children. Mr C was able to tell the police that he had learning disabilities and they contacted the clinical psychologist who had been working with him. They asked the psychologist to sit in on the interview and advise on their questioning. Mr C's sister agreed to act as appropriate adult and his social worker was also in attendance. After introductions and checking Mr C understood his rights the police began interviewing him about the allegations. As these unfolded his sister became agitated and then burst out and called Mr C a range of expletives and needed to be restrained by a police officer and social worker and removed from the interview room. The interview then proceeded but the psychologist had to continue in the role of appropriate adult for Mr C as the social worker had to stay with his sister.

Clearly on this occasion Mr C's sister was not able to fulfil the role of appropriate adult for her brother.

Research on the role of the appropriate adult (Medford *et al.* 2003) found that they contribute very little to police interviews. For example, Mr D was arrested following allegations of rape. The police followed PACE as Mr D was blind but they had not identified that he also had learning disabilities. He was interviewed five times by the police on the same day with very short breaks between the interviews. His appropriate adult was his support worker. During the five interviews the appropriate adult made one intervention which was to correct a police officer's spelling of the detainee's name. Medford *et al.*'s (2003) study of 501 interviews, of which appropriate adults were present at 347, found that family members contribute more than social workers and volunteers and that their presence had several effects. In the case of adult suspects it increased the likelihood of a legal representative being present and of the legal representative taking a more active role. Also, less interrogative pressure was noted in interviews where an appropriate adult was present.

Victims and witnesses with learning disabilities should also be interviewed with an appropriate adult present. Victims of crime and witnesses of crime may be interviewed at the police station, in a special interview suite, at home or elsewhere. These interviews are usually recorded by hand and the police officer writes a statement for the complainant or witness. However, the Youth Justice and Criminal Evidence Act 1999 makes provision for complainant and witness interviews to be video-recorded. This is usual practice for child victims of sexual crime, but is increasingly being adopted with vulnerable adult victims.

Mr B, who agreed to be interviewed by the police, asked the psychologist to act as appropriate adult during his interviews with them. This turned out to be important, as the police officers had never interviewed a witness with learning disabilities before. During the interview they asked several leading and closed questions which caused the appropriate adult to intervene. Mr B also had physical difficulties, which caused tiredness. It was the appropriate adult who checked this with Mr B and ended the sessions. Mr B provided new and corroborating evidence and in particular important evidence that identified the abuser. The police told him that he would most likely be needed as a witness in court. As the matter progressed the appropriate adult for Mr B was also asked to provide a statement on the interviews and was informed that she would also be needed as a witness. This is something that people who take on the role of appropriate adult are often not aware of. It is therefore important that any person who acts in this role should make notes concerning the interview and file them carefully.

Once the police have finished interviewing a suspect they will consider what action needs to be taken. If the police do not think that the person arrested and interviewed did the crime they will release them. If they think the suspect did commit the crime and it is a first and minor offence the police may give the suspect a formal caution. This involves the police talking to the suspect about the crime and about what might happen if they do it again.

Being cautioned means that the suspect is not charged and will not have to attend court. However, the police keep a note of the offence on file.

If the police decide they need to make further enquiries they may let the suspect go home on police bail. This means that they will have to return to the police station on another day. However, if the crime the person is suspected of is serious and may place others at risk then the suspect may be detained further. A suspect can be held for interviewing for six to eight hours. If the interviewing officers need more time, the case has to be reviewed by an inspector. The inspector can extend the period of detention up to 24 hours. Then, after further review, a superintendent can extend the period for a further 12 hours. Thereafter the police must release the suspect on bail, charge them or seek a further period of detention from a magistrate. Whatever action the police take the person with a learning disability will need help and support in understanding what is happening.

If the police feel they have enough evidence they will charge the suspect with the crime. The police will tell the person, 'I am charging you with [and then tell them the offence]'. Once charged the person will have their fingerprints and a photograph taken. Depending on the seriousness of the crime the person may be released on bail or detained further on remand at a prison until the matter comes to court. Throughout this process a person with a learning disability will need some support. They will need things explained to them in terms they can understand and may need emotional support.

Reliability of statements

If the police and the Crown Prosecution Service decide to take a matter to court, defendant, complainant and witness statements will be produced and relied upon. Of concern is the reliability of statements made by people with learning disabilities. Such people are generally more suggestible than people of average ability. This is due to their impaired memory capacity, which makes them more vulnerable to suggestibility, acquiescence and confabulation. They are susceptible to suggestion, particularly to giving in to leading questions. Further they are less able to cope with the uncertainty and expectations of questioning (Gudjonsson and Henry 2003). However, a review of the available evidence concluded that people with learning disabilities can provide accurate accounts of events they have witnessed when interviewed appropriately (Kebbell and Hatton 1999). The research suggests that people with learning disabilities can provide accurate accounts, particularly when questioned using open questions about central information rather than closed questions about peripheral information.

The police interviewed Mr D for over four hours. In that time there were four breaks, but only for a few minutes at most. His appropriate adult made no interventions regarding the police questioning. During the fifth interview Mr D confessed to rape and the interview was terminated. Mr D's solicitor had concerns about the conduct of the interview and the way that the confession was extracted. He also had concerns about Mr D's level of intellectual functioning. Mr D was formally evaluated by a clinical psychologist and found to have learning disabilities. A psychologist was also appointed to evaluate the recordings of the police interviews. In his evidence, the psychologist showed that Mr D had been consistent in his version of events throughout the interviews. The confession was made finally to an account of events given throughout the interview by the police. He resisted police officers' attempts to discredit his account but then after four hours accepted their account of events. His confession was him saying 'yes' to the interviewing officers' version of events. Thus Mr D was able to resist the officers' attempts to alter his account as he remembered it but could not resist material introduced by them. Hence he became suggestible and acquiescent when questioned about a version of events he did not recall.

Suggestibility has been assessed by the Gudjonsson Suggestibility Scales (GSS) (Gudjonsson 1997). These were developed to assess an individual's response to 'leading questions' and being told their answers are wrong ('negative feedback') when being asked to report a factual event from recall. The original scale was devised as a result of the conceptual framework developed to assess the reliability of evidence by way of psychological procedure in the case of Mary – a woman who had learning disabilities – who was the main witness in a criminal trial (Gudjonsson and Gunn 1982). Gudjonsson (1992) argues that unlike other tests of suggestibility, the GSS are particularly applicable in legal contexts, such as police interviews with crime witnesses and interrogation of criminal suspects.

There are two parallel versions of the GSS. Both employ a narrative passage, which is read out to the participant who is then asked to recall all they can remember about the story. This gives a measure of immediate recall. About 50 minutes later, delayed recall is obtained, after which the participant is asked 20 specific questions about the content of the passage. Fifteen of these questions are (mis)leading or present false alternatives. The extent to which the person answers affirmatively or chooses a false alternative is called the 'Yield 1' score. Negative feedback is then given, indicating to the participant that some of their answers were wrong and they need to try harder and be more accurate. The examinee is told, 'You have made a number of errors. It is necessary to go through the questions once more and this time try to be more accurate'. The 20 questions are presented again and scored as before to provide a 'Yield 2' score. The extent to which the examinee changes their answers provides a 'Shift' score.

Beail (2002) has cautioned against the use of the GSS with adults who have learning disabilities because of the very poor memory scores obtained on the memory of the narrative passage and the impact this has on the suggestibility scores. He argues that the memory assessment in the GSS is based on memory for facts (semantic memory) and not memory for an event (episodic or autobiographical event memory). Beail reviewed the evidence, which suggests that people with learning disabilities have better recall of real-life events and therefore can produce sound testimony. He also argued that the high suggestibility scores were in fact a measure of acquiescence as the participants were saying yes to leading questions on a matter of which they had very little recall. Gudjonsson and Henry (2003) have subsequently found that memory and suggestibility are moderately related in adults with learning disabilities on the GSS. They also caution that witnesses who prove to be abnormally suggestible on the GSS may not make bad witnesses when they are testifying about autobiographical events that they recall and are examined carefully. White and Willner (2003) further support this caution. They developed a version of the GSS based on a real-life event that some of their participants had witnessed and some had not. Those who had not witnessed the event were given an account of the event only. They found that the group who witnessed the event had higher recall scores and lower suggestibility scores. Thus, research on the suggestibility of witnesses with learning disabilities is building on the pioneering work of Gudjonsson towards more reliable and valid assessment techniques. However, if we are going to support people with learning disabilities effectively during police interviews then we need to be familiar with the questioning styles that are likely to produce poor evidence and the methods that produce good evidence.

Guidance for appropriate adults and police officers

In order to assist the person with a learning disability the appropriate adult should use their knowledge of the person to help avoid certain hazards in the interview. The police would also improve the accuracy of the statements they produce by following these guidelines, which have been summarized by Tully and Cahill (1984). Interview participants should avoid:

- the person acquiescing to leading questions which contain a suggestion as to the answer being sought;
- the interviewer using undue pressure, leading the witness to confabulate (filling in parts they had not witnessed or could not recall);
- repeated questioning on a particular point causing the person to guess or deviate from what they had already said in response to open questions; repeated questioning suggests to the interviewee that they have not given the right answer and so they shift in response to this negative feedback and pressure;
- the interviewer offering compromised descriptions to the witness having difficulty recalling peripheral information – for example, if it had been established that a person in a witnessed event was wearing a jacket but not its colour, the interviewer may suggest a sort of colour; however, that colour may fit with facts known to the interviewer and not the witness;
- the interviewer offering limited alternatives to the witness or defendant;
- information given in free recall being ignored because it does not fit with the interviewer's assumption of what happened;

- the interviewer misunderstanding or failing to check their understanding of the interviewee's responses.

Going to court

In court proceedings the defendant sits in the dock throughout. Prior to the hearing, professionals who have been supporting the defendant need to make some assessment of how the person with learning disabilities will cope in court. This should be discussed with the defence barrister so that they can take any concerns to the judge with any recommendations to help the defendant. This may include someone being close by or sat by the dock, or frequent breaks to give time for information about the proceedings to be explained to the defendant.

Witnesses go into court to give their evidence when they are called or they may give their evidence under the provisions of the Youth Justice and Criminal Evidence Act 1999. Under this Act the court will make some provision to accommodate witnesses with learning disabilities. Video evidence has become admissible along with provision to give evidence by video link. There are provisions to allow someone who knows the witness well to sit with them during the proceedings. For those who go into open court, screens may be erected to shield them from the defendant and wigs may be removed. For witnesses with learning disabilities the court may provide a separate place to sit and allow the presence of support workers.

In court, each witness is interviewed by the prosecuting counsel and the defence counsel. A study of court transcripts of cases were the complainant has been a person with a learning disability found that lawyers frequently asked questions containing negatives and double negatives, multiple questions, and questions with complex vocabulary and syntax. Leading and closed questions were also frequently used, especially in cross-examination (Kebbell *et al.* 2000). Such an approach is not conducive to eliciting the best possible accounts from adult witnesses with learning disabilities. However, lawyers will use methods of questioning either to secure a conviction or to get their client off. Thus they will use such questioning styles according to how they think they can enhance or reduce the credibility of the witness. While professionals who support people with learning disabilities may not approve of such tactics, the lawyers' only answer is that they are doing their job.

The judge can have an impact on a lawyer's questioning style and therefore witness accuracy. The judge has a general duty to ensure that the trial is conducted fairly and has the discretion to intervene to stop any questioning that is likely to result in the court being misled. However, a study of court transcripts by O'Kelly *et al.* (2003) found that judges did not intervene to modify the examination process. Indeed they found no differences between the treatment of witnesses with or without learning disabilities. O'Kelly *et al.* argue that judges should intervene to ensure that all witnesses are able to give the most complete and accurate evidence possible.

Learning disability as a mitigating factor

Increasingly, learning disability is being accepted as a mitigating factor in crime. A behaviour or its consequences (*actus rea*) do not define crime; the person's state of mind (*mens rea*) when they engage in the behaviour is also a significant defining factor (such as intention, recklessness and so on). Thus the court may require evidence regarding the defendant's learning disability and its impact on their behaviour. When the person with a learning disability is a victim of crime the court may also need evidence regarding the degree of their learning disability. This is especially the case when a sexual crime has been committed. The trial will therefore involve the evidence of expert and professional witnesses. Expert witnesses are professionals who prepare reports for the court on the instructions of the prosecution or the defence. Professional witnesses are those who know the defendant or victim with learning disabilities through their work and are asked to provide statements or reports or release their casenotes to the court. If casenotes are required then the solicitor should make a written request for the defence or Crown Prosecution Service to the professional's employer. The professional needs to consider whether releasing the notes would be harmful to their client. If the professional considers that it would not be in their client's interest then they can refuse to release them. However, the lawyer may disagree and apply to the court for an order for them to be released. If this happens the professional would be called to a court hearing to explain why they believe the notes should not be released. The judge will then make an order on the basis of what he or she has heard from the barrister and the professional. If the judge orders that the notes be released, the professional must do so or be held in contempt of court.

In court proceedings where a decision regarding the person's level of learning disability or mental impairment is to be made, expert testimony may be submitted in evidence. The criteria for the admissibility of expert testimony was stated by Lord Justice Lawton in the case of *R* v. *Turner* (1975), as follows: 'An expert's opinion is admissible to furnish the court with scientific evidence which is likely to be outside the experience and knowledge of the judge or jury'. Commonly, scientific evidence likely to be outside the judge's or jury's experience or knowledge concerns the assessment of intelligence and social functioning by a clinical psychologist. This expert evidence may be supported by evidence from professionals who work with the client. They are able to inform the court on the person's history and current day-to-day functioning and support needs.

In the past the courts have held very rigid views on what constitutes mental impairment. In the case of *R* v. *Masih* (1986), expert testimony was given regarding IQ. In this case the defendant's IQ was found to be 72, which falls at the lower end of the 'borderline' range. In Lord Lane's view, expert testimony in a borderline case was not as a rule necessary and was therefore excluded. The judgement went on to state that an IQ of 69 or below was required for a defendant to be formally classified as being 'significantly mentally impaired' (Gudjonsson 1992). This judgement was made according to a very rigid definition of mental impairment with no account being taken of test error or the individual's level of social functioning. Clinical psychologists should always report the range within which the person's IQ falls and not a single figure. This makes an allowance for individual variation in test performance from day to day and for errors made in testing. A diagnosis of learning disability should also only be made when an examination of social functioning (adaptive behaviour) is also made. Today the courts place less reliance on cut-off scores such as 70 and have broadened the criteria for admissibility of psychological evidence.

In the case of *R* v. *Raghip* (1991) the Court of Appeal placed less reliance on arbitrary cut-off IQ scores and recognized the importance of evidence from other psychological tests and areas of functioning. These may include assessments of the person's social and moral reasoning, memory, suggestibility, acquiescence and tendency to confabulate. The psychologist may also screen for any mental health problems and advise on whether a psychiatric opinion is needed. Where mental health difficulties are apparent, the lawyer may seek the opinion of a psychiatrist. This may be important, as there are provisions under the Mental Health Act 1983 to detain and treat mentally impaired offenders. The court may also hear evidence regarding the potential risk of future offending. This would be established by an expert in risk assessment in relation to offending (for a discussion see Johnson 2002). Unfortunately, there are no standardized approaches to risk evaluation. While many clinicians carry out such assessments for services and the courts their methods have not been adequately described (Fraser 2002).

Expert evidence may be heard to establish facts outside the experience or knowledge of the jury. Thus information on intelligence as measured on a fully standardized intelligence test such as the Wechsler Adult Intelligence Scale-III would be admissible but not opinion on whether someone is mentally impaired or learning disabled. Therefore, the final decision as to whether a person is mentally impaired can only be taken by the court. However, in *R* v. *Robbins* (1988) the Court of Appeal decided that the direction of the judge permitting the jury to decide whether the complainant had a severe mental impairment without expert evidence was unobjectionable. Therefore, expert evidence may not always be sought.

Disposal: custody or diversion

People with learning disabilities are vulnerable and would be especially so in an institution such as a prison. *The Reed Report* (Department of Health 1992) stated that offenders with mental disorder should be diverted from prison and that those with learning disabilities should as far as possible be placed in the community rather than in institutional settings. The Report went on to state that the conditions should be of no greater security than is justified by the degree of danger the offender presents to themselves and others. Hence the need for skills in risk assessment and management.

Within services for people with learning disabilities judgements are often made regarding the alleged offender's state of mind without involving the criminal justice system. For example, professional staff supporting a person with a learning disability who has committed an act that could be seen as an offence may decide that the person did not know that what they did was illegal, or could not anticipate the consequences of their behaviour. As such, many acts which would normally be seen as criminal are seen as 'challenging behaviour'. In such circumstances the police are often not contacted. There are also some police forces that do not proceed with a prosecution against a person with learning disabilities because formal assessment suggests that it is unlikely that they had *mens rea* for the alleged offence or would not be able to plead. However, the frequency of this is unknown. There are also areas where the police work in liaison with health and social care professionals to divert alleged offenders away from the criminal justice system towards a needs assessment and development of a package providing management and treatment in the community or in special provision.

In other cases the matter does go to court. However, there is very little data on the frequency with which this occurs. If the defendant is found guilty the court has several options. They could sent the offender to prison, but if evidence is presented on the learning disability and mental state then the court may alternatively use the provisions under the Mental Health Act to detain the person for assessment and/or treatment.

There are now numerous services which specialize in the inpatient assessment and treatment of offenders with learning disabilities (see Lindsay *et al.* 2002; Taylor *et al.* 2002 for examples). However, the assessment of risk may be such that the court may request further reports from professions and the probation service to establish whether the offender could be rehabilitated in the community. There is some evidence emerging to show that offenders with learning disabilities can be treated and managed successfully in the community. This will involve a package of support from a multi-disciplinary team (Clare and Murphy 1998) including individual therapy such as psycho-dynamic psychotherapy (Beail 2001) or cognitive behavioural therapy (Lindsay *et al.* 1998; Taylor *et al.* 2002). However, despite recommendations for community placements with treatment, the evidence base for this approach is only just developing (Beail 2004).

Victims of crime may also need support and treatment after court appearances. One of the difficulties for victims is that the treatment process for the post-traumatic stress they may experience may be seen as an interference to their recall of the actual event. Thus, many victims have to wait until after the trial before they can undergo active psychological treatment. After Mr B had finished being interviewed by the police he was very distressed by the experience and wanted to talk to someone about it. Fortunately the police provided supportive counselling up until the trial but advised that active psychotherapy should not start until afterwards. A wider range of psychological therapies are now available to people with learning disabilities but the evidence base is still in its infancy (Beail 2003, 2004; Prout and Nowak-Drabik 2003).

Exercise 19.1

The local police have contacted you. They have a young man at the police station that they would like to question regarding certain offences. However, they are concerned that the man may have learning disabilities, as he does not seem to understand what they are saying to him.

How can you assist the police in the short term to determine whether the young man may have a learning disability?

If he has a learning disability, what is he entitled to under PACE?

What factors do those supporting him during a police interview need to be aware of?

What alternatives to continuing in the criminal justice system exist in your area for people with learning disabilities?

Conclusion

The focus of this chapter has been the support needs of people with learning disabilities when they come into contact with the criminal justice system. For most people being accused of a crime or being a victim or witness to crime is a stressful experience. For people with learning disabilities this is even more so. This has been officially recognized and the criminal justice system is beginning to respond. PACE recognized the vulnerability of people with learning disabilities and made provision for support during interviews. Also, victims' needs are now being addressed under the Youth Justice and Criminal Evidence Act 1999 and the publication of guidance on achieving best evidence (Home Office and Department of Health 2002). Booklets with pictures and text reflecting the procedures used by the police and by the courts have been produced to use with people with learning disabilities (Hollins *et al.* 1996). However, the significant issue of identifying those that need support has not been addressed and still needs attention. Key questions still need to be asked: are the police officers in your area given any training in identifying vulnerability factors such as learning disability? Do the local police have the support of court liaison nurses and social workers? Does the community learning disability team have the capacity to respond to urgent requests for help and support when a person with a learning disability has been arrested or become the victim of a crime? Can your service arrange for a formal diagnostic assessment by a clinical psychologist should this be needed? Do you have access to psychiatric services to assist with assessment of any mental health needs under the Mental Health Act 1983?

Whether we are dealing with offenders or victims or witnesses there will be resource issues. If the police want to carry out interviews, are any members of the service willing and able to act as appropriate adults? Can you provide resources to support victims, offenders or witnesses through the court process? Can you put together packages of support to provide management and treatment for any offenders diverted from a custodial sentence? Could you fund a placement in a special facility for offenders with learning disabilities? Also, can you provide the victims of crime and the witnesses of crime with counselling and psychotherapy to address any post-traumatic reaction? These are the practical questions service managers and providers need to ask and assess themselves on.

The research base on people with learning disabilities and the criminal justice system is growing and has done so considerably in the last few years. There have been several special issues of journals devoted to forensic issues and learning disabilities and a book devoted to offenders with learning disabilities has also been published (Lindsay *et al.* 2004). This growing literature has largely focused on offenders and less so on victims and witnesses. But despite the growth in research there are still more questions than answers and research endeavours must continue to help inform clinical practice and social care.

References

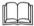

Ammons, R.R. and Ammons, C.H. (1966) The quick test (QT) provisional manual, *Psychological Reports*, 11: 111–61.

Beail, N. (2001) Recidivism following psychodynamic psychotherapy amongst offenders with intellectual disabilities, *The British Journal of Forensic Practice*, 3: 33–7.

Beail, N. (2002) Interrogative suggestibility, memory and intellectual disability, *Journal of Applied Research in Intellectual Disabilities*, 15: 129–37.

Beail, N. (2003) What works for people with mental retardation: critical commentary on cognitive-behavioural and psychodynamic psychotherapy research, *Mental Retardation*, 41: 468–72.

Beail, N. (2004) Approaches to the evaluation of outcomes in work with developmentally disabled offenders, in W.R. Lindsay, J.L. Taylor and P. Strurmey (eds) *Offenders with Developmental Disabilities*. Chichester: Wiley.

Brown, H., Stein, J. and Turk, V. (1995) The sexual abuse of adults with learning disabilities, *Mental Handicap Research*, 8: 3–24.

Clare, I.C.H. and Murphy, G.H. (1998) Working with offenders or alleged offenders with intellectual disabilities, in E. Emerson, C. Hatton, J. Bromley and A. Caine (eds) *Clinical Psychology and People with Intellectual Disabilities*. Chichester: Wiley.

Department of Health (1992) *The Reed Report*. London: HMSO.

Fraser, W.I. (2002) Executive summary, *Journal of Intellectual Disability Research*, 46, Suppl. 1: 1–5.

Gudjonsson, G.H. (1992) *The Psychology of Interrogations, Confessions and Testimony*. Chichester: Wiley.

Gudjonsson, G.H. (1997) *The Gudjonsson Suggestibility Scales Manual*. Hove: Psychology Press.

Gudjonsson, G.H. and Gunn, J. (1982) The competence and reliability of a witness in a criminal court, *British Journal of Psychiatry*, 141: 624–7.

Gudjonsson, G.H. and Henry, L. (2003) Child and adult witnesses with intellectual disability: the importance of suggestibility, *Legal and Criminological Psychology*, 8: 241–52.

Gunn, M.J. (1996) *Sex and the Law: A Brief Guide for Staff Working with People with Learning Disabilities*, 4th edn. London: Family Planning Association.

Hayes, S.C. (2002) Early intervention or early incarceration? Using a screening test for intellectual disability in the criminal justice system, *Journal of Applied Research in Intellectual Disabilities*, 15: 120–8.

Holland, T., Clare, I.C.H. and Mukhopadhyay, T. (2002) Prevalence of 'criminal offending' by men and women with intellectual disability and the characteristics of 'offenders': implications for research and service development, *Journal of Intellectual Disability Research*, 46, Suppl. 1: 6–20.

Hollins, S., Clare, I.C.H. and Murphy, G.H. (1996) *You're Under Arrest*. London: Gaskell.

Home Office (1995) *Police and Criminal Evidence Act Codes of Practice*. London: The Stationery Office.

Home Office & Department of Health (2002) *Achieving Best Evidence: Guidelines for Vulnerable and Intimidated Witnesses*. London: HMSO.

Johnson, S.J. (2002) Risk assessment in offenders with intellectual disabilities: the evidence base, *Journal of Intellectual Disability Research*, 46, Suppl. 1: 47–56.

Kebbell, M.R. and Hatton, C. (1999) People with mental retardation as witnesses in court, *Mental Retardation*, 3: 179–87.

Kebbell, M.R., Hatton, C. and Johnson, S.D. (2000) *Witnesses with Learning Disabilities in Court: Full Report of Research Activities and Results*. Unpublished manuscript: University of Birmingham.

Lindsay, W.R. (2002) Integration of recent reviews on offenders with intellectual disabilities, *Journal of Applied Research in Intellectual Disabilities*, 15: 111–19.

Lindsay, W.R., Neilson, C.Q., Morrison, F. and Smith, A.H.W. (1998) The treatment of six men with a learning disability convicted of sex offences with children, *British Journal of Clinical Psychology*, 37: 83–98.

Lindsay, W.R., Smith, A.H.W., Law, K., Quinn, A., Anderson, A., Smith, T., Overend, T. and Allan, R. (2002) A treatment service for sex offenders and abusers with intellectual disability: characteristics of referrals and evaluation, *Journal of Applied Research in Intellectual Disabilities*, 15: 166–74.

Lindsay, W.R., Taylor, J.L. and Sturmey, P. (eds) (2004) *Offenders with Developmental Disabilities*. Chichester: Wiley.

McBrien, J. (2003) The intellectually disabled offender: methodological problems in identification, *Journal of Applied Research in Intellectual Disabilities*, 16: 95–106.

Medford, S., Gudjonsson, G.H. and Pearse, J. (2003) The efficacy of the appropriate adult safeguard during police interviewing, *Legal and Criminological Psychology*, 8: 253–66.

O'Kelly, C.M.E., Kebbell, M.R., Hatton, C. and Johnson, S.D. (2003) Judicial intervention in court cases involving witnesses with and without learning disabilities, *Legal and Criminological Psychology*, 8: 229–40.

Prout, H.R. and Nowak-Drabik, K.M. (2003) Psychotherapy with persons who have mental retardation: an evaluation of effectiveness, *American Journal of Mental Retardation*, 108: 82–93.

Taylor, J.L., Novaco, R.W., Gilmer, B. and Thorne, I. (2002) Cognitive-behavioural treatment of anger intensity in offenders with intellectual disabilities, *Journal of Applied Research in Intellectual Disabilities*, 15: 151–65.

Tully, B. and Cahill, D. (1984) *Police Interviewing of the Mentally Handicapped: an Experimental Study*. London: The Police Foundation.

White, R. and Willner, P. (2003) Memory as an artefact in the assessment of suggestibility. Paper presented at the Third Seattle Club Conference, Edinburgh.

Wilson, C. and Brewer, N. (1992) The incidence of criminal victimisation of individuals with intellectual disability, *Australian Psychologist*, 27: 114–17.

WHO (World Health Organization) (1992) *ICD-10: International Classification of Diseases and Related Health Problems*, 10th revision. Geneva: WHO.

20

Promoting independence through work

Mark Powell and Margaret Flynn

Introduction

This chapter adopts an evolutionary approach to the subject of work and people with learning disabilities. An introductory context is followed by a brief history of day services – not least because, with some noble exceptions, day services remain the 'core' contribution of local authorities to the day-time occupation of adults with learning disabilities. Further, 'training for independence', including vocational training, are themes that thread through their activities.

The heart of the chapter traces the experiences and influences regarding the development of 'work' alternatives to day services and provides some examples arising from different sectors, as well as capturing people's reflections on these alternatives. This, and the following section, reflect the experiential knowledge of Mark Powell as he has engaged with employment of people with disabilities over the last 15 years in Sheffield and South Yorkshire.

The chapter then seeks to make sense of the tenacity of the day service model, irrespective of current policy, and promising opportunities opening up in the social economy. The social economy is distinctive because it places people before profit, and social benefit before return on investment. It seeks to tackle social, economic and environmental matters with a holistic approach. Examples arising from Sheffield and South Yorkshire's social economy furnish the chapter with glimpses of people's sense of themselves and their independence.

Finally, the chapter outlines ways in which policy and practice have sought to rethink the promotion of independence through work, in part because of the rise and stalling of supported employment. It challenges the assumed interconnectedness of independence and employment. The aims are to consider the policy backdrop to day services; the ways in which vocational training and employment have been de-prioritized in policy and practice; the obstacles to realizing 'real' employment for adults with learning disabilities; and the implications for future generations of school leavers.

Context

From accounts of how the biographical upheavals of unemployment and redundancy are experienced, we know that there is little to commend either. In western capitalist societies, unemployment and redundancy decisively impact on families, relationships, people's experience of time, mental and physical health and financial security, including home ownership, because being employed is a crucial means for achieving personal meaning, status and wealth (Fineman 1990; Alheit 1994). Typically, as adults, we spend a large proportion of our lives at work; many of our friendships arise from our work; and work provides a fixed temporal structure to our days and our lives. Leaving paid work for retirement is similarly a momentous event and currently refers to a life phase which can extend to as many as 40 years. Whether the retired population takes advantage of their freedom hinges on many considerations, not least their use of time and money (Young 1988). The transition from being 'time poor' to 'time rich' can range from being experienced as a 'tragic gift' with grievous consequences (Jahoda *et al.* 1972), to a positive liberation, with a universe of experiences in between.

Exercise 20.1

How do you mark the passage of time in your life?

Each of us has ways of thinking, feeling and acting about, *inter alia*, work, experienced time and independence which we have learned throughout our lives. Our early childhoods and the social environments in which we acquire and make sense of experience comprise our 'mental software' or culture that is partly shared with others who live or lived in the same environments (Hofstede 1994). A mainstream school may be judged on the employability of its students and their performance in examinations. A special school for children and young people with learning disabilities, which legitimizes the distinction between the intelligent and the less intelligent, is more likely to reward effort and personal accomplishment in achieving skills. The whole educational system however has been slow to value the contributions of children with learning disabilities and provide all children with a compelling learning environment (Rioux 1991). Almost 20 years ago it was claimed by disabled people that the special educational system in Britain did not provide young people with the skills to get jobs or to live independently as adults (BCODP 1986). There is associated and well documented concern that special schooling legitimates the discrimination visited upon children and young people with learning disabilities and sets the scene for subsequent disadvantage, most particularly in respect of employment (e.g. Walker 1982; Flynn and Hirst 1992; Barnes 1996).

The 'mental software' associated with an educational system that sorts children and young people into mainstream schools and special schools for those disentitled to the former is glimpsed in the following quotations. They arise from interviews with adults who are looking back over their lives and from a conference presentation. Only one person had limited experience of paid work. The first two were women living independently with a partner and with a friend respectively:

> . . . I don't understand half of the things. See with me being in a special school when I was younger, I never learnt nothing. Me other sisters all went to normal school and because I was slow, they put me in a slow school and I never learned there.

> . . . when I was 17 my mother was told I had a mental age of nine . . . I'll always think like a child, even though I'm 44. So I've got a split personality. I must have. I've got a girl's mind in a woman's body . . . and the psychologist, not long ago said about my IQ [drawing a bell shape in the air] normal people are just there, but you're just below it, here.
>
> (Flynn 1989: 52)

> I know I'm a slow learner . . . What would I be like if I'd been treated better? . . . I was watching my dad to cook, to wash, to clean. 'Cos if you watch, that's how you learn . . . And I said to dad, 'Can I learn how to do that?' And he said, 'Yes, one of these days.' That's how I wanted to learn in the first place, but he was pushing me away, like, 'Go away.'

> [Special schools] are terrible because this is one of the reasons why people pick on you . . . they say, 'Oh look at him, he's backward!' But I wasn't backward. It's just because I was slow picking things up. I wasn't like a normal child. A normal child could just pick it up. I didn't start learning to read and write 'till I was 21 . . . That was because I was slow. I didn't pick it up as quickly as anybody else . . . I went to the normal school but they couldn't control me . . . I ran away from schools a few times . . . I'm an outcast . . .

> [I went to different schools because] I found it hard to pick up.
>
> (Flynn and Bernard 1999: 18–22)

Such views, identities and experiences have been part of the impetus for inclusive schooling – a strengthened right to a mainstream education, albeit not for all children with learning disabilities (DfES 2001). The interviewees did not meet with employment professionals; they were not inspired by men and women who had left their schools for employment and careers; and irrespective of the value they placed on their independence past and present, their pre-placement visits to local day centres confirmed the tenacity of a day care assumption.

Exercise 20.2

Thinking back to your schooldays, do you remember how you experienced (a) having no aptitude for particular subjects and how you experienced the passage of time during these lessons; (b) what ambitions you had for your future?

Young people have their pasts. What is the case for finding out about the pasts of young adults with learning disabilities?

A brief history of day services

Better Services for the Mentally Handicapped (DHSS/Welsh Office 1971) fudged the conceptually distinct experiences of having a paid job and career, and being in a day centre for an unspecified period. It used the language of vocational training, employment and independence, but without any conviction that these outcomes were feasible for the majority. The expansion of day centre places was an explicit aim. The document stated:

> For adults who are unable to benefit from the usual adult training centre programme there are special facilities . . . in the form of units for 'adult special care' or 'pre-vocational training'.

> Adult training centres provide further training, and in many cases permanent daily occupation, for mentally handicapped adults who are not able to work in open or sheltered employment. Although progress has been made in improving and increasing these, many more places are still needed . . . For the long term future . . . a target of 2.4 places per 1,000 population in this age group is suggested. No authority has yet reached this target . . .

> Most mildly handicapped school leavers are able to go directly into open or sheltered employment . . . some need a period of special training in an adult training centre first. Most of the severely handicapped also need to attend an adult training centre . . . the majority need permanently some form of work or occupation specially geared to their limited capabilities . . . The object of this special training and work or occupation is to develop work habits and to increase self reliance generally, so as to help each handicapped person to live a more independent life.

The services in which the greatest expansion is needed are adult training centres or sheltered workshops . . .

(Paras 62, 64, 154, 201)

Almost 20 years later, the National Development Team (1990: 9) submitted evidence to the House of Commons Select Committee on Social Services. They identified the following drawbacks of day services:

. . . many people who have been asked say they would rather have a real job . . . Training centres have come to serve many different and incompatible purposes – training people for jobs, serving as a factory, providing life and academic education, occupying people, serving as a primary health clinic, acting as a sports club and also providing respite care for families. This mixture causes confusion amongst service users and staff, no one is clear about what they should be doing, efforts are diluted and client progress is slow . . . Centres are based on a 'readiness' model of service provision. That is, as people acquire work and social skills they are supposed to progress up through the centre, maybe to an advanced training centre, a sheltered workshop, an enclave scheme and eventually into open employment. In fact, very few people progress from one stage to the next; day centres provide an unchanging routine year after year. A person's material poverty is matched by the narrowness of their experience.

Thus, part of the heritage of the 1971 *Better Services* White Paper included day centres falling short of the known aspirations of adults with learning disabilities and tending to operate a narrow range of programmes, on a part-time basis, leaving many with too much unstructured time. Day centres became very selective about admissions and exclusions (so people whose behaviour was difficult to manage might be excluded, irrespective of the hardship this might cause to their families); they came to accommodate many more people than they were designed for, in segregated groupings, with people spending a great deal of time at the beginning and end of each day on unpredictable and inflexible but expensive transport. Significantly too, the availability of further education to people attending day centres stalled concerns about how to occupy and accommodate the annual graduation of school leavers. There were people attending colleges for years, sometimes repeating courses. For families, the scope for such outcomes as employment, wages and careers was eclipsed by considerations of the reliability and continuity of the day service. The promotion of 'independence' within day services, rather than in employment, appeared to be more palatable to people's relatives and their residential services for a host of reasons, including fears of mistreatment, the risks most particularly faced by women, the loss of a (full-time or part-time) day centre place and the non-recoverable loss of welfare benefits (Flynn and Thomas 1991; Felce *et al.* 1998).

The Department of Health's Local Authority Circular (DoH 1992) trailed different models of day care and while still peddling vocational training, was more circumspect about the links between employment and independence:

> Local authorities should plan to shift away from services based on attendance at the traditional adult training centre, towards an approach to day services based on individual assessment and programmes in which skill learning and vocational preparation are prominent . . .
>
> (Para. 18)

> . . . participation in a paid job will help them to achieve greater social independence and self assurance . . . It should not be assumed that 'self-reliance' in terms of employment is matched by independence in respect of people's living circumstances. Because there are non-vocational areas of people's lives which are essential to employment – getting up on time, being clean, wearing appropriate clothes, handling money to buy lunch, catching a bus etc. – few people with learning disabilities who secure and hold a job do so without reliable assistance from others in the non-vocational areas of their lives.
>
> (Annexe: 20)

After nearly three decades of day service developments there remains an endemic day centre bias (Powell 1996; DoH 1999). In 2001, local authorities spent some £300 million a year on day services, of which more than 80 per cent was spent on day centre places, often focusing on large group activities (DoH 2001). So it is relevant to examine the organizational domains associated with day care. They are the outward and visible rationale for the development of alternatives to day centres (Flynn and Thomas 1991):

- Local authorities have inherited a building-based service response to adults with learning disabilities, not just as a result of Section 29 of the National Assistance Act 1948, but due to the demands of families caring for young adults with extensive support needs and accommodation and support services working with the former residents of long-stay hospitals.
- Day services are not shaped by a unitary system of goals and values.
- Day centres tend to do the kind of forward planning which attends to pressing problems as they arise (e.g. we've added a special care unit, we no longer offer full-time places because the college offers part time placements, we have a compulsory retirement age, we have to exclude people with challenging behaviours).
- Day services are not comprehensive. Pressures to expand and meet increasing demands have not met with pressures to redefine their functions.
- Assessments tend to rely unduly on what is available and existing, low productivity and repetitious programmes.
- Social services have an anomalous lead agency identity in respect of day services. Their history resides in welfare, not in vocational training, employment or education.

- The tasks and roles of day centre officers, instructors, care assistants and support workers do not sit comfortably with the known aspirations of many adults with learning disabilities for real jobs.

- Managerial capacity and culture in day services along with a melting pot of past and present policies, has inhibited their redesign.

- Design and development capacities are further casualties of a system which has witnessed a low rate of change.

- The welfare benefit income of many adults attending day centres supplements the incomes of parents, whose employment may have been constrained by their caregiving. National policy leadership with reference to day services has been limited.

Exercise 20.3

What are the reasons that the overwhelming majority of special school graduates do not enter full-time, paid employment?

What advice would you give to local politicians and parent groups who want to replace a large day centre with an even larger one?

What do day services contribute to the independence of adults with learning disabilities?

The development of 'work' alternatives to day services

Work alternatives managed by statutory providers of day services

When *Caring for People: Community Care in the Next Decade and Beyond* (DoH 1989) (which preceded the passing by parliament of the NHS and Community Care Act 1990) had been digested by local authority social services departments, there was an understandable sense of urgency about developing new work-related initiatives for clients of working age. Joint Investment Plans between social services departments and health authorities included employment targets, and Welfare to Work strategies espoused the philosophy of giving people with learning disabilities the chance to work. Action plans identified who should take forward 'work'-related initiatives, but not necessarily how. As a consequence, development was patchy throughout the 1990s, with some statutory service providers establishing satellite work projects and others contracting with outside agencies to do it for them.

Where local authorities have taken the lead, the common factors have been that the 'workers' have not been paid a wage, and their 'work' has not focused on commercial outputs. Training to nationally accredited standards, such as NVQs, has become commonplace, but there is little evidence to suggest that employers are eagerly awaiting an annual crop of horticultural-ists, kitchen assistants and bookbinders with basic qualifications and a smidgen of non-commercial work experience. The unpaid work trainees of ten plus years ago are still unpaid work trainees today. Further, they are still attached to day centres, giving them, their parents and carers a sense of security alongside a sense of the satisfaction and pride that arises from being a 'worker'.

Day service employees invited to supervise new work schemes are unlikely to turn into business entrepreneurs as a result. They are still day service employees. Encouraged by their 'eternal trainees' and yet reined in by local authority risk aversion, they run work schemes as if they were day centres.

Work alternatives managed by voluntary sector organizations

Voluntary sector organizations have always provided alternatives to statutory day services and, because of their freedom from some public sector con-straints and a tendency towards innovation and pioneering at the margins, they have been developing a vast array of work alternatives for many years.

Until recently, the idea of self-sufficiency and commercial viability has rarely been considered, and service providers have been at the mercy of local and national political trends in grant-giving for their survival. Many have not survived, and others spend so much time raising money for short-term survival that there is neither the energy nor the capacity for longer-term planning. As with the statutory sector, wage payments to 'workers' are rare.

The 'workers' who turn up on the doorstep of voluntary sector pro-viders are likely to have been through the statutory services first. They may have voted with their feet, or they may have been pushed, or something in between the two. If boredom, personality clashes or parental dissatisfaction cause further turbulence, they move on to the next time-limited training programme or work project with vacancies. Even in localities with Case Register assisted tracking of people with learning disabilities, the exercise of identifying outcomes for them bears some of the hallmarks of enthusiastic trainspotting. The circular movement of bodies has little to do with career planning or development – these are not options.

Supported employment

Supported employment agencies proliferated in the UK in the late 1980s and early 1990s (Lister *et al.* 1992; Pozner and Hammond 1993). If a person with a learning disability wanted a job, then an appropriate agency would offer advice and support in identifying a suitable area of work, in applying for the job, in attending the interview and, where necessary, in providing on the job support. A career opportunity opened up for local authority and voluntary sector employees in 'job coaching' and the art and science of 'training in systematic instruction' was imported from the USA and applied to all manner of job tasks (Powell 1991).

Supported employment continues to provide support to hundreds of learning disabled people annually, often utilizing government aid schemes such as 'Workstep' (formerly the Supported Employment Programme, SEP), to subsidize the wage of the disabled worker, and European funding programmes to pay for the agency employees and additional support costs. Referrals come through word of mouth, and typically, those referred have had enough of moving around the system, or are re-entering the public world after a bad day care experience and a period of withdrawal. The high cost of supported employment needs to be weighed against the economic and social benefits of helping learning disabled people to find and keep jobs (Corden 1997; O'Bryan *et al.* 2000).

Two significant external factors have contributed to the slippage and stalling of supported employment in the UK in recent years. Firstly, the European funding regimes that have propped up many agencies have been contingent on 'progression' towards employment, enabling many agencies to thrive on placing people in voluntary work, or 'training' programmes, without ever getting them into employment. This apes the 'train then place' stance of day services and defeats the innovatory 'place then train' characteristic associated with supported employment.

Secondly, the prevailing nature of supported employment has been 'person-centred' and agencies have learned a lot about how to work with clients, but not nearly as much about how to work with employers. Not surprisingly, the number of learning disabled people entering paid employment on the same basis as their non-disabled peers remain very low.

Social firms

In the late 1990s, the NHS Surrey Oaklands Trust was successful in a grant application to a European transnational fund (Helios) for money to explore the extent to which social firms were operating in the UK. A social firm, as defined by the European Confederation of Co-operatives and Social Business (1997), is a business that creates employment for disabled people through the market-oriented production of goods. The term 'social firm' was not in common usage in the UK in the late 1990s, although many community businesses and cooperatives fitted the description well. The result has been the development, over the last five years, of a social firm movement, spear-headed by Social Firms UK, a practitioner-led organization that now boasts 400 members, 45 of which are social firms and 120 of which are committed to becoming so.

For some local authority social services departments who were struggling with rising numbers in day centres, increasing numbers of part-time attendees and serious annual budget deficits, the rhetoric of social firms came as music to their ears. Service managers were tasked with setting social firms up as income-generating alternatives to traditional day centre activity, typically without any additional budget to do so. Despite interest from the Department of Work and Pensions, and from HM Treasury, and a general policy chorus in favour of modernizing day services by skirting day centres and exploring employment and learning opportunities in non-specialist contexts, no significant social firms have yet developed out of day service structures. 'Pack-it' in South Wales is the single example of a successful packaging and distribution social firm, with a turnover in excess of £1 million, that can claim to have local authority roots. The reality has been that the cultural divide between low-risk, non-commercial day centres and high-risk, economically viable social firms has been too great.

Why would local authority employees swap their favourable terms and conditions of employment to set up businesses with a high chance of failure and a workforce of people with learning disabilities who perceive their 'work' as taking place in day centres? Why would parents and carers, for whom the only imaginable alternative to the day centre they have known for years is a bigger day centre, opt for losing out on welfare benefits in the faint hope that their sons and daughters with learning disabilities might survive for a few months on a minimum wage in a doomed enterprise before being flung penniless on the scrap heap? These questions do not require written answers . . .

Despite such overwhelming obstacles to social firm development from within statutory structures, the tide bringing 'social enterprise' to the UK is so strong that social firms are being set up by individuals who have the support of a government-backed enterprise sector, and a vision of a future in which disabled and non-disabled people can live and work alongside each other without anyone being surprised about it.

Summary

- The statutory sector's work-related initiatives and strategies have barely dented the day care assumption or such employment simulations as unpaid jobs and (unduly long-term) training.
- Local authority employees do not have a track record of becoming effective business entrepreneurs attuned to self-sufficiency and commercial viability.
- Securing grant funding plagues the endeavours of those seeking employment for people with learning disabilities.
- Supported employment, as it was originally conceived, is stalling, irrespective of its track record in finding jobs and maintaining people in employment, because of European funding requirements.
- Social firms have inherited the promise once associated with supported employment and face similar challenges.

Opportunities opening up in the social enterprise sector – a credible alternative to day centres?

In 2005, it is difficult to be unaware of a regeneration process that is under-way in almost all of our most deprived communities. Hundreds of millions of pounds are being made available year on year for community development and for neighbourhood renewal programmes.

Historically, people with learning disabilities have been conveniently excluded from such mainstream initiatives by being dubbed 'a community of interest'. The latter cannot be seen as an inclusive measure when all it does is lump together thousands of people who have no more in common than an unspecified degree of assumed intellectual impairment.

The tide is turning. Social firms are accepted as a discrete strand of social enterprise, and a social enterprise development unit such as the Sheffield Community Enterprise Development Unit (SCEDU) or a social enterprise support network such as South Yorkshire Social Enterprise Network (SYSEN) would be incomplete without a disability sector arm as well as a black and minority ethnic community arm, and so on. Wherever the regeneration process is taking place, 'What about disabled people?' is a refrain. Of course, the population of people with learning disabilities is typically no more than 3 per cent of the total population of disabled people in an area, and the possibility for marginalization is still strong, but at least the question is being asked.

One of the key measures for validating the amount of money spent on regeneration and renewal is paid jobs created. At a time of low unemployment, when there are three people on incapacity benefit and severe disablement allowance for every one on job seeker's allowance the case for getting more disabled people into employment as a means of meeting funders' targets is a persuasive one. If it makes good social and economic sense, why not swim with the tide?

In my back yard (IMBY)

In 1996 the leaders of six non-statutory organizations in Sheffield that provided services to learning disabled people came together to consider ways of developing more employment opportunities for their clients. They called themselves IMBY (the defiant opposite of NIMBY – not in my back yard).

IMBY put out to tender work to test out existing training and employment organizations for learning disabled people in Sheffield against community business standards. Tony Phillips' 'realife consultancy' was commissioned to do the work. The report on the work undertaken indicated that not one of the organizations viewed by the consultants was anywhere near being a business, and all of them shared many of the characteristics of day centres. Real wages were not being paid to any workers, and no workers worked a full working day. Starts and finishes were often dictated by the whim of social services transport or by carers' meal times. Workers were involved in work tasks, but none had any significant involvement in planning or organizing the work. Non-disabled people were supervisors and managers and learning disabled people turned up and were kept occupied until it was time to go home.

One of the organizations – a plastics reclamation initiative called 'Reclaim' – took the report on the chin, and started to make plans to pay learning disabled staff and involve them in all aspects of the business. There is no money to spare in a plastics reclamation business, but Reclaim's managers made a commitment to budget for paying wages for three learning disabled workers within 12 months, and to continue the commitment thereafter. Reclaim now boasts 45 paid staff, many of whom have learning disabilities or mental health problems. Currently, it is the third largest plastics reclamation operation in Great Britain.

One of the first learning disabled employees at Reclaim was Paul. He was a well-built man of 21 with boundless energy. He had worked as a volunteer at Reclaim for some months, and took advantage of the arrival of New Deal's Environmental Task Force to try out employment. He did so well that he was signed on for a year as an intermediate labour market employee, and was then retained on improved terms as a reclaimer of construction waste. This was under a contract negotiated by Reclaim with a local waste management company. He has been there for more than three years.

Another employee is Alan. When Reclaim began, he was one of the first volunteers to come from a social services work preparation centre. He cried if you greeted him, because such positive recognition was too much for him to bear. He was a 'Cinderella' at home, used as a babysitter until all hours and treated disrespectfully by his family. Alan was a strong and willing worker, and early in his career at Reclaim he was given the chance to leave to become a council refuse operative. He developed stomach-ache during his trial and ended up in hospital, and then returned to Reclaim. When a job came up for a baling press operator at Reclaim, Alan was coached through the skill training required for the job, supported in the interview and supplied with handkerchiefs to cope with his disbelieving tears of joy when he was offered the job. Almost his entire family was kind enough to accompany him to the bank to cash his first pay cheque. Finally, Reclaim arranged an adult fostering placement for Alan to enable him to keep his money and to live in peace. Six years on, he shows visitors around Reclaim, and takes full responsibility for his baling press and for his expanding social life.

Part of Reclaim went up in flames in 1999, and the training function of the organization – staff, trainees and equipment – found an old school to inhabit. The old school is now a vibrant development trust, with a café, a gym, a boxing arena, a dance studio, a business incubator and a home for dozens of community groups. It employs staff with learning disabilities in a variety of ways. The potential for job creation is enormous and, as one of the agencies housed on the site is a supported employment agency, few opportunities are missed.

Reclaim itself was soon discovered by Social Firms UK and named as a social firm, and IMBY was given the task by Social Firms UK of stimulating the development of more social firms in the Yorkshire and Humber region. This looked easy, as almost every local authority social services department and joint planning team was now obliged to look for employment options for clients. However, although awareness-raising conferences generated great interest and enthusiasm they did not conjure up the social entrepreneurs or 'champions' for social firm ideas. Everybody was watching out for new social firms, but no one was setting them up.

IMBY and business development

It was only in 2004 that real progress began to be made, coming about in South Yorkshire and in other parts of the UK as a result of several harmonizing factors: the belief in the concept of social firms held by a few individuals with vision, passion and drive; low unemployment coupled with high numbers of disabled people receiving welfare benefits; and a tide of social enterprise development. Instead of being seen as a worthy peripheral organization dealing with a charitable cause, IMBY now had a seat at the table of regeneration and renewal bodies insisting that disabled people should be 'included' in their plans. It should be noted that it is IMBY, a business-orientated organization, that is at the table, and not a social services department. When IMBY is looking for start-up funding for a business venture centred on disabled people, it is to the Department of Trade and Industry and to social economy loan finance bodies that it turns, and not the social services.

Buster's Coffee Merchants

An example of a social firm, built around four learning disabled people in Sheffield, is Buster's Coffee Merchants. A social entrepreneur and part-time GP, Paul Hodgkin, came to IMBY in 2002 to see if there were any groups supporting disabled people that might welcome a little extra income through roasting and selling ground coffee. He was offering his 'Get Fresh' coffee idea to a variety of community groups.

IMBY was interested in the business possibility of people with learning disabilities doing the roasting, packaging and distribution of the coffee themselves, and recruited a 'catalyst entrepreneur' to work with a self-selected group of four young adults for a year to bring them to a point where it would be realistic to start the business. Funding for the pre-enterprise phase came from a charitable trust and from the Learning and Skills Council on the condition that the learning undertaken by the potential workers would enable them to act as educators to disabled and non-disabled people alike regarding their experience of setting up a business from a point some considerable distance behind the starting line. What is profit? What is a bank account? What if you don't feel like working? These are just a few of the questions to which the group needed to find answers. They created a business plan, a trading forecast for the coming year and a code of conduct. They are now in great demand as speakers at conferences and seminars.

The key ingredients that led to Buster's early success were: a good, well-researched business idea (in the coffee business, even when fairly traded, the profit margins are high); the one-year time limit on the pre-enterprise phase of the business to avoid drift; the incentive of paid jobs when the business started to trade; sufficient start-up resources to fund the pre-enterprise period; good business advice; and a catalyst or 'champion' to keep them going.

Other social firm brands

There is currently a plan to open a real-ale pub in South Yorkshire where learning disabled people would have the opportunity to work behind and in front of the bar or in the associated brewery and bed & breakfast. IMBY has identified knowledgeable partners and is presently, at the time of writing, putting in bids for suitable premises.

Sceptics may say that few people with learning disabilities could cope behind a busy bar at eleven o'clock on a Saturday night. They may be right, but the whole idea of a social firm is that disabled and non-disabled people should work together in a business, with each doing the job that they can do best, and with each having the opportunity to progress.

Another idea in the same mould is 'Toots' – a new style of laundry experience. People should, it is hoped, welcome the opportunity to drop off their laundry at a convenient layby on their way to work and collect it on their way home.

The branding of social firms, like the branding of fast-food outlets, is likely to hasten the pace of their development in the coming years. Social Firms UK has been researching franchise opportunities from the distribution for sale of greeting cards to manufacturing products from recycled glass. An early success has been a franchise of the manufacture of certain soap products, which has created employment for a number of learning disabled people on Shetland, and will do so elsewhere.

Clusters and networks

Not all social firms start from scratch. 'Indigo' is the new name for the Cudworth and West Green Partnership's Pinfold Community Garden Project – in marketing terms, a succinct improvement. Business and marketing advice has been purchased, through IMBY, to sharpen up the commercial focus of a Barnsley community project that is led by gifted horticulturalists who are committed to creating employment for disabled people. Garden projects offering work experience and therapy to people with learning disabilities are commonplace, but few of them even aspire to making commercial ends meet. This demands a substantial cultural shift to move from 'a project that trades' to 'a business that supports', but Indigo is getting there.

The social firms' sector now boasts a catalogue of products and services available nationally. Not only is there a growing enthusiasm for buying from another social firm, but there is a parallel tendency for members of social firms' networks to identify gaps in provision in their own area – in printing or catering or IT support, for example – and to set about filling them.

Business advice

IMBY has responded to the need to bridge the gap between people with learning disabilities who want to work and generic business support agencies who give advice by running a European-funded training programme for business advisers on giving social firm business advice. The course has raised awareness, but it is clear that such an approach is just one of many steps to creating an expectation on all sides that learning disability and business can and do mix.

IMBY is collaborating with JobCentre Plus in developing training programmes to orientate and motivate people with learning disabilities, with integrated 'action learning' in social firms such as Buster's. Being part of business in action is likely to provide business advisers and potential employees with the best insight into what social firms are all about.

Supported employers

As a percentage, only a small number of people with learning disabilities who want paid work are going to enter businesses specifically geared to their needs and aspirations. The majority are going to find work in more conventional business set-ups – in shops and offices, in cafés and on building sites.

For 20 years or more, there have been agencies helping small numbers of people with learning disabilities to move into employment. In Sheffield in 1997, IMBY invited Reclaim to host a 'supported employment agency' called IMBY Employment. This agency is as successful as most in placing clients into employment, and is now branching out on its own as 'Bridge Employment'. The limitations on an agency like Bridge Employment are that funding relates to numbers of clients, and all the emphasis is on client development. Recruitment to the post of employment adviser is often dependent on the applicant's experience with the client group and commitment to the aims of the agency. There is a gap here, and IMBY has been working with social services and health professionals in Sheffield to develop a new type of employer-focused agency – a social enterprise to be called 'Deploy'.

Deploy staff will get an understanding of how an employer operates – as would any professional employment agency – but more significantly they will explore with an employer how the part-time and full-time employment of disabled people might help their bottom line – not by paying poor wages, but by getting the most reliable and competent people for the job. As with social firm development, success will come when large numbers of employers start to see that employing disabled people makes good business sense rather than regarding it as a tokenistic contribution to corporate social responsibility. It is expected that Deploy staff will learn that, for example, an employer needs five more checkout operatives in a month's time. There will be the opportunity to mobilize service provider agencies to train up five or more willing clients to the employer's standards, and to offer them for interview.

This is a more constructive approach than training shiploads of people with learning disabilities in skills that are not required by local employers, or in areas where jobs are unavailable.

A credible alternative to day centres?

If social firms and employer support organizations blossomed everywhere tomorrow, would day centres close? The answer is an emphatic 'no'. The resistance and fears of people's families and local authority members result in consultation and needs-led assessments which authorize the continuation of day centres and ensure that the status quo prevails (e.g. Powell 1996). A more testing question is, 'What serious alternatives could be provided if day centres had to close tomorrow?' The answer may point to a network of clustered social firms, many with training arms, which could be developed everywhere in the country, alongside supported employment initiatives. However, a transitional fund would be needed to resource the development, not least as the task is as complex as closing a long-stay hospital. The infectiousness of social firm success in terms of people having real wages and credible jobs may be a powerful advocate for persuading families, carers and day centre staff of the benefits of policy and practice change, and the saving from the public purse as day centres reduce their size would make a lot of difference to local authority and HM Treasury thinking on the subject. Past policy has not revolutionized the support and integration of people with learning disabilities in employment, although some halting first steps have been taken. Current policy has not been shaped by the growth of social firms or social enterprise. It follows that initiatives such as those driven by IMBY can play a part in moving hearts and minds.

Summary

- Non-statutory organizations are vulnerable to adopting the habits and routines of day services and unfocused 'vocational training' activities.
- Established social firms are rooted in communities with the potential for mutual gain.
- The scope for further job-creating opportunities is vast, even if caution attends the creation of social firms.
- Excellent products and services are at the heart of social firms, driven by the conviction that people with disabilities and non-disabled people can and should work together. They have no interest in undirected and long-term 'vocational training' or work 'opportunities' without planned employment outcomes.
- The success of social firms has yet to have an impact on day services.

Conclusion: rethinking the promotion of independence through work

Supported employment is to be credited with challenging the conviction that only the most able people can be employed, even though its mission of focusing on the people with the most extensive support needs has been progressively diluted (McIntosh and Whittaker 1998). A focus on Sheffield and South Yorkshire reveals something of the ongoing developments and implementation in employment. These appear well adapted to orient people with learning disabilities to real employment at the going rates. The examples outlined animate the view that people's employment is less contingent on assessments of their independence or their capacity for pre-vocational training than on local responses to opportunities arising in social regeneration. Further, supported employment recasts the aim of employment for people with learning disabilities in an environment quite other than that of the statutory sector. If supported employment is at the interface between social services and employment (McIntosh and Whittaker 1998), then social firms are rooted in the social enterprise and economic mainstream, yet are attuned to the disadvantages arising from being in special education and day services, for example.

In our experience, having a salary does not mean that employees know how to budget or avoid financial exploitation of the kind experienced by Alan. There is even the argument that they will not have time to learn these life skills if they spend all day at work! But such a view leans heavily on the professional 'fix-it' model of goals and programmes directed at unassisted performance. The sense of personal agency that arises from employment is captured in endorsements of supported employment and in our experience of social firm development. Alan's peers and manager were instrumental in supporting him to leave his family and become established in a home of his choosing (i.e. instead of viewing their roles narrowly as his colleagues, they saw that the effectiveness of their operations would be enhanced by ensuring that all employees were supported to perform efficiently) (e.g. Moore 1995). In turn, the assets of the social firm as represented by Reclaim create the additional value of relative independence from social services' efforts to secure employment for people (Beyer *et al.* 2004). Arguably it is such independence that employment should strive to achieve.

Exercise 20.4

What has been your experience of seeking and maintaining work for yourself and someone with a learning disability?

What can social regeneration teach health and social care services about independence and employment?

References

Alheit, P. (1994) *Taking the Knocks: Youth Unemployment and Biography – A Qualitative Analysis*. London: Cassell Education.

Barnes, C. (1996) Institutional discrimination against disabled people and the campaign for anti-discrimination legislation, in D. Taylor (ed.) *Critical Social Policy: A Reader*. London: Sage.

Beyer, S., Grove, B., Schneider, J., Simons, K., Williams, V., Heyman, A., Swift, P. and Krijnen-Kemp, E. (2004) *Working Lives: The Role of Day Centres in Supporting People with Learning Disabilities into Employment*. Research summary. www.dwp.gov.uk, accessed 12 March 2004.

BCODP (British Council of Organizations of Disabled People) (1986) *Disabled Young People Living Independently*. Derbyshire: BCODP.

Corden, A. (1997) *Supported Employment, People and Money: Social Policy Reports, Number 7*. York: The University of York Social Policy Research Unit.

DfES (Department for Education and Skills) (2001) *Inclusive Schooling – Children with Special Educational Needs*. London: DfES.

DHSS (Department of Health and Social Security)/Welsh Office (1971) *Better Services for the Mentally Handicapped*. London: HMSO.

DoH (Department of Health) (1989) *Caring for People: Community Care in the Next Decade and Beyond – Caring for the 1990s*. London: Department of Health.

DoH (Department of Health) (1992) Local Authority Circular (LAC(92)15) *Social Care for Adults with Learning Disabilities (Mental Handicap)*. London: Department of Health.

DoH (Department of Health) (1999) *Facing the Facts – Services for People with Disabilities: A Policy Impact Study of Social Care and Health Services*. London: Department of Health.

DoH (Department of Health) (2001) *Valuing People: A New Strategy for Learning Disability for the 21st Century*. London: Department of Health.

European Confederation of Co-operatives and Social Business (1997) Definition of social firms agreed. The CETEC Conference in Linz, Austria.

Felce, D., Grant, G., Todd, S., Ramcharan, P., Beyer, S., McGrath, M., Perry, J., Shearn, J., Kilsby, M. and Lowe, K. (1998) *Towards a Full Life: Researching Policy Innovation for People with Learning Disabilities*. Oxford: Butterworth Heinmann.

Fineman, S. (1990) *Supporting the Jobless: Doctors, Clergy, Police, Probation Officers*. London: Tavistock.

Flynn, M. (1989) *Independent Living for Adults with Mental Handicap: A Place of My Own*. London: Cassell.

Flynn, M. and Bernard, J. (1999) *Deep Trouble! Adults with Learning Disabilities who Offend*. Manchester: National Development Team.

Flynn, M. and Hirst, M. (1992) *This Year, Next Year, Sometime? Learning Disability and Adulthood*. London: Social Policy Research Unit and the National Development Team.

Flynn, M. and Thomas, D. (1991) *Day Services in the Nineties for People with Learning Difficulties in Northern Ireland*. DHSS for Northern Ireland: Her Majesty's Stationery Office.

Hofstede, G. (1994) *Cultures and Organisations – Software of the Mind: Intercultural Cooperation and its Importance for Survival*. London: HarperCollinsBusiness.

Jahoda, M., Lazarsfeld, P. and Zeisel, H. (1972) *Marienthal: the Sociography of an Unemployed Community*. London: Tavistock.

Lister, T., Ellis, L., Phillips, T., O'Bryan, A., Beyer, S. and Kilsby, M. (1992) *Survey of Supported Employment Services in England.* Manchester: National Development Team.

McIntosh, B. and Whittaker, A. (1998) *Days of Change: A Practical Guide to Developing Better Day Opportunities with People with Learning Difficulties.* London: King's Fund and the National Development Team.

Moore, M.H. (1995) *Creating Public Value: Strategic Management in Government.* Cambridge, MA: Harvard University Press.

National Development Team (1990) *Promises to Keep.* London: National Development Team.

O'Bryan, A., Simons, K., Beyer, S. and Grove, B. (2000) *Economic Security and Supported Employment for the Policy Consortium on Supported Employment.* Manchester: National Development Team and Joseph Rowntree Foundation.

Powell, M. (1996) What's new in day care? MA dissertation, Department of Social Policy and Social Work, University of York.

Powell, T.H. (1991) *Supported Employment: Providing Integrated Employment Opportunities for Persons with Disabilities.* New York: Longman.

Pozner, A. and Hammond, J. (1993) *An Evaluation of Supported Employment Initiatives for Disabled People*, Employment Department Research Series No. 17. Sheffield: Department of Employment.

Rioux, M. (1991) Education: a system of social disempowerment, in G.L. Porter and D. Richler (eds) *Changing Canadian Schools: Perspectives on Disability and Inclusion.* Ontario: The Roeher Institute.

Young, M. (1988) *The Metronomic Society – Natural Rhythms and Human Timetables.* London: Thames & Hudson.

Walker, A. (1982) *Unqualified and Underemployed: Handicapped Young People and the Labour Market*, National Children's Bureau Series. London: Macmillan.

21

Counselling people with a learning disability

Jill Jesper and Jayne Stapleton

Introduction

Counselling for people with learning disabilities has tremendous therapeutic potential if used creatively. Counselling can have many useful functions, not just for the resolution of problems or for the expression of distress, but for personal development, for supported decision-making or resolution of internal conflict (see Box 21.1). Counselling can be an empowering experience for the client. It can enhance communicative ability, personal insight and inspire confidence.

The process, ethical context and potential limitations of counselling will be explored in this chapter, along with some of the core conditions essential to creating a therapeutic environment. The notion of counsellor competence will be addressed, along with some discussion of the use of counselling skills in the delivery of day-to-day care. In particular, emphasis will be placed on the application of counselling approaches to working therapeutically with people who have learning disabilities. This will be achieved by offering case study examples from clients at various stages of the life span.

Box 21.1 A definition of counselling

The overall aim of counselling is to provide an opportunity for the client to work towards living in a more satisfying and resourceful way. Counselling may be concerned with developmental issues, addressing and resolving specific problems, making decisions, coping with crisis, developing personal insight and knowledge, working through feelings of inner conflict, or improving relationships with others. The counsellor's role is to facilitate the client's work in a way which respect the client's values, personal resources and capacity for self determination.

(BACP 1997)

Life experience and its demands

It is acknowledged that people who have learning disabilities experience life and its demands in similar ways to other people. They are really no different to others in being human. They experience moments of celebration and joy, they tackle challenges and seek opportunities, they dream and fantasize and they experience the same tedious routines and moments of insecurity and distress as anyone else. They deal with conflict and difficulties in decision-making and they experience loss and life changes. Many people with learning disabilities cope remarkably well with changing life events, but in some cases adaptation has not been so positive, leaving the individual with worries and anxieties which can, over time, become unmanageable, even pathological.

People generally have a range of resources which can be utilized to solve problems in times of difficulty. However, anyone who has experienced trauma or distress will know that normal coping and the ability to identify and use personal resources can become seriously compromised during that difficult phase. Ability to cope can be clouded by emotion and feelings of helplessness.

What can counselling offer?

In the context of this chapter, counselling is not about giving advice, it is not disciplinary, it is not particularly about being directive (Rogers 1951; Mearns and Thorne 1988; BACP 2002). It is about helping, enabling, creating a therapeutic opportunity, empowering, facilitating choice, supporting and validating. It is based on a fundamental belief that the person with a learning disability is a person first and as such, worthy of respect and value as an individual (Wolfensberger 1972; DoH 2001).

Of course, counselling is not for everyone. People have the right to make choices about the services offered to them. Counselling, therefore, must be presented as an option which can be declined by the individual. When a person is referred to a counselling service, an initial meeting and assessment can serve a very useful purpose. Some counsellors may take a specific approach in their assessment and a variety of assessment tools are available for this purpose. Others take a less structured approach where the assessment offers an opportunity to explore the concept of counselling with the client, answering their questions, identifying their potential needs and exploring the possibilities for therapeutic engagement.

The counsellor should explain any particular model or approach that they might wish to use. Different situations often require different approaches. Confidentiality, record-keeping and practical arrangements regarding appointments are also important issues. The client also needs to understand their own responsibilities towards the counsellor, including attending appointments and conducting any potential 'homework' in which they might be expected to participate. It is also essential to discuss the potential impact of engaging in counselling, for example, acknowledging that people can feel distressed when 'reliving' a personal trauma such as bereavement, physical, sexual or psychological abuse, family separation, bullying and so on.

Contracting

The contracting stage occurs when agreements are reached about how the counsellor and client will work together. The contract, whether written or unwritten, is mutually agreed and should set out each person's responsibilities. Whether accredited or not, counsellors should work within a clear ethical framework, such as that proposed by the BACP (2002) (see Box 21.2). This, in most cases, would include general principles of fidelity, autonomy, beneficence, non-maleficence and justice (Gillon 1985; Sugarman 1992; Bond 1993). These elements relate to the trustworthiness and competence of

---

Box 21.2   The BACP *Ethical Framework* (2002)

Values
The fundamental values of counselling and psychotherapy include a commitment to:

- respecting human rights and dignity;
- ensuring the integrity of practitioner-client relationships;
- enhancing the quality of professional knowledge and its application;
- alleviating personal distress and suffering;
- fostering a sense of self that is meaningful to the person(s) concerned;
- increasing personal effectiveness;
- enhancing the quality of relationships between people;
- appreciating the variety of human experience and culture;
- striving for the fair and adequate provision of counselling and psychotherapy sessions.

Ethical principles

- *Fidelity*: honouring the trust placed in the practitioner;
- *Autonomy*: respect for the client's right to be self-governing;
- *Beneficence*: a commitment to promoting the client's well-being;
- *Non-maleficence*: a commitment to avoiding harm to the client;
- *Justice*: the fair and impartial treatment of all clients and the provision of adequate services;
- *Self-respect*: fostering the practitioner's self-knowledge and care for self.

Personal moral qualities
Empathy, sincerity, integrity, resilience, respect, humility, competence, fairness, wisdom, courage.

the counsellor, their ability to facilitate client autonomy and choice, to provide a climate of privacy and confidentiality (only disclosing information when absolutely essential and with the consent of the client), to always act in the best interests of the client, to work within the limits of counsellor competence, to avoid any form of client exploitation, to uphold the client's human rights, to maintain their personal dignity and to always show a commitment to fairness.

The ways in which these principles are interpreted must always relate to the communication needs and conceptual ability of the client and their capacity for exploring and exhibiting emotions. For example, clients who have limited verbal communication skills may respond better to written language, symbols or visual images. Some counsellors may use tape recordings for the client to replay in the privacy of their own home. This can help them to recall information given by the counsellor and perhaps stimulate questions to address in their next meeting. It should not be assumed that a client's limited communication implies an inability to think or solve problems. Many clients may have an understanding of their problem or situation, but do not possess the vocabulary or the functional ability to communicate this verbally.

Beginning to engage

Assessment and contracting are essential precursors to the counselling process. They demarcate boundaries, expectations and limitations and set the scene for engagement. Once counselling commences, a therapeutic process should begin. Some theorists identify a series of stages through which a form of 'agenda' evolves (e.g. Egan 1982) (see Box 21.3). Essentially the client begins to tell their story, to reveal in a variety of ways the issues of significance to them. Priorities may emerge; the client may disclose information they did not expect to reveal; issues may arise that supersede the initial 'referring problem'. The therapeutic process is fluid and dynamic. The counsellor needs to be receptive and responsive and to demonstrate certain

---

Box 21.3   The helping model (Egan 1982)

STAGE I
Helping the client to explore and clarify their problem/issues

STAGE II
Setting goals

STAGE III
Facilitating action

qualities and skills in order to maximize the experience and the evolving opportunities for deeper exploration.

Human qualities and core conditions

Some of the personal/professional qualities expected of a 'good' counsellor can be interpreted as 'core conditions' of counselling (Rogers 1951; Truax and Carkhuff 1967; Egan 1982; Thorne 1987; Mearns and Thorne 1988). These core conditions provide a fundamental basis from which the therapeutic relationship can develop. They include human warmth, empathy and sincerity, evidence of trustworthiness and honesty, integrity, commitment and competence. They can promote trust and help to develop a safe environment in which the client can relax, explore and grow. Warmth, sincerity, honesty and integrity may naturally exist as human qualities within many individuals. Other qualities may need to be developed or enhanced. For example, many individuals are naturally empathic, but may have difficulty supporting people through deeply emotional experiences. Empathy is often misunderstood as sympathy or total understanding ('I know exactly how you feel . . .'). Empathy as a responding skill provides a means of acknowledging and identifying with the emotions expressed by the client. It can help to facilitate understanding and can clarify issues for both client and counsellor.

Trustworthiness is also assumed to be a natural human quality. However, people engaging in counselling may feel insecure or may have lost the ability to trust others, so trust may need to be re-established in their lives. The gradual development of a counselling relationship can provide an opportunity for trust-building through the provision of mutual respect and a non-judgemental atmosphere, the establishment of emotional boundaries, the maintenance of confidentiality and an overtly person-centred approach. Every counselling situation is unique, and thus no specific time limit can be allocated to the development of a therapeutic relationship. Generally, counsellor and client may have established a level of rapport within the first few meetings, but the potential for trust-building depends largely upon the dynamics of the relationship and the level of comfort experienced by both participants.

It is essential that practising counsellors are competent. Competence is more than a human quality. It involves the application of specific knowledge and skills to a particular context. Counsellors have a responsibility to ensure that they are appropriately equipped to provide a service and to acknowledge their personal and professional limitations. They must also ensure that their work does not become detrimental to their personal health and well-being and that their professional role does not become compromised. Educational programmes leading to a qualification in counselling, at the level of diploma or degree, normally have criteria for performance and assessment. Attainment of criteria is usually measured by appropriately qualified persons such as educationalists, qualified counsellors and counselling supervisors. Educational programmes generally offer academic credits, and while not all programmes are accredited by the British Association for Counselling and Psychotherapy (BACP), most acknowledge the BACP (2002) *Ethical Framework* in their guidelines for practice.

Counselling can be a personally demanding experience and it is important that support strategies exist in order to help the counsellor to function effectively. For example, practising counsellors are generally expected to engage in personal supervision on a regular basis. Employers and professional organizations wanting to regulate the practice of those offering human services generally insist on this. Counselling supervision provides a confidential environment in which professional issues and concerns about practice can be discussed and explored. Sometimes a counsellor may need advice on how to proceed with a particular client or issue, sometimes they may be confronted with issues that effect them on a personal level. In order to provide the best service for clients, counsellors need their own support and guidance. Counsellors are also recommended to engage in their own personal therapy. This can be particularly important when the counsellor is experiencing life traumas or distress themselves. This is something that counsellors would need to organize, and generally pay for, themselves.

Counselling skills

There are a vast range of skills necessary for effective counselling. A novice practitioner would need to practise these skills rigorously and systematically in order to discover their potential in therapeutic work. As the skills become more comfortable to work with, they become internalized and are demonstrated in more natural ways. They are selected according to requirements and become the competent counsellor's 'toolkit'.

It is not possible within the confines of this chapter to identify or examine all the skills required for effective counselling. For ease of reference, brief examples of listening and observing, questioning and responding skills are shown in Boxes 21.4–6. The order in which these skills are presented does not imply level of importance or sequential position in the counselling process. For additional information on counselling skills, please refer to the reference section on p. 432.

Exercise 21.1

'Counselling' is a complex concept. Consider how you would explain counselling to a person who has learning disabilities and limited communication.

Box 21.4   Listening and observing

Passive listening
Indicates attentiveness but does not interfere
Accompanied by facial expressions, gestures and nods
Helpful when clients are deeply emotional or when needing time to think

Active listening
Attentive but more interactive
May involve summarizing and clarification of points raised by the client

Observation
What we observe often communicates feelings more powerfully than what we hear.
   Observation includes noticing body language and movement (e.g. arms/legs crossed, level and nature of eye contact, movements of the head, use of gestures, physical distance, evidence of physical barriers).
   May also include evidence of trembling, sweating, nervous hand gestures, nail biting or skin picking, possibility of diminished self care/personal neglect.

Box 21.5   Questioning

Open questions
Enable development of issues, expansion by the client
Can help to identify and clarify feelings
Facilitate 'flow' and development of the relationship
Help to avoid 'yes' and 'no' answers
Examples include: 'How do you feel about . . .?', 'What did you think about . . .?', 'When did this happen . . .?'

Closed questions
Can help to clarify issues
Enable confirmation by the client
Examples include: 'Did you feel angry about that . . .?', 'Are you unhappy now . . .?'

Exercise 21.2

Please answer the following questions:

Empathy

What does empathy mean to you?

How would you demonstrate it?

Communicating feelings

What communication methods, other than the spoken word, might help a person with learning disability to express their emotions?

How would you use these to help the person?

Ethical issues

What do you feel are the main ethical considerations in counselling practice?

Box 21.6 Responding

Empathy

Attempting to see the client's world through their eyes/within their frame of reference

Feeling, with the client

but also

Acknowledging that, as the helper, one occupies a separate world to the client

Probing

Not being invasive, but using questions/statements that may help to:

Clarify

Define problems more clearly

Prioritize

Establish congruency

Silence

Used in a way to 'hold' the moment

To avoid inappropriate interruption

To facilitate catharsis (expression of emotion)

To communicate time and patience

To create a powerful space for the client

Counselling people who have a learning disability

There are many models and tools that counsellors can use in their work. When working with people with learning disabilities it is essential to be intuitive. When the counsellor has knowledge of this particular client group it is apparent that more than verbal interaction is needed. The development of theoretical approaches in the field of learning disabilities has shifted from the view of Freud in 1905 that talking treatments were not appropriate. This view changed slowly alongside other developments including Wolfensberger's (1972) work on normalization and advocacy groups such as People First (Hodges 2003).

Some people may still underestimate the potential of counselling for people who have learning disabilities. This may be due to assumptions about their level of understanding, their ability to engage with others, their ability to concentrate and participate, to problem-solve and to explore their self-concept. However, many clients, given the opportunity and time, will develop positive relationships in which their shared perception of life and experience will lead to new insight and meaning.

On the other hand, for many clients, the expectation of engaging in an intensive, one-to-one situation dependent largely upon verbal exchange can be daunting and intimidating, rather than empowering. Therefore, counselling skills need to be flexible and accommodating. They need to be applied creatively to facilitate communication and expression of feeling and to enable the client to use the opportunity in a way that has meaning for them. This may include art work, diaries, life maps, life story books, audio/visual work, mirrors, music, drama, relaxation therapy and guided fantasy. The opportunities are endless. Individual counsellors tend to have a specified therapeutic approach and thus may not be qualified to use all these methods. They may, however, be able to access specialist practitioners who can provide these skills.

The case studies that follow demonstrate how theoretical approaches and diverse practical skills can be combined to meet the needs of individuals with learning disabilities. Examples from different stages of the life span are offered as an illustration of the range of circumstances that might lead an individual toward counselling as a therapeutic intervention.

In each scenario a personal picture is drawn, the counselling approach used is summarized and its theoretical base is acknowledged. The intention of these illustrations is to show how different counselling approaches and skills can be tailored to meet the needs of individuals.

Case study: working in school

Mark is 12 and has a learning disability. He was referred to counselling by his GP and the teacher from his special school. Mark had disclosed that he had been abused by his grandfather, but then refused to communicate. Although his grandfather had died he seemed afraid of men and in particular of his mother's boyfriend. Mark came out of his lessons for the counselling sessions and seemed pleased to be singled out to be special. His verbal communication was limited and he had a stammer. However, by using books and objects, he began to engage and appeared at ease. In the second session, the counsellor asked him about his grandfather. Mark began to model sexualized behaviour and started to drop his trousers. The counsellor asked him to stop and gave him a pencil and paper saying, 'Can you draw it for me?' He drew a picture of the act of sexual abuse. The counsellor realized that he had no language for body parts and therefore went through the names for these. This made Mark laugh and he was eager to tell his classmates, so went back to his lesson. This work went on for some time. The counsellor had to bear in mind the impact not only on Mark but also his family, teacher and classmates. By making people aware of the possible changes and responses that might occur after the counselling sessions, they worked out strategies to help and support Mark.

Sources of influence

Mark's beliefs about people were generated from his abusive past. Not only his grandfather, but also his mother and her limited ability to protect him, had created his 'model of the world'. The counsellor worked with Mark's mother who also had a learning disability and had been a victim of abuse. This helped her to be more assertive with her partner, who had mental health problems. She was able to work on her own past and in addition manage Mark's behaviour more effectively. Mark had good role models at school. Moreover, positive beliefs started to emerge. Philips and Buncher (1997) state that other sources of belief can be cartoons, magazines, films or even games we play at school. Mark often took things literally, as with others who have learning disabilities. During a session, the counsellor noticed that he was acting out a computer game while talking to her. Mark's mother had also commented that he was kicking her and being quite nasty. Mark was modelling the behaviour of the person in the game. Therefore, the game needed exchanging for something more suitable and work needed to be undertaken regarding Mark's behaviour.

The models used for the work with Mark were psychodynamic, person-centred, learning and systems theory, alongside teaching social and sexual education. Psychodynamic models relate to the 'dynamic interplay of psychological processes' (Colman 2003) whereas person-centred therapy is more focused on the client and their felt experience of the world as they perceive it (Rogers 1951; Egan 1982; Colman 2003). Much of the early work on learning theory provides the theoretical basis for the behavioural approach. However, as learning theory has continued to evolve, it now takes account of mind and language as important shapers of behaviour and is more frequently found integrated with systems and interactional theory (Pierson 1996). Systems theory is drawn from industrial relations but also applies to 'family therapy and group therapy, in which organisations, families and other groups resemble organisms composed of interdependent parts, each with its own function and pattern of interrelationships with the others' (Colman 2003: 727).

Dryden (1993) suggests that learning and systems theory help us to understand the role of shaping, modelling, generalization, *in vivo* learning (an internal process) and cognitions in determining human behaviour; the importance of problem definition and behavioural analysis in making a diagnostic assessment; and how behavioural, system and dynamic processing operates in marriage and families and can result in disturbed functioning.

Mark's family suffered from a multitude of dysfunctions. Unless the counsellor could begin to understand the complexity of this family, any changes would be difficult to effect. The contribution of psychological theory on cognitive dissonance (inconsistent thoughts), attribution theory, which explains how people perceive, infer, or ascribe causes to their own and other people's behaviour (Colman 2003) and crisis theory all enabled the counsellor to have a greater understanding of change and the family's resistance to it. Crisis management in particular responds to the needs of the individual who is not coping with crisis, aiming to relieve distress, maintain and restore function, enable readjustment and reconstruct long-term patterns of thinking and behaviour (Nelson-Jones 1993; Gelder *et al.* 1994).

In addition to the complex dynamics within the family system, it became apparent that Mark, by the age of 15, had begun to develop sexually abusive behaviours and was accused of sexual assault on two young girls. Abuse in childhood is a risk factor in developing abusive behaviours later on in life, especially for men (Glasser *et al.* 2001). When it was suspected that Mark could be abusing others, he was properly assessed and managed through appropriate risk assessment and treatment. Abuse toward people with learning disability is unfortunately very common and can take many forms including physical, sexual, emotional, financial, neglect and discrimination (Emerson *et al.* 2001). It is essential that counsellors are prepared for this type of work, and that they receive appropriate supervision and support to enable them to work effectively. Often a disclosure of abuse comes unexpectedly and can be made to nurses, teachers or friends. Policies, procedures and training need to be available to support professionals in this process.

Case study: working with adolescents in care

Megan is a 16-year-old girl who has Down's syndrome. She was referred for counselling because of her residential care staff's concerns about her sexual behaviour. This took the form of exposure of her breasts in shops, masturbating while watching television and inserting objects into her vagina.

Megan uses Makaton sign language to communicate and has some words in her vocabulary. Occasional words seem to make little sense in the context in which they are used. By working with the staff team and her mother, the counsellor managed to gather a good history of Megan's life experiences. She had been in care from the age of 3 and had attended residential special school. Her mother felt that her behaviour was not sexual and commented that her pants were too tight or that she was hot. Some of the staff at the home said that she 'should be stopped', using punitive behavioural methods, and others wanted to explore ways of helping her to satisfy her frustrations. One of the words Megan often used was 'ridiculous' which she said after she was observed with her hand down her pants. She would then stand up and run herself a cold bath. The counsellor visited the residential school to gather more information. During this visit she asked if Megan had masturbated at school. It became apparent that Megan had on many occasions disturbed the rest of the children in her dormitory due to getting herself 'into a lather' while masturbating during the night. The night staff had removed her, saying 'this is ridiculous'. The counsellor wondered if they had also given her a cold bath to calm her down, as Megan had learnt this behavioural response from somewhere.

Taking into account Megan's sexual needs, risks, responses from her family and the staff team, the counsellor undertook some group sessions with key people on a need to know basis. After a very intense debate, it was identified that Megan's sexual needs could be met in safety by purchasing a sex aid (vibrator). The counsellor, alongside Megan's key worker, undertook a programme of work with Megan to sensitively introduce this. Signs and pictures were of great help to get the message across to Megan and for her to demonstrate her understanding. Staff and their beliefs were a great challenge to the counsellor. This needed addressing in supervision.

When working in the field of learning disabilities, it is common to find people with fixed beliefs about sexuality. These span from people thinking that learning disabled people have no sexual feelings to those who think that all learning disabled people are deviant in some way. People who have learning disabilities should have the same rights and opportunities as anyone else in society (DoH 2001).

The models used in this case were: person-centred, systemic, group counselling and behavioural approaches which were based on differential reinforcement (e.g. rewarding all positive behaviours that are different to the ones that need to be changed).

Case study: independence

Steven is aged 30 and was a great strain on his parents. The community nurse had been involved with the family for some time and wanted the counsellor to get involved. It took many months for the parents, Bob and Jan, to allow the counsellor to visit. When they eventually agreed they were desperate and commented that they felt like killing their son. The counsellor undertook work with the parents and also helped them with some interventions with Steven. During many sessions the counsellor found that Bob and Jan had never come to terms with their son's disability. They were both living in the past and wanted Steven to be 'normal'. His brother had moved out into his own house and since that time Steven's behaviour had become worse. Not only was he grieving but he also appeared to want to move out too. Bob and Jan were afraid to allow this and when the counsellor explored their reasons it was apparent that they were afraid of potential abuse. They also communicated with Steven as though he was a child, which made him very angry. Steven's speech was not clear and therefore a speech and language therapist worked alongside the counsellor and the parents to devise a communication book. Language patterns were learnt by the parents and modelled to encourage Steven in a more adult manner. Neurolinguistic programming (NLP) and transactional analysis (TA) were used. NLP is a form of psychotherapy and a model of interpersonal communication in the tradition of humanistic psychology, based on elements of transformational grammar and preferred sensory representations for learning and self-expression (Bandler and Grinder 1979; O'Connor and McDermott 1996). TA is both a theory of personality and a form of psychotherapy, originated by the Canadian-born psychoanalyst Eric Berne (1910–70). It aims primarily at improving interpersonal relationships by adjusting the balance between the child, adult and parent ego states that are assumed to coexist within the same personality (Berne 1961, 1964). The parent/child states are learned in childhood and each has positive and negative attributes (nurturing parent, controlling parent, free child, adaptive child). Although we might move in and out of all these states from time to time, the most healthy state for all parties is the adult state – behaviours, thoughts and feelings which are direct responses to the here and now. Problems arise when adults get 'stuck' in habitual ways of behaving. Adaptive child and controlling parent are rarely appropriate states for healthy adult communication (Joines and Stewart 1987).

Work continues with Bob and Jan and each have tried to use the strategies devised in their counselling sessions. This helps to a degree, but the biggest hurdle for them will be to let Steven live away from home. This brings up the argument that Steven should be able to enjoy a 'normal' life, according to his parents. Unfortunately, his parents feel that they cannot accept Steven for who he is. Steven himself is very happy mixing with his peers and professionals feel that he could move on and develop his life in the community.

Case study: working with a couple

Molly and Jack were referred by the courts and social services for a learning disability assessment and an 'ability to parent' assessment. Molly had served time in prison for the abuse of her first child. She was now with a new partner, married and due to give birth to their baby in six months. On meeting Molly, the counsellor realized that she had problems with her hearing. The counsellor immediately referred Molly to a speech and language therapist for a hearing assessment. Molly did have significant hearing loss and therefore needed a hearing aid. During the assessment, the counsellor uncovered a large amount of information. Molly had suffered abuse from her father as a child and then she became involved with a drug user who also abused her. Her first child was in danger from her boyfriend and she would often pull the child away from him in an effort to protect her. However, this behaviour caused the child injuries, which were mainly twist fractures. The counsellor worked with Molly to come to terms with her past and the loss of her child, who had been adopted. Molly needed to be assertive and her new husband was a little overpowering, although he was generally a good person. The counsellor undertook some work with them both as a couple while continuing to assess their knowledge of child care. Jack would often use threats about 'child protection' coming to remove their baby if Molly did not do as he said. This tactic was used in everyday family arguments. Due to their compliance with the work, social services allowed them to take their new baby daughter home. Careful monitoring took place and the counselling work continued to address the couple's understanding of power relations within a family. Molly became more assertive and Jack more understanding. They worked hard to do everything that was asked of them and soon became comfortable with key people with whom they felt they could relate. This enabled them to choose a team of professionals who met their needs and negotiate the times of their visits. Both parents were loving and willing to learn. Molly often took things literally and professionals needed guidance from the counsellor on their communication with her.

In this case there was a successful conclusion, unlike many parents with learning disability who have their children removed. Molly and Jack went on to have a little boy two years later. They now have little contact with professionals and care for their children very well. Molly has good coping strategies and if Jack 'gets on at her', she says she switches her hearing aid off. The models used in this case were: person-centred, systemic, NLP and modelling behaviours as part of the teaching programme. Work with other professionals (e.g. health visitors, midwives and social workers) was undertaken in groups and on an individual basis.

Working with someone who has a sensory problem may be a challenge. However, counsellors and other professionals need to be aware of the way each individual processes information and how best we can communicate with that individual. By calibrating a person's response to questions or information, the counsellor can make an assessment of the individual's learning and processing style. New information needs to be presented using a range of sensory techniques. We experience the world through our five senses, known as VAKOG: visual (what we see), auditory (what we hear), kinaesthetic (movement), olfactory (what we smell) and gustatory (what we taste).

Molly had many disadvantages in life and slipped through the educational net due to many factors. One was obviously her undiagnosed hearing problem. Molly was labelled as inattentive or ignorant at school. Another reason was her strong kinaesthetic preference, and since Molly needed to move in order to learn, it made sense to incorporate movement whenever she was presented with new information. Although most people can learn through any of their senses, some people who have a very strong preference for one can find it difficult or impossible to take in information unless it is presented in this mode. Therefore, telling Molly how to do something, even when she was wearing her hearing aid, seemed useless at times. The midwife would often say, 'I have told her lots of times and she hasn't understood.' The counsellor would suggest *showing* her, and then letting her demonstrate her understanding. This process needed to be modelled and reinforced many times.

Case study: moving out in a crisis

Jean was 50 when the community nurse referred her in a crisis. The day centre had initially referred Jean, who has Down's syndrome, after they had seen her kissing another service user. The community nurse began to assess her sexual knowledge using the 'Not a Child Any More' assessment pack. Jean was a very vulnerable and naïve lady who lived with her 90-year-old father. During the assessment, the community nurse displayed different forms of contraception on a tray. She asked Jean is she knew what they were. Jean said that you took the pill when you were poorly. She thought the coil would be used to measure things with but she knew what the plastic thing was (condom). She went on to say, 'It's what he uses on his long thing when he puts it up my bottom.' 'He' was her brother-in-law. The community nurse immediately contacted the social worker and the counsellor. Jean was going home that night to her brother-in-law's house as her father was away. Jean's life was about to turn upside down, as she was whisked off to be examined at the hospital and not allowed to go home after that day. The police were informed and an investigation was carried out. Jean was placed in a safe house. Moreover, her father was shocked on his return. Her sister stopped speaking to her and she was very distressed. The counselling would need to be handled carefully as it could be seen as interfering with, or leading, the witness. It therefore took the form of support and someone to talk to, rather than making therapeutic changes. Everyone had to be careful not to put words in Jean's mouth, even though she had no language for body parts.

This support continued but Jean's mental and physical state deteriorated. She began to lose her skills and fell over quite a lot. Her memory was impaired and she was showing signs of possible dementia. The counsellor was sure that this was more likely to be a manifestation of post-traumatic stress and was concerned that if the defence were to suspect that Jean was suffering from dementia they would say that she was unfit to stand as a witness. Fortunately, the trial took place and Jean made a very good witness. The barrister did try to use simple language, but at times he confused Jean and she would say, 'I'm confused'. The counsellor was worried that the court would think that Jean was not a reliable witness. During lunch, the counsellor worked with Jean to help her respond appropriately to questioning. She said to Jean that it was the barrister's fault, not hers. They then practised what to say. The counsellor would use some big words to Jean and then Jean would say, 'You are confusing me'. After lunch, the barrister started to question Jean again using big words and she told him that he was confusing her. Jean made a great witness and even though she could not remember the dates and times, she did remember that her father was on holiday in Skegness. The brother-in-law was convicted and served a long prison sentence. Jean moved into appropriate accommodation, received counselling and now lives a happy life.

Working with Jean through the trauma and helping her to make some sense of her experience needed a great deal of patience and understanding of how she interpreted her world and experiences. Jean's eye movements indicated how she was thinking. When individuals are trying to imagine or remember something, they literally look around inside their heads. When their eyes stop before they focus back on you is the point at which they have found that information. Looking up usually indicates someone visualizing, while looking to one side (or putting one's head on one side or touching one's ear) can indicate listening to an internal voice or sound. Looking down usually indicates someone accessing feelings or having an internal dialogue. Some people misinterpret this as ignorance and not wanting to give eye contact. However, it generally means that the person is experiencing emotion or recalling a feeling. In Jean's case, 'visual' was her predominant preference, followed by some 'auditory' experience when trying to remember events. However, she became stuck in 'kinaesthetic', looking down and not being able to move from the overwhelming feelings that gripped her. To help her, the counsellor reminded her to look up and focus on something high to enable visual recall. This enabled the counsellor to undertake visual change work with Jean.

Conclusion

It is important that the psychological well-being of people with learning disabilities is recognized throughout their lives. Counselling can be a great help during challenging times, enabling people to process events, stress or trauma more effectively. Hence, carers and professionals need to actively respond to the needs of learning disabled people who may not themselves be aware that such help is available.

References

BACP (British Association for Counselling and Psychotherapy) (1997) *Code of Ethics for Practice for Counsellors*. London: BACP.

BACP (British Association for Counselling and Psychotherapy) (2002) *Ethical Framework for Good Practice in Counselling and Psychotherapy*. Rugby: BACP.

Bandler, R. and Grinder, J. (1979) *Frogs into Princes*. Moab, UT: Real People Press.

Berne, E. (1961) *Transactional Analysis in Psychotherapy*. New York: Grove Press.

Berne, E. (1964) *Games People Play*. New York: Grove Press.

Bond, T. (1993) *Standards and Ethics for Counselling in Action*. London: Sage.

Colman, A.M. (2003) *Oxford Dictionary of Psychology*. Oxford: Oxford University Press.

DoH (Department of Health) (2001) *Valuing People: A New Strategy for Learning Disability for the 21st Century*. London: Department of Health.

Dryden, W. (ed.) (1993) *Individual Therapy: A Handbook*. Buckingham: Open University Press.

Egan, G. (1982) *The Skilled Helper*, 2nd edn. Monterey, CA: Brooks/Cole.

Emerson, E., Hatton, C., Felce, D. and Murphy, G. (2001) *Learning Disabilities: The Fundamental Facts*. London: The Mental Health Foundation.

Freud, S. (1905) *Fragment of an Analysis of a case of Hysteria*. Standard edition 7, pp. 3–122.

Gelder, M., Gath, D. and Mayou, R. (1994) *Concise Textbook of Psychiatry*. Oxford: Oxford University Press.

Gillon, R. (1985) Autonomy and consent, in M. Lockwood (ed.) *Moral Dilemmas in Modern Medicine*. Oxford: Oxford University Press.

Glasser, M., Kolvin, I., Campbell, D. and Glasser, A. (2001) Cycle of child sexual abuse; links between being a victim and becoming a perpetrator, *British Journal of Psychiatry*, 179: 482–94.

Hodges, S. with contributions from Nancy Sheppard (2003) *Counselling Adults with Learning Disabilities: Basic text in Counselling and Psychotherapy*. London: Macmillan.

Joines, V. and Stewart, I. (1987) *TA Today*. London: Sage.

Mearns, D. and Thorne, B. (1988) *Person-Centred Counselling in Action*. London: Sage.

Nelson-Jones, R. (1993) *The Theory and Practice of Counselling and Psychology*. London: Cassell.

O'Connor, J. and McDermott, I. (1996) *Principles of NLP*. London: Thorsons.

Pierson, J. (1996) The behavioural approach to social work, in C. Harvey and T. Philpot (eds) *Practising Social Work*. London: Routledge.

Philips, G. and Buncher, L. with Stevenson, B. (1997) *Gold Counselling: A Practical Psychology with NLP*. Camarthen: The Anglo American Book Company Ltd.

Rogers, C.R. (1951) *Client-Centered Therapy: Its Current Practice, Implications and Theory*. Boston, MA: Houghton Mifflin.

Sugarman, L. (1992) Ethical issues in counselling at work, *British Journal of Guidance and Counselling*, 20(1): 64–74.

Thorne, B. (1987) Beyond the core conditions, in W. Dryden (ed.) *Key Cases in Psychotherapy*. London: Croom Helm.

Truax, C.B. and Carkhuff, R.R. (1967) *Toward Effective Counseling and Psychotherapy*. Chicago: Aldine Publishers.

Wolfensberger, W. (1972) *The Principle of Normalisation in Human Services*. Toronto: National Institute of Mental Retardation.

PART FOUR
Social inclusion and adulthood

In the fourth part of the book we continue to follow the life cycle by moving from adolescence towards a focus on adulthood. When this shift occurs it is relative and differs from person to person, family to family and culture to culture. For example, in many Gypsy and Traveller communities it is common for people to take on adult responsibilities from around 14 years of age, whereas in more sedentary societies it appears permissible to avoid adulthood at least until 18, or even later.

The nature of adulthood is similarly variable as some people view the move towards adulthood as a 'loss', as giving things up. Such people speak of lost innocence, the passing of youth and the end of freedom. However, others view it more positively and welcome an adult's ability to take responsibility, make decisions and contribute to the society of which they are a part.

Central to this more positive view of adulthood, and a significant factor in social inclusion, is the ability and opportunity to engage with work and leisure pursuits; to broaden the scope of social networks, friends and acquaintances; and to establish independent and culturally congruent patterns of living.

Grappling with such issues of potential loss and the prospect of increasing autonomy can be rewarding but is also challenging and daunting for everyone, no matter what gender, culture, ethnicity or social class. Not so many years ago some people, such as those with learning disabilities, were excluded from this challenge and consigned to a lifetime of near total dependency and isolation from the larger society. Although marked progress has been made in recent years, the chapters within this section demonstrate that there is still a long way to go and give some indication of how you can help.

In Chapter 22, Gwynnyth Llewellyn and David McConnell challenge the presumption that people with learning disabilities cannot be adequate parents by showing how in many ways the joys and problems of child rearing are shared by all parents, with or without disability. However, like all families, those featured in the five stories are unique and face different and diverse challenges, so few generalizations can, or should, be drawn. As the chapter unfolds we see repeated examples of how parents with a learning disability have not only to contend with new babies and growing children but also the barriers that arise from stereotypical views and misconceptions within society and service agencies regarding their capabilities as parents. Despite having their competency questioned and their ability to learn and to cope challenged, the narratives demonstrate a remarkable resilience that allows parents with learning disabilities to achieve, with support, successful quality lives for themselves and their families. The chapter will help the reader to better understand:

- the major themes and areas of concern that arise from the literature on parents with learning disabilities;
- the range of challenges and the diversity of potential solutions;
- the scope of coping strategies and the efficacy of factors that promote resilience;
- the implications for practitioners and service delivery in providing appropriate and sensitive support.

Chapter 23 by Roy McConkey highlights the centrality of friendships to the quality of life of us all, but especially those people with learning disabilities. The potential for such people to lead relatively impoverished lives because of derogatory and stigmatized views on capacity and risk-taking highlights the increased need to pay attention to forming friendships, rather than just having acquaintances. However, studies across a range of settings show that little emphasis is placed by carers and service personnel on developing the skills and strategies that promote friendships. This is seen as particularly unfortunate as developing and maintaining friendships requires a considerable level of social skills. By articulating specific areas of potential need and helpful strategies to support people to develop a wider network of social relationships and friendships the reader is encouraged to consider:

- the extent of loneliness, its origins and causes, and the effects on the lives of people with learning disabilities;
- the rewards and benefits that friendships bring to people's lives;
- the personal, social and attitudinal issues involved in promoting and sustaining relationships and friendships;
- the role of carers in supporting people to widen their social networks, relationships and friendships.

Person-centred planning (PCP) is the focus of Chapter 24. In exploring the important differences between individual programme planning (IPP) and PCP, Jacqui Brewster and Paul Ramcharan identify the importance of locating power and control with the individual and their family. By teasing out the relationship of needs and wishes it is suggested that PCP opens up care to encompass not only individuals but also neighbourhoods and communities alongside service provision. Utilizing examples, Brewster and Ramcharan provide insights into how PCP might be operationalized within the present policy context. Through this the reader is helped to gain a greater understanding of:

- what being person-centred entails;
- listening and hearing what people with learning disabilities want and value;
- ways of eliciting support from family, friends and associates within PCP;
- the strengths and potential weaknesses of this particular approach.

In Chapter 25, Ghazala Mir and Raghu Raghavan draw attention to the systematic discrimination that contributes to the higher levels of ill health in some minority ethnic communities. They also highlight that belonging to such a community can confer a degree of strength, support and resilience. Using examples from the lives of people with learning disabilities from South Asian and African Caribbean backgrounds, the chapter identifies a deficit in the level of cultural competency demonstrated by some service professionals. This is all the more disappointing in that the need for substantial amounts of support in order for people to access health and social care services is supported by research. In exploring the relationship between integrated or specialist services for those from minority ethnic communities, a parallel is drawn with similar debates relating to specific or generic services for people with learning disabilities, which in turn begs the question of the needs of people from an ethnic minority with a learning disability. In pointing to some possible answers, the chapter seeks to provide the reader with an appreciation of:

- the need to view all communities as diverse and all individuals as unique;
- the importance of advocacy and the role played by key individuals and support groups;
- the absence of targets and monitoring systems in relation to cultural competence that create ambiguity;
- ways in which individuals and existing services can develop more effective services.

The importance of work, learning and leisure is the focus of Chapter 26. In this chapter, Nick Fripp provides a review of the historical context of work, learning and leisure in order to identify its segregationist legacy. This chapter draws from the views expressed by people with learning disabilities and uses them to critically appraise current policy initiatives in relation to some fundamental needs and values that apply to people with learning disabilities just as much as the rest of society. In this chapter the reader is encouraged to consider:

- the nature and meaning of work, learning and leisure;
- the role of national policy in setting the context within which people operate;
- the barriers to access that are encountered by people with learning disabilities;
- current initiatives in the light of national policy.

In Chapter 27, Chris Hatton and John Taylor explore the nature of mental health and grapple with fundamental questions concerning the nature of mental health and mental illness. In doing so there is a recognition that life circumstances, life events and a range of other factors can challenge, but also strengthen, mental equilibrium. People with learning disabilities, because of prejudice and stereotyping, are as likely, if not more so, to encounter a range of potentially challenging circumstances as anyone else. Additionally the factors that may support the resilience of people with learning disabilities may be less accessible. This chapter will assist the reader to better appreciate the problematic nature of mental health and the significant obstacles that people who have a learning disability as well as a mental health problem can face in accessing support and appropriate assistance. In particular the reader's attention is drawn to the following:

- mental health and its relationship to people with learning disabilities;
- the barriers to recognizing mental health problems and accessing services for people with learning disabilities;
- diagnostic and assessment issues;
- the range of possible interventions including biological and psychosocial treatment modalities.

Drawing extensively from two detailed case studies, in Chapter 28, Gordon Grant and Paul Ramcharan address the issue of whether intensive personalized support is sufficient. In describing the complexities of people's lives, this chapter notes the potential for superficial social contact to mask the presence of loneliness and lack of inclusion. The emphasis by service providers on risk and protection, whilst important, can be seen as having the potential to stifle access to meaningful things such as work, wealth and friendships. The chapter concludes by identifying some ways in which communities can contribute to enhancing the lives of people with learning disabilities and areas in which service provision can be strengthened. The narratives and helpful commentary and analysis provide the reader with an appreciation of:

- different models of service provision;
- the need to listen to the voices of those who are 'living the life';
- the potential for greater community involvement;
- the need to address social and economic barriers as well as individually-generated ones.

In the final chapter of this section, Paul Ramcharan and Malcolm Richardson take a critical view of community support in relation to person-centred approaches to supporting people with learning disabilities. They argue that a community development approach, in tandem with PCP and intensive personalized support discussed in the previous chapter, is necessary for sustained success, as defined by people with learning disabilities. Utilizing two case examples and a range of exercises, the reader is encouraged to develop a critical awareness of the nature and mechanisms of support networks, social relationships and the fulfilment of human needs. In particular the reader's attention is drawn to:

- ecological approaches to communities of interest;
- social policy and theoretical dimensions;
- community development issues;
- establishing, developing and sustaining approaches over protracted periods of time.

22

You have to prove yourself all the time

People with learning disabilities as parents

Gwynnyth Llewellyn and David McConnell

With Lynne, Debbie, Kylie, Joy & Shirley, and Robert & Julie

Introduction

This chapter is about people with learning disabilities being parents. Before you read further take a moment to think about how society regards parents and parenting on the one hand and on the other how people with learning disabilities are usually portrayed.

Exercise 22.1

As the first exercise in this chapter, write down in one column a list of terms or phrases that come to mind when you think about parents and parenting. Write down words or phrases that are commonly used about people with learning disabilities in a second column. Are the two lists similar or different?

For some people, parenting by those with learning disabilities is controversial. This is not surprising. In our society, parenting is an important marker of adulthood and social status. Being a parent implies maturity and responsibility. In contrast, the popular view of people with learning disabilities is that they are childlike or childish. This implies that they are unlikely to become adult and therefore are not capable of taking on adult roles like parenting. This stereotypical view about people with learning disabilities makes it hard for others to imagine they could be parents. It is as if people with learning disabilities, being viewed as children themselves, could not possibly be responsible for their own children. This pessimistic view has led to many challenges for people with learning disabilities becoming or wanting to become parents.

The stories of five families headed by parents with learning disabilities are central to this chapter. Their narratives illustrate the challenges and the achievements typically found in the lives of parents with learning disabilities. Their stories also speak to the particularity of each parent and their family's circumstances. From their individual and collective experience we can begin to understand the place of parenthood in achieving successful, quality lives.

Prior to introducing the family narratives, we identify major themes in the literature concerning parenting by people with learning disabilities. The emphasis placed on particular topics at different times illustrates the changing nature of beliefs about whether people with learning disabilities should or could be parents. From the narratives we draw lessons that challenge the presumption that people with learning disabilities cannot be adequate parents. We invite you to explore the literature in the resources section (see p. 464) which is arranged around the major themes discussed in the next section.

A word of caution is necessary in relation to the literature about parenting by people with learning disabilities. First, various terms are used to describe parents reflecting the differences in acceptable terminology across countries. These terms include mentally retarded or intellectually handicapped parents, parents with intellectual disability and parents with learning disabilities or learning difficulties. Second, the parents included in research studies rarely represent all parents with learning disabilities. For practical reasons, the parents studied are generally those already known to social care or disability agencies. We therefore know much less about parents with learning disabilities who have not been identified and referred to the service system. Third, although the literature refers to parents with learning disabilities, in reality studies typically only include mothers. There is a very large gap in the literature, and we know almost nothing about fathers with learning disabilities.

Themes in the literature on parenting for people with learning disabilities

Preventing conception

Until the middle of the twentieth century, concern about people with learning disabilities becoming parents was a major reason for segregating young men and women with such disabilities from the rest of the community. Young women were often placed in institutional 'care' on the presumption that they were (or would become) promiscuous. Within the institutional walls, men and women were separated from each other. Young women and to a lesser extent men with learning disabilities were routinely sterilized to prevent another generation of 'feeble-minded' people. This eugenic fear that people with learning disabilities would reproduce a large number of genetically inferior offspring was eventually discredited. Research has demonstrated that the majority of children born to parents with learning disabilities do not experience such disabilities themselves. References for review articles can be found on page 465.

The question of competence

As institutions closed, the possibility of people with learning disabilities becoming parents again came under close scrutiny. As younger people with learning disabilities were now out and about in their local community there was growing concern that they too, in similar vein to their peers, may want to become parents. One of the first questions to be asked was whether they would be able to be adequate parents. Interestingly, a study conducted by Mickelson as early as 1947 concluded that many people with learning disabilities were capable of looking after their children. This study was the first of many to investigate this question of parental competence, also covered in the review articles.

Parents' ability to learn

During the 1970s the emphasis changed from questioning parental competence to questioning whether parents had the capacity to learn. Alexander Tymchuk and Maurice Feldman in North America pioneered the use of applied behavioural techniques to teach parenting tasks to parents with learning disabilities. These techniques include the opportunity to learn skills in the situation where these will be applied; use of illustrated material and demonstration; and practice opportunities with positive reinforcement. Together the studies on parent learning demonstrated that parents with learning disabilities can and do learn child care, home safety, child health and parent-child interaction skills. Over the next two decades, parent education programmes broadened the skills to be taught and expanded the range of techniques for learning (see 'Parent learning' in the resources section, p. 464).

A focus on children

At around the same time that parent education programmes were being developed, interest was growing in how the children of parents with learning disabilities fared. Earlier, as we have seen, the primary concern was that the children would inherit defective genes (the 'nature' argument). With the demise of the eugenics movement, attention was redirected to the quality of care that their parents provided (the 'nurture' argument). In the earlier research, parental neglect was defined primarily as poor household organization and low standards of cleanliness. Commentators explained parents' deficiencies in this area as due to their knowing no better (an act of omission) rather than purposeful neglect of their children. Although household cleanliness remained a key factor in determining neglect, by the late 1980s inadequate stimulation had become the defining feature.

The key question at this time was: what are the outcomes for children reared by parents with learning disabilities? Investigators focused mostly on outcomes for younger children. The clear message from these studies is of substantial variation among children of parents with learning disabilities, with most children meeting age-norm expectations. An influential factor appears to be the presence of at least one consistent and supportive adult in children's lives, an indicator of resilience also found in the lives of children in other potentially vulnerable situations (see 'Outcomes for children' in the resources section, p. 465).

Despite this evidence, family and children's court studies in Australia, the USA and the UK suggest that parents with learning disabilities are 15 to 50 times more likely than other parents in the community to have their children removed and placed in care. These studies also demonstrate that allegations of abuse by parents with learning disabilities are rare. Children are removed more often on the grounds that they are 'at risk' of harm due to neglect – that is, their parents' presumed inability to provide a safe, healthy and nurturing environment. Many authors have noted that the prejudicial belief that people with learning disabilities cannot learn is a major factor in court decisions to remove children. Another factor influencing court decisions is the lack of support services that are able and/or willing to support parents in their parenting role (see 'Court studies' in the resources section, p. 465).

Support to parents in their parenting role

The well-documented relationship between social support and maternal health led researchers to explore the influence of support on outcomes for parents with learning disabilities and their children. The findings from quantitative and qualitative studies demonstrate substantial variations in the type of support offered and the way it is provided. As Tucker and Johnson noted in 1989, support to parents with learning disabilities fell into one of two types: competence-promoting or competence-inhibiting. People offering the competence-promoting type of support helped parents to learn and achieve by themselves. In contrast, those offering competence-inhibiting support 'did for' the parent rather than helping the parent to do for themselves. Competence-inhibiting support denied parents the opportunity to learn, undermined their confidence and made their situation worse. A key factor in determining the effectiveness of support is how parents perceive the support they are offered. Several practice tools for assessing the nature, type and frequency of support are now available (see 'Maternal health and social support' in the resources section, p. 466).

Service delivery

With the growing number of referrals of parents with learning disabilities to health and social care agencies in the 1990s, the emphasis changed to issues of service delivery and practice. The key question became which services, either community-based or specialist disability, are most appropriate to meet the needs of parents with learning disabilities and their children. Building up to a recent series of reports in the UK and elsewhere, most commentators favour parents with learning disabilities being included in community-based services and offered specialist disability services only when appropriate adaptations cannot be made (see 'Service delivery and family support' and 'Reports' in the resources section, p. 466). Principles to guide development and delivery of support include:

- services need to be family-centred in contrast to a parent-only or child-only focus;
- services need to emphasize prevention as a priority rather than crisis intervention;
- services need to take a strengths-based rather than deficit approach to intervention;
- services need to be tailored to meet the individual support needs of each parent and family;
- services need to provide support for parents with learning disabilities over the long term;
- services need to provide flexible support, recognizing that the intensity of support required waxes and wanes as children develop and life circumstances change.

Parent voices

A new development in the literature pays attention to parents' voices to understand their experiences of parenting. The seminal work of Tim and Wendy Booth in the UK gave credit for the first time to parents with learning disabilities as experts on their own lives. The increasing recognition and documentation of parents' voices provides a dramatic counterpoint to the mostly negative portrayal of their lives in the literature and popular press (see 'Voices of parents' in the resources section, p. 467).

The family stories that follow are constructed from interview material we have gathered over many years and our personal knowledge of the parents and their families. Wherever possible the parents' own words are used. We ask you to place yourself imaginatively in their shoes. While reading each family story, note down particular points that strike you. Before going on to the next story, note down how the issues raised illustrate more generally societal beliefs about parenting or learning disabilities, service philosophies or practices.

A little joy: *Lynne's story*

The first story is Lynne's. She is 38. Her 5-year-old daughter Joy was removed by child protection services shortly after her birth. Lynne did not have the opportunity to take her daughter home. Only recently could she bring herself to part with the cot that stood ready but unused. Three or four times a year Lynne travels nine hours by train to be with her daughter for several hours. This occurs on scheduled access visits that are supervised by child protection staff.

On loss

I nearly lost Joy. I had an infection and very high blood pressure, and she was born very early. I didn't know what the heck was going on. I had tubes in my nose, and there were doctors and nurses around watching me like a hawk. I said, 'Can I visit my daughter?' They said, 'No, you are too sick and she is too sick as well.' They were telling me to sleep, to go to sleep, but I just wanted to see her. I don't know how long I was in intensive care. When I finally got to see her I just broke down. She was so small. There were tubes in her nose. I was scared and sad when I saw her. I felt hopeless. I just wished I could do more for her. She was fighting for her life.

Craig and his family wanted me to 'get rid of the kid', but I wanted to have a go. I wasn't planning to get pregnant, I just did. He denied being the father. He wouldn't put his name down on the birth certificate. He didn't want anything to do with her. If I had my time over I wouldn't get involved with a person like that. We met when I was working at a sheltered workshop. We started off as friends at first, but he turned out to be a ratbag. I thought we were friends, but it was a funny friendship. He was basically just using me for sex. He wouldn't take no for an answer. In a way I am blaming myself for that.

Little Joy spent quite a few months in hospital. I just hated leaving her there. I went back and forwards from the hospital to visit her each day. When they said, yeah, you can take your daughter home, I was so excited, and scared, all at the same time. Little Joy and I took a taxi from the hospital to Karitane, a place where you can live while you learn how to take care of your baby. We spent two weeks there. They treated me just like everyone else, and everyone was a big help to little Joy, and it was OK. They said I could take my daughter home, but they were worried because I was alone.

The staff at Karitane wanted to organize some support for me so I could take Joy home. They called DOCS [social services] because there are not many services around so that people with disabilities can take their kids home. The DOCS workers came, they said yeah I could take my daughter home, and I thought OK, they are really nice people. But the more they came out they started to look down on me as a disability person.

To be treated like a disability person is to be treated like you got something wrong with you. As if I am dumb as anything, a total idiot. I don't know how to behave like a disability person. I only behave like a normal person. Sometimes I make mistakes, but who doesn't? To me there is no such thing as disabilities really. To me that is just a tag. I want to be treated just like everyone else, like a normal person, a person who can do things and learn things. To me everyone is normal, no matter what they got wrong with them, I mean, the way I see it, no one is perfect.

Looking back, I think DOCS knew what they were doing right from the word go. They told me I could take my daughter home, but they were probably thinking, 'we are going to take her baby away, here is why, because her family don't want nothing to do with her, they want nothing to do with her child, she has no family support at all, she is a disability person, and what with her epilepsy, she hasn't a hope in heck of being able to look after her baby'. I asked them to give me a go; they said, 'No, our boss won't let us.' I even asked the boss. She said, 'No, because our main concern is the baby, and look we are not saying you are an unfit mother or anything, it is just that our first priority has to be the baby.' They reckoned I wouldn't cope, but how could they know? All I needed was a chance and someone to help me.

What ended up happening was the fire alarm went off twice on one day and DOCS were putting the pressure on me. That is when I went to the bathroom, locked the door and just broke down. In other words, I cried, I went hysterical. Well who wouldn't? I said look, take her, I don't want her. I said that but I didn't really mean it. They took her then and there. They took little Joy away from me. I took it very hard. I was feeling numb, scared and confused. To be frank I think the way they did it was hitting below the belt, and wasn't called for really. They called the police! They probably thought 'we will get the police just in case things turn nasty'. Don't worry; I didn't threaten them or anything like that.

On trial

At first I was allowed to see little Joy every week, but it had to be supervised at the DOCS office. I was going back and forth to the court. I wanted to have a go at being a mum. I am a trier not a quitter. After three or four months they stuck Joy and me in a refuge together. The refuge was noisy with other people's troubles. I don't think it was a good place for Joy and me. We didn't fit in. I mean I am no Einstein, but for crying out loud, you don't put a parent in a refuge to learn parenting skills!

Then what happened was, I got taught so many different ways how to care for Joy it was confusing. I was trying my best to have a go at being a mum. But I was on tenterhooks, and thinking 'what are they going to do next?'. I was going back and forth to court, and what with hearing all the problems in the refuge, and with DOCS coming and putting the pressure on me, it was all too much. I snapped. And that is when DOCS took Joy to the foster carers where she has been ever since. The day they took her away, for the second time, I couldn't bear to see her go. I just had to turn my back. They said, 'You sure you don't want to give her a goodbye kiss or anything like that?' I said, 'Just take her away.' I wish I had given her that kiss now.

The court case went on for more than one year. There were tests, tests and more tests. I saw a psychologist. She made me put blocks together and say what was missing from the pictures. I think the questions were dumb. She said she was on my side. But when she got in the stand she said something like, 'Lynne is a lovely person, but because of her disability I don't think she can manage without a lot of support.' And she didn't think that kind of support would be there for me. DOCS won the case. I was upset, but I was glad it was over. I mean I had been suicidal. I had wanted to destroy myself. It might sound weird, but just coming out of that court case knowing I didn't actually kill myself has made me stronger. I survived.

On love

Joy is now 4 turning 5 years old. The foster carers moved away, so Joy is a nine-hour train trip from home. I love Joy. And I will admit I miss her like anything. Sometimes she calls me mummy, but mostly she calls the foster carers mummy and daddy. That makes me feel sad really. The last time I saw her she came running up behind me and put her arms around me. I said, 'I love you Joy.' The woman who was supervising the access visit said she knows who her mother is, which I am glad about really because I wasn't sure if she knew who her mother was or not.

I have nothing against the foster carers. They are spoiling her. I can see why. Joy is the baby of all the kids, and they get on really well together. There have been some very difficult times though. I remember the first time I met the foster carers. It was during the court case. Apparently they didn't want Joy at first, but they took her anyway. The first thing they said to me was, 'She is good', and they said, 'We love her to death and treat her as part of the family'. I thought 'What? My daughter? In your dreams. You are not going to adopt her sweetie!'

I told myself, 'Lynne, don't you dare put her up for adoption.' A lady said to me I might as well. I thought no, I can't. I mean I just can't. I would never forgive myself. She might come back and say, 'Why did you give me up for adoption? What happened? Mum why? I mean you are supposed to be my mother.' I couldn't do it. I mean OK, this might sound stupid, but I would rather lose the roof over my head than I would my daughter.

On hope

I live for my visits with Joy. Deciding what we might do together is the hardest part. I don't know the town very well, and what the possibilities are. But we always have fun together. Sometimes we go to a park or to the movies, but we always seem to end up at Kids World. There have been hard times. Like when Joy told me she didn't want to see me the next day. I think she was going to miss out on doing something with her friends. I said that was OK, even though it hurt like heck. And not only that, another time Joy asked me to read her a book. She ended up reading it to me! I was so embarrassed. When I got back home I enrolled in a literacy course to improve my reading and writing. Now I am a much better reader. I can almost read a whole book to Joy!

The fight goes on. But do you know what? DOCS has just agreed to unsupervised access! This means that I can spend time with Joy without anyone looking over my shoulder. And they gave me some encouragement a few weeks back. They said, 'Lynne, you are not so tense, you are more comfortable with Joy.' DOCS have treated me better since I dropped the appeal.

And what if they returned Joy now? Well I would welcome her with open arms. I would hug her. I might never let her go! I think I would be an overprotective mother. I'd make sure she gets to school safely and on time for that matter. But getting her back would take a miracle. I will always love little Joy. So if she says, 'Mum, let's live together,' I will say OK. A lady told me that when she is 18 years old she has to move on from the foster carers and she can live where she wants. Maybe she will want to live with me.

Cutting the cord: *Debbie's story*

The second story comes from Debbie. She has four children, all boys, the youngest of whom is 9 months of age. Debbie is happily married to Glen, who has a good job and makes a good living. She has a wide network of friends, a home of her own, and loves being a mother. Now life is good. But this was not always the case. When we first met Debbie in 1995 she was struggling to be free from a controlling mother and abusive partner.

On school and work

I had a hard life. In high school I was teased and bullied. One day some older students threw chairs at me. I had to get stitches in my head. My mother took me out of school. I was sent to a special school. It was like a workshop. I learned reading, writing and maths. I even learned to tell the time. I was 15 and one half before I could tell the time!

When I left school I got a job in a 'disability workshop'. I mostly did office work, which I really liked doing. But if you ask me, it was a bit of slave labour. The best thing about that job was meeting Marie. She was my supervisor. We got on really well together. She became my best friend, and we used to go out together after work. Marie was with me when I met my husband Glen, and she was the maid of honour at my wedding.

I just started going to TAFE [technical and further education college]. I'm getting my reading and writing better. We also do maths and get to use the computers. At TAFE my teacher is helping me to write the story of my fourth son's birth. One day, when all the kids are at school, I might want to go back to work.

About my mother

My mother made my life miserable. She never thought I could do anything. She'd never let me do things in the kitchen when I was growing up.
I was never allowed to have my own money, she used to keep it and
control what I could spend it on. She did this even when I was on my
own looking after Nathan! She made all my decisions for me. I was never
in control of my own life. My sisters always had their own money and
they were allowed to do things. I was the one she saw as stupid and
dumb. She never thought I'd be able to look after myself, or look after
my children.

When I got pregnant with Nathan she was on at me to get an abortion. She told me I'd never be able to look after a baby. When I refused
to have an abortion she told me she'd ring up welfare and put my baby
up for adoption. She couldn't do that, because I had to agree to it. After
Nathan was born and after I had kicked my partner out, I was on my
own for just two days when 'the welfare' turned up at the door to check
that everything was going alright. I'm sure my mother phoned them and
told them to go and check on me. But I proved her wrong. For five years
I looked after Nathan by myself. People used to say to me, 'You do a
good job with your son.'

Whenever I got pregnant mum always gets on at me to have an
abortion. Only once was she happy when I told her I was pregnant.
When Glen and I had Zachary, my third son, she was pleased, because
he was Glen's and she realized he was sticking around. When I fell
pregnant with our next son though, it was the same old story. She said
we couldn't afford it and I couldn't cope with four kids. Glen said he
would really tell her what he thought if she ever said that in front of him!
She doesn't understand that Glen and I raise these kids together. I don't
have to cope on my own!

On meeting her husband

I was pregnant with my second child when I met Glen. He told me it
didn't matter. I had a hard time believing him. Lots of people I knew
also thought he was just using me for sex and would leave when the baby
was due. But Glen treated me properly, and he said he was ready for a
family. He took on a 5-year-old and me being pregnant, and he was all
excited that he was going to become a dad. Even though the baby wasn't
his I moved into Glen's house and he was with me when the baby was
born. He cut the cord! Then he had the video camera on Jacob, he was
just hysterical. I named my son after him: Jacob Glen. Glen cried when I
told him that's what I was going to call the baby.

The week we got engaged so many things happened. It was one good
thing after another. First I got my driver's licence. Then Glen proposed
to me. And he did it in the right romantic way. He took me out to dinner
in the city and we stayed at a hotel with a spa bath. He even got the

photographer in the restaurant to take photos of him proposing! The only bad part was I was pregnant with our son, and I was sick! I couldn't eat my dinner! But it was such a lovely night.

Glen is a wonderful husband. I wouldn't be able to manage with these kids without him. He helps me with the kids and does things for me. Sometimes we ask one of our friends to baby-sit so we can go out for dinner together. We have been on holidays once without the kids since we got married. They stayed with Glen's mum and dad so we could go to his best mate's wedding in Melbourne. We had a great time, but I missed the kids so much, I was glad to get back to them.

We didn't plan to have four. When I told Glen I thought I was pregnant the last time he just said, oh well, if you are you are and we'll just manage. We had to sell the house and buy another one. Now we live in a much bigger house with more room for the kids to play.

On being the mother of a child with a disability

Recently, two of our sons were diagnosed with a disability. It is hard having a disabled child. Jacob has behavioural problems, and they told us that Zach had autism. Glen said he didn't have autism, because he was very interactive with us and with his brothers. He told the doctor that, and it turned out he was right. But he is behind with his development. Jacob and Zachary are both going to have speech therapy, and Zach is starting to say words now. We have noticed with our fourth son that he is much further ahead than Jacob or Zach were – so we can see what the doctor is talking about.

With any kid it's not easy being a mum. My eldest, Nathan, has trouble at school because he gets bullied. We have to go up to the school to talk to the principal. I love all my kids, and I love being a mum. It is so exciting watching them grow and learn and do new things all the time.

Living up to expectations: *Kylie's story*

This is Kylie's story. Kylie is 20 and has three children; however, the first two are in care. Kylie and her partner Vuna married before the birth of their third child, William. Their relationship has a turbulent past but they have managed to turn things around. William is a happy baby who is meeting all his developmental milestones.

On feeling bad

My first boy Edward was born three years ago. I was 17. Things weren't great then. Vuna and I hadn't been together for long and DOCS [social services] made me live in a place for teenage mums, with the family support service. The place was okay but I felt everyone was telling me what to do and deep down questioned whether I could look after my son. Things got worse when I found out I was pregnant again. Edward was only 6 months when this happened. So being a mum at 17, having a baby and another on the way was really hard.

When Edward was born I wanted to go back to live with my family. Things were not great between Vuna and me. DOCS said no and came and took Edward off me. That was heartbreaking because he was my first son and I loved him. Others couldn't see that. They only saw me as having a disability and as someone who couldn't do things.

I had a hard upbringing and nobody was really there for me when I was growing up. Growing up like this makes learning and going to school hard. So I didn't do well at school. When I was in Year 8 (13 years old) I had to go to a special school. Even though I had to go to this school, I didn't see myself as having a disability. I just think I have some problems learning. When people say I have a disability they think I can't do a lot of things and that is definitely not true. This makes me feel bad. See on the inside I just feel normal and I just want people to treat me that way. In many ways when people treat me like I can't do things they are the one's that create problems for me. Their attitudes really suck and make me angry and frustrated. Because people have thought I can't do things I have lost confidence in myself.

If it wasn't bad enough having Edward taken away from me, when my second son, Gilead was born, DOCS came into the hospital and took him from me. I had him on the Friday. The DOCS workers came in that same day and said they were coming back on the Monday to take Gilead into care. What these workers did was the cruellest thing. I had to stay in a hospital ward with all these other mothers who had their babies and who were celebrating, knowing that in two days my baby was going to be taken away from me. These workers had no idea. Because they just saw me as a person with a disability they assumed I didn't have feelings or that I cared about things. They knew stuff all. My heart broke the day my son was born. My heart is still broken. On the Tuesday I went to court. I wanted to go back to the hospital to say goodbye to my son and the DOCS workers said, 'Don't bother, he won't be there.' I just broke down and cried. They didn't try and comfort me, they just walked away.

After that I had a hormone implant. I didn't want to go through the pain of having any more children removed from me again. But a month after having the implant I fell pregnant. When the doctor told me I felt shocked. I was happy but I was also scared – scared they would come and take this baby too. Vuna and I decided we were going to do things differently. We got married and got everything ready for William. I did a child care course as part of 'work for the dole', a government programme for people without jobs. Vuna did a father's programme.

On hope and trust

On 10 March 2003, William was born. Vuna and I thought everything was fine. The doctor said I could go home within 24 hours. I was ready to go and the social worker came and said, 'No, no, no you can't go until DOCS has come.' I just thought, 'Oh no, not again.' I wanted to throttle her. First they said the reason why they were calling DOCS was because they were worried I wasn't feeding William enough. DOCS and the hospital staff put me on a one-week trial to see if I was a good enough mother. Vuna got the idea of us keeping a book and writing down every time I fed, bathed or changed William. When the week was up they had a meeting. Now they said that they were concerned I was doing things for William by the clock and that I wasn't bonding to my baby. I couldn't win. Because DOCS had removed our other children we were in a 'lose, lose' situation. We couldn't do anything right.

We went to court and we bumped into Margaret, a social worker who trains family support workers about parents with disabilities. She sat and talked with us. And she became our advocate. After the first court hearing Vuna and I talked and we decided we just needed to get help. So we rang people we felt understood us. At first I found it so hard to talk to people and tell them how I felt and what I thought. Because up until this time nobody seemed to care that my heart was breaking, and because I felt shy and uncomfortable. I had no self-esteem left. Margaret and Renee, my outreach worker from the family support service, helped me put words to my feelings and encouraged me to tell people. Up until then I had just drawn the curtain and didn't want to let anyone in.

DOCS backed off. They gave us a chance. And things are different this time around. Even though I am only 20 I am a lot more mature now than when I was 17. When William was born, DOCS weren't prepared to believe I was different. They just judged me on how I was three years ago. The family support service was different. The staff were prepared to put their past ideas about me aside and support me. It is important to remember that people change – even people with learning problems!

On help from other people

This time round, people believed in me. Even when I felt I couldn't do things, my worker Renee from the family support service and Margaret and Vuna told me I could. I saw they got really excited and were proud of me when I tried to do things and that made me feel good about myself. Vuna and the workers work with me. They don't just do things for me nor do they tell me what to do. They don't lecture me. They help me solve problems and reassure me that all mothers need support and help. It is not just me because I have learning problems. They also don't act like they have all the answers and they listen to my ideas.

When they need to explain things they do it in a way that I can understand. Sometimes they draw pictures. They also take my questions seriously and don't treat me like I am dumb for asking questions. They also don't try to teach me things before I needed to know them. When the time is right and William is starting to do new things, the workers help me out with the information I need, like what food to feed William at what stage and things like that.

Their sense of humour also helps. Renee and Margaret make fun of things, which relaxes me. This helps me to be more myself. They also make mistakes, which helped me. Margaret, Renee and Vuna sometimes have trouble doing things or forget things. Showing me that they aren't perfect makes me feel better about myself and makes me realize I can do some things better than them.

I have other supports too. I have a good local doctor. I feel I can talk to her and she gives me time. If William gets sick I know I can rely on her to help me. She loves William and cares about us as a family. Vuna and I have also joined a church. The church community helps me believe in myself. They don't treat me like I am dumb or different. They treat me just like anybody else. They also encourage me and tell me I am a good mum.

Vuna has stood by me through thick and thin and is a really good dad. Vuna does more for me than I do for him and I love him for this. William makes it easier too. He has a lovely little nature. He is very clever and meets all his milestones. This makes me feel I am doing the right thing. He seems to be really enjoying being part of our family.

I feel like things have all fallen in my lap now and I am happy. If only those people who didn't believe in me could see me now. Our next goal is to have our other boys returned to us . . . then we can be the family and parents we want to be.

Taking one day at a time: *Joy and Shirley's story*

The next story comes from Joy and her mother Shirley. Joy lives with Shirley. Their lives are intertwined. Andrew, Joy's teenage son, is beginning to assert his independence and they are careful to give him the space he needs. Joy and Shirley are private people, even shy. Nevertheless they are involved in a range of community activities and make important contributions through their volunteer work.

On starting a family

Shirley: Joy didn't plan to get pregnant. She and David had been friends for quite a while and I think they were planning to get married, maybe in a year or so. The staff at the workshop didn't think that they could possibly cope with the demands of a baby. But I supported Joy's decision to go ahead with the pregnancy. My philosophy is that slow learners like Joy and David should be given a chance, and with encouragement and family support, there is no reason why they can't succeed.

Joy: David never had a family. He grew up in institutions and group homes. Me and mum wanted to be his family, so David moved in with us. It was hard though because he didn't know how to be part of a family. We were living here when Andrew was born. It was good having mum here to help. Mum and me took it in turns.

Shirley: Andrew was born early and he had a lot of problems. Joy was so good with him, and so eager to learn. We had to see the doctor regularly and we had all kinds of therapists coming here. Joy made every effort to follow all their instructions. I was here to help and to offer guidance, but really Joy grew into the responsibility. Joy really matured. I always say that watching Joy at the time was like watching a rose bud open. Becoming a mother is the best thing that could have happened for Joy.

Joy: We lived with mum, then we got our own place. It was just down the road. I looked after Andrew. David wasn't much help. But mum was there to help me when I needed it. I could call her every day. David never did much of the looking after, and he also had trouble with his temper. He used to get angry and shout a lot. When he got angry I took Andrew and we went for a walk until he calmed down. But then one day David got angry and hit me. Andrew was 5 then, and he called mum on the phone and told her. Mum came and got me and Andrew and we came back to live with her. This is where we have been ever since. We don't see David much any more.

Shirley: Joy and I share the load. She is not a burden at all. Like I do the washing and Joy does the ironing and we share the cooking. For a few years my mother was living here too. She was old and frail and we looked after her together. We had four generations all living under the same roof! Joy also does the grocery shopping. Before Andrew came along Joy was very shy. She didn't want to go outside the door on her own, not even to the shop. Now she is more confident. They all know her down the shops. She is always running in to someone she knows. It might be someone she used to know from the workshop, or it might be someone from church, or it might be one of our neighbours. We have good neighbours. We look out for each other here.

On volunteering

Joy: When Andrew was in junior school I used to go there twice a week to do reading with the children in kindergarten and first class. I also helped in the library. I like to sort things. But now Andrew is at high school. The only volunteering I can do there is in the canteen. But I am not good with handling money.

Shirley: Joy helps out a lot down at the church now. Like, every second Friday there is a group called MOPS, mothers of preschoolers. I was asked to help look after the babies, so Joy comes with me and we look after them together. There are about 15 little babies there. We like looking after them, but looking after older children is too much responsibility. There are so many rules, spoken and unspoken about how to handle and how to talk to children, and the rules have changed. It is hard for both of us to get used to the new rules. But babies are easier to handle. Joy is good at rocking the babies to sleep in their prams. The other mums there really trust Joy.

Joy: On Sundays we go to church. I like the music. Andrew goes to Sunday school. He also goes to night church. Sometimes he is a steward. That's the person who collects the offering. He doesn't want me to go with him on Sunday nights. He wants to be more independent now. I like going to church, but I don't always under-stand the Bible very well. Mum says that doesn't matter. The important thing is just being there. And I like the music.

Shirley: On a Saturday morning Joy also helps the little ones at T-Ball. That is before her own game. Joy and Andrew play in a team together. I usually go down and help prepare the morning tea. They call me 'the cook'.

Joy: I heard about T-Ball from a lady down the street. Me and Andrew walked down to the field. We were standing there watching when Harry [the coach] asked us if we would like to come and join in. I didn't know if I could play it. We have been playing for seven years now. Me and Andrew we love playing it. We even went to Japan to play in a tournament! We might even go to New Zealand to play. That is what the coach said, if we can get the money.

On friendship

Joy: Every week I go to a group at the church. We do craft activities together. I do my fabric painting. I like listening to the other women talk. They talk about all sorts of things, like what is hap-pening in the world, and what they heard on the news. They tell jokes too. They make jokes about men and sex! There is one mum there who has a daughter with a disability. I knew her from the workshop. But I don't speak much. I tell them about T-Ball. But I don't talk much when I'm down there. I haven't got much to say. Mum says it is because we are one-to-one people.

Shirley: We do a lot of things together. It's all about sharing experiences.

Juggling work and family: *Robert and Julie's story*

Robert and Julie tell the final story. They are well-known activists who have championed the cause of self-advocacy for people with learning disabilities in Australia and particularly in New South Wales. They have three children: the eldest is 13 and the youngest is 9. Robert and Julie have recently separated yet they continue to 'work as a team' when it comes to the children. Their children always come first.

On getting married and starting a family

Julie: My life could have been so different! I grew up in a country town and my parents were very protective. My life was pretty much restricted to home, the disability workshop, and occasionally tagging along with my brother and his girlfriend. I think life would have been more of the same if it wasn't for a teacher at the local community college. I was doing a typewriting course, and I had to write a story. The teacher read my story and took a real interest in me. She talked to me about another life, and encouraged me to join a social group. This group became Self-Advocacy: an organization to help people with learning disabilities speak-up for themselves. I met Robert there.

Robert: Julie approached me, and she liked me a heck of a lot, you could see it. We got to be good friends and one thing just led to another. Julie and I got to talking: we talked about Julie moving to Sydney and us getting a flat together, we talked about getting married then having children. But it didn't work out quite the way we planned. Julie got pregnant. I asked her, 'What do you want to do?' and she said, 'I want to have the child.' I said, 'We will do the right thing then and get married.' This friend of ours got some information for us about abortion and started talking to us about it. We told him that we were getting married and we were having the baby. He said, 'OK, I'll support you in any way you like.' He was the best man at our wedding.

Julie: Other people were no support at all. Some workers were telling me not to have the baby. It was very upsetting. But Robert and I talked about it. I also talked to my mum. She was worried about how we would manage, but she decided to support us. She said, 'We need to discuss wedding plans.' We got married in my home town.

Robert: It was a great wedding, 140 people came. Julie and I decided together who was going to do what. Julie got the dresses organized for the bridesmaids and I got the suits for the groomsmen. Julie's mum and my best man helped out a lot. We got married in a church. I remember Julie kicking off her high heels as she walked down the aisle! I think the hairdresser had given her some champagne. We held the reception at a local club. One of Julie's old school teachers was the MC [master of ceremonies]. I made a speech, my brother made a speech and my best man made a speech. Julie met the rest of my family and they got on like a house on fire.

On learning to be a parent

Julie: Our baby came early. They had to do an emergency C-section. I remember waking up and she wasn't there. My first reaction was, 'What have you done with my baby?' Until I saw my baby girl I was panicking. It was the worst thing I have ever gone through. She was so small, just 3 pounds and 3 ounces. And she had a heart murmur. But she is OK now. Now she is fine, growing up a real young lady. We learned heaps at the hospital. But then we had to go to a special live-in clinic to learn parenting skills. We didn't like it there. They showed us different ways of looking after our baby, different to what the hospital had showed us, and it was confusing. We preferred the ways we learned at the hospital.

Robert: You don't learn how to be a dad growing up in institutions. My parents gave me up when I was just 3 years old. I had a lot of problems. I was born with hydrocephalus, with a harelip, cleft palate, webbed fingers and other deformities. I had lots of operations. I was in and out of hospital. I think it was very stressful for my parents and the doctor suggested that they put me in an institution and forget about me. Most of my childhood was spent within the walls of an institution. I learnt a lot of things there. I learnt to be wary of people. But I was basically raised by nurses. I never had a role model. For most of my life I have never had a father.

Julie: Friends and family helped us a lot, especially my aunty. She has always been there for us. Robert had a falling out with his family, so we never see much of them. We learned a lot from listening to and watching other people. But that is not to say we have simply followed directions. Robert and I listen and carefully consider the advice we get. Often it is conflicting! Then we try out different strategies before deciding what works best for us. For example, people told us lots of different things to do when our baby was teething. We tried different things before we found the best solution. We have also learned a lot from experience. Like everyone else, we have learned from our mistakes.

On sharing responsibility

Robert: We now have three beautiful children: Amanda-Lee (13), Bradley (11) and Cassandra (9). None of our children has learning disabilities, but they do need a bit of extra help in school. Bradley likes school, and he does his homework. Amanda-Lee doesn't! Cassie now goes to a special school. She was born with heaps of medical problems. Like, she had to have a colostomy bag. They have now done surgery and fixed it up, but we are still toilet training her. We use a star-chart system to encourage her.

Julie: Robert and I have always shared the responsibility for the children. We make the decisions together. And between us we have managed to have a career as well. When we first met, we were both involved in Self-Advocacy; we helped set it up. And since Self-Advocacy got funding, one or both of us has had a job there. At first I stayed home to look after the kids, and Robert went to work. But we swapped roles after Cassie was born.

Robert: I think we were both shocked when we learned about Cassie's medical problems. Julie had a bit of a breakdown. We talked about it and decided that the best thing to do was for me to resign from my job. Cassie needed constant care, and we decided that I should be the one to give it. Julie applied for my position and got it. She has been working for Self-Advocacy ever since.

On separation

Robert: Julie and I separated about two years ago. It was a hard decision, and one that I think surprised a lot of people. But it was the right decision for our family. So many people have problems with their children because they are divorced. I am not going to let that get me down, and it hasn't and it won't. I try to think positive all the time. Julie and I share the care: we still work together as a team when it comes to the children. I moved out and found a place in the same area. The kids live with me four days each week, from Mondays through to Thursdays. Julie picks them up from school on a Thursday and they stay with her over the weekend.

   Julie and I regularly talk about the kids, and she knows she can call me any time. Like sometimes, if Julie has to go into work early, she will call me up and I will pick the kids up and walk them to school. And we still do stuff together as a family. Like sometimes Julie wants to take the kids to the pool. It is hard when there is just one of you because Cassie has to go to the toilet every hour. So sometimes I go with Julie: one of us looks after Cassie, while the other keeps an eye on the other two. Julie and I agree that the kids come first.

On work

Julie: I love my work. With Robert and I sharing custody I am able to keep working. It is a stretch though. I have to be very organized and stick to routines. I almost never have nothing to do! I have a duty statement that is three pages long! I have to support individual consumers, train staff about the rights of people with learning disabilities and visit workplaces. When people come in and we ask them who they would like as their advocate, they usually ask for me! I like making a difference in people's lives. Sometimes they are people who haven't had an opportunity, or feel they cannot go against their parents, or people who are wanting to do something more in their lives. I help them brainstorm all the possibilities and I help them develop a consumer action plan. I want to be the next manager of Self-Advocacy. That is my goal. I have even done a course on work assessment and training. I am one of only two people with learning disabilities in New South Wales who have completed that course!

Robert: Nowadays I only do casual work. I do it when I get a call, when I am asked to do it, maybe once, twice, three times a month. It depends. I know a heck of a lot of people, and a lot of people know me! I get asked to give talks and training – disability awareness training mostly. It's because people don't know how to talk to you. They think you are different. I have given talks at courts, workplaces, schools, universities and loads of other places. I loved teaching the children, but I have never given a talk at the school my kids go to. Amanda-Lee gets teased for having a father like me. I try to help people see that everybody has a disability – mine is just easier to see. And nobody should think that disability is not their business. Anything can happen, like a car accident. I also want to show that people with disabilities can do things. They can be parents!

On keeping up with the kids

Robert: It is tough being a parent though. I am quite strict with my kids. Being a good parent is about setting limits for children. I will not take any crap from them. But it is also important to listen. I will listen to them, I will question and I will find out. It is important to find out before we take actions. I never hit my children or yell at them (well maybe sometimes I yell). They know the tone of my voice.

I try to teach them. There are different ways of behaving and some are more accepted in the community. But sometimes they embarrass themselves, sometimes they embarrass me with their manners! But they are good kids really. I also think it is important to know what is happening in their lives. Like if one of the kids gets a bruise, I want to know how it happened. I'll call Julie, and if necessary the school.

Years ago, my daughter was touched the wrong way. I reported it and the school did nothing. So I went to DOCS. Then something was done about it. The school punished the boy. I took my daughter to hospital and to have counselling. It is important that people see that I am a responsible father. You have to prove yourself all the time. People are always watching you because you have got a disability.

I think it is safe to say that our children don't see us as parents with learning disabilities. To them we are just mum and dad. Julie and I have proven that together, and with the right support, people with learning disabilities can raise a normal happy family. We have also proven that people with learning disabilities can have successful careers and run an organization together!

Lessons from parents' lives

We draw three major lessons from the family stories. The first is that parents with learning disabilities are as diverse a group of parents as you could hope to find. Some years ago, Taylor (1994) suggested that practitioners must treat parents with learning disabilities as individuals and not as members of a category. Earlier, Budd and Greenspan (1984) had reached a similar conclusion. They observed that: 'if few generalizations can be made about parenting abilities of "mentally retarded" women, then each family deserves to be examined on an individual basis for specific child-rearing strengths and weaknesses' (p. 488).

The learning disabilities label continues to evoke a stereotyped response. This seduces us to focus on the qualities that labelled people are thought to have in common. The stories in this chapter emphasize how parents with learning disabilities are different from each other in many ways: in their personalities, life experiences, living situations, the people in their lives, and the ways in which they learn and adapt to parenthood. Importantly, parents with learning disabilities change and develop as they respond to the dynamic and ever-changing demands of their children growing up.

Exercise 22.2

A useful exercise is to reread the stories to identify significant differences. Try to pay attention to each family's particularity. The following questions will help guide your review:

What do parents say about their childhood experiences?

Who do the parents talk about as being supportive and 'there for them'?

There are ups and downs in each family's life. What significant turning points do the parents identify?

The second lesson is that, as a group, parents with learning disabilities face predictable challenges. These come from the 'place' of people with learning disabilities in society. This place is one of being thought less able, less capable than others. Parents with learning disabilities face low expectations about their abilities, capacity and potential to take on parenting. These low expectations translate for many parents into an ever-present threat that the welfare authorities will step in and remove their children. In addition, many parents with learning disabilities live in difficult socioeconomic and personal circumstances. These may include being on social security benefits and living in less than desirable neighbourhoods with little opportunity to access appropriate or useful support to raise their children.

There are many challenges facing parents with learning disabilities, illustrated by the family stories in this chapter. The motion picture *I am Sam* (New Line Cinema 2001) in similar vein presented the challenges facing Sam, a single father with learning disabilities, as he fought to retain custody of his daughter. Taken together family stories and movies such as *I am Sam* can alert practitioners to the sociopolitical context, the 'bigger picture' in which parents with learning disabilities raise their children.

Exercise 22.3

Think about the societal factors that present significant barriers to people with learning disabilities being parents. The family stories bring these challenges 'alive'. You may also wish to reflect on material in the earlier chapters of this book to identify some of these barriers.

Identify several major challenges faced by people with learning disabilities wanting to be parents.

What barriers arise out of the low expectations of others and how do these barriers effect parents' lives?

Competence promoting support has been shown to be more effective. What are the features of competence promoting support and competence inhibiting support? Provide examples of both types of support from the family stories.

The third lesson that we can draw from the family stories is that parents with learning disabilities share remarkable achievements in common. In becoming parents and raising children they contribute to society and in so doing defy others' expectations. They achieve this under circumstances that would deter or defeat the sturdiest of people wanting to become parents. These achievements confront and overturn the stereotyped view that people with learning disabilities should not be parents.

The family stories demonstrate a shared resilience among these parents in the face of adversity. A dominant theme is each parent's ongoing struggle to show that they are just like everyone else. They struggle against the oppression of the disability label; they work hard to show that they are no different or less than others. Their battle against the disability label emerges frequently in their talk of doing things 'normally'. Having a white wedding and getting married emerge as symbols of their achievement in meeting societal expectations of a normal rhythm of adult life. Parents with learning disabilities also struggle against the systemic barriers which flow on from beliefs that learning disability means 'less than'. They achieve, for example, by succeeding in the face of child protection scrutiny and intervention.

The family stories also demonstrate achievements at an individual level – for example, in overcoming parental control or learning new skills never thought possible. Parents with learning disabilities also achieve by taking on and seeking out opportunities unlikely to come their way in the natural course of things.

Exercise 22.4

The final exercise requires the reader to locate shared and individual achievements evident in the stories. The following questions guide this task:

Are there major achievements in common in these family stories? If so, what are they and how did each parent reach their achievements?

Identify new activities that parents have taken up or skills learnt or tasks undertaken in response to being parents.

Labels such as learning disability suggest a static condition, yet the family stories suggest ongoing development and change. Identify at least one instance of change in each story and draw out the circumstances in which this change occurred.

Conclusion

There have always been some people with learning disabilities who became parents. However, the eugenics movement and the era of institutionalization generated a pervasive belief that people with learning disabilities must not be allowed to take on the role of parenting. Contradicting this belief, people with learning disabilities became parents and more are doing so and achieving successful, quality lives as the narratives in this chapter demonstrate. Research across several continents has contributed to our understanding of the challenges faced by these parents in 'having to prove themselves all the time'. No one in any place would suggest seriously that the task of parenting is an easy one. All parents need support to raise healthy, happy children in safe environments. Some parents benefit from additional support. All parents benefit from having at least one person who believes in and works with them to help achieve their goals for themselves and their children. The lessons we have drawn here from the family stories and the literature serve to illustrate the way forward for practitioners in providing support and services to parents with learning disabilities.

Acknowledgement

We acknowledge the contributions made by our colleagues, Rachel Mayes and Margaret Spencer, who supported Debbie and Kylie as these mothers shared their stories for inclusion in this book.

Resources

Literature reviews

Booth, T. and Booth, W. (1993) Parenting with learning difficulties: lessons for practitioners, *British Journal of Social Work*, 23: 459–80.

Feldman, M.A. (1994) Parenting education for parents with intellectual disabilities: a review of the literature, *Research in Developmental Disabilities*, 15: 229–332.

Llewellyn, G. (1990) People with intellectual disability as parents: perspectives from the professional literature, *Australia and New Zealand Journal of Developmental Disabilities*, 16: 369–80.

McGaw, S. (2000) *What Works for Parents with Learning Difficulties?* Essex: Barnardos.

Tymchuk, A.J. and Feldman, M.A. (1991) Parents with mental retardation and their children: review of research relevant to professional practice, *Canadian Psychology*, 32: 486–94.

Parent learning

Feldman, M.A. (2004) Self-directed learning of child care skills by parents with intellectual disabilities, *Infants & Young Children*, 17: 17–31.

Feldman, M.A., Case, L., Rincover, A., Towns, F. and Betel, J. (1989) Parent education project III: increasing affection and responsivity in developmentally handicapped mothers: component analysis, generalization, and effects on child language, *Journal of Applied Behavior Analysis*, 22: 211–22.

Llewellyn, G. (1997) Parents with intellectual disability learning to parent: the role of experience and informal learning, *International Journal of Disability, Development and Education*, 44(3): 243–61.

Llewellyn, G., McConnell, D., Honey, A., Mayes, R. and Russo, D. (2003) Promoting health and home safety for children of parents with intellectual disability: a randomised controlled trial, *Research in Developmental Disabilities*, 24: 405–31.

Tymchuk, A.J. and Andron, L. (1992) Project parenting: child interactional training with mothers who are mentally handicapped, *Mental Handicap Research*, 5(1): 4–32.

Outcomes for children

Booth, T. and Booth, W. (1998) *Growing Up with Parents who have Learning Difficulties*. London: Routledge.

Feldman, M.A. and Walton-Allen, N. (1997) Effects of maternal mental retardation and poverty on intellectual, academic and behavioral status of school-age children, *American Journal on Mental Retardation*, 101: 352–64.

Keltner, B., Wise, L.A. and Taylor, G. (1999) Mothers with intellectual limitations and their 2-year-old children's developmental outcomes, *Journal of Intellectual and Developmental Disability*, 24(1): 45–57.

McConnell, D., Llewellyn, G., Mayes, R., Russo, D. and Honey, A. (2003) Developmental profiles of children born to mothers with intellectual disability, *Journal of Intellectual and Developmental Disability*, 28(2): 122–34.

Perkins, T.S., Holburn, S., Deaux, K., Flory, M. and Vietze, P.M. (2002) Children of mothers with intellectual disability: stigma, mother-child relationship and self-esteem, *Journal of Applied Research in Intellectual Disabilities*, 15: 297–313.

Pixa-Kettner, U. (1998) Parents with intellectual disability in Germany: results of a nationwide study, *Journal of Applied Research in Intellectual Disabilities*, 11(4): 355–64.

Court studies

Bishop, S.J., Murphy, J.M., Hicks, R., Quinn, D., Lewis, P.J., Grace, M. and Jellinek, M.S. (2000) What progress has been made in meeting the needs of seriously maltreated children? The course of 200 cases through the Boston Juvenile Court, *Child Abuse and Neglect*, 3: 599–610.

Booth, T., Booth, W. and McConnell, D. (in press) The prevalence and outcomes of care proceedings involving parents with learning difficulties in the family courts, *Journal of Intellectual Disability Research*.

Llewellyn, G., McConnell, D. and Ferronato, L. (2002) Prevalence and outcomes for parents with disabilities and their children in an Australian court sample, *Child Abuse and Neglect*, 27: 235–51.

McConnell, D., Llewellyn, G. and Ferronato, L. (2000) Disability and decision-making in Australian care proceedings, *International Journal of Law, Policy and the Family*, 16: 270–99.

Taylor, C.G., Norman, D.K., Murphy, J.M., Jellinek, M., Quinn, D., Poitrast, F.G. and Goshko, M. (1991) Diagnosed intellectual and emotional impairment among parents who seriously mistreat their children: prevalence, type, and outcome in a court sample, *Child Abuse & Neglect*, 15: 389–401.

Maternal health and social support

Feldman, M.A., Varghsea, J., Ramsay, J. and Rajsa, D. (2002) Relationships between social support, stress and mother-child interactions in mothers with intellectual disabilities, *Journal of Applied Research in Intellectual Disabilities*, 15: 314–23.

Kroese, B.S., Hussein, H., Clifford, C. and Ahmed, N. (2002) Social support networks and psychological well-being of mothers with intellectual disabilities, *Journal of Applied Research in Intellectual Disabilities*, 15: 324–40.

Llewellyn, G. and McConnell, D. (1995) *Support Interview Guide.* www.fhs.usyd.edu.au/fssp/.

Llewellyn, G. and McConnell, D. (2002) Mothers with learning difficulties and their support networks, *Journal of Intellectual Disability Research*, 46(1): 17–34.

Llewellyn, G., McConnell, D. and Mayes, R. (2003) Health of mothers with intellectual limitations, *Australian and New Zealand Journal of Public Health*, 27(1): 17–19.

McGaw, S. (1995) *I Want to be a Good Parent: The BILD Parenting Series*, www.bild.org.uk/index.htm.

Service delivery and family support

Aunos, M. and Feldman, M.A. (2002) Attitudes towards sexuality, sterilization and parenting rights of persons with intellectual disabilities, *Journal of Applied Research in Intellectual Disabilities*, 15: 285–96.

Booth, T. and Booth, W. (2003) Self-advocacy and supported learning for mothers with learning difficulties, *Journal of Learning Disabilities*, 7: 165–93.

Espe-Sherwindt, M. and Kerlin, S. (1990) Early intervention with parents with mental retardation: do we empower or impair? *Infants and Young Children*, 2: 21–8.

Llewellyn, G., McConnell, D. and Bye, R. (1998) Perception of service needs by parents with intellectual disability, their significant others and their service workers, *Research in Developmental Disabilities*, 19(3): 245–60.

Llewellyn, G., McConnell, D., Russo, D., Mayes, R. and Honey, A. (2002) Home-based programmes for parents with intellectual disabilities: lessons from practice, *Journal of Applied Research in Intellectual Disabilities*, 15: 341–53.

McGaw, S., Ball, K. and Clark, A. (2002) The effect of group intervention on the relationships of parents with intellectual disabilities, *Journal of Applied Research in Intellectual Disabilities*, 15: 354–66.

Ray, N.K., Rubenstein, H. and Russo, N.J. (1994) Understanding the parents who are mentally retarded: guidelines for family preservation programs, *Child Welfare*, LXXIII(6): 725–43.

Tymchuk, A.J. (1999) Moving towards integration of services for parents with intellectual disabilities, *Journal of Intellectual and Developmental Disability*, 24(1): 59–74.

Reports

Genders, N. (1998) *The Role of the Community Nurse (Learning Disability): Parenting by People with Learning Disabilities*, London: The Maternity Alliance.

Goodinge, S. (2000) *A Jigsaw of Services: Inspection of Services to Support Disabled Adults in their Parenting Role*, London: Social Services Inspectorate, Department of Health.

Wates, M. (2003) *It Shouldn't be Down to Luck: Results of a DPN Consultation with Disabled Parents on Access to Information and Services to Support Parenting*, United Kingdom: Disabled Parents Network.

Voices of parents

Booth, T. and Booth, W. (1994) *Parenting under Pressure: Mothers and Fathers with Learning Difficulties*, Buckingham: Open University Press.

Olsen, R. and Clarke, H. (2003) *Parenting and Disability: Disabled Parents' Experiences of Raising Children*, Bristol: The Policy Press.

Strike, R. and McConnell, D. (2002) Look at me, listen to me, I have something important to say, *Sexuality and Disability*, 20(1): 53–63.

Traustadottir, R. and Johnson, K. (2000) *Women with Intellectual Disabilities: Finding a Place in the World*, London: Jessica Kingsley.

Websites

Australian Family and Disability Studies Research Centre: www.afdsrc.org/.
British Institute of Learning Disabilities: www.bild.org.uk/.
Disability, Pregnancy and Parenthood *International* www.dppi.org.uk/.
Disabled Parents Network: www.disabledparentsnetwork.org.uk/.
Supported Parenting: www.supported-parenting.com/.
Through the Looking Glass: lookingglass.org/index.php.

References

Budd, J. and Greenspan, S. (1984) Mentally retarded mothers, in E.A., Blechman (ed.) *Behaviour Modification with Women*. New York: Guildford Press.

Mickelson, P. (1947). The feeble-minded parent: a study of 90 family cases, *American Journal of Mental Deficiency*, 51: 644–53

Taylor, S.J. (1994) Children's division is coming to take pictures: family life and parenting in a family with disabilities, in S.J. Taylor, R. Bogdan and Z.M. Lutfiyya (eds) *The Variety of Community Experience: Qualitative Studies if Family and Community Life*. Baltimore, MD: Paul H. Brookes.

Tucker, B.M. and Johnson, O. (1989) Competence promoting versus competence inhibiting social support for mentally retarded mothers, *Human Organisation*, 48: 95–107.

23

Promoting friendships and developing social networks

Roy McConkey

Introduction

Many people with learning disabilities lead lonely lives. In this chapter you will read the evidence for this, think about why this is so, ponder the consequences of it and consider what can be done about it.

Building relationships among people is a daunting task. Support staff might teach a person the necessary communication and social skills; they may organize leisure activities for them and perhaps even arrange social gatherings such as parties, but as Firth and Rapley (1990: 21) noted, 'It is not possible to provide friendship, or to make friends for other people . . . friendships can only be chosen'. Thus staff cannot rely on their usual 'organizing strategies' when it comes to enabling people with learning disabilities to find and cement their own friendships. They need to adopt different strategies, but often these fall outside of their present roles and job descriptions.

Promoting friendships has its risks. What if the person in your care chooses the 'wrong' people' – as you see it? Could they be taken advantage of? Will they get hurt if the friendship is not reciprocated? All the same fears that your parents probably had about your choice of friends when you were a teenager going on 40! Yet you and they managed to find a way through and so too can staff and parents who are responsible for people with learning disabilities. But it means managing the risk rather than trying to eliminate it, as so often happens with service policies and procedures.

People with learning disabilities are often faced with stigmatized, discriminatory and hurtful attitudes from other members of the community such as health professionals, employers and neighbours. Thus societal attitudes can act as a strong barrier to social inclusion, especially if they remain unchallenged. Often, specialist services have left it to family carers and people themselves to confront negative attitudes, but should this continue?

The rewards that come from having a network of friends are great. It means having the company of others, laughter and adventure, people to give you advice and guidance, practical help, emotional support and protection, and above all, friends to whom you can show love and affection and who will do the same for you. Quality of life studies constantly stress the importance of friendships and this is no less so for people with learning disabilities. For example, Atkinson and Ward (1987: 242) concluded from their pioneering study of around 50 individuals living in their own homes after having been resettled from hospital that, 'the quality of their lives was to a great extent determined by the range and type of their social relationships'. They found that individuals with learning disabilities described their lives and lifestyles in terms of the people they shared a house with, members of their family, their friends and workmates, and people in their neighbourhood.

Indeed it could be argued that people with learning disabilities have even more need for friends than those without a disability, as their lives are often more impoverished. To deny them opportunities for friendships only compounds their handicap. Yet as we shall see, this is precisely what happens in many of our existing services.

Friendships and people with learning disabilities

Of all the assessments done on people with learning disabilities, the one least likely to be carried out is an examination of their friendships! Perhaps busy professionals see this as not being relevant to their work; or maybe they think it is too intrusive to enquire; or perhaps they feel that it's not very important for people with learning disabilities to have friends.

But if they did take the time to enquire, they would probably confirm the evidence from a growing number of research studies, namely that people with disabilities have few close friends. Here are some examples from across the age range and for people living in different settings.

Teenagers

Smyth and McConkey (2003) interviewed the parents of over 50 school leavers from two special schools for pupils with severe learning difficulties in Northern Ireland. Three in five of the young people (58 per cent) were reported to have no friends of their own. Of those reported to have friends (16 students in all), 12 were from the same school or centre the young person attended, although two of these also lived in the neighbourhood of the young person. Only one young person had a weekly meeting with her school/centre friends outside of the school setting; more often it was fortnightly (3), monthly (4) or occasionally (4).

Four students were reported to have non-disabled friends from the neighbourhood (11 per cent), although only one person met his friend weekly, usually in clubs or pubs. In all, 90 per cent of parents would like their son or daughter to be more involved with friends of their own age and they mentioned the need for more clubs (10) and for more sports and leisure activities (6).

Similar findings have been reported by Buckley and Sacks (1987) for Down's syndrome teenagers in the south of England and by Redmond (1996) for young people in Dublin.

Adult persons living with family carers

McConkey *et al.* (1981) interviewed over 200 parents in Dublin city who had a son or daughter living with them at home – average age 23 years. Previous Irish studies with non-disabled samples of comparable age found that three-quarters of young people regularly shared their leisure time with friends. But of those who had learning disabilities, only two in five spent any time with a friend and as many as one in five were reported to have no one with whom they shared their leisure time. Some of the comments made by the young people sum up their plight: 'I need a friendship. I wish I had a companion I could go out with and chat to. I have nobody and it hurts me.' 'I would like to have friends although my mammy might not like friends coming in all the time to the house.' Similar findings have been reported by Jobling and Cuskelly (2002) for adults with Down's syndrome in Australia and by Rosen and Burchard (1990) in the USA.

People in residential settings

Robertson *et al.* (2001) obtained information on the social networks of over 500 people (average age 45 years) presently living in three types of residential accommodation: dispersed community houses; NHS-run residential campus settings consisting of a cluster of houses; and village communities run by voluntary organizations, usually in rural settings. The services in this English study were nominated by key informants as being 'good exemplars' of that type of provision. Robertson *et al.* found the median size of each person's networks was two persons (once staff were excluded) but a quarter only had one or no persons in their networks.

Staff, family members and other people with learning disabilities featured in the networks of most people, but fewer than one-third had a person from outside these categories in their network. These findings held irrespective of the type of setting the person resided in, but service practices did have an influence on network size and composition. People living in less institution-like services had larger social networks and they were more likely to have a relative or non-disabled person in their networks.

Similar findings have been reported by Jahoda *et al.* (1990) in Scotland, Lowe and de Paiva (1991) in Wales; Donnelly *et al.* (1994) in Northern Ireland and McConkey *et al.* (2003b) in the Republic of Ireland.

Charting friendships

It is easy to dismiss these findings by thinking they don't apply to the people with whom you work. But how do you know unless you take the trouble to find out? Two findings I can almost guarantee.

First, the people they name will often be staff and fellow service-users. Probe a little deeper and you may find that the amount of time and the types of contact they have with their so-called 'friends' is very different to what you expect and get from your own friends. Also, if you were to ask the people they name who their friends are, many may never mention the person who gave you their name in the first place. An unreciprocated friendship is no friendship at all.

Second, most people will tell you about the friend or friends they used to have. This starts with teenagers and goes on throughout people's lives. The fewer friends one presently has, the more precious become the memories of those you once knew. Probe further and you may discover that some friendships were broken because service personnel decided that a person had to move from a hospital, home, school or centre with no consideration given to the social networks the person had forged and no support given to them to maintain contact with old friends. Studies of people moving from long-stay hospitals found that they did not have contact with those remaining in hospital (McConkey *et al.* 2003a). Perhaps such practices still go on, but taking time to listen to people talk about their friendships is one way of questioning them.

This analysis should lead us on to ask if anything can be done to help people to form friendships. First though, we need to appreciate the complex web of processes that underpins the development of human friendships (Duck 1992).

How friendships develop

Despite the centrality of friendships to human well-being, there is no prescription for their successful development. You will know from your experience that some friendships spring up rapidly from an initial meeting while others evolve over a long period of time. Some of your friends have a lot in common; others are very different from each other. You may have friendships that have lasted a long time, whereas others have faded after a short time.

But underlying this variation there do appear to be some common elements in the development of friendships based on research findings, personal experiences and outcomes of service interventions. As Figure 23.1 shows, these fall into two groups: the social opportunities and the personal skills and attributes required by the individual. However, these groups are interlinked and interactive. For example, self-confidence grows as people

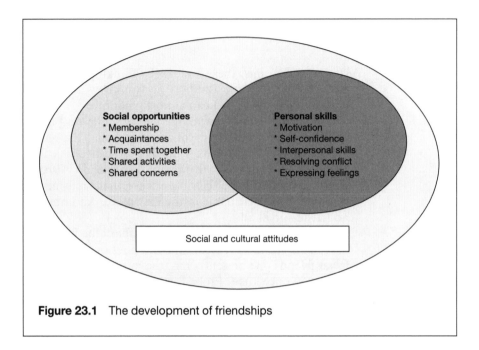

Figure 23.1   The development of friendships

avail themselves of social opportunities, yet some self-confidence is needed to join with others in social activities.

Friendship formation is also influenced to a greater or lesser degree by the prevailing social and cultural attitudes within the communities in which people live. This is most obviously felt in so-called 'divided societies' in which Jews and Muslims, Catholics or Protestants, black and fair-skinned persons will find many subtle and sometimes not so subtle influences that affect their choice of friendships. Arguably, these influences are just as potent in a society that separates people into the 'able' and the 'disabled'.

We can use the framework of Figure 23.1 to better understand why people with learning disabilities can find it so difficult to make and keep friends – particularly with people who are not learning disabled.

Social opportunities

Membership

Babies are born into a world of social opportunities: first within their family but gradually extending into the wider society as they visit other homes, attend crèches and playgroups and become 'members' in other social groupings, such as neighbourhood playmates, schools and youth organizations. These opportunities introduce the person to others and others to the individual. Although such introductions are first determined by the child's carers, later their siblings, peers and the person themselves will begin to make their own introductions.

However, from an early age, children with learning disabilities can become segregated from their non-disabled peers. This may be for the best of reasons, such as special schools offering teaching and support better suited to their disabilities. Nonetheless, a consequence is that their opportunities to belong to the same social groupings as other children is often curtailed. This pattern is then continued into the teenage and adult years.

Acquaintances

Acquaintances can start to develop from within our membership groupings. This is a crucial step in the growth of friendships as our close friends are likely to emerge from acquaintances or else it is through our acquaintances that we are introduced to others who may become our friends (Firth and Rapley 1990).

Building acquaintances is dependent on factors such as physical attractiveness, similarity in appearance and ease of communication, which may be perceived by others to be lacking in people with disabilities. For example, Farrell and Scales (1995) reported that non-disabled preschoolers were more likely to name other non-disabled peers in their integrated playgroups as friends rather than those with learning disabilities.

Time spent together

Some friendships may develop rapidly but more usually it is a case of 'getting to know one another' by spending time together. This is the time for testing out if you share interests, values and attitudes; for example, as you gossip about others, recount past experiences and make suggestions for activities you might do together.

The fact that people with learning disabilities develop close personal friendships with their peers in special schools, centres and residences is testimony to the importance of spending time together. However, this contact is often denied to people who are not disabled as their meetings with disabled people tend to be restricted to social greetings on the streets (McConkey 1987). Nevertheless, when they do get the opportunity to spend time together, notably when people with learning disabilities are placed in ordinary work settings, then increased numbers of friendships are reported (Jobling and Cuskelly 2002).

Moreover, it can take longer to get a fuller picture of a person with a disability, as many staff will testify. For instance, staff often comment that they see a different side to the person when they are with them outside of the usual workplace – such as on holiday together. However, people who are non-disabled may be reluctant to invest the extra time if they are receiving little back from their contacts.

Shared activities

Various shared activities help to forge closer relationships, especially if they involve the sharing of feelings and emotions such as those engendered by sports, drama and religious celebrations. Equally, participation in a variety of social pursuits helps to build a network of acquaintances and creates more opportunities for friendships.

This brings us to a real vicious circle. The more acquaintances and friends you have, the easier it is to join in a range of social pursuits which in turn help to consolidate and sustain friendships. But the opposite is then also true. Fewer acquaintances means less opportunities to engage in social pursuits. Indeed, the lives of people with learning disabilities tend to be dominated by watching television and listening to music (Smyth and McConkey 2003).

Shared concerns

Friendships are often nurtured through working together on common concerns. Membership of self-help groups and residents' associations can bring people together as can sharing adversities such as discrimination and grief (Pennington *et al.* 1999). The latter may impel people to share many feelings, thoughts and values which otherwise they might not have done and in so doing they discover their 'soul mates'.

However, people with learning disabilities are usually perceived as a concern in their own right rather than people who can share emotions and support other people in their times of need. This mutuality factor more than others explains why staff usually cannot be considered friends of their clients in the fullest sense of the word 'friends', although it may happen in some instances and certainly does occur when staff leave the work setting and relinquish the role of caregiver.

As you reflect on the above, it quickly becomes apparent how important it is for people with learning disabilities to be given opportunities to be in the company of other people – both disabled and non-disabled. This is the foundation on which acquaintances and friendships develop. It's as simple as that. Yet for many decades in the last century people were denied these opportunities – paradoxically on the grounds that it was in their best interests. A more haunting question remains: is social isolation still happening in the twenty-first century?

Personal skills and attributes

Social opportunities are not sufficient on their own. People need to actively contribute to the process of making friends.

Motivation

'Without a desire to develop a relationship, no relationship is likely', wrote Firth and Rapley (1990: 15). Lack of motivation may be because people want to be alone; they may feel they have sufficient friends already; or they could be ambivalent about what a relationship may bring – unwilling to risk rejection or undertake obligations. However, people's motivation is strongly affected by their past experience. Those who have experienced repeated or traumatic rejection may themselves openly reject people who offer friendship (Vanier 1991). Also, people with autistic spectrum disorders can show little interest in other people. Likewise, some people may have mental health problems such as depression and as a result are hard to get to know.

A challenge for staff and families is therefore to keep people motivated to be sociable, for them to find laughter and fun in the company of other people and for them to experience having their particular 'wants' met through, and with, other people.

Self-confidence

This is needed throughout all social activities, from greeting people to keeping in contact with them. People who are shy, retiring or taciturn therefore have difficulty in making friends. Self-confidence is also influenced by people's upbringing and their past experiences as well as their feelings and beliefs about themselves – 'I'm ugly – nobody will want to be my friend.' Ironically, successful social interchange builds self-confidence, but how does this get started if there is little self-confidence in the first place?

Once again, a key role for staff and family carers is to promote and encourage the person's self-confidence by accentuating their positive features and compensating for their weaknesses. However, this often goes against the culture that pervades their lives, namely these people are helpless – they need to have things done for them!

Interpersonal skills

This covers a multitude of diverse skills including 'body language', communication skills, social conventions, and judging people's moods and attitudes and acting accordingly. Young children are often excused for their lack of interpersonal skills but only up to a point. It takes a great deal of observation, imitation and feedback to master all the subtle skills that oil our interactions with other people and convey our willingness for friendships. However, these skills take longer to develop when people have disabilities and indeed many may never be realized. In these instances, the more able communicators have to be prepared to adjust their communications but many find this very hard to do (McConkey *et al.* 1999).

Resolving conflict

For some people the problem is not making friends, it is keeping them. The skills involved in avoiding and resolving conflict are difficult for people to learn if they are not able to 'put themselves in another's shoes'. Often they cannot appreciate or anticipate the hurt they might cause to their erstwhile friend through misjudged words or actions.

Such insights cannot be directly taught, but people do benefit from reflecting on their experiences in one-to-one sessions or through role-playing with video playback so that they can be helped to identify the specific behaviours that may be causing the problems.

Expressing feelings

Many people are poor at expressing their feelings to others. They may be reluctant to give praise, to say sorry, to express their hurt, even to say thanks. This failure may cause relationships to stagnate and even break down. However, as in other domains of their life, people with learning disabilities can benefit from social skills training, although surprisingly this often does not feature among the priorities of staff working in services – possibly because these behaviours are thought to be *part* of their disability.

The complexity of the skills required to make and sustain friendships is all too apparent. Little wonder children take some ten years before they become adept at these skills. It is not surprising that people with learning disabilities may struggle to acquire some or all of these high-level social skills. However, this difficulty is *not* an inherent feature of their disability. Rather, the lack of social opportunities that many have experienced allied with the dearth of educational programmes focused on communication and interpersonal skills are far more to blame.

Exercise 23.1

Pick a friend you know well. Use the above framework to identify his or her strengths when it comes to making friends. What do you feel are his or her main weaknesses?

Now repeat this for a person with learning disabilities you know well. What are his or her strengths when it comes to making friends? What do you feel are his or her main weaknesses? How might these be overcome?

Social and cultural attitudes

The prevailing social and cultural attitudes within a community often influence the pattern of friendships that form – put crudely, people prefer their 'own kind' and outsiders may be ignored, shunned or abused. In many senses, people with a learning disability (or mental handicap as the condition was previously known) are still outsiders within our society. They continue to experience discrimination and hurtful attitudes from their fellow citizens (see Box 23.1). These include family carers and professionals as well as the 'general public'. Likewise, parents describe being refused admission to restaurants with their profoundly handicapped child and service managers have had to deal with protests from neighbours opposed to a new facility for people with learning disabilities in their area.

Box 23.1 Hurtful attitudes reported by people with learning disabilities (McConkey 1994)

- Name-calling from children
- Teenagers who try to take money off you
- People staring at you in shops
- Trouble from GPs; they talk to the staff but not us
- Trouble from churches; no one talks to us or makes us welcome
- Bad neighbours – always complaining and blaming us for things which are not our fault
- Staff in centres who smoke in your face and boss you around
- People who mean well but get it all wrong – 'patronizers'
- Youngsters knocking on your door and running away
- Parents who mean well but who treat us like children
- Shop assistants don't take time to listen if we can't make ourselves understood

---

A growing number of research studies undertaken in various countries have identified several truisms about society's attitudes (McConkey 1994). The majority of people – usually around 75 per cent – have had no personal contact with people who have learning disabilities. Hence their images of them are likely to be stereotyped and possibly mistaken. Locating people with disabilities in community settings is no guarantee that they will meet and get to know local people. Less than 10 per cent of people living close to a day centre had met any of the attenders. People anticipate many more problems in terms of having contact with people with learning disabilities than is borne out by the reality of the experience. This has been shown in studies with neighbours of group homes, employers, teachers, nurses, therapists and GPs (e.g. McConkey 1994).

Personal contact with people who have learning disabilities has consistently been found to lead to more positively disposed attitudes and increased confidence. Personal contact, rather than putting people off, appears to win them over. Hence the priority should be to create even more opportunities for people to meet. Although most people in the community have no interest in meeting people with learning disabilities, there are a minority (around 25 per cent) who are willing, and often they report having had previous contact with this group so they do know what they may be taking on. Certain neighbourhoods are more welcoming than others to groups of people with learning disabilities. Taking time to determine the characteristics of neighbourhoods through community consultations would help services seek out those districts where the risks of active opposition are lower and the chances for social integration higher.

But the most crucial conclusion about attitude change is also the most hopeful. It is so much easier to change attitudes to specific individuals than it is to an indeterminate group of people know as the 'handicapped'. This is why media campaigns, political lobbying and information leaflets have all proven to be relatively ineffective in changing attitudes. Far more powerful is the opportunity to meet and get to know people as people, not as patients, residents or service-users. Such meetings should take place in ordinary locations such as pubs, churches and shopping malls rather than in special centres.

The need for go-betweens

However, these encounters will not happen if left to chance. 'Go-betweens' are needed. As the name implies their strength derives from knowing both parties. They know the needs, interests and talents of the person with a learning disability but unlike them, they are connected with various community groups. They are well placed to identify possible connections either with individuals or groups. Indeed their job is often easier if small groups are involved of, say, two or three people. In order to achieve anything, of course, a go-between has to be prepared to ask! Schwartz (1992) identifies this simple task as one of the most crucial weapons in the armoury of community integrators. Equally he notes the reluctance of some professional staff and carers to ask favours of others. Why? Perhaps because they are afraid of being rejected – people may say no. Yet experience and research suggests that the majority of people are disposed to be of assistance and very few would ever be rude and critical. Or maybe they feel no one can quite measure up to the task or that there are too many risks involved – hence they have to continue shouldering the responsibility. Again, experience shows that professional staff and carers tend to overestimate the risk involved and do not consider that the person with the learning disability may respond differently to the 'new' person. More worryingly, could it be that they feel there is nothing in it for the other person – that there are no benefits to befriending a person with learning disabilities? Interestingly, family carers and voluntary helpers seem much more adept at naming these benefits than are paid staff (Stainton and Besser 1998).

The next stage is that of introductions. Like a good host or hostess, the go-between needs to put the strangers at their ease by facilitating the conversation, modelling interactions, finding joint activities for them to do and, when the opportunity arises, discreetly withdrawing for a time so that they take on the responsibility for maintaining the interaction.

Finally, the go-between needs to be supportive of the blooming partnership by keeping in touch with both parties, checking how things are going and making discreet suggestions, while subtly praising them for how well they are coping with the challenge.

The contribution of such go-betweens to the lives of people with disabilities has been best captured in the work of Edgerton *et al.* (1984) who describe the crucial role of people they termed 'benefactors' in helping people with learning disabilities discharged from long-stay hospitals to socially integrate into local communities. However, this dependence decreased over time as people merged into society.

Rarely are these connecting tasks written into the job descriptions of professional workers; nor are people recruited for their 'people-making' skills. Paradoxically, most of us acquire these skills and utilize them in our personal lives so perhaps their deployment in the service of people with learning disabilities could be readily promoted if only the will to do so was there.

Friendly with whom?

This is an apposite juncture to think a little more about a challenging issue: namely, are people with a disability 'happier with their own kind' or should they find friendships predominantly with non-disabled people?

In the heyday of the normalization movement, a premium was placed on people with learning disabilities being integrated into mainstream society. Specialist, segregated settings only served to devalue their humanity and perpetuate the low status that society placed on such individuals. Implicitly the message was: don't congregate people with disabilities.

This was also the wish of some people with learning disabilities – especially those who were more mildly affected. Edgerton *et al.*'s (1984) research for example, identified a strong wish to lose the label of 'mentally retarded' and to pass as non-disabled within their community.

With hindsight, this idealistic thinking was naïve for a number of reasons. Not least, it discounted the express wish of many people with learning disabilities who value their friendships with similar people (e.g. Bayley 1993). Many of the advances in social policy have resulted from marginalized groups banding together, promoting solidarity and advocating their rights. This has been equally true for the disabled movement, led predominantly by those with physical and sensory disabilities, but it is also emerging for people with learning disabilities (Bersani 1998). Social integration has been very slow to achieve. People who have moved into dispersed community housing still have few non-learning disabled people in their social networks and those who report most satisfaction with their existing level of relationships tend to be those with a greater proportion of other learning disabled people in their networks (Gregory *et al.* 2001).

In our society, intimate relationships tend to occur among people who are matched in terms of age, background and interests. Indeed, legal prohibitions exist preventing men having sexual intercourse with women who have 'mental impairment'. These are likely to be ignored if both parties are deemed to have a learning disability and are thought capable of giving consent. Hence those seeking an intimate relationship are more likely to find it among friends who are similarly labelled. We will return to this issue later.

In sum, a more reasonable stance is to promote both types of friendship; it is not an either-or situation. However, there is an important provision: it depends on the person. In a group home for instance, one person may be reluctant to socialize with the other residents as they are keen to escape what they see as the stigmatizing label of learning disability. However, other residents may prefer to be in the company of their fellow housemates as they may feel threatened and uneasy in the company of people who are more able communicators than they are. Hence the importance of person-centred planning which takes account of people's talents and preferences and the need to find ways of providing a range of opportunities suited to that particular person's needs and aspirations.

Nurturing friendships

In this section we examine various strategies that can be used with people who have learning disabilities to widen their network of acquaintances and to nurture their friendships. Before exploring these in more detail, three basic principles need to be stressed:

- Friendships cannot be made for other people; people choose their friends. At best we can build up a network of acquaintances out of which friendships may develop.
- Friendships usually grow out of shared interests and activities and from among people already known to the person. This is the starting point.
- Choice and self-determination are key elements in friendships. Hence you need to constantly consult and listen to the people you are trying to help. We must not impose our values and desires onto another.

Befrienders

These principles are at odds with the popular idea in services and with family carers of finding a person (usually a volunteer) to befriend a person with learning disabilities. Experience suggests that such schemes can be done and that they do offer benefits for both parties (e.g. Walsh *et al.* 1988), but they are risky for a number of reasons.

The matching of 'friends' is often done by a professional worker or scheme coordinator; hence the person with learning disabilities has very limited scope for choosing and developing their own friendships. The 'friendship' that develops runs the risk of being artificial in the sense that the able-bodied person is invariably cast in the role of helper and supervisor.

Through time this can place quite a strain on the relationship. If the able-bodied person is no longer able or willing to continue, there is the added problem of finding a replacement while dealing with possible feelings of disappointment and loss in the person left behind.

In sum, the befriender approach is another example of adopting a specialist solution to a disability issue. Therein lies the biggest risk of all: a befriender absolves everyone else – busy support staff and social workers for example – from their responsibilities for nurturing friendships.

The four-stranded approach

Newton *et al.* (1994) start from a different perspective entirely. Their proposition is that the focus of all staff involved with disabled persons should not be on the person with the disability *per se* but rather on the relationships between the person and the other members of his and her communities. (Note the term 'communities' can include a family community, a service community such as a day centre, a work community as well as neighbourhood communities.) Newton *et al.* identified four interrelated elements to nurturing relationships (see Figure 23.2). These are examined in turn below.

Social support

Among the many definitions of social support in the literature, the original conceptualization by Cobb (1976) is particularly apposite for those of us working with individuals who have a learning disability. He viewed social support as telling people they are cared for and loved, showing them they are valued and esteemed and helping them to find a place in a network of

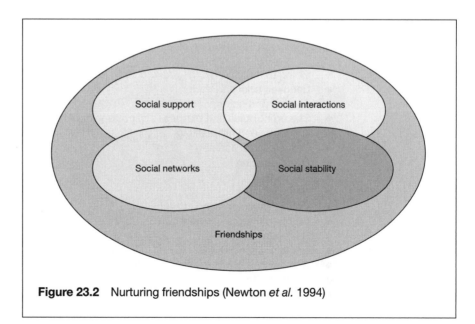

Figure 23.2   Nurturing friendships (Newton *et al.* 1994)

communication and mutual obligation. The goal of social support is to make people feel good about themselves and to feel needed.

Numerous studies have documented the stress-buffering and health-promoting influences of social support across a wide variety of societal groups (Sarason and Sarason 1985) and it is a concept that has been extensively investigated with parents of children with disabilities (Dunst and Trivette 1990).

Others (e.g. Sarason and Sarason 1985) have described the practical outworking of social support by creating typologies of different forms of support such as material support (e.g. providing them with money and loan of equipment); emotional support (e.g. listening if they have problems); information support (e.g. naming other people they could contact); and instrumental support (e.g. practical assistance such as escorting a person on a bus).

Of course many staff in services will recognize this as a summary of their job descriptions but there is a crucial difference. People with learning disabilities need to be seen as sources of support to others and not just as receivers of support. It is the mutuality of support that is a hallmark of friendships. This is the basis on which many advocacy groups function.

Social interactions

Here the focus is on what happens when two or more people meet and jointly engage in activities, be it conversing, celebrating a birthday, attending a meeting or painting a room. As noted earlier, people with learning disabilities can experience particular difficulties in holding their own in such settings. However, certain settings are more conducive for promoting social interactions than others (see Box 23.2). As you read through the list you might

---

Box 23.2   Activities for developing relationships (Firth and Rapley 1990)

- Going to the cinema, theatre and concerts
- Snooker, pool and darts
- Singing and acting
- Shared hobbies and classes (e.g. pottery, cooking)
- Rambling and hill-walking
- Folk/old-time dancing
- Disco dancing
- Camping
- Holidays
- Visiting museums and attractions
- Going to the pub or meal out
- Religious events
- Tenants' associations
- Self-advocacy groups
- Team sports
- Part of a team helping others in need

consider why these have been chosen rather than other activities such as watching television or listening to music – the most commonly reported pastimes of people with learning disabilities. Some of the common features you might have noted are:

- *couples*: there are opportunities for people to 'pair-off' for the activity;
- *relaxation*: people meet in relaxed and enjoyable situations;
- *privacy*: people can have private times together;
- *shared feelings and values*: people are given the opportunity to share their views and beliefs;
- *common cause*: it was noted earlier how friends are often forged in adversity or for a common cause – advocacy groups can be an important setting to acquire the skills required for social interaction.

Of course some of the above features can still be incorporated into watching television and listening to music. For example, by having privacy at home for friends to do this together or by talking together about films and TV programmes with a strong emotional content.

Another approach has been to provide education programmes that aim to develop the communication and social skills of people with learning disabilities. Although research reports are broadly positive, there is less convincing evidence of their widespread application in practice (Chadsey-Rusch 1992). One reason is that the staff who are in the best position to provide this guidance (namely those who are with the individual most frequently and consistently) are also those who are least likely to be trained in skill development. Rather, social skills courses tend to be run by specialist staff in 'classrooms' with possibly little carry-over into the person's everyday life.

Similar strategies have been used with communication, particularly the development of alternative and augmentative communication systems based around signs and pictures. However, these approaches perpetuate a focus on the individual with a problem. If the perspective becomes one of relationships, then the alternative strategy is to focus on the more able person and encourage him or her to adapt their interactions to become better attuned to the person with the disability. This is the approach increasingly promoted for enhancing communication (Purcell *et al.* 2000). Box 23.3 summarizes the ways in which people should change the way they talk to people with learning disabilities. Equally, able communicators – including staff – must become more adept at using sign systems such as Makaton.

Box 23.3 Adapting communication (Purcell *et al.* 2000)

- *Slow down*: leave more time for client initiations and responses.
- *Respond*: be more responsive to clients during interactions, with more use of non-verbal feedback in particular, such as head nods, facial expression and gestures.

- *Fewer questions*: reduce their use of closed questions (e.g. Do you want tea?) and increase the use of open questions (e.g. What do you want to drink?).
- *Comment*: increase the use of comments about yourself, what is happening and so on.
- *Simplify*: reduce the complexity and amount of the verbal language you use, with shorter sentences and simpler words.
- *Attention*: get and maintain the person's attention on shared activities through use of gestures and verbal prompts.

Social networks

A social network is composed of people who socially interact. This broad definition is useful as it reminds us that we all belong to many different networks and we enter and leave various networks in the course of any day.

That said, our networks vary in terms of size, intimacy and longevity. But for most people with learning disabilities, their networks tend to be smaller, more dense (the same people feature) and have more unreciprocated relationships. Many learning disabled individuals are overly reliant on one or two people (usually a family or staff member for companionship), and in fact there are some who are friendless. Some have argued that the advent of dispersed community housing has resulted in more loneliness for tenants with fewer opportunities to join with others in communal pursuits compared to residential homes and long-stay hospitals (Srivastava 2001).

One solution has been the concept of a community for people with disabilities living together with able-bodied helpers on a life-sharing basis. The Camphill communities begun by Rudolf Steiner or the L'Arche communities founded by Jean Vanier are two examples of international practices also found in Britain and Ireland (Jackson 1999). These 'intentional communities' have been the subject of much debate. However, recent research focusing on the outcomes for people living in such settings found they had greater satisfaction with their friendships and relationships than those living in dispersed community housing, although the size of their networks were similar (Gregory *et al.* 2001).

Another approach attracting much interest of late is that of creating 'circles of support' or a 'circle of friends' (Neville 1996). There is no prescription for the form and format these take as they will be guided very much by the wishes and needs of the person with a learning disability as identified in their person-centred plan (see also Chapter 24). That said, there are some common strands in such circles. They might include family members such as siblings, cousins, aunts and uncles, neighbours and acquaintances, co-workers for people in work settings, members of clubs, churches and suchlike who know the person. The size does not matter; a few interested people can make a start. The circle does *not* have to include professional workers although they can have a key role as facilitators or go-betweens, as noted earlier.

It is likely that the depth of friendship will vary across the members of the circle. Some may be prepared to be intimately involved, others will continue as acquaintances, but they will be better informed than previously. The circle might meet from time to time to explore with the person and each other the contributions they are making to each other's lives. Activity plans might develop as to how the circle could change or develop. 'In all circles of support people are encouraged to dream' (Neville *et al.* 2000: 151). Without a vision of what might be possible, the old routines and disappointments persist. Fulfilling these dreams often involves taking risks, but 'the circle itself is a safety-net and each time a new risk is safely negotiated greater encouragement is generated to renew the risk-taking effort' (Neville *et al.* 2000: 151).

This idea can find expression in different ways. For example, Key Ring is a housing provider for people with learning disabilities that works by building up mutually supportive networks among the tenants living within a geographical area as well as linking them into the communities where they live (Simons and Watson 1999). Likewise, new forms of day provision often operate on the basis of creating social networks for their clients by slotting them into educational, employment and recreational opportunities in the community (Towell 2000).

Social stability

The final element is probably the least investigated among people with learning disabilities, namely the continuity and stability of their social relationships. Undoubtedly there are many examples of lifelong friendships but we have an imperfect understanding of why this happens for some and not for others. Equally, change is a feature of everyone's friendships and sometimes this can be good for all concerned. Yet there have been few studies on the impact on people with learning disabilities when they loose friends.

The dimension of social stability is particularly challenging for services as the lower-paid staff they employ have a high turnover rate. This makes it very difficult for staff to assist people to sustain any relationships that have been forged. This reality is unlikely to change for the foreseeable future, which again emphasizes the need to promote friendships among service-users and to build circles of support.

Exercise 23.2

Pick one person with learning disabilities who you know well. Make a list of the different ways you think their social networks might be widened. What would staff need to do differently to make this happen?

Intimate relationships

In this final section we explore the responsibilities of staff in supporting people who are in intimate relationships.

Given all that we have said before, such relationships must be the choice of the people involved, and they will have developed over time. Hence the key role of staff is to respect the person's choice and help them to enjoy and develop their friendship. This will mean treating the people as a couple when it comes to planning activities, giving them times for privacy and taking pleasure in the benefits which the friendship brings to them rather than becoming preoccupied with the risks, which professional staff are wont to do.

Equally, you may need to help them work through the problems or difficulties that such a relationship will encounter from time to time. In particular, they may need assistance with the 'negotiation' skills needed to repair disputes and disagreements such as trying to see the other's view-point, being prepared to listen to their hurt, apologizing and finding ways of showing respect and love for their partner.

However, service staff also need to be aware of their limitations. There may come a point when it is necessary to encourage the couple to seek help from other sources, such as specialist workers or organizations, for example, Relate or the Family Planning Association.

Challenges and dilemmas

Undoubtedly, intimate relationships bring particular challenges and dilemmas for service staff with their 'duty to care' responsibilities:

- Have the couple received sex education? Are they aware of contraceptives? If the answer is no to one or both questions, then whose responsibility is it to ensure this happens?
- Is the relationship lawful? As noted earlier, this is a grey area with outmoded laws. The risk is that people's happiness can be sacrificed unnecessarily by simply keeping to the letter rather than the spirit of the law. Who will give you an informed and credible opinion if you encounter these issues?
- Does the relationship offend your morals? You may not want to condone physical relationships between people of the same sex, or outside marriage. This is an issue you must share with your co-workers and all come to an agreed course of action. To do otherwise is to risk harming your relationship with the person and with your colleagues.
- Could the relationship be abusive or is it in danger of becoming so? This can include financial, emotional, physical and sexual abuse. You need to sensitively check out your suspicions; record them factually and be especially vigilant for any signs that are indicative of abuse.
- Are the couple having a fling? Sexual activity between couples need not imply a lasting emotional relationship. This is sometimes referred to as

'recreational sex' and modern society offers many opportunities for it. Some would argue that people with learning disabilities have the same rights to partake in such relationships as their peers. But given the degree of supervision these people experience in their lives, it is unlikely to happen without someone turning a blind eye. Can paid staff afford to do this without the backing of their superiors? Is this likely to be forthcoming?

These challenges and dilemmas will continue to reverberate in our services for many years to come. Meantime it is helpful if:

- clear guidelines are prepared for staff who deal with the above issues;
- time is given over at team meetings to discuss the implementation of the guidelines;
- staff supervision is used to assist front-line workers to deal with the issues noted;
- key workers have particular responsibilities to provide non-judgemental support in intimate relationships;
- people with learning disabilities are actively taught assertiveness and self-protection skills so that there is less danger of exploitation and abuse;
- people with learning disabilities have a circle of support who will look out for them as well as assist them;
- people are given opportunities for privacy and to get to know one another – this may mean opportunities for weekend breaks, going on holiday together and perhaps living together.

Conclusion

A few themes have re-echoed throughout this chapter. Friendships can take a long time to grow, the ground needs to be well prepared and a plentiful supply of fertilizer is required! Even so, the harvest is still variable and may be disappointing. Support staff have to be gardeners.

Friendships can take many forms. We need to look beyond the immediate contacts in people's lives and try to build a circle of support for each person that will root them more firmly within their local community and society. Support staff have to be intermediaries.

Friendships enrich lives and sexual fulfilment is most often found in intimate relationships. But intimate relationships involving people with learning disabilities bring particular challenges to services and to a society. New styles of services are needed along with new ways of managing them and defining staff responsibilities. Support staff have to be inventors.

Nevertheless, services remain as they always have been because we continue to mistakenly try to isolate, care for or 'fix' the individual with the disability rather than nuture his or her relationships with other people. Who knows what would result if relationships became the focus of all our endeavours? Perhaps the time has come to find out.

References

Atkinson, D. and Ward, L. (1987) Friends & neighbours: relationships and opportunities in the community for people with a mental handicap, in N. Malin (ed.) *Reassessing Community Care*. London: Croom Helm.

Bayley, M. (1993) The personal friendships of people with learning difficulties, *Social Care Findings*, 39.

Bersani, H.R. (1998) From social clubs to social movement: landmarks in the development of the international self-advocacy movement, in L. Ward (ed.) *Innovations in Advocacy and Empowerment for People with Intellectual Disabilities*. Chorley: Lisieux Hall.

Buckley, S. and Sacks, B. (1987) *The Adolescent with Down's Syndrome: Life for the Teenager and for the Family*. Portsmouth: Portsmouth Polytechnic.

Chadsey-Rusch, J. (1992) Towards defining and measuring social skills in employment settings, *American Journal on Mental Retardation*, 96: 405–18.

Cobb, S. (1976) Social support as a moderator of life stress, *Psychosomatic Medicine*, 38: 300–14.

Donnelly, M., McGilloway, S., Mays, N., Perry, S., Knapp, M., Kavangh, S., Beecham, J., Fenyo, A. and Astin, J. (1994) *Opening Doors: An Evaluation of Community Care for People Discharged from Psychiatric and Mental Handicap Hospitals*. London: HMSO.

Duck, S.W. (1992) *Human Relationship*, 2nd edn. London: Sage.

Dunst, C.J. and Trivette, C.M. (1990) Assessment of social support in early intervention programs, in S.J. Meisels and J.P. Shonkoff (eds) *Handbook of Early Childhood Intervention*. Cambridge: Cambridge University Press.

Edgerton, R.B., Bollinger, M. and Herr, B. (1984) The cloak of competence: years later, *American Journal of Mental Deficiency*, 88: 345–51.

Farrell, P. and Scales, A. (1995) Who likes to be with whom in an integrated nursery? *British Journal of Learning Disabilities*, 23: 156–9.

Firth, H. and Rapley, M. (1990) *From Acquaintance to Friendship: Issues for People with Learning Disabilities*. Worcester: British Institute of Mental Handicap.

Gregory, N., Roberston, J., Kessissoglou, S., Emerson, E. and Hatton, C. (2001) Factors associated with expressed satisfaction among people with intellectual disability receiving residential supports, *Journal of Intellectual Disability Research*, 45: 279–91.

Jackson, R. (1999) The case for village communities for adults with learning disabilities: an exploration of the concept, *Journal of Learning Disabilities*, 3: 110–17.

Jahoda, A., Cattermole, M. and Markova, I. (1990) Moving out: an opportunity for friendship and broadening of social horizons? *Journal of Mental Deficiency Research*, 34: 127–39.

Jobling, A. and Cuskelly, M. (2002) Life styles of adults with Down syndrome living at home, in M. Cuskelly, A. Jobling and S. Buckley (eds) *Down Syndrome across the Life Span*. London: Whurr.

Lowe, K. and de Paiva, S. (1991) Clients' community and social contacts: results of a 5-year longitudinal study, *Journal of Mental Deficiency Research*, 35: 308–23.

McConkey, R. (1987) *Who cares? Community Involvement with Mental Handicap*. London: Souvenir Press.

McConkey, R. (1994) *Innovations in Educating Communities about Learning Disabilities*. Chorley: Lisieux Hall.

McConkey, R., Walsh, J. and Mulcahy, M. (1981) The recreational pursuits of mentally handicapped adults, *International Journal of Rehabilitation Research*, 4: 493–9.

McConkey, R., Morris, I. and Purcell, M. (1999) Communications between staff and adult persons with intellectual disabilities in naturally occurring settings, *Journal of Intellectual Disability Research*, 43(3), 194–205.

McConkey, R., McConaghie, J., Mezza, F. and Wilson, J. (2003a) Moving from long-stay hospitals: the views of Northern Irish patients and relatives, *Journal of Learning Disabilities*, 7: 78–93.

McConkey, R., Walsh, D. and Sinclair, M. (2003b) The social inclusion of people with intellectual disabilities living in community and campus settings. Paper submitted for publication.

Neville, M. (1996) Around in a circle, *Commuity Care*, February/March: 4–5.

Neville, M., Baylis, L., Boldison, S.J., Cox, A., Cox, L., Gilliand, D., Laird, M., McIver, B. and Williams, C. (2000) *Building Inclusive Communities*. Rugby: Circles Network.

Newton, J.S., Horner, R.H., Ard, W.R., LeBaron, N. and Sappington, G. (1994) A conceptual model for improving the social life of individuals with mental retardation, *Mental Retardation*, 32: 393–402.

Pennington, D.C., Gillen, K. and Hill, P. (1999) *Social Psychology*. London: Arnold.

Purcell, M., McConkey, R. and Morris, I. (2000) Staff communication with people with intellectual disabilities: the impact of a work-based training programme, *International Journal of Language and Communication Disorders*, 35: 147–58.

Redmond, B. (1996) *Listening to Parents: The Aspirations, Expectations and Anxieties of Parents about their Teenager with Learning Disabilities*. Dublin: Family Studies Centre – UCD.

Roberston, J., Emerson, E., Gregory, N., Hatton, C., Kessissoglou, S., Hallam, A. and Linehan, C. (2001) Social networks of people with mental retardation in residential settings, *Mental Retardation*, 39: 201–14.

Rosen, J.W. and Burchard, S.N. (1990) Community activities and social support networks: a social comparison of adults with and without mental retardation, *Education and Training in Mental Retardation*, 25: 193–204.

Sarason, I.G. and Sarason, B.R. (1985) *Social Support: Theory, Research and Application*. Dordrecht: Martinus Nijhoff Publishers.

Schwartz, D.B. (1992) *Crossing the River: Creating a Conceptual Revolution in Community and Disability*. Cambrdge, MA: Brookline Books.

Simons, K. and Watson, D. (1999) *The View from Arthur's Seat: Review of Services for People with Learning Disabilities – A Literature Review of Housing and Support Options Beyond Scotland*. Edinburgh: Scottish Executive Central Research Unit.

Smyth, M. and McConkey, R. (2003) Future aspirations of parents and students with severe learning difficulties on leaving special schooling, *British Journal of Learning Disabilities*, 31: 54–9.

Srivastava, A. (2001) Developing friendships and social integration through leisure for people with moderate, severe and profound learning disabilities transferred from hospital to community care, *Tizard Learning Disability Review*, 6(4): 19–27.

Stainton, T. and Besser, H. (1998) The positive impact of children with intellectual disability on the family, *Journal of Intellectual and Developmental Disability*, 23: 57–70.

Towell, D. (2000) Achieving positive change in people's lives through the national learning disabilities strategy: lessons from an American Experience, *Tizard Learning Disability Review*, 5(3): 30–6.

Vanier, J. (1991) *Community and Growth*. London: Longman & Todd.

Walsh, P.N., Coyle, K. and Lynch, C. (1988) The partners project: part 1, *Mental Handicap*, 16: 122–5.

24

Enabling and supporting person-centred approaches

Jacqui Brewster and Paul Ramcharan

Introduction

The commitment to person-centred planning (PCP) as the foundation for changing the lives of people with learning disabilities in the UK (Department of Health 2001a, 2001b) makes it vital that nurses and other support and service workers are aware of its history and operation. However, Sanderson *et al.* (2000: 1) have pointed out that 'there is a wealth of material on Person-Centred Planning that is hidden from the usual places where we search for information'.

You will therefore need to access more publications than can be covered in this chapter. As will be seen, the use of PCP in practice will also require you to attend relevant training events to expand both your expertise and your understanding of your place as a professional within person-centred approaches as a whole. The lack of literature on PCP is, we would argue, also accompanied by a lack of empirical research evidence.

The idea of being 'person-centred' has a warm ring to it. Like 'community care' it is a fortunate term. Indeed, it has been suggested of community care that it was '. . . substantiated not on the basis of its merits, but on the basis that the alternative was unthinkable' (Bean and Mouncer 1993). In this chapter we will therefore seek to identify the key features of PCP and its operation. We will comparatively examine PCP against its predecessor in the UK, individual programme planning (IPP), discuss the meaning of person-centredness, and then assess the merits of the PCP approach. This will be undertaken by using case examples to demonstrate the points being made.

What is PCP?

Some have argued that PCP is a natural evolution from previous IPP systems. For example, the All Wales Strategy saw that the person with a learning disability and their families were involved in preparing, implementing and reviewing individual programme plans. As Felce *et al.* (1998: 16) note, 'Co-ordination of the individual planning system was to be done by multi-disciplinary teams . . . each person with a learning disability was to have a nominated key worker in addition to providing specialist professional input in the multi-disciplinary team and was to act as a single point of contact for individuals, families and generic services alike'. Contrast this with the official UK definition of PCP: 'Person Centred Planning is a process for continual listening and learning, focusing on what is important to someone now and in the future, and acting upon this in alliance with their family and friends' (Department of Health 2001b: 12). To understand how these two systems differ we compare them in Table 24.1 along five well-established dimensions (Sanderson 2000; Department of Health 2001a, 2001b).

Table 24.1   Comparison of the IPP and PCP process along the five PCP dimensions

Dimension of PCP	The IPP process	The PCP process
1 Person at the centre		
Person's place in planning process	Involved as participant	Control
The planning group	Professionally convened	Person, advocates and supporters, i.e. circle
Membership of group	Professionals with user/carer	Chosen by the person, relationship-oriented
Ethos of planning meeting	Participative	Person in control and ownership
2 Family members and friends as partners in planning		
Ethos	Participation of carer and user in identifying professionally assessed need	Partnership with family, friends and community. Professionals invited as necessary
Resolution of conflict	Professional knows best	Creative management of conflict through negotiation. The person and his/her circle knows best

Table 24.1 *(continued)*

Dimension of PCP	The IPP process	The PCP process
3 Using the person's gifts, capacities and aspirations to judge the relevant support they need		
Ethos	Takes a deficit perspective in assessing needs	Is artful, creative and innovative in responding to wishes and dreams
Approach	Quantitative, concentrating on training the person to be more independent and keeping them safe	A qualitative approach concentrating on total quality of life from the person's perspective
Information-holding and collecting	Information and decisions held by professionals and presented in ways that can be inaccessible to the person. File on shelf	Information presented in ways which are accessible and meaningful to the person and accessed by those involved in the planning
4 Planning for action		
Focus	Service- and professionally-oriented. Assumes services can meet all needs	A shared commitment to action in family, relationships and community as well as in services to support these changes
Resources mobilized	Service resources to promote inclusion	A focus on mobilizing those with a commitment to the person, i.e. communities of interest
Provision	'Off-the-shelf' service packages	Demand for a made-to-measure response from services and others
5 The planning process		
Meetings	IPP meeting and six-monthly review	Plan is not the outcome. Circle of support meets as often as necessary. A continuous process of listening and responding to wishes as the person grows

Table 24.1 (*continued*)

Dimension of PCP	The IPP process	The PCP process
Coordination	Professional coordinates the service response through purchaser	A continual process with the circle facilitator prompting relevant parties to act. This may also involve assessment for services under the NHS and Community Care Act 1991
Service orientation	Person as recipient of what is available	Reflects what is possible. Still limited by service availability, but able to push for new services to cover an unmet need. A variety of formats running from the artistic and personal history right through to formal plans for action
Product	A completed and locally standardized pro forma usually split into specific sections to reflect quality of life issues and specialist health and other needs	

Case study: *Jane*

Jane is a young woman of 19 years who has just left school. She lives at home with her parents and her 10-year-old brother. Jane loved school, had many friends, and is a real extrovert. Her favourite subjects at school were music and art. Jane has Down's syndrome and when she was at school lost a lot of time due to her asthma and epilepsy. She and her family have recently moved to another part of the country due to her father's new job. The whole family are trying to find their feet. Jane has enrolled on a special needs literacy and numeracy course at the local further education college but she is unhappy there and wants to do something else. She tells her newly-appointed social worker that she is sick of feeling 'poorly'. When asked what she wants, Jane is very clear . . . she wants a job where she can help people; she has always wanted to sing on stage; she wants a boyfriend and some space away from her little brother.

> **Exercise 24.1**
>
> Think about Jane's wishes and aspirations for the future and her practical day-to-day needs. Write a description of how you would see a planning meeting for Jane under the IPP process and then under a PCP process. Which do you feel would produce a better outcome and why? Who might lead the process? Who else would be involved? Which process would you prefer if you were to make a plan for a time of change in your own life?

The IPP system was innovative in seeking the participation of the person and their families in planning services but it did not wrest power from the professionals to assess and provide services off a rather 'dusty shelf'. The natural evolution would seem to be represented by locating control with the person and their allies. Hence, the PCP system also represents the melding of ideas of normalization and of support groups (e.g. circles of support) (Brandon 1991). Table 24.1 graphically illustrates the contrasting features of the IPP and PCP approaches, but also shows lines of similarity. Clearly, power and control within the PCP system have migrated to the individual and their families and friends. In this sense the PCP model represents the bringing into being of a community that cares. This is 'community care with service support' as opposed to a 'community service model'.

Sanderson (2002) states that PCP has not simply appeared but has naturally 'evolved' from the 'most progressive' philosophies and care practices of the last three decades. PCP is part of a wider move towards person-centred care that has increasingly come to characterize a central underlying value of human services within medical, health and social welfare.

It used to be said that IPP was person-focused and indeed there were a number of arguments about the ways in which 'needs-led' services represented the ultimate balance between professional and user interests, placing the user at the very heart of decision-making (McGrath and Grant 1992). So, while there has been a movement in several aspects of IPP, it is the circles of support that mark out PCP. Here, the responsibility for making connections with, and planning for, inclusion in the community (see also Chapters 23 and 29) is left to the circle of support. Most importantly, PCP marks a movement from the person as the focus in a professional, needs-led assessment to a situation in which the person and their circle of support prompt those professionals who assess under the NHS and Community Care Act 1991 the person's needs.

This does not mean that under the PCP system there are no professionals assessing the person's needs. This still has to be undertaken by a care manager under the provisions of the NHS and Community Care Act 1991. The guidance on PCP exhorts care managers to ensure under the provisions of the NHS and Community Care Act that 'people's goals and choices are powerfully reflected in care planning and design, and in the purchase and review of services' (Routledge and Sanderson 2001: 45). There remain issues about how a system of PCP might be 'tripped up' by a system that is the ultimate policy representative of the ascendancy of a needs-led rather than a person-centred ideal. In this light, 'buying' the right services (rather than relying on a care manager to do so) is well addressed by the direct payments system. This represents a further move towards the circle of support and users themselves assessing and organizing their own provision.

In many ways, the PCP system represents an intended transfer of responsibility from the professional to the person. In the PCP model, the circle of support establishes the dreams, wishes and aspirations of the person as the vital centrepiece of both assessment and provision. Dowson (1990) has argued that when I want something, say a holiday, I need to save, to go through brochures, to go to a travel agent, to buy the right clothes and so forth. Needs are therefore a practical means to achieve wishes. They are the practical part of 'getting to where I want to be'. Unlike in the past where services assumed responsibility but were unable to measure up, now that responsibility is taken on by those who care about the person enough to help them with the practical aspects of meeting needs through services, circles, neighbourhood and community. Services in this conception are but a small and supportive part of a person's life and not life's centrepiece as often seemed the case in the past. This frees the person from service dependency and unshackles them from the service system as representing who they are.

But how can person-centredness be achieved in practice? Below we outline the key features of person-centredness and provide some worked examples of how it might be organized within the PCP system.

Person-centred care

It is important to identify the specific meaning of person-centred care as conceptualized under the present policy framework of *Valuing People* (Department of Health 2001a, 2001b). At its very heart Coyle and Williams (2000: 452) make the suggestion that person-centred care is about 'valuing people as individuals', an interesting definition given the title of the learning disability White Paper in England and Wales and the fact that Coyle and Williams' work was in a different care sector.

However, as is often the case within professional, academic and service settings, such terms are adopted and used in a variety of ways. The resultant arguments about how an ideal might be thought about or operationalized in practice therefore lead to little agreement. Such is the case with person-centredness where, in their systematic review of quantitative studies on patient-centredness, Mead and Bower (2000) point out that there is very little consensus on its meaning. Person-centred care has therefore been categorized and defined in a number of ways:

- *By its 'constituent parts'*: in this approach a number of characterizing features are variously identified. For example, involvement in decision-making (Grol *et al.* 1990; Winefield *et al.* 1996); 'responsiveness to need' (Laine and Davidoff 1996); sharing of power and responsibility (May and Mead 1999); communication and partnership, empathy, health promotion, clarity and representing personal interests (Little *et al.* 2001); user choice (Barclay 1998); and patient-as-person (Kitwood 1997).

- *In terms of perspective and discipline*: in relation to primary care there is a move towards person-centred care and away from the traditional doctor-patient relationship and doctors seeing the individual solely in terms of biological pathology (see e.g. Gerteis *et al.* 1993; Little *et al.* 2001). Others have similarly written about its applicability in secondary health care settings (e.g. Coyle and Williams 2000). Different perspectives have been brought to understanding how person-centred care might operate. Coyle and Williams (2000) see it in terms of 'a personal identity threat'; others see it in terms of a 'biosocial model', emphasizing the 'experiencing individual' as the centre of decision-making (Smith and Hoppe 1991) or in terms of a model of 'egalitarianism' between doctor, service worker and patient/client or user (May and Mead 1999).

- *In relation to its outcomes*: there are a growing number of studies in this area following on from the different approaches taken in practice settings, (see e.g. Martin and Younger 2000; Mead and Bower 2000; Parley 2001).

The mish-mash of competing perspectives therefore suffers a recurrent academic fate. The concept is dismembered and then one part is taken to define it (e.g. out of all the possible things it might be there is a focus on, say, 'responsivness to need' or 'involvement in decision-making'), or it is applied in different settings and loses its specific meaning to the area under discussion (e.g. in relation to the doctor-patient relationship).

We would argue, however, that there are some rather specific and unique intentions in adopting the idea of person-centredness within contemporary learning disability policy. These are perhaps best understood by working through some examples of the ways in which such an approach might be operationalized within the present policy context.

Valuing People (Department of Health 2001a), which represents current policy for England and Wales, places PCP at the heart of service provision and objectives. In later guidance (Department of Health 2001b: 12), person-centred planning is defined as:

A process of continually listening and learning, focusing on what is important to someone now and in the future, and acting upon this alliance with their family and friends. The listening is used to understand a person's capacities and choices. Person-centred planning is the basis for problem-solving and negotiation to mobilise the necessary resources to pursue a person's aspirations. These resources may be obtained from someone's own network, service providers or from non-specialist and non-service sources.

It is rare now to see, for example, an advert for a position in learning disability services which does not ask for an understanding of and a commitment to person-centred care and PCP. It is the fulcrum around which nurses and other service personnel will be organizing to support clients to achieve independence, inclusion, dignity and respect in the coming years.

PCP is seen as a 'process' rather than an event. It is not a one-off meeting with a review every six months but, rather, a way of thinking and acting together. It is based on a number of assumptions that have been set out in texts on person-centred care (see Sanderson 2000 for a review). For Sheard (2004: 2), '. . . person centred care is a life philosophy – an aspiration about being human, about pursuing the meaning of self, respecting difference, valuing equality, facing the anxieties, threats and guilts in our own lives, emphasising the strengths in others and celebrating uniqueness and our own 'personhood'. Sheard's definition highlights the importance of working with people in a way which recognizes and acknowledges their unique identity as people of value whatever label they have been given because of their 'difference'. It also recognizes that person-centred care and support is important for everybody – we all need support in life, we all need to feel recognized, 'celebrated', loved and respected for what we do and who we are.

We will now proceed by seeking to outline key elements of the person-centred approach and appropriate ways to accomplish such an approach. Key points are highlighted as the text proceeds.

Person-centred tasks

Celebrating uniqueness and learning to value the person

At the heart of person-centred approaches is the belief that each person is a valuable human being and deserves to be valued and treated with respect and dignity. One of us (JB), in discussing her own experiences as a student nurse with current students, was asked if any of the people with whom she had worked stood out in her mind. Despite this being over 20 years ago the memories of many people with whom time was shared and enjoyed came flooding back. Each of these people had gifts to offer – honesty, humour, warmth, openness, an ability to show concern and love for others, enthusiasm, energy, passion, patience, practical skills and abilities – yet often they were only known for their 'impairments' and the given labels that went with them: severe learning disability, challenging behaviour, autistic spectrum disorder, cerebral palsy and so on.

- **A person-centred approach means helping people to recognize their unique qualities and abilities, looking beyond impairments, showing people that we recognize their gifts and enjoy being with them.**

To recognize a person's qualities assumes at least two things. Firstly that we are able to communicate with that person and secondly that we know the person well enough to be able to recognize their own unique gifts and talents.

Often this will involve not only meeting and knowing the person, but knowing others who care about and for them. The group of people who care about and for the person, who support them and know them best, can be called a 'circle of support' (see Perske and Perske 1988; Brandon 1991) and that circle may change over time. Service workers working in a PCP system are therefore less likely to be on their own in knowing the person and can learn a lot more about the person through those in the circle.

- **Learning about the person implies knowing them, listening to them, learning from them, listening and learning from others in their circle and, as a group, being there with them so that we can observe their life experiences.**

One of the strengths of learning with the person and their circle is that, particularly for those whose communication we find hard to understand, we can learn about the best ways to communicate with them. We can learn from the circle how to share a system of communication and hence to value the experience of their main carers, whether family or service personnel, or be inventive as a circle about the best ways to learn from them.

But that leaves open *what* we should be learning from the person. If we think about our own relationships we expect those around us to know the things we like, our dreams, nightmares and so forth. It is no different for people with learning disabilities. Perhaps the central difference is that in order to provide a consistent approach, the circle needs to meet as a group to share their understanding with the person.

- **The circle should meet to ensure that they share a view about the person based upon the person's own preferences, whether verbalized or reported as their responses to previous experiences.**

But what is the circle looking for in listening, talking or experiencing? At the centre of the person-centred process is listening to the person and/or observing the things which give them pleasure as well as the things that drive them crazy; talking to people about the things they love, the things that comfort them when they are down, the things that make them feel cherished; and sharing activities which reflect the things that they love. For some circles this is more a matter of sharing ideas rather than of discovery, though there are always new things to learn. However, where the circle do not know the person well, Sanderson (2002) recommends a more detailed approach such as essential lifestyles planning (see Table 24.2 for a summary).

- **Circles should focus on dreams, aspirations and wishes.**

Essential lifestyle planning does not only look at hopes, dreams and aspirations through storytelling, discussion and sharing histories. It also focuses on the mundane everyday 'stuff of life'. Consider how annoying it would be for someone you know to continue to make your coffee in a way you did not like, to get you out of bed early when you do not have to, to help you to get dressed when you do not need that help, to make meals they know you do not like. These everyday experiences contribute to your quality of life as much as moving towards your dreams. They define your present-day

Table 24.2   A summary of person-centred planning approaches

Type of PCP	Cues to use and predominant focus	Approach
Essential lifestyle planning (Smull *et al.* (undated)	Where the circle does not know the person well Where it is difficult to understand what the person wants	Listening to the person's story, getting to know their unique skills and qualities, how they communicate, what support is needed for them to stay fit and healthy and to make plans about who will do what, when and how. It may involve storytelling, learning logs, discussion of incidents, routines and rituals. It is perhaps the most comprehensive PCP approach
MAPS (Forest and Lusthaus 1989)	When a person can communicate their dreams Where the person already has support to work towards their dreams	The group: finds a way together; explores the person's story and history; explores what the 'best life' would be; explores nightmares and worries; brainstorms who the person is and who she or he wants to be. By picture-building it provides a way of planning action
Personal futures planning (*see* Mount and Zwernik 1988; Mount 2000)	To give an overview of the person's life as it is To focus on the future and on dreams	Provides a means of drawing up maps of key areas in the person's life, for example a community map, health map or a choices map. It specifically addresses areas of concern. It outlines personal accomplishments and provides tools to implement six key tasks associated with planning a personal future
PATH (*see* O'Brien *et al.* 1993)	To develop and plan for action and change	A way of developing a series of actions that can achieve a person's dream. It helps identify who does what, when they do it and how they do it. The approach also explains the role of the circle facilitator

experiences and your quality of life. The same is true for all people including people with learning disabilities. This experience means that people respect your 'non-negotiables' (Smull and Burke-Harrison 1992) and that they provide competency-enhancing support (Booth and Booth 1994) without creating dependency.

Exercise 24.2

Take a few minutes to think about the place of a chosen routine in your own life. Write down the answers to each of these questions.

Morning routines: what do you do when you get up in the morning? Dress straight away or slob about in your nightwear for a while? Jump out of bed immediately with a smile on your face or does it take lots of caffeine to get you going? Take a bath or a shower? What shower gel, toothpaste, cosmetics, teabags etc. do you use? Is it important to leave the house tidy before you leave or are you not bothered?

Other rituals: what are your comfort rituals when you've had a bad day? Glass of wine, hot bath, go to the gym, go out for dinner, phone a friend? Which side of the bed do you sleep on?

More rituals: How do you spend Sundays? At church, cleaning the house or just chilling out? Do you do anything special each year for your birthday or for anniversaries and Christmas? What's your idea of a great holiday?

Now compare and contrast these answers with those of a friend. What do your rituals say about the things in life that are important to you? Examples might be 'I'm not a morning person and like to wake up slowly and quietly' or 'When I'm in a bad mood I like to be left alone'.

In *Positive Rituals and Quality of Life* Michael Smull (2004) reiterates the importance of finding out what people want their days to be like:

> Our efforts need to begin with these daily rituals. We have found that some of the people referred to us because of 'non-compliant' or aggressive behaviours simply have daily rituals that were not recognised. Our obsession with implementing program plans and continuous training has resulted in ignoring, suppressing, and trying to replace rituals that are positive, individual adaptations to the rhythms of life.

Smull points out that the routines of many people living in residential care settings may change according to which member of staff is on duty. He also points out that our comfort rituals are not just something we allow ourselves when we have been 'good' – we will still have that bottle of wine even if it was our fault that we had a bad day, whereas people with learning disabilities are often expected to 'earn' these indulgences. The sense of control over my rituals is therefore a vital part of experiencing a life that is 'good to and for me'. So it is for all individuals.

- **It is vital to consider how present life experiences respect routine, ordinary and day-to-day choices.**

Getting to know the person therefore incorporates their future dreams and their present life experiences. But our present personal identity is also shaped by our past. Helping people explore their biography can be a powerful means of self-expression and an important ingredient in appreciating constituents of successful ageing and adaptation (see Chapter 33).

Case study: *George*

George has lived in service settings from being a teenager after the death of his parents. George has moved many times and he has never had a key worker move with him. Now George is elderly and physically frail. Through a support group George was recently invited to talk about himself and his past and express this by making a personal poster using paint and magazine images. George shared with the group that he was the son of a Northumbrian farmer and he moved the group with stories of feeding chickens, fetching eggs and bringing the sheep in with a beloved sheepdog. The care worker attending with George was fascinated. Despite having worked with George for six months and having a great deal of information in the form of care plans and risk assessments, she had not got to know George as a person with a past and a future.

Case study: *Dean*

Through dreams we can often get to what is essentially important to a person. Dean explored his dreams through art as he found words difficult. Dean's drawings and paintings were of open fields and mountains with birds and animals and of himself driving caravans and motorbikes. When exploring these images with Dean and thinking about his history, the team realized that Dean had spent much of his life in confined overcrowded places, starting with prison in his teens and then a constant series of small group homes. Dean desired open spaces where he could feel free. The wild outdoors and being on his own, at least some of the time, really appealed to somebody with this type of background.

Life story work, personal posters, art work, poetry, diaries, scrapbooks and photo albums can be powerful ways of helping people express their identity. Perhaps one way to start this work with people is to look at the examples published by other people with learning disabilities. One text which broke the mould in these terms was *Know Me as I Am*, an anthology of poetry and prose by people with learning disabilities (Atkinson and Williams 1990). It has been followed by several others (see Ramcharan and Grant 2001 for a review of 'testaments of life').

As Atkinson and Walmsley (1999) point out, life history work can serve several purposes: understanding personal identity; recapturing ownership of one's life; comparing the past with present circumstances; dealing with the experiences of a difficult history; and planning ahead. Exploring the past is often a necessary step towards planning for the future and it can sometimes be painful and take a long time.

In the ordinary course of our own lives we would find it very hard to share information about ourselves with a large group. We all have things about us which we share with very few people, if anybody at all. Often this privacy has been denied people with learning disabilities and very personal details such as embarrassing health problems, bowel movements, personal relationships and things they may not feel particularly proud of have been shared in quite public settings without their express permission, such as in care planning meetings. We therefore need to realize that people may not want to tell us everything about their lives or, indeed, to share their lives in the ways suggested above.

We must also be aware that for many people with learning disabilities there may be some very painful memories to share. Memories may reflect a lifetime of exclusion, isolation and loneliness, and sometimes abuse. Some people may find it cathartic to share this information, others may find it all too painful or difficult to share, or may not have the words. We must therefore be sensitive about asking people to share memories with us, watch for signs that the person may be distressed and give support and/or get further support to help the person where necessary.

- **Exploring the past is very often as important as knowing the present and dreaming about the future.**

Being person-centred requires that any circle collectively understands the core of a person's ideals, values and emotional strengths and frailties as described above. But, given the emphasis on community inclusion in present policy, it also places a responsibility on the members to be 'mapping' inclusion and becoming involved in direct action to support the person to make such inclusion meaningful to them. Personal futures planning (*see* Mount and Zwernik 1988; Mount 2000) and MAPS (see Falvey *et al.* 1997) focus on these issues (see Table 24.2) though not to the exclusion of other approaches.

In considering a person's life we might address: where the person wants to spend their days – at work, in day activities, doing voluntary work; involvement in hobbies and personal interests; the clothes they choose to wear or the fragrance they use; the possessions they enjoy; the way they decorate their home; and the people the person wishes to share these things with. We also need to know more about the person's health needs and how they choose to stay healthy. This may involve creating a map of their choices in relation to community and health, as in personal futures planning or planning how to accomplish what they choose. A central task of being person-centred therefore involves ensuring that plans for a person's future are inclusive and that their identity is, over time, seen as an included rather than an excluded identity.

- **Inclusion in the community may involve having an overview or a map of a person's choices, their present experiences and a plan of action to move towards meaningful inclusion in their own community.**

In this section key areas of person-centredness have been identified and tied to the actions of a circle of friends. It is, however, vital that this circle do not simply take over the person's life. There are also issues about the membership of the circle itself.

Person-centred interaction

So far consideration has been given to the parameters of person-centredness and how these are translated into forms of PCP. But there is also a 'how'. The ways in which people are brought together and how they treat one another are vital elements in ensuring a group works together with and for the person concerned. These are reviewed in more detail below.

Welcoming family and friends

Family and friends provide an abundance of shared memories and experiences and a depth of emotion which means that they often care in a way which is different to the paid caregiver. Our relationships with family and friends help us to form a view of ourselves as lovable and loving human beings. It is true that many people with learning disabilities have lost contact with their families or that these relationships have been damaged, sometimes after many years of struggling with an under-resourced service which fails to understand their needs and concerns. A person-centred approach to care welcomes family and friends as individuals with special knowledge and insight into the person. It calls for a more honest and open way of working with families and supports these relationships in enthusiastic and non-judgemental ways.

As with any family there are always power struggles and relationship difficulties and there will be times when relatives and friends have a different view of what is best for the person than the person themselves. At these times it is important to acknowledge that these conflicts are often based on real fears for the person. It is a time to discuss these fears with those involved, ensuring that as care workers we do not come across as the 'experts who make the decisions' but as advocates and equals looking for a positive solution which meets the wishes of the person concerned.

Interaction based on demonstrable respect, partnership and power sharing

The way we speak to a person, including the words we use, our tone of voice, the inflection used and the body language that accompanies our verbal expression, strongly reflect the way we see that person and the level of respect we have for them.

Exercise 24.3

Consider the difference between these two interactions:

'My mum used to make porridge.'
'Did she? We don't have time this morning. We're going to be late for day care if we don't hurry up.'

'My mum used to make porridge.'
'Did she John? My mum did too. What was it like? Tell me about it as we get ready to go out. We could make some tomorrow if you like.'

Identify the differences between the two. Which is better and why?

Writing about the development of person-centred standards for care homes, Mo Ray (1999) describes how communication in such homes can become 'relegated to the status of an activity' rather than 'a constant and consistent process of interaction' which involves partnership, companionship and respect: 'Personhood becomes denied as the task becomes the most important part of the interaction. In this way a person needing skilled and special support at mealtimes can become labeled as a "choker", and a group of people who need help to eat can be labeled "feeders" (p. 17). A person-centred approach to care recognizes that people with learning disabilities often have problems communicating. It approaches all attempts at communication, be they making noises, walking away, singing, laughing, crying, or getting angry and aggressive, as a serious attempt to express self, to participate, to make choices and to be a social person. We need to find ways to maximize individuals' communication abilities, recognizing that all individuals communicate. It is often as much a matter of us learning the person's communication repertoire as the person developing more communication strategies (see Chapter 13).

In addition to the way we communicate with people, the things we share with them and the ways we involve them in all aspects of their lives are also an indication of how we value them as people. Consider the difference between the following tales of moving house. The tales may be thought of in terms of the idea that 'Being consulted means being respected'.

Case study: *Liz, Henry and Joe*

Liz and her partner Henry and their son Joe have just moved house. The move has taken two years of planning – two years of thinking, talking, saving, getting help, making decisions and taking action. Friends and family gave support which was practical, emotional and financial. They needed to consult with professionals: estate agents, mortgage advisers and solicitors. The professionals helped them through the maze of different mortgage deals and the legal necessities involved in moving house. At times it was all very confusing and stressful. The decision to move reflected a change in the family's circumstances which, in turn, was based on the life choices they had made. The family love their new home. Its rural setting is just right for a family who enjoy the great outdoors. Joe has started at his new school and the family have made new friends among their neighbours, at the local pub and by visiting the local church.

Case study: *Bob, Peter and James*

Bob, Peter and James have also just moved house. Unlike Liz, Joe and Henry they are not a family – they only met four months ago when their local social services department made the decision that, as three elderly men with physical and learning disabilities, they would get on well with each other. The decision to move was based on government policy which led to the homes they were living in being closed. The men themselves did not choose the home. It was chosen for them: a large bungalow which was chosen to meet their physical impairments. Unlike Liz and her family, the men's friends and families had nothing to do with the move and the consultations with estate agents and other professionals were done for them as it was felt that the men would be incompetent in this task.

For Liz and her family, moving home was exciting, scary, stressful but, ultimately, a positive experience. The decisions taken reflect what is important to the family now and their hopes, dreams and aspirations. For Bob, Peter and James moving home was yet another experience of exclusion, of being ignored and of powerful others making decisions for them based on 'policy' and their similarities based on age and professional views about their impairments.

Person-centred care means that the person is at the centre of his or her life. What does being at the centre mean? It means that what happens in your life depends on you in partnership with the people who love and care for you. Being at the centre of your life is therefore very much the same as being in control of your life. All of us struggle with issues of control in our lives. We may have managers who make decisions about us rather than with us; we may lack money that stops us living where we wish. Yet for many people with learning disabilities this struggle is continuous and oppressive. Others who are more powerful make decisions about where they live, with whom, how they spend their days, how they dress, what they eat, how their money is spent and even what they are allowed to say. To experience this level of oppression can amount to an emotional strait-jacket which people often find their way out of through challenging behaviour or by withdrawing into themselves.

Care where the carer shares of themselves

David Brandon (1989) describes how staff often lose their way when working with people and become overwhelmed by the demands of the organization they work in. Brandon describes this as 'learning a few crude techniques' and losing the 'easy giving of self'. This 'easy giving of self', Sheard (2004) argues, is often undervalued in our services, yet the people who give of themselves in this way make a huge and positive impact on the lives of those with whom they are involved: 'they have developed themselves into people who instinctively live their lives with the ability to connect to others' feelings who use their instincts and gut feelings, who feel person-centred care rather than just practise it' (Sheard 2004: 23). Sanderson (2002) points out that to make PCP a reality, services need to work in person-centred ways towards staff. Support staff working with people with learning disabilities are often poorly paid, and have very little control over their working lives; they also work very unsocial hours which has an effect on family life. Sanderson argues that often PCP fails because support staff are unsupported themselves and become 'burnt out' at work, going through the motions of care and becoming more controlling over those for whom they provide support. Person-centred care calls for a rethink of the way services act towards the paid carers of people with learning disabilities: it calls for a process of getting to know staff as unique individuals with unique gifts to offer and not as numbers to be managed.

PCP in practice

A number of person-centred approaches have been developed. You might want to look at MAPS (Forest and Lusthaus 1989), PATH (O'Brien *et al.* 1993), personal futures planning (Mount and Zwernik, 1988), essential life-style planning (Smull and Burke-Harrison 1992) and life review (Kropf and Greene 1993). Table 24.2 summarizes aspects of the different approaches to PCP. None are meant to be exclusive. Guidance (Routledge and Sanderson 2001) points to the need to adopt strategies to fit different situations and to be 'artful' and 'inventive' in how each approach is used. Column 2 of Table 24.2 also helps to identify cues for the use of different approaches (see p. 500).

Five characterizing features of PCP were identified and compared to the previously existing IPP system in Table 24.1 while some of the main approaches to PCP are outlined in Table 24.2. As has already been said, there are many different planning styles, each looking at who the person is, their unique gifts, skills and needs, along with their personal history. Each style also finds out what is important to the person while identifying who are the people who love and care for the person. Each different style also explores how the person can take part in their community and how they can be helped to live a life outside the service system.

PCP meetings should be conducted using language and communication methods which are accessible and enjoyable for the person. Methods used therefore might include photos, pictures, drawings, computer images and graphics, role play, Makaton and music. In fact, the meetings should use anything that is meaningful to the person which makes the meeting friendly, accessible and uplifting, using language and approaches which are qualitatively different from those generally heard in service settings. Each of the planning styles comes with a graphic which leads the planning team through a more creative, person-centred way of looking at a person's life.

The PCP process starts with the creation of a 'circle of support' around the person. The circle will involve people who love and care for the person, chosen by the person themselves, and it is the circle who will help the person to make plans for change in their lives based on the things the person sees as important. This approach is therefore not about what the service thinks the person should do and the support they should have. The circle will also have a plan of action seeking to support the person in changing their lives, getting the appropriate resources to do so and mobilizing the right people to become involved.

A facilitator will typically coordinate the group in the above activities and ensure that the group monitors how things are going over time. Planning meetings should take place in a setting chosen by the person and the facilitator should also ensure that meetings are conducted in an atmosphere of support, enthusiasm and positive respect. The facilitator's role is therefore essential (*see* Mount 1991; Joyce 1997) but you may not be in that role. Knowing the role you occupy in the circle and the tasks that fall to you will be a key part of making the circle a success. Indeed, in many instances professionals will not be invited to the planning meeting but may be consulted for their specialist knowledge which will be put to use in a way that the person and his or her supporters think appropriate.

PCP has the potential to change the very fabric of people's lives by placing at their disposal the resources, skills and commitment of those people who are closest to the person. The process provides an inventive array of resources which can be drawn upon imaginatively to make essential links between the persons' past and present in a plan set out to achieve their stated future dreams and aspirations. However, there may, as outlined in the final section to follow, be some real difficulties with the PCP approach.

Criticisms of PCP

In *Guidance for Partnership Boards* (Department of Health 2001b) there is a recognition that a second aspect of PCP is 'To provide a means through which commissioners and providers . . . can learn how their services and systems need to change in order to respond positively to the aspirations of people with learning disabilities and their families' (p. 6). This implies that information in PCP at an individual level needs to move into the strategic arena so that the supply of services might better reflect the collective demand for each service as expressed in all PCP (for any one Partnership Board area). There are important issues with the ownership of the PCP, that it is sometimes not documented in formal ways and that it is often held and owned by the person with learning disabilities themselves. In this sense the flow of information may not reflect the reality of people's plans. This relates to resources in two distinct but related ways. A similar system of using individual plans to develop appropriate services was engineered as part of the All Wales Strategy over two decades ago. But it was found that there was, 'considerable variation in the prevalence of IPs between counties (from 3% to 30%), reflecting both the priority accorded to IPs . . . and the available staffing levels' (Felce *et al.* 1998: 56). This raised questions about how the county planning groups (the equivalent of the Partnership Boards) were actually making their decisions about service priorities.

The IPP system required several professionals to meet with the person and their carer. This represented a huge draw on the resources of the professionals involved. This may explain why not every person had an individual plan under the IPP system. The same inability to facilitate PCP to the numbers of people envisaged in *Valuing People* has been noted by Mansell and Beadle-Brown (2004). The resources of staff would very quickly be soaked up were they to be playing a key role in several PCP initiatives, especially since the meetings are likely to be more frequent than the IPP meetings and their six-monthly reviews. Indeed, the actual number of reviews undertaken in Wales under the IPP system was very small, leaving the statutory services to respond to emergencies only, except in the minority of cases.

At the same time as these demands, professionals are also undergoing increasing demands in relation to quality and standards of care (see Chapter 7). Sheard (2004), discussing PCP in elderly care homes, points to a continued overemphasis on disability and dependency, and an obsession with risk assessments, care standards, care plans, quality assurance, rules and regulations. The constant checking of fridge temperatures for example not only stifles the person with learning disability but the people giving care as well. All of the above create mountains of paperwork which takes people who care away from the people they want to care for and leads to a culture of apathy and weariness. This places even further strain on an already scarce resource. Alongside this, and despite a formal system of training under the Learning Disability Awards Framework (LDAF), there remains low pay and low status for people providing direct care, leaving a group of devalued staff to offer care which is based on valuing the person they are supporting while providing love and respect. Over time this can lead to compromises over best intentions, with respectful support being supplanted by an emphasis on tasks to be done.

Packer (2001: 28) asserts that we must keep on trying to implement a person-centred approach to care but recognizes that in so doing carers can get very worn down: 'As long as we continue to struggle to implement "new culture" ideals in the face of "old culture" resource management, our personal stockpile of coping strategies, however extensive, will remain under constant pressure'. It may seem strange for a strategy adopted as national policy but there remains very little systematic or empirical evidence supporting PCP. There is little evidence about how person-centred approaches help to improve people's lives, and the evaluation studies available are small in scale so generalizations are difficult (Malette *et al.* 1992; Hagner *et al.* 1996; Heller *et al.* 1996; Dumas *et al.* 2002). In their review of qualitative evidence on the use of lifestyle planning, Rudkin and Rowe (1999) concluded that there are few reports with outcome data. However, it was accepted that lifestyle planning does seem to lead to processes which would be experienced as enabling people to express preferences and make choices, reinforcing a sense of ownership and inclusion. The question is whether this helps to create conditions that positively and materially alter the (quality of) lives of service users and families. In a separate report, Rudkin and Rowe (1999) concluded that there is as yet no quantitative evidence to support the use of lifestyle planning in general or in any individual form. For the most part we are therefore left with anecdotal reports or with largely descriptive, process-oriented accounts that offer rather mixed results (Parley 2001). Thus far there seem to have been no studies that have systematically evaluated one person-centred approach against others in process, cost and outcome terms. However, Holburn *et al.* (2000) have begun the task of developing validated measures of PCP processes and outcomes. Replication work would now be timely.

Mansell and Beadle-Brown (2004) argue that to expect service staff to take on the role of planner calls for a level of communication skill, especially in terms of facilitating non-verbal communication for choice and decision-making, which years of research suggests that they do not possess. Like normalization before it, the acceptance of PCP seems to have occurred without a great deal of questioning or criticism: 'It epitomised the way forward for the design of services: anything progressive could be achieved only by adopting the Normalisation principle. It had moved from being ridiculous and naïve to become the accepted wisdom. To criticise it was tantamount to heresy' (Chappell 1997: 47).

Many of the people identified in *Valuing People* as needing a plan, for example those still living in long-stay hospital, do not have allies and supporters outside the service system and because of the nature of their problems and impairments (i.e. severe learning disability, aggression and challenging behaviour as well as chronic health conditions), it is very difficult to build on any naturally occurring support network (Mansell and

Beadle-Brown 2004). The authors also point out that there is still a 'lack of an accepting community' upon which the circles are likely to be able to draw (see Chapter 29). They also feel that there is concern that in expecting the family and friends of people with learning disabilities, particularly female carers, to create plans which do not rely on the service system, local authorities are opting out of their responsibility to put resources into responsive, high-quality services.

The PCP system seems to have placed the responsibility for organizing a person's life firmly at the door of those closest to them. For many carers already struggling with recalcitrant services, fighting while tired and stressed for a person's rights, the idea of accommodating the interests of other parties in a coordinated circle may represent just one step too far. Indeed, spending copious resources on training people to do planning using specific tools and approaches, a requirement of the PCP system, may create an 'activity trap'. In this trap, carers unable to undertake such training may feel somehow sidelined. In contrast, further pressure is placed on services since time which could be spent with service users creating person-centred approaches to care is spent instead on training.

Conclusion

When talking to a student recently about her experiences of what she found to be a very difficult placement in a group home, we discovered that she dealt with the problems by talking to members of staff, making suggestions for change, challenging negative attitudes and by making sure, as she put it, that she made a positive difference each day, in some small way. We can all make these 'differences', challenge attitudes and talk to others as people of value. Packer (2000: 30) puts it well: '. . . every little bit counts. Small ripples can make big waves, but only if enough of those involved in direct care are prepared to be proactive in spite of these limitations, and to accept the psychological conflict this involves'.

We might also challenge 'old service models' by questioning how services are designed, by getting involved in supporting people with learning disabilities through self-advocacy activities or by attending service planning or Partnership Board meetings and advocating the rights of service users. Adopting a person-centred approach in the face of traditional services is not easy and requires us to find others to talk to who understand, as well as looking after our physical and psychological health.

We need to be aware of the barriers to adopting person-centred approaches and helping people create person-centred plans for their lives. If we are not aware of the difficulties and are not prepared for them then these approaches are more likely to fail. We need to question and reflect on these approaches in a positive but well-informed way while continuing to work towards a more positive future for people with learning disabilities.

In replying to the criticisms of PCP raised by Mansell and Beadle-Brown

(2004), O'Brien (2004: 15) states that we must guard against cynicism and pessimism and see PCP as an opportunity to help people live better lives:

> There is no need nor justification to look at person centred planning through rose-coloured glasses. There is good reason to look with clear eyes at the possibilities for a significantly greater measure of choice and inclusion and to make an energetic commitment to the hard work of making those possibilities real at whatever scale the local and national environment can support.

References

Atkinson, D. and Walmsley, J. (1999) Using autobiographical approaches with people with learning difficulties, *Disability and Society*, 14(2): 203–16.

Atkinson, D. and Williams, F. (eds) (1990) '*Know me as I am*'. London: Hodder & Stoughton.

Barclay, J. (1998) People, plans and possibilities: exploring person-centred planning, *Community Living*, 12(2): 9–10.

Bean, P. and Mouncer, P. (1993) *Discharged from Hospitals*. London: MIND.

Booth, T. and Booth, W. (1994) *Parenting Under Pressure: Mothers and Fathers with Learning Disabilities*. Buckingham: Open University Press.

Brandon, D. (1989) Professional behaviours, in D. Brandon (ed.) *Mutual Respect*. London: Good Impressions Publishing.

Brandon, D. (1991) *Direct Power: A Handbook on Service Brokerage*. Preston: Tao.

Chappell, A.L. (1997) From normalisation to where? in L. Barton and M. Oliver (eds) *Disability Studies: Past, Present and Future*. Leeds: The Disability Press.

Coyle, J. and Williams, B. (2000) Valuing people as individuals: development of an instrument through a survey of person-centredness in secondary care, *Journal of Advanced Nursing*, 36(3): 450–9.

Department of Health (2001a) *Valuing People: A New Strategy for Learning Disability for the 21st Century*. London: Department of Health.

Department of Health (2001b) *Valuing People: A New Strategy for Learning Disability for the 21st Century. Towards Person Centred Approaches. Planning with People: Guidance for Partnership Boards*. London: Department of Health.

Dowson, S. (1990) *Who Does What? The Process of Enabling People with Learning Difficulties to Achieve What They Need and Want*. London: Values into Action.

Dumas, S., de la Garza, D., Seay, P. and Becker, H. (2002) I don't know how they made it happen but they did: efficacy perceptions in using a person-centred planning process, in S. Holburn and P. Vietze (eds) *Person-Centred Planning: Research, Practice and Future Directions*, Baltimore, MD: Paul H. Brookes.

Falvey, M.A., Forest, M., Pearpoint, J. and Rosenberg, R.L. (1997) *All My Life's a Circle. Using the Tools: Circles, MAPS and PATHS*. Toronto: Inclusion Press.

Felce, D., Grant, G., Todd, S., Ramcharan, P., Beyer, S., McGrath, M., Perry, J., Shearn, J., Kilsby, M. and Lowe, K. (1998) *Towards a Full Life: Researching Policy Innovation for People with Learning Disabilities*. Oxford: Butterworth Heinemann.

Forest, M. and Lusthaus, E. (1989) Promoting educational equality for all students:

circles and maps, in S. Stainback, W. Stainback and M. Forest (eds) *Educating all Students in the Mainstream of Regular Education*. Baltimore, MD: Paul H. Brookes.

Gerteis, M., Edgeman-Levitan, S., Daley, A. and Delbanco, J. (1993) *Through the Patient's Eyes*. San Francisco: Jossey Bass.

Grol, R., de Maeseneer, J., Whitfield, M. and Mokkink, H. (1990) Disease-centred versus patient-centred attitudes: comparison of general practitioners in Belgium, Britain and the Netherlands, *Family Practitioner*, 7: 100.

Hagner, D., Helm, D.T. and Butterworth, J. (1996) This is your meeting: a qualitative study of PCP, *Mental Retardation*, 34: 151–71.

Heller, T., Factor, A., Sterns, H. and Sutton, E. (1996) Impact of person-centred later life planning training program for older adults with mental retardation, *Mental Retardation*, 35: 364–72.

Holburn, S., Jacobson, J., Vietze, P., Schwartz, A. and Sersen, E. (2000) Quantifying the process and outcomes of person-centred planning, *American Journal on Mental Retardation*, 105: 402–16.

Joyce, S. (1997) *Planning On: A Resource Book for Facilitators*. Ontario: Realizations.

Kitwood, T. (1997) *Dementia Reconsidered*. Buckingham: Open University Press.

Kropf, N.P. and Greene, R.R. (1993) Life review with families who care for developmentally disabled members: a model, *Journal of Gerontological Social Work*, 21(1/2): 25–40.

Laine, C. and Davidoff, F. (1996) Patient-centred medicine: a professional evolution, *Journal of the American Medical Association*, 275: 152–6.

Little, P., Everitt, H., Wiliamson, I., Warner, G., Moore, M., Gould, C., Ferrier, K. and Payne, S. (2001) Observational study of the effect of patient centredness and positive approach on outcomes of general practice consultations, *British Medical Journal*, 323: 908–11.

McGrath, M. and Grant, G. (1992) Supporting needs-led services: implications for planning and management, *Journal of Social Policy*, 21: 71–97.

Malette, P., Mirenda, P., Kandborg, T., Jones, P., Bunz, T. and Rogow, S. (1992) Application of a lifestyle development process for persons with severe intellectual disabilities, *Journal of the Association of Persons with Severe Handicaps*, 17: 179–91.

Mansell, J. and Beadle-Brown, J. (2004) Person-centred planning or person-centred action: policy and practice in intellectual disability services, *Journal of Applied Research in Intellectual Disabilities*, 17: 1–9.

Martin, G. and Younger, D. (2000) Anti-oppressive practice: empowerment of people with dementia through choice and control, *Journal of Psychiatric and Mental Health Nursing*, 7: 59–67.

May, C. and Mead, N. (1999) Patient-centredness: a history, in C. Dowrick and L. Frith (eds) *General Practice and Ethics: Uncertainty and Responsibility*. London: Routledge.

Mead, N. and Bower, P. (2000) Patient-centredness: a conceptual framework and review of the empirical literature, *Social Science and Medicine*, 51(7): 1087–110.

Mount, B. (1991) *Dare to Dream: An Analysis of the Conditions Leading to Personal Change for People with Disabilities*. Manchester, CT: Communitas.

Mount, B. (2000) *Personal Futures Planning: Finding Directions for Change Using Personal Futures Planning. A Sourcebook of Values, Ideals and Methods to Encourage Person Centred Development*: Manchester, CT: Capacity Works.

Mount, B. and Zwernik, K. (1988) *It's Never Too Early, It's Never Too Late: A*

Booklet about Personal Futures Planning. St Paul, MN: Governor's Planning Council on Developmental Disabilities.

O'Brien, J. (2004) If person centred planning did not exist, *Valuing People* would require its invention, *Journal of Applied Research in Intellectual Disabilities*, 17: 11–15.

O'Brien, J., Pearpoint, J. and Forest, M. (1993) *PATH: A Workbook for Planning Positive Possible Futures*. Toronto: Inclusion Press.

Packer, T. (2000) Facing up to the Bills, *Journal of Dementia Care*, 8(4): 30–3.

Packer, T. (2001) Everybody wants something: recognising your own needs, *Journal of Dementia Care*. 9(1): 26–7.

Parley, F.F. (2001) Person-centred outcomes: are outcomes improved where a person-centred care model is used? *Journal of Learning Disabilities*, 5(4): 299–308.

Perke, R. and Perske, M. (1988) *Circles of Friends: People with Learning Disabilities and their Friends Enrich the Lives of One Another*. Nashville, TN: Abingdon Press.

Ramcharan, P. and Grant, G. (2001) Views and experiences of people with intellectual disabilities and their families. (1) The user perspective, *Journal of Applied Research in Intellectual Disabilities*, 14: 348–63.

Ray, M. (1999) Developing person centred standards for care homes, *Journal of Dementia Care*, 11(6): 16–18.

Routledge, M. and Sanderson, H. (2001) *Valuing People: A New Strategy for Learning Disability for the 21st Century: Towards Person-Centred Approaches. Planning with People: Guidance for Implementation Groups*. London: Department of Health.

Rudkin, A. and Rowe, D. (1999) A systematic review of the evidence base for lifestyle planning in adults with learning disabilities: implications for other disabled populations. *Clinical Rehabilitation*, 13: 363–72.

Sanderson, H. (2000) *Person Centred Planning: Key Features and Approaches*. York: Joseph Rowntree Foundation.

Sanderson, H. (2002) A plan is not enough: exploring the development of person centred teams, in S. Holborn and P. Vietze (eds) *Person Centred Planning: Research, Practice and Future Directions*. Baltimore, MD: Paul H. Brookes.

Sanderson, H., Kilbane, J. and Gitsham, N. (2000) *Person-centred Planning (PCP): A Resource Guide*. www.valuingpeople.gov.uk/documents/PCPResource.pdf.

Sheard, D. (2004) Person centred care: the emperor's new clothes? *Journal of Dementia Care*, 12(2): 22–5.

Smith, R. and Hoppe, R. (1991) The patient's story; integrating the patient- and physician-centred approaches to interviewing, *Annals of Internal Medicine*, 115: 470–7.

Smull, M., Sanderson, H. and Allen, B. (undated) *Essential Lifestyle Planning: A Handbook for Facilitators*. Manchester: North West Training and Development Team.

Smull, M. (2004) *Positive Rituals and Quality of Life*. www.paradigm-uk.org, accessed 10 May 2004.

Smull, M.W. and Burke-Harrison, S. (1992) *Supporting People with Severe Reputations in the Community*. Alexandria, VA: National Association of State Directors of Developmental Disabilities Services Inc.

Winefield, H.R., Murrell, T., Clifford, J. and Farmer, E.A. (1996) The search for reliable and valid measures of patient-centredness, *Psychology and Public Health*, 11: 811–24.

25

Culture and ethnicity

Developing accessible and appropriate services for health and social care

Ghazala Mir and Raghu Raghavan

Introduction

The health of people from minority ethnic communities is of growing concern as a social policy issue. Research has shown higher levels of ill health, limited access to health and social care and disadvantage in areas related to health indicators such as housing and employment (Modood *et al.* 1997; Acheson 1998). Higher levels of poverty are also implicated in the greater incidence of chronic conditions within these communities (Nazroo 1997). Studies of disability have highlighted later diagnosis, poor levels of information to service users and low take-up of service provision alongside systematic discrimination in the allocation of welfare benefits (Chamba *et al.* 1999; Ahmad 2000).

Minority ethnic communities are diverse and internally differentiated in relation to age, gender and socioeconomic experiences. The notion of 'cultural competence' has been promoted as a way of addressing diversity. This involves acquiring the skills to understand and be sensitive to cultural differences and to ensure that services respect the values of all people (Acheson 1998). Evidence suggests that 'cultural competency' among service professionals is often disturbingly inadequate and professional uncertainty about how to meet the needs of service users from minority ethnic communities is widespread (ibid). For example, stereotypical views of South Asian families 'looking after their own' and barriers in communication often result in services failing to meet minimum acceptable standards (Chamba *et al.* 1998). It is not surprising, therefore, that South Asian carers are reported to suffer from high levels of stress and poorer mental and physical health than their white peers (Hatton *et al.* 1998).

The younger age profile of people within some, particularly South Asian, communities has been highlighted as an important factor in the future planning of services for people with learning disabilities and their carers (Emerson and Hatton 1998). Current projections show that the number of

South Asian adults with learning disabilities will have more than doubled by 2007 (Emerson and Hatton 1998) and in some areas will form an ethnic majority among people with learning disabilities. Demand for primary health care services is already high within these communities (Nazroo 1997), yet there remains a considerable level of unmet need for health and social care services generally (Chamba *et al.* 1998).

This chapter is based on a review commissioned by the Department of Health to accompany *Valuing People*, the English learning disability policy (Mir *et al.* 2001) and the preliminary findings from two research projects with young people with learning disabilities and their carers (Raghavan *et al.* 2004a, 2004b). The studies used a review of existing literature, supplemented by interviews with key respondents in groups of users and carers, statutory and voluntary service organizations and research units. The studies focus on particular minority ethnic communities which have been shown to experience high levels of unmet need, but they draw out general lessons about how to develop cultural competence in services. As will be seen in what follows, such competence is often missing from the social supports through which health and social care may be accessed. Because of this, much of the chapter looks at how the organization of such supports might be developed and maintained. It is only by getting these right that healthy lifestyles, health and good quality health services can be developed and delivered.

Access to health and social care

The importance of service support for minority ethnic families has been highlighted by research into the experience of carers and disabled people themselves. Studies have highlighted a number of problems with access to such support. Poor awareness of existing services, lack of bilingual staff, culturally inappropriate activities and diet, and racial discrimination within services all contribute to low take-up and poor service development (Baxter 1998; CVS Consultants 1998; Hatton *et al.* 1998).

A 'colour-blind' approach, or assertion that 'we treat everyone the same', is often operated within health and social care organizations. Such statements may, however, disguise the fact that the needs of minority ethnic communities have either not been considered or have been ignored (Alexander 1999). The resulting lack of attention has the consequence of underdeveloped policies and the absence of any mechanisms by which needs can be explored and service development effected. This approach has been also been shown to foster stereotypes and racist attitudes towards minority ethnic communities. At a grass-roots level, such attitudes may influence the use of discretionary decision-making and deprive communities of their rights to services (Ahmad 2000).

A second service response has been that of specialist services, provided solely for individuals from minority ethnic communities. These initiatives have acted as valuable access points within these communities; attention to the beliefs and perceptions of service users can contribute to service development and positively influence take-up. Faith beliefs, for example, have been shown to act as a positive force in treating mental illness and may suggest innovative ways of providing support (Cinnirella and Loewenthal 1999; Mir and Tovey 2003). However, specialist services can promote a surrogate form of racism if they are inadequately funded but used nevertheless to absolve mainstream services of responsibility (Ahmad 2000). Specialist services also run the risk of failing to address individual needs, for example needs relating to age, nature of disability or diverse interests. People in such groups may feel uncomfortable if they do not have much in common with other members. Furthermore, the range of activities that some specialist support groups offer can be limited and if there is no progression to other provision this can lead to underachievement (Mir *et al.* 2001).

Integrated services are likely to be better resourced and given a higher priority than specialist services. Although the ideal may be a quality mainstream service that is sensitive to the needs of all users, the cultural needs of some minority ethnic service users are currently more likely to be met in specialist provision, though this is generally under-resourced and insecure (Mir *et al.* 2001). Specialist services do not, of course, eliminate the need to remove racist practices and attitudes from mainstream provision and to develop accessible and appropriate integrated services that will meet the needs of all members of the community.

Many people involved in community groups feel there is a continuing need for specialist services alongside improvements in general service provision. Integrated services are seen as a long-term aim that would not be possible without great improvements in mainstream services (Mir *et al.* 2001). Some people may always feel a need for specific services that would reinforce personal identity and provide a familiar and safe setting. In such cases, targeted services could provide a more acceptable focus than would be likely in a more integrated setting.

Groups which are based on cultural and ethnic identity enable members to become involved in political activity and to challenge inequity in services, whether voluntary or statutory. In the face of external hostility and concerns about institutional racism, members of ethnic groups may become more insular, but such challenges also foster identity formation. 'Culture' can become a means of constructing a 'positive collective identity' (Priestley 1995). There is evidence that this may differ between groups: African Caribbean groups emphasize ethnicity as the most important aspect of group identity, whereas South Asian groups place more emphasis on having a common language and culture (Mir *et al.* 2001).

The debate about whether specialist or integrated services are the ideal echoes wider debates relating to disability and to ethnicity. Similar arguments are put forward about whether there should be specific services for learning disabilities rather than more general disability services for everyone. Generally, people with learning disabilities and their carers feel that generic services cannot offer the same quality of service. A wider remit means that less attention can be paid to the specific needs of people with learning disabilities and that mistakes which have a huge impact on the lives of individuals can be made when a specialist service is not available.

The parallel with specific and generic services for disabled people is an important one. If separate groups and facilities are seen as necessary to an adequate service for different types of impairment, the same justification may be used for an extra layer of provision relating to ethnicity. It could be argued that pursuing integrated services for minority ethnic communities as a principle should also have implications for other groups with differing needs – generic services should then become the ideal for other services which are based on different needs and experiences.

Debates about the recognition of diversity have also taken place in the field of ethnicity. Proponents for the use of 'black' as a self-definition of all minority ethnic groups have argued that the common experience of racism ought to lead to a common identity. Echoing the views of some within debates about disability, a lack of differentiation has been promoted as a means of mobilizing support and enabling greater resistance to discrimination. This argument has lost support within more recent sociological literature which accepts the benefits of recognizing the diversity of cultural identities within the UK and the different ways in which racism may be experienced (Modood *et al.* 1997; Mason 2000).

Among communities themselves, different attitudes exist towards the question of specialist or integrated services. Service providers within mainstream services sometimes feel that as a matter of policy, integrated services must be pursued. This is expressed as a statement of principle however, rather than as a view based on the wishes of service users themselves (Mir *et al.* 2001). Among people with learning disabilities and carers, both kinds of provision are valued and strong views are expressed in favour of both. Specialist services are felt to be easily accessible and to offer familiar, appropriate and comfortable environments. Integrated services, on the other hand, offer wider opportunities and the ability to meet a wider range of people. The problems are also recognized: people with learning disabilities complain of not being listened to and of experiencing racism in mainstream services. Carers feel they have little access to services or information that would help them; appropriate facilities with which they feel comfortable are often not provided and staff with the necessary skills to communicate and involve them are often not available.

Tait *et al.* (1998) found that South Asian people in Leicester wanted an integrated service, not a specialist one. Other studies have found positive responses to specialist services (Butt and Mirza 1996; CVS Consultants 1998). The key issue appears to be the quality of the services available. Where inclusive services are sensitive to cultural and religious needs, there is likely to be no need for specialist services. For that to occur, mainstream services and organizations need to address their own shortcomings (whether or not specialist provision exists) in order to remove racist and insensitive practices and attitudes from provision. At the same time, recognition and resources will be needed to enable separate provision where this provides a more effective service. The need for specialist services will remain to a greater or lesser extent so long as they represent the only available means of addressing issues of identity and access for people from minority ethnic communities. The evidence suggests that decisions about the extent and nature of any specialist services need to be made at a local level in consultation with service users and carers.

The kind of services that should be offered must be considered alongside how to inform communities about their existence and how to make them relevant to the needs of services users. Chamba *et al.* (1999) report that African Caribbean and Asian parents of severely impaired children are less likely than white parents to know about support groups in their areas and are less likely to be members of such groups. The lack of parental support groups has been highlighted in our own research (Raghavan *et al.* 2004b). Emerson and Robertson (2002) found that these and other community groups played a very small role in the support of South Asian families. A lack of transport and funding can also be barriers to access and to a support group's development (Pawson *et al.* in press).

Access to emotional support appears even more restricted. Many people with learning disabilities from minority ethnic communities experience isolation as a result of family restrictions and a lack of opportunity for social contact (Butt and Mirza 1996; Bignall and Butt 2000). Racism and harassment in everyday settings may further increase feelings of isolation and emotional stress (Butt and Mirza 1996). Studies show that the initial diagnosis and continuing effects of impairment or chronic illness have a strong impact on many already disadvantaged families. Carers and people with learning disabilities often refer to depression when they think about their situation and there is evidence of high levels of stress among South Asian carers (Azmi *et al.* 1996a). However, concerns about worrying others may often lead to both parents and family members concealing their distress from each other (Ahmad 2000).

Studies show that socioeconomic disadvantage and financial insecurity may add significantly to the stress that carers experience (Chamba *et al.* 1999). Caring obligations affect employment opportunities and consequently reduce family income. This situation is compounded by the additional costs which may be associated with caring for a disabled person, for example in relation to transport, clothing and heating (Baldwin 1994). Inequalities in income mean that the financial impact of caring may be even greater on minority ethnic families (Chamba *et al.* 1999).

The simultaneous disadvantage experienced by individuals in relation to race, disability and gender has been termed 'double disadvantage' or 'triple jeopardy' in some research studies (Baxter *et al.* 1990; Butt and Mirza 1996). However, Begum (1995) argues that the specific nature of this experience must be recognized as comprising more than a number of superimposed layers of discrimination. The interaction of multiple kinds of discrimination produces its own particular effect on individuals and social groups, which is more than the sum of its parts.

Exercise 25.1

Think of your contact with people with learning disabilities and their carers from black and minority ethnic communities. How confident did you feel about how to interact? Do you feel that you were able to respond to their needs in the same way as others? If your experience was different, how might any of the problems be overcome?

Developing networks of support

Above we have shown that health and a healthy community need to be backed up by services sensitive to the needs of people from ethnic minority groups. Most importantly, whatever services are available they need to be of high quality. However, for many people with learning disabilities who live in a family home and where families play a major part in their care the importance of responding to the needs of family carers is highlighted. Research evidence shows that the concerns of minority ethnic carers are often not taken seriously, for example when reporting developmental delay and abuse (Mir and Tovey 2003; Raghavan and Small 2004). Advocacy support can play an important role in such situations by ensuring that people with learning disabilities and their carers are heard and that they receive feedback about promised action to meet their needs (Morris 1998). Advocacy support has also been identified as a particular issue for people with challenging behaviour who may be placed out of their locality and disconnected from their own community, with little practical or emotional help (Downer and Ferns 1993; Lewis 1996). A general shortage of advocates has been identified however (Lewis 1996), and our own field work revealed an acute shortage of minority ethnic advocates in particular (Mir *et al.* 2001).

As a concept, advocacy is not necessarily understood or accepted by all communities. The model of advocacy offered can therefore do much to encourage or deter take-up of advocacy services by people with learning disabilities and their carers.

Exercise 25.2

Read the following case study and try to identify why the attempt to work with minority ethnic communities was not successful.

Case study: *Advocacy (1)*

An inner-city advocacy group found that the employment of a South Asian worker on a part-time contract did not result in any significant increase in caseload of service users from minority ethnic communities. The organization promoted self-referral as central to their model of citizen advocacy and advocates felt accountable solely to the person with learning disabilities. Very few people with learning disabilities from these communities or their families had approached the organization for advocacy services during its history. The worker who was appointed had no previous experience of disability work and had not been able to identify individuals who required advocates.

A pilot research project to assess the feasibility of specific advocacy services drew on the experiences of local community groups which addressed ethnicity but did not have a focus on disability generally or on learning disabilities specifically. These organizations had no contact with individuals with learning disabilities and were unable to make referrals. They perceived minority ethnic families as being hostile to the idea of advocacy for cultural reasons and due to a failure to understand or accept the clinical diagnosis of the person with learning disabilities. As a result, no further work was considered viable in this area. Once the worker left the organization she was replaced with a member of staff whose remit did not include a focus on minority ethnic users.

The above case study raises a number of issues. It highlights the need for relevant training about disability and ethnicity, which may not be available within an organization and may have to be sought from further afield. In addition, it is important to recognize that minority ethnic community organizations cannot act as a 'catch-all' for all issues relating to these communities. Lessons will need to be drawn from organizations that focus specifically on both disability and ethnicity if service development is to actually take place. Their experience is vital to finding ways of identifying individuals who might benefit from an advocacy service.

The model of advocacy operated by this project also appears to work against the development of an appropriate service. Self-referral is seen as central to the concept of citizen advocacy in some organizations and actively recruiting people for the service is not therefore viewed as a course which should be followed. This would seem to preclude attempts to enhance take-up through direct approaches to individuals or families for whom advocacy is a new concept.

In addition, the advocate's role is focused on empowering the individual with learning disabilities, which might provoke or exacerbate conflicts with family and professionals. Where carers' needs or roles are not considered this can be difficult for the family of a person with learning disabilities to accept. For communities that place a high value on collectivity and interdependence, it could well be alienating and seen to consciously undermine the principles on which a family structure is based. The case study also highlights the fact that, without actually speaking to people with learning disabilities or their carers from minority ethnic communities, assumptions about their reasons for not using a service are likely to be inaccurate.

Case study: *Advocacy (2)*

Sheffield Citizen Advocacy also identified low take-up by South Asian service users as a problem which it needed to address. It established a joint project with the Youth Service, with a focus on working with young South Asian women to increase confidence, independence and participation in a range of activities. It recognized, however, that in order to enable this particular group to participate there was a need to work with families in the first instance. The South Asian worker who was appointed was vital to this aspect of the project; at the same time, other workers used their broader experience of advocacy work to support her. Home visits were used to strengthen her existing familiarity with families' beliefs and cultures and family members were invited to attend with the young women with learning disabilities if they wished. In this way, parents were encouraged to build up a relationship of trust with workers. Through their participation in the group they were also able to appreciate the skills their daughters already had and were developing. Parents valued these skills and approved of the group activities. They also gained opportunities for support from other parents: this helped them to increase their own support network.

Exercise 25.3

Discuss why the above case study provides a successful advocacy input.

The above example highlights the need to adopt an approach which, by involving family carers, runs counter to the argument that carers' needs and views should not influence the way that disabled people decide to lead their lives. Such an argument can be both simplistic and potentially detrimental to the well-being of people with learning disabilities.

Minority ethnic communities are not necessarily resistant to the idea of advocacy and a number of self-advocacy groups have been set up by people from these communities themselves. However, the role of the advocate may need to include work with families rather than be independent of them. Considering the importance of family to many disabled people (Priestley 1995; Bignall and Butt 2000; Ward 2001), outcomes which do not alienate family members will most often accord with the wishes and interests of individuals with learning disabilities themselves.

'Key workers' may take on the role of advocate as well as providing information and a gateway to services (Mukherjee *et al.* 1999). Chamba *et al.* (1999) noted that the availability of a key worker was associated with fewer unmet needs, though the availability of such a service is often ad hoc and depends on the initiative of individual professionals (JRF 1999). Moreover, not all professionals identified as key workers had truly taken on that role.

Access to support networks can be further facilitated through non-traditional publicity about services. Routes through community centres and on community radio and TV may be more effective than traditional methods, especially as not all carers or people with learning disabilities are literate (Nothard 1993). Video and audio tapes and face-to-face communication may also be effective means of passing on information orally.

Translated literature provided in a vacuum and not linked to staff who can respond to queries is not entirely useful, however, if language remains a barrier to applying for services. Moreover, some concepts such as 'carer' are not as meaningful in some communities as they have become within the ethnic majority. Translations that try to include such concepts without explanation ignore the cultural and linguistic realities of groups. Attempts to promote such concepts within communities will need to ensure that the roles and expectations of the parties involved are made clear (Baxter *et al.* 1990).

Good practice examples

Refugees, who have different needs to people who are established in the UK, are even less aware of services and entitlements than other minority ethnic groups, and creative ways of outreach need to be found. In Kensington and Chelsea, outreach workers used a video-recording to communicate information about registering with a GP. The video used images and drama to overcome the problem of catering for a potential 80 to 90 different languages (Lewis 1996).

The Parvaaz Project has secured funds for a South Asian development officer to work with families and other agencies to effect change in mainstream services. The job will involve holding seminars, meetings and generally creating awareness among South Asian parents about entitlements, benefits, rights and equipment that could be of benefit to them. It was envisaged that the development officer would work with national and local organizations to help them become more sensitive and responsive to the needs of South Asian people with learning disabilities and their carers.

An example of good communication practice involved a touring exhibition in Bradford using South Asian staff in places used by and well known to South Asian people. The exhibition, which aimed to increase awareness of short-term breaks visited the Bradford Mela, the city centre, mosques, community centres, temples, street corners and open events. Photographs (especially of South Asian users with South Asian staff) were used as well as a video in Urdu. The display was advertised on a local South Asian radio station, in the local press and in local South Asian publications. The initiative showed that families do come forward when contact methods are relevant to their background and experiences. The result was not only a considerable increase in South Asian referrals to the services publicized but increased awareness of disability within local communities, especially as media images of disabled people are currently missing from both the minority and majority media (Begum *et al.* 1994).

Family, friends and the wider community

The evidence shows that members of South Asian communities often perceive kinship-based groups as an important source of identity and support (Priestley 1995; Ahmad 2000). The importance of these relationships can mean that family expectations about the social roles of people with learning disabilities are significant in the decision-making of individuals.

The roles of women and girls, in particular, are interpreted differently in different communities and across generations. Parents who restrict the activities of their daughters may feel they are safeguarding them from situations in which they are vulnerable to abuse or more exposed to unacceptable behaviour, such as mixed gender environments. Parents may also feel under social pressure from within their communities to uphold such restrictions and to maintain the existing boundaries of appropriate behaviour between (particularly younger) men and women (Kelleher and Hillier 1996; Dwyer 1998). There may be a feeling within some communities that traditional values and beliefs are undermined by services which attempt to encourage young women to spend more time out of their homes in environments that are considered unsuitable (Dwyer 1998; Jacobson 1998).

Support from families, friends and community members may be restricted by negative attitudes to disability. Studies have shown that these have not been specifically addressed within minority ethnic communities (Hatton *et al.* 2002), while within the ethnic majority negative attitudes have been strongly challenged. Thus greater stigma may be attached to disability in cultures where the social model of disability has not been promoted (Mir and Tovey 2003). There is evidence that in some communities people may feel greater shame in respect of a disabled family member and attempts may be made to keep the existence of such members a secret (Westbrook *et al.* 1993).

At a broader level, a study of deaf South Asian children found that many South Asian families reported less acceptance of their deaf child by the South Asian community than by members of the white community (Chamba *et al.* 1998). Bignall and Butt (2000) report that young disabled people feel such prejudice must be dealt with if individuals are to receive enough support to develop more independent lives. Carers, too, suffer from these negative attitudes and are often left unsupported by both services and their extended families (Katbamna *et al.* 2000). Low take-up of services may in part be a consequence of negative attitudes towards disability – this does not, however, remove the responsibility of service providers to address such attitudes (Begum 1992, 1995).

Negative attitudes are compounded by a lack of information about the facilities and opportunities that are available to people with learning disabilities. The absence of such opportunities reinforces the notion that individuals with impairments are a 'burden'. Failure by service providers to offer adequate support to individuals and families can reinforce the notion that disability is 'tragic' – people are more likely to move away from this conception of disability when they have information that promotes a positive approach and when they are able to manage their circumstances without struggling (Mir and Tovey 2003; Raghavan and Small 2004).

There may be diversity between individual families within a community in terms of appropriate roles for people with learning disabilities. Within South Asian communities, for example, some parents may strongly support and be involved in marriage plans for their son or daughter with learning disabilities, while others may not see marriage as an option or may resist the idea of marriage between two people with learning disabilities (CVS Consultants 1998; Mir *et al.* 2001). Equally, marriage may be more easily accommodated where the aptitude or skills of the marriage partner are only one part of the whole equation. If marriages are a key part of reaffirming or reflecting kin relationships rather than emotional involvement or attraction between the couple, then South Asian cultures may be more accommodating of disabled people. The extent of support for each of these perceptions about marriage has yet to be explored.

The role of service workers in developing and sustaining networks of support

Working with families

The significance of family relationships can mean that their active involvement may be seen as vital to the success of support services by some disabled people (Priestley 1995). Particular skills are needed in services that interact with a range of family structures and value frameworks to avoid according primacy to any one, to the detriment of another.

Services organized for people from minority ethnic communities often recognize the need to involve families in order to build up trust, but the motives for doing this may differ according to how much status is given to a collectivist culture. One advocacy scheme for young women with learning disabilities undertook work with families in the first five to six months of their involvement. However, the aim of such work was to build up trust and eventually discourage attendance by family members so that the group could then work exclusively with the young women. Primacy was therefore ultimately given to an individualistic concept of advocacy (Mir *et al.* 2001).

Independent living schemes may also ignore the importance of family connections and base supported housing away from areas in which family members live. This can result in individuals with learning disabilities having to face the dilemma of living far away from the family in supported housing or living nearby without adequate support (Begum 1995). Bignall and Butt's (2000) study of young people shows that although some wish to move away and live in their own homes, many want to stay with their families but be able to do more for themselves and have increased control over decision-making. Bignall and Butt suggest that total self-sufficiency is an unrealistic concept: interdependence may be a more appropriate and cross-cultural notion. The issue to be resolved by service professionals, then, is how such interdependence can be harnessed to everyone's benefit.

Options that are acceptable to families would appear to be the key to improving opportunities for (particularly young) people with learning disabilities. Negotiated provision seems more effective than attempts to push parents reluctantly into avenues in which they feel uncomfortable or trying to ease them out of the picture altogether. Addressing attitudes within families and communities towards the opportunities provided by projects is thus seen as a significant part of the work with young disabled people.

As already highlighted, social restrictions on people with learning disabilities from their families are often based on fears for their safety and on cultural views about acceptable behaviour (Mir *et al.* 2001). They may, however, be interpreted as oppressive and stifling by service professionals, and sometimes by people with learning disabilities themselves. Media attacks on the role of South Asian (particularly Muslim) women contribute to the way this situation is interpreted. Stereotyped images of young South Asian women suffering from 'culture clash' may be reinforced when staff promoting independent living skills feel obstructed by family members. Where single gender settings have been provided for South Asian women to learn such skills however, parents value such opportunities for their daughters (Mir *et al.* 2001).

Widening opportunities for young women would seem to lie in respecting their cultural identity and the values and beliefs of their families, rather than in persuading them that the majority culture is necessarily better. Whereas respecting young people's rights is important, it has sometimes proved to be a convenient pretext for undermining non-white cultures (Ahmad 2000). Pursuing a balanced approach will be far from easy for professionals; not appearing to be balanced will risk alienating young people or parents, or perhaps both.

Engaging minority ethnic groups and individuals in partnerships

Community groups can act as a gateway to support services. However, studies show that links between local authorities and minority ethnic community groups in a number of areas are often poor. There is evidence of inadequate consultation over needs and services through such groups, despite the knowledge that available services are not being used (Azmi *et al.* 1996c; Butt and Mirza 1996; Lewis 1996). The absence of these links means that need is currently determined by service providers rather than by users and their families, despite moves towards user-centred assessment (Tait *et al.* 1998; Bignall and Butt 2000).

Traditional methods of consultation are not recommended in the literature. Baxter *et al.* (1990) note that consultation should be carried out at local level with community organizations rather than through public meetings. Such links improve understanding of the experiences that are common to different minority ethnic communities, highlight any differences from majority needs, and provide an opportunity to develop proposals for specific action. The drive for partnership working assumes to some extent that groups of service users will already be established or easily formed. This may only be true of some areas in which minority ethnic communities live and partnership activity may involve facilitating the development and progression of community groups (Mir *et al.* 2001).

Community organizations may need support initially to form and then to become involved in planning and managing services, and perhaps to secure contracts to offer services themselves. Such groups often provide a range of services that do not mesh well with the structures of local authorities or other purchasing agencies. The bidding process works against small organizations and they may need assistance to apply for such contracts effectively. It has been suggested that service contracts should require funded organizations to ensure the involvement of all ethnic groups at all levels and that such contracts should be evaluated and monitored by people who are representative of the local population (Lewis 1996).

Good practice: developing and sustaining inclusive services

Winn and Chotai (1992), writing about the work of an ethnic minorities development worker in Haringey Health Authority, recommend community development as a means of gaining regular and systematic information about needs rather than the snapshot pictures obtained through one-off consultations. The worker's role involved initiating and sustaining contact with local minority ethnic community groups and involving them in health service planning. This led not just to informal consultation but to membership of formal mechanisms such as planning committees and sub-committees. Managers and relevant staff within the health authority were encouraged to make links with community groups as part of their work so that dependency on one or two health professionals was avoided. The development worker had access to key decision-makers and planners in the district and could feed directly into decision-making where needed.

The Asian Disability Joint Planning Team (ADJPT) in Bradford is an example of partnership working involving community groups as well as statutory agencies (including education as well as health and social services). Consultation with users and carers is a key component of its approach; all plans made by any of its constituent members are required to include support for South Asian disabled people. Some meetings are open to the public, and public participation is enhanced through community confer-ences and bilingual workshops. To ensure that all partners have their views heard, ADJPT has an independent chairperson and has been supported by a worker jointly funded by the local authority and Barnardo's. ADJPT has played an important role in the development of the local South Asian voluntary sector.

Exercise 25.4

You have been asked to develop an inclusive service for an area that includes a large Somali population. What do you now know about the Somali culture? How can you develop the best form of inclusion? Find out as much about Somali culture as you can. Are your initial views still the same?

Developing cultural competence

Appropriate skills and attitudes in relation to service users from minority ethnic communities are often the focus of any strategy to help professionals develop inclusive approaches in their work. Such competence has most commonly been found within services run by and for people from particular communities themselves. This suggests that partnerships and interaction with such community-based services will be an important element of any strategy.

However, cultural sensitivity is only one element of quality in service provision, and many service users feel that what is actually being provided is more important than who is providing it. An emphasis is also needed on well-resourced schemes offering a variety of activities and opportunities. Schemes that are subject to cuts in funding are limited not only in the scope of their activities but also in their ability to build on previous work. The withdrawal of funding after a year, for example, can result in the loss of regular contact with many families of disabled children, which has taken around six months to develop (Mir *et al.* 2001).

Staff and training

For managers, the recruitment and retention of skilled staff is clearly an important strategy for inclusive service provision. The availability of minor-ity ethnic staff helps to improve access to services and helps users and carers to make informed choices; these staff members can also advise service organizations on appropriate policy and practice to meet service users' needs. Appropriate publicity is needed to attract workers to health and social care work and to ensure their proportional representation (Baxter *et al.* 1990; Emerson and Hatton 1998). While qualifications and the opportunity for training are essential ingredients in a quality service (Department of

Health 2000a), strict adherence to qualification requirements at entry can impede the appointment of appropriate staff (Ganguly 1995). The lack of minority ethnic staff in such settings sends negative messages to staff and service users alike about the status of people from these communities within the organization (Baxter *et al.* 1990; Azmi *et al.* 1996a).

Staff from minority ethnic communities may feel caught between the different expectations of colleagues and carers from their own community (Mir *et al.* 2001). Appropriate support is not always available, nor is there training to equip staff with the skills needed in such a situation (Baxter 1998). One solution has been to establish minority ethnic workers' support groups and to consult these on major policy issues (Lewis 1996).

A further issue relates to the shortage of volunteers from minority ethnic communities. Efforts to recruit minority ethnic advocates are often unsuccessful and may be related to inappropriate publicity. However, there may be other factors too, related to the ability and motivation to volunteer. Atkinson (1999) points out that lack of funding is a barrier to the recruitment of advocates and that secure funding makes it possible to invest in training, support and payment. Payment for such services and accredited training may be particularly important for people from disadvantaged communities who face greater barriers to employment and education. The skills that such volunteers could bring to organizations are often central to the success of work envisaged with these communities, which cannot effectively be carried out without them. Such a pivotal role may need special resourcing to ensure that it is carried out.

At the same time, it should not be assumed that families will necessarily want support from someone from their own community. Some families may prefer white advocates, for example, as this may feel less intrusive and they may wish to keep some distance between themselves and the professionals with whom they have contact (Mir *et al.* 2001). White professionals need to be aware of their own prejudices, however, and these can be particularly damaging in the dynamics of transcultural work.

Many professionals currently feel ill-equipped to respond to people from a different culture and often rely on specialist workers who share the same linguistic and cultural background (Mir and Tovey 2003). Minority ethnic professionals play a vital role in enabling access to services for many families; however, studies have recommended that all professionals should increase their competence in this area by improving their awareness of the cultural backgrounds of the population they serve (Acheson 1998; Hatton *et al.* 1998; Chamba *et al.* 1999). This would also have positive consequences for minority ethnic staff. A culture of joint responsibility towards non-English speaking service users could prevent them, and bilingual staff members, from being marginalized within service organizations. It would also ensure that they had full access to the same opportunities offered to mainstream users and staff (Azmi *et al.* 1996b). Hatton *et al.*'s (1998) study, for example, suggests that language training for a wide range of front-line staff, such as receptionists, could increase the confidence of carers when accessing services.

Areas specified for the development of cultural competence within a staff group have included:

- increased awareness of organizational policies on anti-racist practice and how these are to be implemented;
- dealing with racial harassment;
- training in language issues for relevant staff, which would include the training needs of interpreters and of staff who work with them;
- opportunities and training for minority ethnic staff to gain qualifications and move into more senior positions;
- cultural competence training, including an awareness of relevant conceptual differences between different ethnic groups (Azmi *et al.* 1996a; Lewis 1996; Baxter 1998; CVS Consultants 1998; Bignall and Butt 2000).

Funding and resources

Insufficient resource allocation often mean that services aimed at improving delivery are not local to many people and do not have the resources to provide an adequate service. Studies suggest that current resource allocations need to be reviewed in order to meet the service needs of individuals with learning disabilities from minority groups and their carers. Studies recommend that budgets should reflect local demographic profiles and allow for resources to undertake ethnic monitoring of service use, employment of minority ethnic staff and training relevant to achieving improved services (Hatton *et al.* 1997; Tait *et al.* 1998).

In addition, procedures for the allocation of funds need to be more flexible if they are to encompass the services needed. Non-traditional purchasing sources may need to be considered, for instance to cater for different diets or to produce appropriate publicity. The pooling of budgets, as outlined in the Health Act 1999 and *NHS Plan* (Department of Health 2000b, 2000c), should, for its part, provide a mechanism to ensure the better coordination of services.

The agenda for research and practice

Developing the social model

Research on learning disabilities and ethnicity has emphasized unmet need and the consequent implications for social policy and practice. However, the theoretical implications of this research have been less well developed. Our approach in this chapter is grounded in an appreciation of the value of a social model framework. The conventional approach to disability has been to see it as a personal tragedy, with solution through medical intervention. A social model of disability stresses that the impact of impairment is 'mediated, to a degree, by social and cultural circumstances' (Mercer and Barnes 2000: 83). Thus, attitudes towards people with impairments can have a greater impact on individuals than the impairment itself and can affect access to a range of opportunities enjoyed by those without impairments.

We argue that the potentially disabling effects of specific attitudes and professional practices require explicit recognition. The social model allows us to analyse and explain the experiences of service users and carers with reference to social injustice and discrimination rather than as personal misfortune alone.

However, in utilizing this approach we are conscious that a failure to acknowledge the diversity of disabled people's experience has led minority ethnic communities and women to question the relevance of the social model to their experience (Mir and Tovey 2003). The interaction of ethnicity and gender with disability to further disadvantage individuals and social groups requires specific attention within this model. Without such attention the social model of disability itself becomes discriminatory through marginalizing these other areas of disadvantage and failing to recognize the multiple discrimination that some people with disabilities experience. Developing the model to address multiple disadvantage is important as a means of questioning established patterns of service delivery and of providing insights into how these interacting dimensions of inequality in health and social care might be addressed.

Developing service provision and performance management

Areas of concern in current services for people from minority ethnic communities include:

- communication between service users and service providers and access to relevant information;
- attitudes towards cultural sensitivity and flexibility;
- personnel recruitment and training;
- availability of adequate funding and other resources;
- whether services should be specialized for particular communities or integrated into general service provision.

Studies have highlighted a need for conceptual shifts in the values underlying service provision to allow more inclusive approaches that would work against the current exclusion of people from minority ethnic groups (Mir *et al.* 2001; Raghavan and Small 2004). Inconsistency in the approaches adopted by services in different geographical areas or even within the same locality was highlighted by our research (Mir and Tovey 2003; Raghavan *et al.* 2004b) and indicates a need for national leadership to set quality standards in service provision for people from these communities. The evidence suggests the need to move away from the notion of 'an average citizen', to acknowledge diversity of need and required services at all levels of service provision, and to provide resources to meet these needs (Alexander 1999).

At a local level, for example, flexible ways of involving service users and carers and enabling them to express their views, if necessary in languages other than English, need to be developed (CVS Consultants 1998). At a broader level, statistical information about people from minority ethnic groups is needed to deliver services equitably. Proactive attempts to identify families currently unknown to services have been recommended, for example through GP surgeries and multi-ethnic support groups. Studies suggest that monitoring service take-up and minority ethnic staff numbers at different levels would increase awareness and potentially lead to targeted action on the part of service planners (Chamba *et al.* 1998; Hatton *et al.* 1998, 2002). Studies show that current monitoring procedures are inadequate for such purposes (Butt and Mirza 1996; Mir *et al.* 2001). Records generally fail to identify who is getting which service, or general patterns of use and experience.

Lewis (1996) suggests that there is considerable scope for service contracts to include a requirement that funded organizations should not only inform all communities about provision offered but also monitor the ethnic origin of users and workers and ensure that this is representative of the local population. User feedback is considered by those active in the field as an essential tool in performance management: some argue further that the criteria for monitoring performance should be set by those receiving the services (Lewis 1996).

Exercise 25.5

You are managing a service in an area with a substantial mix of ethnic groups. How would you ensure that your staff were organized to provide an appropriate standard of care? How would you make sure that services meet the needs of people from all cultures?

The extent of unmet need within minority ethnic communities has, understandably, led to an emphasis on difficulties faced by people with learning disabilities and their carers, with far less documentation of positive features of their experience. Within service provision, examples of good practice are increasingly being identified as role models for future service development. There is a need to build on these and consider how the expertise developed, particularly in community-based services, can be linked into other parts of learning disability provision. The development of formal links that could contribute to staff training and service development is likely to raise the quality of provision in both areas (Mir and Din 2003). At the level of family and other non-professional networks, these examples of good practice have yet to be explored and disseminated.

Good practice: developing conceptual shifts in service principles

An example of a creative approach to the specific needs of people from minority ethnic communities can be seen in the work of Shared Care

(Bradford), which has moved away from the traditional idea that relatives should not be used as providers of short-term breaks within a statutory framework. The scheme recognizes the importance of trust and familiarity to families and is open to the nomination of family members. Take-up of shared care arrangements has been very high and the scheme has been successful in recruiting large numbers of volunteer carers, particularly from South Asian communities. As yet, siblings are excluded from the scheme even if they live in separate households. However, in view of fostering guidelines, which encourage the use of close family members as carers, this has been reviewed. A decision to include siblings living outside the household would appear to be supported by research which shows that practical and ongoing family support in South Asian communities is generally limited to household members (Chamba *et al.* 1998; Mir *et al.* 2000).

▋ Conclusion

In referring to 'minority ethnic communities', we are aware of the risk of introducing a degree of homogeneity where none exists. The traditions and cultural heritage of different communities will inevitably differ; different communities may well experience disadvantage, service provision and racism in different ways, but some of those experiences may be similar. This chapter argues for sensitivity and appropriate responses to the needs of the particular communities with which service providers will be in contact. We have sought to draw out common themes as well as the views and experiences of particular groups.

The literature itself focuses more on the needs of people with learning difficulties from South Asian communities than those from African Caribbean backgrounds; little is available about the needs of those from other groups, such as the African and Chinese communities or refugees or Travellers. The gaps in the literature indicate areas to which further attention needs to be given.

The need for cultural competence has been significantly promoted by a number of national policy documents and is echoed in the learning disabilities White Paper, *Valuing People* (Department of Health 2001). However, raising awareness about the needs of minority ethnic communities is not the same as setting targets that aim to meet those needs or implementing monitoring systems that measure how effectively such needs are being met. Such aims are conspicuously absent from *Valuing People*. Even the sparse references to targeted action have not been followed through: to date no information has been gathered about the numbers of service users from minority ethnic communities even though this was the single performance indicator that could have acted as a monitoring mechanism for improvements in access to provision.

Not surprisingly, therefore, the Learning Disability Task Force in England reports continued concerns about services for people with learning disabilities from minority ethnic groups and their carers (Learning Disability Task Force 2003; 2004). While urging learning disability Partnership Boards (responsible for implementing *Valuing People*) to comply with the Race Relations (Amendment) Act 2000 and proactively ensure race equality in service provision, the government's own instructions and guidance to implement *Valuing People* have often failed to address these very issues.

Some positive action has been taken. A toolkit designed to help Partnership Boards deliver *Valuing People* has been circulated and is leading to pockets of change around the country. Work to include minority ethnic communities has been made a priority for the Learning Disability Development Fund. Formal monitoring and continued support for this work may help to break the pattern of piecemeal approaches to addressing current inequities in service provision.

Given that highlighting needs has, in itself, failed to result in policy that influences widespread and consistent changes in practice, the agenda for future research and practice must focus on what many government departments have failed to do: providing models for inclusive services and ways of measuring take-up by people from minority ethnic communities. Strategies and service models that ensure the needs of people from minority ethnic communities are considered throughout learning disability services and consistently built into service developments are central to future progress.

One way forward might be to implement and evaluate small-scale service interventions that could be replicated on a national scale. Using research in this way could help develop existing services in the research locality and add to knowledge about what works in practice – rather than simply repeating the findings of unmet need from previous studies. This would not only be a more effective use of research funds but would also, importantly, be of immediate benefit to people from minority ethnic communities who are helped by the intervention itself. People from socially disadvantaged groups are often exploited by the research process and may receive little, if any, benefit for their contribution (Barnes 1996).

Research that works hand in hand with practice may come closer to bridging the gap that often exists between research findings and service developments that translate these into practice. At worst, this type of study would provide additional, though short-term, support to a small number of people from minority ethnic communities. At best it could provide a stimulus to effective interventions being adopted on a wider scale and higher national standards of cultural competence.

| References

Acheson, D. (Chair) (1998) *Independent Inquiry into Inequalities in Health*. London: The Stationery Office.

Ahmad, W. (ed.) (2000) *Ethnicity, Disability and Chronic Illness*, Buckingham: Open University Press.

Alexander, Z. (1999) *The Department of Health: Study of Black, Asian and Ethnic Minority Issues*. London: Department of Health.

Atkinson, D. (1999) *Advocacy: A Review*. Brighton: Pavilion Publishing/Joseph Rowntree Foundation.

Azmi, S., Hatton, C., Caine, A. and Emerson, E. (1996a) *Improving Services for Asian People with Learning Disabilities: The Views of Users and Carers*. Manchester: Hester Adrian Research Centre/Mental Health Foundation.

Azmi, S., Hatton, C., Emerson, E. and Caine, A. (1996b) *Asian Staff in Services for People with Learning Disabilities*. Manchester: Hester Adrian Research Centre/ Mental Health Foundation.

Azmi, S., Emerson, E., Caine, A. and Hatton, C. (1996c) *Improving Services for Asian People with Learning Disabilities and Their Families*. Manchester: Hester Adrian Research Centre/Mental Health Foundation.

Baldwin, S. (1994) Needs assessment for people from Black and minority ethnic groups, *Care in Place*, 1 (2).

Barnes, C. (1996) Disability and the myth of the independent researcher, *Disability and Society*, 11(1): 107–10.

Baxter, C. (1998) Learning difficulties, in S. Rawaf and V. Bahl (eds) *Assessing Health Needs of People from Minority Ethnic Groups*. London: Royal College of Physicians/Faculty of Public Health Medicine.

Baxter, C., Poonia, K., Ward, L. and Nadirshaw, Z. (1990) *Double Discrimination*. London: King's Fund Centre/Commission for Racial Equality.

Begum, N. (1992) *Something to be Proud of*. London: Waltham Forest Race Relations Unit.

Begum, N. (1995) *Beyond Samosas and Reggae: A Guide to Developing Services for Black Disabled People*. London: King's Fund.

Begum, N., Hill, M. and Stevens, A. (eds) (1994) *Reflections: The Views of Black Disabled People on their Lives and Community Care*. London: Central Council for Education and Training in Social Work.

Bignall, T. and Butt, J. (2000) *Between Ambition and Achievement: Young Black Disabled People's Views and Experiences of Independence and Independent Living*. Bristol: Policy Press/Joseph Rowntree Foundation.

Butt, J. and Mirza, K. (1996) *Social Care and Black Communities*. London: HMSO.

Chamba, R., Ahmad, W. and Jones, L. (1998) *Improving Services for Asian Deaf Children*. Bristol: Policy Press.

Chamba, R., Ahmad, W., Hirst, M., Lawton, D. and Beresford, B. (1999) *On the Edge: Minority Ethnic Families Caring for a Severely Disabled Child*. Bristol: Policy Press.

Cinnirella, M. and Loewenthal, K.M. (1999) Religious and Ethnic Group Influences on Beliefs about Mental Illness: A qualitative interview study, *British Journal of Medical Psychology*, 72: 505–24.

CVS Consultants/Asian People with Disabilities Alliance (1998) *Ethnicity and Learning Difficulties: Moving Towards Equity in Service Provision*. London: CVS Consultants.

Department of Health (2000a) *A Quality Strategy for Social Care*. London: Department of Health.

Department of Health (2000b) *Implementation of Health Act Partnership Arrangements*. London: Department of Health.

Department of Health (2000c) *The NHS Plan*. London: The Stationery Office.

Department of Health (2001) *Valuing People: A New Strategy for Learning Disability for the 21st Century*. London: Department of Health.

Department of Health (2002) *Key to Partnerships: Working to Make a Difference in People's Lives.* London: The Stationery Office.

Downer, J. and Ferns, P. (1993) Self-advocacy by black people with learning difficulties, in P. Beresford and T. Harding (eds) *A Challenge to Change: Practical Experiences of Building User-Led Services.* London: National Institute for Social Work.

Dwyer, C. (1998) Contested identities: challenging dominant representations of young British Muslim women, in T. Skelton and G. Valentine (eds) *Cool Places.* London: Routledge.

Emerson, E. and Hatton, C. (1998) Residential provision for people with intellectual disabilities in England, Wales and Scotland, *Journal of Applied Research in Intellectual Disabilities,* 11: 1–14.

Emerson, E. and Robertson, J. (2002) *Future Demand for Services for Young Adults with Learning Disabilities from South Asian and Black Communities in Birmingham.* Lancaster University: Institute of Health Research.

Ganguly, I. (1995) Promoting the health of women of non-English-speaking backgrounds in Australia, *World Health Forum,* 16: 157–63.

Hatton, C., Azmi, S., Emerson, E. and Caine, A. (1997) Researching the needs of South Asian people with learning difficulties and their families, *Mental Health Care,* 1: 91–4.

Hatton, C., Azmi, S., Caine, A. and Emerson, E. (1998) Informal carers of adolescents and adults with learning disabilities from South Asian communities, *British Journal of Social Work,* 28: 821–37.

Hatton, C., Akram, Y., Shah, R., Robertson, J. and Emerson, E. (2002) *Supporting South Asian Families with a Child with Severe Disabilities: A Report to the Department of Health.* Lancaster University: Institute for Health Research.

Jacobson, J. (1998) *Islam in Transition: Religion and Identity among British Pakistani Youth.* London: Routledge.

JRF (1999) *Implementing Key Worker Services: A Case Study of Promoting Evidence-based Practice.* York: Joseph Rowntree Foundation.

Katbamna, S., Bhakta, P. and Parker, G. (2000) Perceptions of disability and relationships in South Asian communities, in W. Ahmad (ed.) *Ethnicity, Disability and Chronic Illness.* Buckingham: Open University Press.

Kelleher, D. and Hillier, S. (eds) (1996) *Researching Cultural Differences in Health.* London: Routledge.

Learning Disability Task Force (2004) Report: Rights, independence, choice and inclusion http://www.valuingpeople.gov.uk/documents/TaskForceReport2004.pdf

Learning Disability Task Force (2003) *Making Things Happen: First Annual Report of the Learning Disability Task Force.* London: Learning Disability Task Force.

Lewis, J. (1996) *Give Us a Voice.* London: Choice Press.

Mason, D. (2000) *Race and Ethnicity in Modern Britain.* Oxford: Oxford University Press.

Mercer, G. and Barnes, C. (2000) Disability: from medical needs to social rights, in P. Tovey (ed.) *Contemporary Primary Care: The Challenges of Change.* Buckingham: Open University Press.

Mir, G. and Din, I. (2003) Communication, knowledge and chronic illness in the Pakistani community. Leeds: Centre for Research in Primary Care, University of Leeds.

Mir, G. and Tovey, P. (2003) Asian carers' experiences of medical and social care: the case of cerebral palsy, *British Journal of Social Work,* 33(4): 465–79.

Mir, G., Tovey, P. and Ahmad, W. (2000) *Cerebral Palsy and South Asian Communities*. Leeds: Centre for Research in Primary Care, University of Leeds.

Mir, G., Nocon, A. and Ahmad, W. with Jones, L. (2001) *Learning Difficulties and Ethnicity*, London: Department of Health.

Modood, T, Berthoud, R., Lakey, J., Nazroo, J., Smith, P., Virdee, S. and Beishon, S. (1997) *Ethnic Minorities in Britain: Diversity and Disadvantage*. London: Policy Studies Institute.

Morris, J. (1998) *Still Missing?* The WhoCares? London: Trust/Joseph Rowntree Foundation.

Mukherjee, S., Beresford, B. and Sloper, P. (1999) *Unlocking Key Working: An Analysis and Evaluation of Key Worker Services for Families with Disabled Children*. Bristol: Policy Press.

Nazroo, J. (1997) *The Health of Britain's Ethnic Minorities*. London: Policy Studies Institute.

Nothard, A. (1993) *Uptake of Services for People with Learning Disabilities from Black and Minority Ethnic Communities in Leeds*. Leeds: Information and Resources Section, St Mary's Hospital, Leeds Community and Mental Health Unit.

Pawson, N., Raghavan, R. and Small, N. (in press) Social inclusion, social networks and ethnicity: the development of the social inclusion. Interview schedule for young people with learning disabilities. *British Journal of Learning Disabilities*.

Priestley, M. (1995) Commonality and difference in the movement: an 'Association of Blind Asians' in Leeds, *Disability and Society*, 10: 157–69.

Raghavan, R. and Small, N. (2004) Cultural diversity and intellectual disability, *Current Opinion in Psychiatry*, 17: 371–5.

Raghavan, R., Small, N. and Pawson, N. (2004a) Transition, ethnicity and social networks for young people with intellectual disabilities, *Journal of Intellectual Disability Research*, 48: 483.

Raghavan, R., Small, N., Newell, J. and Waseem, F. (2004b) Mapping of service for young people with intellectual disabilities and mental health problems, *Journal of Intellectual Disability Research*, 48: 306.

Tait, T., Chavannes, M., Dooher, J. and Miles, M. (1998) *A Study to Consider the Accommodation Support and Care Needs of Individuals with Learning Disabilities from the Asian Community in the City and County of Leicester*. Leicester: de Montfort University/The Housing Corporation.

Ward, C. (2001) *Family Carers: Counting Families In*. London: Department of Health.

Westbrook, M.T., Legge, V. and Pennay, M. (1993) Attitudes towards disabilities in a multicultural society, *Social Science and Medicine*, 36: 615–23.

Winn, L. and Chotai, N. (1992) Community development: working with black and minority ethnic groups, in L. Winn (ed.) *Power to the People: The Key to Responsive Services in Health and Social Care*. London: King's Fund Centre.

26

Work, learning and leisure

The journey towards fulfilling lives

Nick Fripp

Introduction

Education and employment are at the heart of government rhetoric in the early twenty-first century, and policy for developing education and employment is designed to meet the challenges of that century. Leisure is becoming a central concern for many people as a result of post-war economic development in the UK and similar western economies, resulting in decreased hours spent at work accompanied by increasing disposable income (Bull *et al.* 2003). People with learning disabilities and their families face continuing social exclusion in respect of their access to work, learning and leisure (DoH 2001a; Mencap 2001; Pearlman and Holzhausen 2002).

Work, learning and leisure opportunities for people with learning disabilities have in the past been provided by specialist staff in segregated settings. Traditionally these life areas have been the concern of people working in services collectively called day services. The current challenge faced by these services is summed up by Wertheimer (1996: 1): 'We are on a journey: from the artificial world we have created for people with learning difficulties towards the real world where we dream of supporting them in ordinary lives in inclusive communities'.

Many people with learning disabilities are clear that they want to work (DoH 2001b) and there is a developing service design consensus that employment and education will be important in the process of modernizing day services (Ritchie *et al.* 1996; Wertheimer 1996; McIntosh and Whittaker 1998; Simons and Watson 1999). Policy in respect of work, learning and leisure is skewed towards promoting access to and use of mainstream services. There is guidance in the form of *The Day Services Modernisation Tool Kit*, Parts 1 and 2 (NDT 2002, 2003) and the *Framework for Developing an Employment Strategy* (Institute for Applied Health and Social Policy 2002). Objectives 7 and 8 of *Valuing People* (DoH 2001a: 26) provide the central focus for the development of service to people with learning disabilities:

Objective 7: fulfilling lives

To enable people with learning disabilities to live full and purposeful lives in their communities and to develop a range of friendships, activities and relationships.

Objective 8: moving into employment

To enable more people with learning disabilities to participate in all forms of employment, wherever possible in paid work and to make a valuable contribution to the world of work.

This chapter looks at the gap between the rhetoric of lifelong learning, full employment and the growing importance of leisure, and the reality for people with learning disabilities and their families in the context of the policy and practice that impacts on their lives. Issues of adult identity and citizenship provide a backdrop for the discussion.

What will I be when I grow up?

Work, learning and leisure help to define us both in terms of self-image and of how we are perceived by others. In Shakespeare's *As You Like It* Jacques presents a view of adult life:

> . . . And then the lover,
> Sighing like furnace, with a woeful ballad
> Made to his mistress' eyebrow. Then a soldier,
> Full of strange oaths, and bearded like the pard,
> Jealous in honour, sudden and quick in quarrel,
> Seeking the bubble reputation
> Even in the cannon's mouth. And then the justice,
> In fair round belly with good capon lin'd,
> With eyes severe, and beard of formal cut,
> Full of wise saws and modern instances;
> And so he plays his part . . .

His adult is defined by their leisure time, their prowess as a lover or musician, by their occupation and by their learned wisdom. All this defines the person who plays their full part in the world.

Argyris (cited by Egan 1994: 67) proposed the personal journeys that need to be undertaken to move to adult maturity:

- assume an active rather than a passive role in life;
- change from a strategy of dependency on others to relative independence;
- widen your range of behaviours – act in many ways rather than few ways;
- develop a wider range of interests – moving from erratic, shallow and casual interests to mature, strong and enduring interests;
- change from a present-oriented time perspective to a perspective encompassing past, present and future;

- move from solely subordinate relationships with others to relations as equals or superiors;
- change from merely understanding yourself to some kind of control over your destiny.

Argyris conveys a sense of self-awareness and self-determination in the mature person. The journeys from dependence to independence, from subordinate to leader and the development of strong and enduring interests are all areas of development that would be difficult to achieve without participation in work, learning and leisure. This journey to adulthood helps us to satisfy needs we have as human beings.

Argyris' view of becoming who you can be is congruent with that of Maslow. Maslow (cited by Gross 1992: 903) presents his hierarchy of needs. These needs are divided into two domains: D-motives – physiological, safety, love and belonging and esteem needs which are satisfied as a means to an end, and B-motives – relating to self-actualization, which are engaged in because they are intrinsically satisfying.

Work, learning and leisure have a part to play in all elements of Maslow's hierarchy and in the journey to adulthood described by Argyris. They may provide the means to ensure food, shelter and safety, the opportunity to make friends and fall in love or the environment, activity or role that facilitates one becoming everything that one is capable of. Work, learning and leisure do not exist in isolation from each other – we can learn at work, meet our partner at college or find work through developing a leisure interest. While our needs unite us as human beings, experience of life may be very different for people with learning disabilities. *Valuing People* (DoH 2001a: 19) outlines the social exclusion faced by people with learning disabilities and their families:

- Families with disabled children have higher costs as a result of the child's disability coupled with diminished employment prospects. Their housing needs may not be adequately met. There is little evidence of a flexible and co-ordinated approach to support by health, education and social services, and there is significant unmet need for short breaks.

- Young disabled people at the point of transition to adult life often leave school without a clear route towards a fulfilling and productive adult life.

- Carers can feel undervalued by public services, lacking the right information and enough support to meet their lifelong caring responsibilities.

- Choice and Control. Many people with learning disabilities have little choice or control in their lives. Recent research shows only 6% of people with learning disabilities having control over who they lived with and 1% over choice of carer. Advocacy services are patchy and inconsistent. Direct payments have been slow to take off for people with learning disabilities.

- Health Care. The substantial health care needs of people with learning disabilities too often go unmet. They can experience avoidable illness and die prematurely.

- Housing can be the key to achieving social inclusion, but the number supported to live independently in the community, for example, remains small. Many have no real choice and receive little advice about possible housing options.

- Day services frequently fail to provide sufficiently flexible and individual support. Some large day centres offer little more than warehousing and do not help people with learning disabilities undertake a wider range of individually tailored activities.

- Social isolation remains a problem for too many people with learning disabilities. A recent study found that only 30% had a friend who was not either learning disabled, or part of their family or paid to care for them.

- Employment is a major aspiration for people with learning disabilities, but less than 10% nationally are in work, so most people remain heavily dependent on social security benefits.

The needs of people from minority ethnic communities with learning disabilities are too often overlooked. Key findings from a study by the Centre for Research in Primary Care at the University of Leeds (Ahmad 2001), published alongside *Valuing People*, included:

- prevalence of learning disability in some South Asian communities can be up to three times greater than in the general population;

- diagnosis is often made at a later age than for the population as a whole and parents receive less information about their child's condition and the support available;

- social exclusion is made more severe by language barriers and racism, and negative stereotypes and attitudes contribute to disadvantage;

- carers who do not speak English receive less information about their support role and experience high levels of stress;

- agencies often underestimate people's attachments to cultural traditions and religious beliefs.

This detailing of the shocking range of exclusion is a measure of the challenges that face services, communities, government and of course people with learning disabilities and their families.

Exercise 26.1

Find out what happened to a long-stay institution near you. What was it like just before it closed? What happened to it when it closed? Compare investment while people with learning disabilities lived there with the investment made in the site when they moved out. What does this say about how people are valued in our society?

The citizenship club – are people with learning disabilities allowed in?

In services for people with learning disabilities, citizenship is often proposed as the goal of service supports and indeed of adults with learning disabilities. Marshall (1950) sees citizenship as having three elements: civil, political and social. This framework is reflected in the four key principles of *Valuing People*: rights, choice, independence and inclusion. O'Brien (1986) identifies five service accomplishments – community presence, choice, competence, respect and community participation – which are the objective of human services in order to promote the full citizenship of people with learning disabilities. Duffy (2003) suggests that full citizenship is still a distant dream for many people with learning disabilities, due to a lack of self-determination and equal civil rights. Duffy identifies six keys to citizenship: self-determination, direction, money, home, support and community life. This chapter is concerned with community life (working, playing and learning with fellow community members) without which Duffy (2003: 135) states, 'You could have achieved all the first five keys to citizenship and yet not really be living a full life'.

Bayley (1997) warns that service-based solutions are not enough. He tells the story of Stan. Stan lives in his own home, uses public transport, socializes in integrated settings and has a full weekly timetable of activities in ordinary community settings. A care management triumph, a picture of community integration, surely. Yet, 'sometimes, having visited him, and without his suggesting any problems or difficulties, I want to cry. His deep sense of loneliness or aloneness is nearly unbearable: no soulmate, close companion or sexual partner, no love' (p. 2). It is clear that Stan could not be provided with what he really wanted by service supports alone. In the same way, citizenship is not something that can be given.

New Labour recognized that many disabled people have been overlooked and made a commitment that 'The Government will work to ensure that they are not left on society's sidelines' (DSS 1998: 51). Despite this commitment, Scott (2000: 58) explores recent welfare reforms and concludes that, 'The notion of citizenship that seems to be emerging with New Labour reforms is one that is largely tied to the interests of paid workers'.

Statistics relating to the number of people with learning disabilities not in work demonstrate the scale of the work ahead: in 1999, 46 per cent of disabled people were unemployed and less than 10 per cent of people with learning difficulties were in jobs (Institute of Applied Health and Social Policy 2002). If the New Labour vision is really tied to the interests of paid workers, then the levels of unemployment for people with learning disabilities place them firmly on the margins of society.

Exercise 26.2

If you are part of a group of people who have an unemployment level of over 90 per cent or are the subject of the social exclusion detailed, would you aspire to being a citizen in the society that let this happen or would you want to transform society?

Work – is there a new deal for people with learning disabilities?

Objective 8 of *Valuing People* is supported by guidance for local authorities to produce strategies for developing employment-related services. The *Framework for Developing an Employment Strategy* (Institute of Applied Health and Social Policy 2002) proposes two key performance indicators: a local measure of people with learning disabilities in work as a proportion of people with learning difficulties known to the council; and a national measure of the proportion of people with learning difficulties in work as compared to the percentage of disabled people in work. The guidance offers a broad range of forms of employment-related activity and involvement. This reflects the *Valuing People* objective which considers not only the aim of getting jobs in open employment but also making a 'valuable contribution to the world of work' (DoH 2001a: 26). Support for people with learning disabilities to get work and the removal of barriers which stand in their way is part of a wider context of welfare policy.

A new contract for welfare?

New Labour proposes that the economic forces of globalization are 'driving the future' (Blair 1999) with lifelong learning seen as a way of adapting to the new economic challenges. 'Education is our best economic policy' (DfEE 1998). New Labour addressed the modernization of welfare in the Green Paper, *New Ambitions for Our Country: A New Contract for Welfare* (DSS 1998). At the heart of the paper is the mantra, 'Work for those who can; security for those who cannot' (p. iii).

Exercise 26.3

'Work for those who can; security for those who cannot' (DSS 1998: iii). Who do the government mean when they talk about 'those who cannot'? What is the nature of security? What do the answers to these questions mean for the citizenship of people with learning disabilities?

Does this 'Third Way' (Blair 1998) break the mould of social policy in the twentieth century or is it simply a new way of excluding people from the mainstream? The paradox at the heart of the government's approach to the modernization of welfare is the suggestion that the contributory citizen is independent of support and in employment, paying taxes to enable the state to organize education, social and health care. In this context, Burke (2002: 27) notes, 'Social exclusion is understood as a threat to the Nation, weakening the labour market and "our" competitive position against the rest of the world'. How can those 'who cannot' be part of this vision unless the vision leaves room for contributory citizens to have a currency of worth that is something other than the creation of wealth/payment of taxes? A vision of the independent citizen must accommodate difference and the requirements of disabled people, not least as 'Independence does not mean not having support' (Beresford and Holden 2000: 982).

Support and dignity or participation?

In the years since *New Ambitions for our Country: A New Contract for Welfare* (DSS 1998) was published, much has changed. Unemployment fell to under 1 million people in early 2001 (Nathan 2001) and full employment was again a political goal that could be openly supported by a Green Paper, *Towards Full Employment in a Modern Society* (DfEE 2001). There remain, however, groups of people who continue to exist at the margins of our society. There are geographical areas suffering low employment and older unemployed people, lone parents and disabled people continue to show a much higher than average rate of unemployment. Johnstone (1994) suggests that 'The evidence that disabled people are denied the full rights to citizenship as a result of the demands of the labour market is overwhelming'. There is evidence of this exclusion in the parameters that organizations such as Job Centre Plus (focusing on getting people off benefit and thereby deploying limited resources for people with learning difficulties who have no immediate prospect of coming off benefit) and the Learning and Skills Council (focusing on targets relating to basic skills and vocational training which again exclude many people with learning difficulties) work within. There are radical perspectives that challenge the notion of Welfare to Work and seek a more radical and inclusive view of the currency of worth in our society (Holman *et al.* 1997).

Necessarily, initiatives such as Welfare to Work address the majority of people. Squeezing people with learning disabilities into a Welfare to Work model contrasts their experience of unemployment with the first duty of citizenship for non-disabled people: paid work. For disabled people, policy means work can be both a duty *and* a right (Williams 1999) or as Powell (2000: 47) sees it, 'disabled people are positioned [as citizens] by their actual or potential relationship to work'. In addition to the social exclusion of people with learning disabilities that is the reality of not having a job, the situation is compounded in many cases by barriers to getting and keeping work faced by many family carers. Mencap (2001) found that 78 per cent of carers who had worked prior to the birth of their son or daughter had been unable to return to work afterwards.

What can and is being done?

There are examples of legislation that can be seen as steps on the road to inclusion. The government (DSS 1998) introduced the New Deal for Disabled People which launched innovative schemes aimed at supporting people to move into work. A new Disabled Person's Tax Credit replaced the Disability Working Allowance in October 1999 with the aim of reducing disincentives to work caused by the benefit trap. The Department for Work and Pensions has made changes in the Permitted Work rules (DWP 2002) and within these changes the ability of someone in receipt of ongoing support from publicly-funded agencies to retain the upper permitted earnings limit indefinitely is a genuine step forward for people with learning difficulties who have no immediate prospect of earning enough money to come off high levels of benefit. The Connexions partnerships are working with young people with learning difficulties in order to support their aspirations in the context of employment and education as they go through the transition from school to adult life. Connexions accommodates the support requirements of people with learning difficulties by extending support to the age of 25 years. A review of the early work of Connexions partnerships since their formation in 2001 found transition from school to adult life being made easier for people with learning disabilities. The partnerships have the potential to influence schools, colleges, employers and the Learning and Skills Council in the interests of the people being served (Giraud-Saunders 2002), although there was an all too familiar cautionary note that this could not be done effectively without the commitment of other mainstream agencies.

While the policy rhetoric regarding employment promotes the use of mainstream agencies, the majority of employment support for people with severe learning disabilities is provided by specialist agencies. These ways of helping people to get jobs fall into two broad categories: supported employment and social economic development (see also Chapter 20).

Supported employment, as defined by O'Bryan *et al.* (2000) and Brooke *et al.* (1997) aims to support people into 'real' jobs in open employment. The values base of supported employment differs from some generic mainstream employment support approaches in terms of one its key values, 'The presumption of employment – a conviction that everyone, regardless of the level or the type of disability, has the capability and right to a job' (Brooke *et al.* 1997: 4). The service delivery process of supported employment in this context (O'Bryan *et al.* 2000) starts with vocational profiling – person-centred planning focusing on employment – and moves through support for job development – interview skills and employer liaison in recruitment; job analysis – finding out about job roles and natural (those which are naturally present in the workplace as opposed to those provided by the supported employment specialist) supports available. There are also job site supports – minimum supports in the workplace that focus on the employee using natural workplace supports. Ongoing support is offered to both employee and employer and also focuses on career development. Research into this model of support shows that when compared to traditional day activity it is far more effective in terms of outcomes for people such as engagement, social interaction and natural supports (Beyer *et al.* 2001). Research also suggests that welfare benefit regulations continue to restrict the number of hours people could work (O'Bryan *et al.* 2000; Beyer *et al.* 2001).

There is growing social economic activity in the UK. The government believes that the social economy is about 'business with primarily social objectives whose surpluses are principally reinvested for that purpose in the business or in the community, rather than being driven by the need to maximise profits for shareholders or owners' (DTI 2002: 8). The government uses social enterprise as a collective term to include the full range of social economic projects. In some UK services to people with learning disabilities a distinction has been made between social enterprises, where objectives of care and/or education are equal to or of greater importance than commercial goals, and social firms, where the primary objective is commercial – 'businesses that support rather than projects that trade' (Social Firms UK 2002). It is important to note that the performance indicators associated with *Valuing People* (DoH 2001a) and detailed above are not accompanied by rigorous monitoring or by extra resources to provide the means to achieve them. Given unemployment rates of over 90 per cent for people with learning difficulties, this represents an inadequate response to a situation which is at odds with the vision and principles of *Valuing People* and would in any other population be considered a national scandal. The views of people who have got work give some indication of the loss of opportunities that results from being excluded from work.

On work in the public sector

We have a bit of a laugh while we work. I like getting paid and it's easy to get to and from my house.

It has given me a purpose to come out of the house and have a job. I receive all the help and support I need and there is always someone to ask if I require anything. While working on Reception at the civic office it has been very interesting to hear what people come in for and it has given me an awareness of what people need in community.

(Griffin 2003: 12)

On open employment

It's a genuine job that I quite adore . . . I feel really alive.

Just because I was handicapped they didn't think I could work but I proved them wrong.

(Spectrum Day Services 2000)

On social firms and enterprises

Feel strong, got friends.

I can do things for myself, have the independence and not worry about the future, we can help each other out.

When I left work and all that I was really down in the dumps . . . since I have had this job it has been brilliant.

It gives me a lot of power and sensation. People don't think I can do things but I can.

(Spectrum Day Services 2000)

Learning – education for all?

This section explores the general policy background and the nature of provision for adults with learning disabilities, and then seeks relevant and meaningful education and learning approaches.

In some ways it is in adult education that we see a rare congruence of rhetoric and associated funding. The outcome of recent developments for adults with learning disabilities is broadly increased provision. In a general context, further education has moved in recent years towards a vocationally-led curriculum (Johnstone 1994). Much of the access-related legislation addresses the needs of people with 'specific learning difficulties'. This is taken to mean '. . . that a person does not find learning in general to be difficult. Rather it is difficult to learn, perform or demonstrate knowledge and understanding under certain conditions for certain types of task' (Cottrell 2003: 121). The updating of the Disability Discrimination Act 1995 by the Special Educational Needs and Disability Act 2001 seeks to ensure that universities and colleges make reasonable adjustments to their teaching and learning strategies and environment. This leads to a goal of '. . . reasonable adjustments to ensure that people who are disabled are not substantially disadvantaged in gaining access to the education on offer' (Powell 2003: 8). The key issue for people with learning disabilities is that the education on offer may not address their learning goals or styles and enabling access to existing programmes is not necessarily the answer.

The Further and Higher Education Act 1992 created the Further Education Funding Council (FEFC) and colleges were given the duty of having regard to services to people with learning disabilities. Progress in this respect was reviewed in *Inclusive Learning* (FEFC 1996). The report promotes the belief that an 'inclusive learning' approach '. . . will improve the education of those with learning difficulties, but believe that it is also true that such an approach would benefit all and indeed, represents the best approach to learning and teaching yet articulated' (p. 4). *Inclusive Learning* goes on to identify the key issues for developing truly inclusive adult education for people with learning disabilities:

> There is a world of difference between, on the one hand, offering courses of education and training and then giving some students who have learning difficulties some additional human or physical aids to gain access to those courses and, on the other hand, redesigning the very processes of learning, assessment and organisation so as to fit the objectives and learning styles of the students. But only the second philosophy can claim to be inclusive, to have as its central purpose the opening of opportunity to those whose disability means that they learn differently from others. It may mean introducing new content into courses or it may mean differentiated access to the same content or both.
>
> (FEFC 1996: 4)

The Learning and Skills Act 2000 created the Learning and Skills Council in April 2001 following the amalgamation of Training and Enterprise Councils and the Further Education Funding Council. *Valuing People* (DoH 2001a: 78) notes that the Learning and Skills Council needs to 'have regard to the needs of young people and adults with learning difficulties when securing post 16 education and training'. In doing so it needs to consider equality of opportunity, additional support and work experience for people with learning disabilities.

There have been attempts to create approaches to lifelong learning that more readily accommodate people with learning disabilities. In general, the approaches broaden the learning areas to reflect the fact that vocational programmes are not always relevant to the current experience of people with learning disabilities. Wilcox and Bellamy (1987) present a curriculum that overlays all areas of life in three domains: leisure, work and personal management. This carries the danger of someone's whole life being considered as an educational programme and Sutcliffe (1991: 36) reminds us that learning for adults is a choice but that 'adults with learning difficulties have often been distanced from the processes of choice and decision making on the question of whether and what to learn'. The reality of this view is illustrated by Rustemier (2002: 5) who records the experience of a student interviewed about his college experience:

What made you come on this course then?

Student: That's what I'd like to know . . .

Can you remember how it happened?

Student: No. I asked [the curriculum manager] and he says it's because I went to a special school but I've asked other people who were at the same school as me and they didn't have to go through this . . .

An approach to adult learning for people with profound learning disabilities is described in *Learning for Life* (FEU 1994) through a series of pen pictures of individuals, for example:

During his hand massage Dennis has learned to indicate that he wants this to continue by lifting his arm slightly, in the direction of the person providing the massage.

Gillian refused to join in the drama session at the leisure club. She wanted to finish her painting. She enjoys paints. She shook her head and kept pointing to her paper and paint until she was allowed to continue her painting. She has learned to value her own wishes and to make them clear to others.

Learning for Life blends curriculum development with an informal choice-based approach to participation. Mahoney (2001) sees informal education as using the environment – physical, emotional, social and political – for the purposes of learning. The approach is recommended for workers engaged in community-based support and addresses the issue of avoiding institutional-izing the learning process or 'forcing' education on someone in their home, place of work or leisure time.

People with learning difficulties have a mixed experience of their time at college (NIACE 1996). They liked:

- getting certificates;
- friendly staff and people;
- wide choice of courses;
- good lunch food;
- improvements to the building;
- giving suggestions on courses;
- staff listening to complaints and taking action.

They disliked:

- noisy refectory;
- verbal abuse;
- poor access;
- overcrowded rooms;
- poor transport.

Exercise 26.4
What is your role in relation to a person with learning disabilities? Tutor, friend, employer, nurse, social worker, employee? Consider you role using the diagram below, adapted for the purpose of this chapter from McGee *et al.* (1987), which illustrates a range of interactional postures (ways of building relationships with people). Which posture would you adopt?

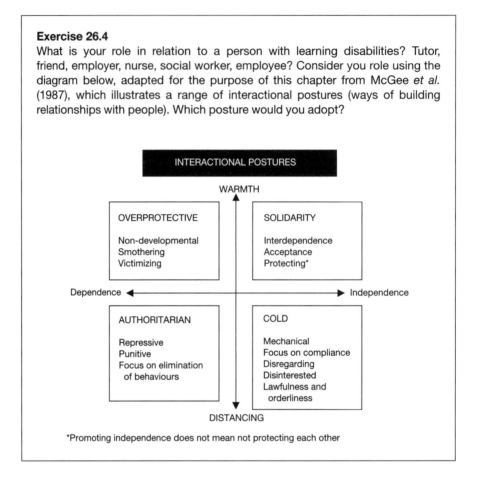

*Promoting independence does not mean not protecting each other

Leisure – the journey from presence to participation

'We need friends. We should have more places where we can meet people and make friends and do things. We want to mix with all sorts of people. We believe people shouldn't just stay at home and feel sorry for themselves and ask for pity; there's a beautiful world out there and we want to be part of it' (Bayley 1997: 63). Leisure is becoming a central concern of the lives of many people because of decreasing time spent at work and increasing disposable income. Bull *et al.* (2003) identify four major approaches to defining leisure:

- *Time-based approaches* – see leisure as the time not spent at work or meeting basic needs for survival (e.g. sleep, eating).

- *Activity-based approaches* – define leisure in terms of activities that are not daily necessities or obligations in the context of family, social or employment responsibilities.

- *Attitude-based approaches* – informed by the varying definitions of individuals about what leisure is. This approach sees leisure in terms of how a person perceives what is going on rather than in terms of location, time or activity.

- *Quality-based approaches* – attribute affective characteristics to activities. An activity could be described as leisure if it is associated with freedom, physical activity, pleasure, relaxation or creativity.

If the first two approaches are used, the majority of people with learning difficulties would be leisure participants for most of their lives. When viewed from a quality-based approach, leisure has sometimes been turned into little more than an occupation that is programmed and controlled rather than something characterized by choice and freedom.

There are further difficulties with approaches based on an acceptance that work is a key element of people's lives, given the fact that the majority of people with learning disabilities are unemployed. Many people with learning disabilities have a solitary and lonely experience of time passing without purpose (McConkey *et al.* 1981 cited by Cavet 1995). Bayley (1997: 32) found during his study of friendship that:

> An overwhelming impression from the project was that many people with learning difficulties find time a burden not a gift – whether it was Arthur Needles watching television all day in the sitting room at his parent's house, Christopher Johnson lying on the sitting room floor playing with his sock, or Philip Brindley and Jason Havering in their pleasant house watching television programmes that did not interest them . . .

Exercise 26.5

What would you do if you had a year off?

When Nash (1953 cited in Hogg and Cavet 1995) was studying leisure he asked people what they would do with a year off. He recorded some of the things people told him: 'Here they are writing poetry, building a cabin, making a piece of poetry, singing a song, playing the ukulele, painting a picture, sailing a boat ... They go to ends of the earth to see canyons, climb mountains, chase caribou, follow migratory birds, dig dinosaur eggs in the Gobi desert . . .'

Imagine a year not doing the things that get in the way of ambitions and dreams. Ask a person with learning disabilities what they would do and also what they would stop doing. Ask with words, ask by sharing experiences and when you have heard what somebody wants, try to do something about it.

Hogg and Cavet (1995) explore definitions of leisure for people with profound learning and multiple disabilities and seek definitions that are based on choice and the non-obligatory nature of leisure instead of definitions of leisure as the converse of work. Hogg reviews Nash's 1957 hierarchical scheme of leisure participation which runs through a numerical scale from sub zero which represents acts against society through zero (injury or detriment to self or others), 1 (killing time, amusement, entertainment and escape from monotony), 2 (emotional participation, watching, appreciating), 3 (active participation, playing the part, copying the model), to 4 (creative participation, the maker of the model, composer, artist, inventor). Hogg and Cavet (1995) develop a non-hierarchical model retaining the four above zero activity areas but move away from attaching relative value or status to any of them. They acknowledge that in the case of some people with profound learning disabilities and multiple impairments, all forms of activity can have non-adaptive consequences in terms of injury or detriment to others or self, but see this as being less likely in the context of creative participation than in activities which are merely an antidote to boredom. Hogg and Cavet's ecology of leisure for people includes carers and for many people with learning difficulties the mapping of relationships will mean that leisure today will need to be considered in the context of a world that has been created for people rather than chosen by them. Like a good PATH (planning alternative tomorrows with hope) process (Sanderson *et al.* 1997) (see also Chapter 24), the vision is the starting point but the outcome is positive. In this context, wishing away the service-created environment that people live in is to ignore people's reality.

Dowson (1998: 20) reviews the role of leisure in day centres and concludes that 'days spent in leisure pursuits do not represent "living like other people" – especially when low income is a bar to many activities'. One service cited by Dowson justified introducing people with learning difficulties to community leisure activities by promoting a move from the stigmatizing label of 'day centre user' to the more 'normal' label of 'unemployed'. This is leisure activity imposed by dogma rather than leisure based on freedom and choice.

There are current, more positive, examples of initiatives that start from the position of equal access to leisure. Easton (2002) describes the Inclusive Fitness Initiative which is designed to support leisure centres to adopt and put into practice policies that will enable all disabled people to be included. The initiative offers training to staff working in leisure centres and guidance on marketing the benefits and availability of fitness to disabled people. The sophisticated, evidence-based approach aims to ensure that mainstream amenities can accommodate the support requirements of disabled people. This is achieved through both changing the equipment and physical environment and also the culture, so as to welcome disabled people: 'Negative attitudes and culture are perhaps the greatest bars to participation in this type of leisure pursuit' (Easton 2002: 19). Livesey (2003) records the experiences of the Bringing Leisure Alive project in Glasgow. Following consultation with people with learning disabilities, families and carers, access to leisure was identified as a priority. Training is offered to staff working with people with learning disabilities and the aim of the project is to work towards a vision that foresees that 'people with learning difficulties will be able to access leisure in the same way as other citizens, having open and accessible facilities, being treated with dignity and respect and being included'.

A positive example of exploring life outside a segregated setting as part of day service modernization is presented by Nielsen and Porter (2002) who recorded the experience of a group of people with learning disabilities who tried activities in their local community as an alternative to their day centre. Paul's story demonstrates that joining in with community life is not about labels but choices, relationships and enjoyment.

Case study: *Paul*

Paul is a 42-year-old man with Down's syndrome who had attended a day centre for more than ten years. He participated in most activities, particularly sports and art and craft groups, but was less engaged in less structured times during his day there. He did try local colleges but chose not to attend. Paul was one of three service users who took part in the project full time, so did not go to the day centre at all. Instead he met the group outside and went off with them to a variety of community-based activities. These included voluntary work for '60+' and Notting Hill Housing Trust. As a result of the project, Paul's confidence increased and he seemed less dependent on staff. He was more able to make clear choices without prompting. He began to build positive relationships with his peers, and people in the community got to know and recognize him. When asked for his comments on the project and how he felt about returning to the centre, Paul chose the 'angry' picture face. He said he would rather still be on the project.

Alongside improving access to mainstream facilities there continue to be a range of specialist arrangements for people with learning disabilities to have their leisure made appropriate for them – Snoezelen, Gateway Clubs, befriending schemes, community use sessions in day service programmes. There are particular issues for people with profound learning disabilities and multiple impairments that will not be addressed by disability awareness sessions and improved equipment. Hogg and Cavet (1995) provide a thorough review of research, approaches and practice in this respect. They note that people with profound learning disabilities and multiple impairments are often not addressed by inclusion initiatives and set about remedying the situation. However, it is not the case that this group of people need to be served in segregated settings, despite one of the attitudinal barriers identified in *Making it Happen* (Mencap 1997: 16): 'severely disabled people are best left to the professionals because they know what they are doing'. This rings true within specialist services as well as with the general public. *Making it Happen* identifies means of overcoming such barriers and makes practical recommendations for action for inclusion, for example a central information resource, national standards for accessibility and calls for leisure organizations to consider and address the requirements and interests of people with profound learning disabilities.

People with learning disabilities are not just waiting for leisure providers to get it right – they are increasingly taking on the job of sorting out their own events. There are a growing number of club nights run by and for people with learning disabilities. There are also a growing number of drop-in clubs run by and for people with learning disabilities, for example the Meeting Place in South Gloucestershire: a place for people with learning difficulties to meet up with friends and be able to have somewhere to get support through having choice and control.

Finally, when we spend a lot of time considering the costs of services, the following balance sheet recording participation in a local community carnival is one which offers an alternative to a simple financial criteria for success:

Expenditure
- £20 materials
- £5 chicken suit hire
- 4 hours meeting attendance

Outcomes (and income!)
- 1500 hours involvement in preparation and the event itself
- Links with new organizations – hauliers, scouts, nursery, wild west society!
- Team-building
- Being seen by the local community giving our bit too and not just receiving
- £250 share of the profits
- Some happy memories: eventually we moved off for the procession around the streets and we were all singing and dancing and having a brilliant time. To make it all worthwhile we took second place with a cup from the Lord Mayoress. Maybe next year it will be first place, who knows?

Conclusion

Full citizenship is a long way off for people with learning disabilities. The current policy context for employment and education presents an ambiguous picture of the place of people with learning difficulties in higher and further education. The ambiguity is sustained by policy that is described by Burke (2002) as 'a neo liberal logic that serves to reproduce social, cultural and economic inequalities while claiming to be against social exclusion'. Williams (1999) proposes that 'good enough principles for welfare' should include interdependence in the sense that we all need to recognize that 'We are all necessarily dependent on others' (Williams 1999: 677). With that recognition comes a responsibility to challenge institutions that leave some groups of people 'unnecessarily dependent' (Williams 1999: 677). This is a very different form of radically aware social responsibility than that of the duty to pay taxes having taken up paid work. O'Brien (2001: 6) proposed that there will be no real change in the status of people with learning disabilities without 'political organizers, lobbyists, participants in civil disobedience, plaintiffs, and officially observed victims of conditions that violate funder's rules'.

There is great potential for the development of new models of inclusive learning within the further education sector. The opportunity for this development exists in the form of funding mechanisms that accommodate the support requirements of people with learning disabilities. What is missing in terms of a vision of true inclusion and citizenship is the development of more ways of providing learning and achievement status in our society. Only a radical reappraisal of the currency of worth will achieve this.

In the flurry of changing legislation and political debate relating to the modernization of welfare it is worth reflecting on the fact that the most inclusive noise is silence. If service providers and purchasers can learn to be quiet more often, then they will be more likely to hear and learn from the people they serve. The challenge for professionals is to be part of the solution, not the problem. The challenge for people with learning disabilities is to continue to find the courage and strength to live, learn and work in environments which are rarely inclusive.

Resources

Employment

Association for Supported Employment: www.afse.org.uk.
Department for Work and Pensions: www.dwp.gov.uk.
Learning and Skills Council: www.lsc.gov.uk.
Social Enterprise Unit: www.dti.gov.uk/socialenterprise.
Social Firms UK: www.socialfirms.co.uk/.
Valuing People Support Team: www.doh.gov.uk/vpst/employment.htm.

Learning

Learning and Skills Council: www.lsc.gov.uk.
Lifelong learning: www.lifelonglearning.dfee.gov.uk.
National Institute of Continuing Education: www.niace.org.uk/Publications/Subject/learning_diffs.htm.
Skill – National Bureau for Students With Disabilities: www.skill.org.uk.

References

Ahmad, W. (2001) *Learning Difficulties and Ethnicity*. Leeds: Centre for Research in Primary Care, University of Leeds.

Bayley, M. (1997) *What Price Friendship? Encouraging the Relationships of People with Learning Difficulties*. Minehead: Hexagon.

Beresford, P. and Holden, C. (2000) We have choices: globalization and welfare user movements, *Disability and Society*, 15(7): 973–89.

Beyer, S., Shearn, J. and Thomas, J. (2001) *The Cost Effectiveness of Supported Employment for People with Severe Learning Difficulties and High Support Needs: Final Report*. Cardiff: Welsh Centre for Learning Disabilities.

Blair, T. (1998) *The Third Way: New Politics for a New Century*. London: The Fabian Society.

Blair, T. (1999) Conference speech (Labour Party Conference, Bournemouth, 28 September), in P. Beresford and C. Holden (2000) We have choices: globalization and welfare user movements, *Disability and Society*, 15(7): 973–89.

Brooke, V., Inge, K.J., Armstrong, A.J. and Wehman, P. (1997) *Supported Employment Handbook: A Customer Driven Approach for Persons with Significant Disabilities*. Richmond, VA: Rehabilitation Research and Training Center on Supported Employment, Virginia Commonwealth University.

Bull, C., Hoose, J. and Weed, M. (2003) *An Introduction to Leisure Studies*. Harlow: Pearson Education.

Burke, P.J. (2002) *Accessing Education: Effectively Widening Participation*. Stoke-on-Trent: Trentham Books.

Cavet, J. (1995) Sources of information about the leisure of people with profound and multiple disabilities, in J. Hogg and J. Cavet (eds) *Making Leisure Provision for People with Profound Learning and Multiple Disabilities*. London: Chapman & Hall.

Cottrell, S. (2003) Students with dyslexia and other specific learning difficulties, in S. Powell (ed.) *Special Teaching in Higher Education: Successful Strategies for Access and Inclusion*. London: Cogan Page.

DfEE (Department for Education and Employment) (1998) *The Learning Age*. London: The Stationery Office.

DfEE (Department for Education and Employment) (2001) *Towards Full Employment in a Modern Society*. London: The Stationery Office.

DoH (Department of Health) (2001a) *Valuing People: A New Strategy for Learning Disability for the 21st Century*. London: Department of Health.

DoH (Department of Health) (2001b) *Nothing About Us Without Us*. London: Department of Health.

Dowson, S. (1998) *Certainties Without Centres? A Discussion Paper on Day Services for People Who Have Learning Difficulties*. London: Values Into Action.

DSS (Department of Social Security) (1998) *New Ambitions for Our Country: A New Contract for Welfare*. London: The Stationery Office.

DTI (Department for Trade and Industry) (2002) *Social Enterprise: A Strategy for Success*. London: The Stationery Office.

Duffy, S. (2003) *Keys to Citizenship: A Guide to Getting Good Support for People with Learning Difficulties*. Birkenhead: Paradigm.

DWP (Department for Work and Pensions) (2002) *Permitted Work: Procedural Information for Disability Organisations*. London: DWP.

Easton, C. (2002) Fitness for all, *Living Well*, 2(2): 17–22.

Egan, G. (1994) *The Skilled Helper*, 5th edn. Pacific Grove, CA: Brooks/Cole.

FEFC (Further Education Funding Council) (1996) *Inclusive Learning: Principles and Recommendations – A Summary of the Findings of the Learning Difficulties Committee*. Coventry: FEFC.

FEU (1994) *Learning for Life*. London: Mencap.

Giraud-Saunders, A. (2002) Connexions – a better start in life? *Living Well*, 2(2): 23–5.

Griffin, H. (2003) Extending employment opportunities, *Living Well*, 3(2): 10–13.

Gross, R. D. (1992) *Psychology: The Science of Mind and Behaviour*, 2nd edn. London: Hodder & Stoughton.

Hogg, J. and Cavet, J. (eds) (1995) *Making Leisure Provision for People with Profound Learning and Multiple Disabilities*. London: Chapman & Hall.

Holman, A., Steele, D., Aspis, S., Letts, P., Crowhurst, G. and Brandon, D. (1997) Our agenda for change, *Community Living*, 10(4): 4–8.

Institute of Applied Health and Social Policy (2002) *Framework for Developing an Employment Strategy*. London: DoH.

Johnstone, D. (1994) *Further Opportunities: Learning Difficulties and Disabilities in Further Education*. London: Cassell.

Livesey, C. (2003) Bringing leisure alive: improving access to leisure for people with learning difficulties in Glasgow, *Living Well*, 3(2): 27–30.

Mahoney, J. (2001) What is informal education, in D. Richardson, M. Wolfe (eds) *Principles and Practice of Informal Education: Learning Through Life*. London: Routledge.

Marshall, T.H. (1950) *Citizenship and Social Class*. Cambridge: Cambridge University Press.

McIntosh, B. and Whittaker, A. (1998) *Days of Change*. London: King's Fund.

McGee, J.J., Menolascino, F.J., Hobbs, D.C. and Menousek, P.E. (1987) *Gentle Teaching*. New York: Human Sciences Press.

Mencap (1997) *Making it Happen: Community Leisure and Recreation for People with Profound Learning and Multiple Disabilities*. London: Mencap.

Mencap (2001) *No Ordinary Life*. London: Mencap.

Nathan, M. (2001) *Getting Attached: New Routes to Full Employment*. London: The Fabian Society.

NDT (2002) *The Day Services Modernisation Tool Kit*, Part 1. London: DoH.

NDT (2003) *The Day Services Modernisation Tool Kit*, Part 2. London: DoH.

Neilsen, P. and Porter, S. (2002) Without walls – not without opportunities, *Living Well*, 2(4): 14–18.

NIACE (1996) *Still a Chance To Learn?* Leicester: NIACE.

O'Brien, J. (1986) A guide to personal futures planning, in G.G. Bellamy and B. Wilcox (eds) *A Comprehensive Guide to the Activities Catalogue: An Alternative Curriculum for Youth and Adults with Severe Disabilities*. Baltimore, MD: Paul H. Brookes.

O'Brien, J. (2001) *Paying Customers are not Enough: The Dynamics of Individualized Funding*. Madison, WI: Wisconsin Council on Developmental Disabilities.

O'Bryan, A., Simons, K., Beyer, S. and Grove, B. (2000) *A Framework for Supported Employment*. York: Joseph Rowntree Foundation/ YPS.

Pearlman, V. and Holzhausen, E. (2002) *Adding Value: Carers as Drivers of Social Change*. London: Carers UK.

Powell, M. (2000) New Labour and the third way in British welfare state: a new and distinctive approach? *Critical Social Policy*, 20(1): 39–60.

Powell, S. (ed.) (2003) *Special Teaching in Higher Education*. London: Kogan Page.

Ritchie, P., Jones, C. and Broderick, L. (1996) *Ways To Work: Converting Day Services*. Edinburgh: SHS.

Rustemier, S. (2002) Inclusion in further education for students designated as having learning difficulties and/or disabilities. Paper presented at the Bolton Institute as part of the 'Action Research and the Struggle for Inclusive Education' series, 1 March. Available from http://homepages.phonecoop.coop/markbolton/boltonsharon.html.

Sanderson, H., Kennedy, J., Ritchie, P. and Goodwin, G. (1997) *People Plans and Possibilities*. Edinburgh: Scottish Human Services.

Scott, G. (2000) New Labour and the restructuring of welfare – what's in it for women, *International Journal of Sociology and Social Policy*, 20(6): 51–65.

Simons, K. and Watson, D. (1999) *New Directions? Day Services for People in the 1990s*. Exeter: The Centre for Evidence Based Social Services.

Social Firms UK (2002) *Employment, Empowerment and Enterprise*. Redhill: Social Firms UK.

Spectrum Day Services (now Brandon Trust Work Learning and Leisure) (2000) *Going to Work*. Brighton: Pavillion Publishing.

Sutcliffe, J. (1991) *Adults with Learning Difficulties: Education for Choice and Empowerment*. Leicester: NIACE.

Wertheimer, A. (1996) *Changing Days: Developing New Day Opportunities with People who have Learning Difficulties*. London: King's Fund.

Wilcox, B. and Bellamy, G.G. (eds) (1987) *A Comprehensive Guide to the Activities Catalogue: An Alternative Curriculum for Youth and Adults with Severe Disabilities*. Baltimore, MD: Paul H. Brookes.

Williams, F. (1999) Good enough principles for welfare, *Journal of Social Policy*, 28(4): 667–87.

27

Promoting healthy lifestyles
Mental health and illness

Chris Hatton and John Taylor

Introduction

Most professionals working in services for people with learning disabilities are likely to be working with a person who also has mental health problems (Quigley *et al.* 2001). Interest in mental health problems among people with learning disabilities has increased exponentially in the past 20 years, from a starting position of almost complete indifference. The gap between the patent mental health needs of many people with learning disabilities and the virtual absence of research or treatment by professionals was noted by many authors throughout the 1980s and early 1990s, with the term 'therapeutic disdain' often used (Bender 1993; Stenfert Kroese 1998). Such disdain has been described as being caused by a lack of interest in the problems of people seen as different; people with learning disabilities being considered not clever enough to benefit from psychological therapies; and therapists' reluctance to offer therapy to people who are unattractive because of their disabilities.

The picture is now quite different, with an explosion of interest in the mental health needs of people with learning disabilities. The quantity of research in this area is increasing, although still at a rudimentary level compared to mainstream mental health research. Professional interest in terms of developing effective interventions for people with learning disabilities and mental health problems is also increasing, although the published evidence base here is still largely at the level of case studies, case series and small trials.

In this chapter we aim to explore issues relating to the causes and prevalence of mental health problems among people with learning disabilities, as well as difficulties involved in the identification, assessment and treatment of these problems. This is done within a framework that sets out the prevailing models for understanding these phenomena, the evidence available to support different types of treatment approaches, and ethical and professional considerations when working in this area.

What is mental health?

Exercise 27.1

Quickly write down your own idea of what you mean by mental health and mental health problem. Ask other people to do the same and compare your definitions.

Are your definitions consistent?

How do they distinguish a mentally healthy person from a person with a mental health problem?

How would your definition apply to people with learning disabilities?

What problems are there with your definition?

How easy or difficult was it to try and write a definition?

Terms like 'mental health', 'mental illness', 'mental disorder' and 'psychopathology' are commonly used as if everyone has a common understanding of what they mean. However, the fundamental question of what mental health is, and how it may be distinguished from mental illness, is still being hotly debated with no consensus in sight (Sims 1988). This is not (only) a rarefied academic discussion; definitions of mental health and mental illness have real consequences for people with learning disabilities. Some influential ideas about health and mental health include the following.

The biomedical model

This model (see Nettleton and Gustafsson 2002) sees mental health as being the absence of disease, where disease is created by physical causal agents (genes, biochemicals, damage to the body), leading to changes in the structure and function of the brain. Changes in thoughts, emotions and behaviour are seen as being caused by these physical agents, and interventions (typically medication or surgery) are directed to these physical agents. One of the many problems with this model for people with learning disabilities is that a person's learning disability can itself be viewed as a 'disease of the brain' (Sims 1988). This view, and the therapeutic pessimism that goes with it, was partly responsible for the large-scale institutionalization and social devaluation of people with learning disabilities in many countries from the nineteenth century onwards (Trent 1994; Wright and Digby 1996).

Illness as variation from the norm

In this view, experiences can be placed on a continuum, and people with an illness are defined as those at the extremes of this continuum (Kendell 1975). The term 'psychopathology' has been defined as 'abnormal experience, cognition and behaviour' (Sims 1988). The view of mental illness as variation from the norm raises several questions, including: who decides what the relevant dimensions of mental health are and how they are measured, and can all experiences be placed on a continuum? Of course, people with learning disabilities in most classification systems are already partly defined in these terms, as being at the wrong end of the continuum labelled 'intelligence' (Luckasson *et al.* 2002), with profound negative consequences (Trent 1994; Wright and Digby 1996).

Mental illness as a mismatch of ideas to external realities

First proposed by John Locke in the seventeenth century, this view suggests that mental illness involves the application of intact reasoning powers to unhelpful or bizarre beliefs: Locke himself contrasted this with his view of a person without reasoning capacity, i.e. a person now labelled as having a learning disability (Goodey 1996). This contrast assumes that people with learning disabilities will not have the capacity to develop mental health problems, resulting in distress among people with learning disabilities being ignored and left untreated by clinicians (Bender 1993).

A holistic view of health

'Health is a state of complete physical, mental and social well-being and not merely the absence of disease or infirmity' (World Health Organization 1946). This definition emphasizes health as positive well-being within a broad social context, rather than health as being the absence of disease within an individual. The definition is helpful in two ways: it emphasizes well-being as the crucial indicator of health rather than physical signs of brain disease; and it emphasizes the social context within which mental health is experienced. However, it can be seen as over-inclusive (can anyone be said to be in a state of mental health in this definition?) and somewhat woolly.

Mental health as social construction

This view suggests that mental health is whatever powerful people (such as psychiatrists) say it is. This position takes the view that there are no fixed experiences that can be called mental health problems; instead societies use terms such as mental health to license methods of dealing with people viewed as problematic for the smooth functioning of society (Parker *et al.* 1995). Certainly, historical studies have shown that frameworks for describing mental illness and the populations of people identified as having mental illness have varied tremendously over time (Porter 1990; Scull 1993; Kutchins and Kirk 1997). However, some authors have argued that some experiences labelled as 'mental health problems' have occurred consistently throughout history and that some have clear biological causes (Berrios 1996). It is also worth noting that even if mental health problems are socially constructed, they are often still real to the people experiencing them and the society in which they live.

Mental disorder

To avoid some of the murky waters associated with using labels such as 'mental health' or 'mental illness', international psychiatric classification systems have instead adopted the term 'mental disorder' (World Health Organization 1993; American Psychiatric Association 1994; see also Chapter 3). Although recognized as a fuzzy term, mental disorder has been defined in the following way:

> Each of the mental disorders is conceptualised as a clinically significant behavioral or psychological syndrome or pattern that occurs in an individual and that is associated with present distress or disability or with a significantly increased risk of suffering death, pain, disability, or an important loss of freedom. In addition, this syndrome or pattern must not be merely an expectable and culturally sanctioned response to a particular event, for example, the death of a loved one.
>
> (American Psychiatric Association 1994: xxi)

This definition includes aspects of many of the (sometimes conflicting) views outlined above. For example, clinical judgement and cultural norms are highlighted, to some extent recognizing that mental disorders occur within a social context. However, the definition also locates mental disorders firmly within individuals, as well as assuming that there are patterns of experience that fall into coherent clinical syndromes, much like physical disease categories. On closer inspection, the term 'mental disorder' seems as problematic as the health-based terms it is intended to replace.

For the purposes of this chapter, the holistic view of mental health will be used as a basic framework, for the following reasons:

- it allows for multiple explanations of the causes of mental health problems, including biological, psychological and social explanations;
- it emphasizes well-being as the fundamental marker of mental health;
- it emphasizes the social context within which people live.

Applying a mental health framework to people with learning disabilities

As other chapters in this book have demonstrated, the living circumstances of people with learning disabilities as a group can be quite different to the general population, with welfare services often having a greatly increased role. These differences can have a profound impact on the degree and nature of mental health problems experienced by people with learning disabilities, and also on the way that services understand and respond to their mental health problems.

Living circumstances, life events and other risk factors

Exercise 27.2

Quickly write down your ideas about what life circumstances are risk factors for mental health problems and which are protective factors. Do you think people with learning disabilities are more or less likely to experience each of the life circumstances you have written down?

As a group, people with learning disabilities are likely to experience several living circumstances and life events associated with an increased risk of mental health problems in the general population (Brown 2000). These include birth trauma, stressful family circumstances, poverty, unemployment, stigmatization, lack of self-determination, and a lack of meaningful friendships and intimate relationships (Emerson *et al.* 2001; Hastings *et al.* 2004). Brown (2000) suggests that the meaning of these life events can be crucial in triggering mental health problems; particularly important are feelings of humiliation (feeling put down or devalued), entrapment (feeling imprisoned in a punishing situation for some time), loss (death or separation from important other people) and danger (feeling the threat of a potential future loss). A strong argument can be made that people with learning disabilities are more likely than the general population to experience humiliation, entrapment, loss and danger in the course of their daily lives. Certainly, people with learning disabilities do report experiencing stigma, linked to feelings of being different and negative beliefs about themselves and their social attractiveness (Dagnan and Waring 2004).

People with learning disabilities may also be at greater risk of developing mental health problems due to psychological factors such as a reduced capacity for coping productively with stressful circumstances, poorer memory and poorer problem-solving and planning skills (van den Hout *et al.* 2000).

Accessing services

Exercise 27.3

Quickly write down your ideas about how most people with mental health problems get help.

How is the person's mental health problem recognized?

How do people get access to services?

Which services do they access and what help do they get?

Is this likely to be the same for people with learning disabilities?

Despite the rapid pace of hospital closure for people with learning disabilities throughout the UK in the past 30 years (Emerson *et al.* 2001), such people are still largely supported by specialist learning disability health and welfare services rather than accessing mainstream health services designed for the general population (Elliott *et al.* 2003). This can cause real problems, including mental health problems.

Services for people with learning disabilities and people with mental health problems are largely separate and have quite distinct service cultures, with relatively few specialist mental health services for people with learning disabilities (Bailey and Cooper 1997: Hassiotis *et al.* 2000). For example, support staff in social services may be quite hostile to seeing a person's behaviour as symptomatic of a mental health problem (Costello 2004).

Support staff may also be using a conceptual framework of challenging behaviour rather than mental health to understand problematic behaviours. Challenging behaviour is commonly defined in the following way (Emerson 2001: 3): 'culturally abnormal behaviour(s) of such an intensity, frequency or duration that the physical safety of the person or others is likely to be placed in serious jeopardy, or behaviour which is likely to seriously limit use of, or result in the person being denied access to, ordinary community facilities'. Although the challenging behaviour definition does not include any reference to well-being, and mental health problems do not necessarily involve the person or others being in serious jeopardy or denial of access to community facilities, there are clear overlaps. There are also overlaps in assumptions about cause; while most challenging behaviours are assumed to be immediately functional responses to particular social environments (e.g. aggression may be more effective in gaining staff attention than polite requests for a conversation), it is likely that some challenging behaviours are maintained neurobiologically (Emerson 2001). As yet, the relationship between mental health problems and challenging behaviours in people with learning disabilities is unclear (Emerson *et al.* 1999).

'Diagnostic overshadowing' (Reiss *et al.* 1982) may also occur, where carers and professionals misattribute signs of a mental health problem as being due to a person's intellectual disabilities. For example, poor self-care symptomatic of depression may be attributed to a person being incapable of self-care due to his or her learning disabilities.

Typical referral pathways to mental health services, through a GP due to a person having problems fulfilling social roles (e.g. spouse, parent, employee) (Goldberg and Huxley 1980) may also be less accessible to people with learning disabilities. First, such people are less likely to be in social roles where problems would be apparent. Second, environments for people with learning disabilities may be so restricted that a mental health problem may not be activated or displayed (e.g. a specific phobia). Third, some mental health problems may not manifest themselves in behaviours that are seen as problematic by carers or professionals (e.g. depression manifesting in social withdrawal and loss of energy) (Edelstein and Glenwick 2001). In contrast, people with learning disabilities may be referred to mental health services when their behaviour is construed as a problem by other people rather than being a problem for the person themselves (e.g. anger in response to restrictions on autonomy and choice).

Finally, training programmes helping care staff to work effectively with people with learning disabilities and mental health problems are relatively rare (Bouras and Holt 1997; Quigley *et al.* 2001) and limited in their effectiveness (Costello 2004).

Identifying mental health problems

Exercise 27.4

Imagine you are trying to interview a person speaking a language different to yours about their mental health problems.

How would you tell them what you were doing?

How would you communicate important ideas?

How would you understand what the person was telling you?

Since most professionals will work with people with learning disabilities who also have mental health problems (Quigley *et al.* 2001) it is vital that professionals are sensitive to the possibility of mental health problems in people with learning disabilities, including having the awareness and skills to identify *potential* problems. It will not surprise you to discover that identifying mental health problems in people with learning disabilities is far from straightforward, with a number of difficult questions arising.

Question 1: do standard psychiatric diagnostic criteria apply to (some or all) people with learning disabilities?

Difficulties in identifying mental health problems have been around as long as there have been mental health professionals (Berrios 1996), with some studies reporting that psychiatrists form a strong opinion about their diagnosis within the first three minutes of a clinical interview (Sandifer *et al.* 1970). Indeed, the unreliability of clinical judgement has been one of the driving forces behind the development of the two standard psychiatric classification systems currently dominant in the UK: the *Diagnostic and Statistical Manual of Mental Disorders DSM-4* (4th edition), produced by the American Psychiatric Association (1994), and the *International Classification of Diseases Classification of Mental and Behavioural Disorders* (*ICD-10*) (10th edition), produced by the World Health Organization (1993). Both of these are designed to be comprehensive systems for reliably classifying experiences into a set of 'mental disorders' according to particular criteria, using accompanying standardized interview schedules (Cooper and Oates 2000). While these classification systems may have increased the reliability of psychiatric diagnoses for the general population (their validity is another matter; see Kutchins and Kirk 1997), it is unclear how applicable they are to people with learning disabilities (Sturmey 1999). First, it is possible that these ways of classifying mental health problems may not be applicable to the experiences of people with severe and complex learning disabilities, who frequently have little or no symbolic language skills (Sturmey 1999). For example, can a person with no symbolic language experience auditory hallucinations, or have the cognitive skills necessary to conceptualize and plan a suicide attempt?

Second, these classification systems are categorical; that is, they seek to establish whether a person is experiencing a mental health problem or not. To reach a threshold for a mental health problem, a person needs to experience a pattern of symptoms at a certain level of frequency and severity. Many people with learning disabilities may show clear signs of a particular mental health problem, but not show a sufficient range of signs to reach the threshold to trigger a diagnosis (e.g. psychotic experiences and schizophrenia; see Moss *et al.* 1996a; Hatton *et al.* under review). There are also broader questions about how useful categorical diagnostic systems are in guiding clinical work with people with mental health problems (Bentall 2004). For example, is knowing that a person has a label of schizophrenia enough to guide a clinical intervention, or is it more important to discover which experiences are a problem for the person and how they might be managed?

Third, these classification systems contain some assumptions that might be difficult to apply to people with learning disabilities. For example, they often diagnose a mental health problem as a change from the usual. This can be a problem for a person with learning disabilities and unrecognized mental health problems, where their mental health difficulties may not have changed for months or years. These systems also assume a usual level of functioning that may be difficult to apply to all people with learning disabilities – for example, criteria for depression include a diminished ability to think or concentrate.

Within the *ICD-10* system, there have already been modified diagnostic criteria produced for people with mild learning disabilities (World Health Organization 1996) and people with moderate to severe learning disabilities (Royal College of Psychiatrists 2001). However, both of these modifications have been the subject of some debate (Einfeld and Tonge 1999; Cooper 2003) and are based on informal expert consensus methods with limited validity.

Question 2: is it possible to accurately assess mental states in people with learning disabilities?

What we call mental health problems are typically complex patterns of behaviours and experiences, expressed individually from person to person. Although the full range of mental health problems encompasses very different behaviours and experiences, identifying a mental health problem almost always involves gaining some access to the mental state of the person (Sims 1988). Many mental states, whether they involve perceptions (e.g. I can hear a voice), emotions (e.g. I feel really down) or beliefs (e.g. I believe there is a neo-conservative plot to take over the oilfields of the Middle East under the guise of removing weapons of mass destruction), can really only be accessed by the person describing what their mental state is; inferring a mental state from a person's behaviour can be highly questionable.

Research evidence suggests that most people with learning disabilities and good functional communication skills can give accurate descriptions of their own mental states, as long as interview schedules are sensitively adapted and potential response biases such as acquiescence (saying yes to a question), suggestibility (saying what the person thinks the interviewer wants to hear) and confabulation (making up a response to fill gaps in memory or uncertainty) are assessed (Finlay and Lyons 2001; Dagnan and Lindsay 2004). There are also many examples of self-report mental health measures that have been successfully developed or adapted for people with mild or moderate learning disabilities (see Table 27.1).

However, there is little or no research evidence demonstrating that asking people with more severe and complex learning disabilities about their mental states produces reliable or valid responses (Ross and Oliver 2003a). Some of these problems in gaining descriptions of mental states seem to be a function of the person's skills – for example, many people with learning disabilities have difficulties in recognizing and describing emotions, often using restricted or idiosyncratic emotional vocabularies (Reed and Clements 1989; Rojahn *et al.* 1995a). It is also the case that many of the ideas involved when assessing mental states are abstract and complex (e.g. distinguishing between a voice, a thought and a dream), and are likely to be imperfectly understood by large sections of the population, including people with learning disabilities.

Question 3: to what extent can we use information from other people to assess mental health problems in people with learning disabilities?

Because of potential problems in gaining information from the person with learning disabilities directly, many measures to assess mental health problems in people with learning disabilities have been designed to be used with an informant (typically a paid carer or a family member) rather than with the person themselves (see Table 27.1). There is some convergence between the self-reports of people with mild or moderate learning disabilities and informants using highly structured clinical interview schedules, with informants more likely to pick up behavioural signs and unlikely to reliably report mental state (Moss *et al.* 1996b). However, people with learning disabilities and carers are less likely to agree using less structured interviews concerning emotional distress (Bramston and Fogarty 2000). Even high levels of agreement would not, however, demonstrate that informant reports of mental health problems were valid for people without formal communication skills.

*Question 4: to what extent can we use observational information to
assess mental health problems in people with learning disabilities?*

Many mental health problems are considered to have distinctive patterns of
behaviour associated with them, although many of these behavioural patterns are less distinctive on close inspection (e.g. criteria for major depressive
disorder include significant weight loss or weight gain and insomnia or
hypersomnia; American Psychiatric Association 1994). Relying on
behavioural observations is unlikely to yield sufficient information to reliably identify most mental health problems. For example, self-reports and
behavioural observations often do not agree (Rojahn *et al.* 1995b). Moreover,
the frequent reporting of 'atypical' behavioural symptoms in people with
severe and complex learning disabilities suggests that reliable behavioural
markers of mental health problems are unlikely in this group (Ross and
Oliver 2003a).

Above we have seen how the problems of establishing a clear understanding
of thoughts, ideas and behaviours create difficulties in recognizing mental
health problems in people with learning disabilities. These problems are also
important in relation to making the right service inputs, not least in terms of
consent and capacity.

Informed consent and capacity

Consent to treatment is an important ethical issue for clinical professionals
(American Psychological Association 2002; Sturmey and Gaubatz 2002).
People with learning disabilities, particularly those living in institutional
settings, have been subject to various forms of abuse, including dangerous
interventions that have resulted in injury and harm. Although some people
with learning disabilities can understand the elements necessary for participation in treatment, many cannot (Arscott *et al.* 1999). In any case, many
people with learning disabilities living in institutional or hospital settings
have been placed there because they are judged to be legally incompetent. In
such cases it is unclear who can consent either to treatment or participation
in treatment outcome research. However, this is probably not very different
for people without learning disabilities (e.g. Featherstone and Donovan
2002). Therefore, we need to avoid the situation where discriminatory
decisions to exclude people with learning disabilities from potentially beneficial treatments are made on the basis of erroneous assumptions about their
capacity to give consent compared with members of the general population.
A balance is required in order to protect potentially vulnerable individuals
and promote self-determination.

According to the Lord Chancellor's Department (1999), valid consent
requires: that clients are provided with sufficient accurate information concerning the treatment; that they have capacity to make a decision about
accepting treatment and to understand the consequences of the decision;
and that their decision to accept treatment is voluntary (see also Chapter 5).

Making information about treatment understandable and accessible to people with cognitive limitations is challenging for clinicians, but not insurmountable (Arscott *et al.* 1999). One helpful approach is to include a psycho-educational preparatory phase following which participants will be better informed and able to give or withhold valid consent (e.g. Taylor *et al.* 2002a).

Further enquiry is needed concerning the evaluation of people's capacity to give valid consent. Capacity involves the ability to comprehend information about the treatment, to be able to assimilate and recall the information, and to be able to make a decision about accepting the treatment being offered (Wong *et al.* 1999). However, the extent to which consent-giving by people with learning disabilities can ever be totally free, and so voluntary, given issues concerning acquiescence and suggestibility, is questionable. This is a debate that needs to be brought into the open and not avoided or ignored. In that way clinicians, clients and their supporters can be clear about the ethical issues in this difficult area of work.

If consent cannot be given and the client would have benefited from a particular treatment, then another ethical dilemma is the denial of the benefits of particular treatment interventions to people for whom adequate consent cannot be obtained. In England and Wales this issue is addressed in the Department of Health (2001) guidance document, *Seeking Consent: Working with People with Learning Disabilities*. This guidance suggests that individuals who do not have the capacity to give consent can be given treatment if it is judged to be in the person's best interests. Treatments for mental health problems, including those for people with learning disabilities, have been subject to fashions and fads that sometimes are not harmless (Sturmey *et al.* 2004). Facilitated communication, for example, has been considered not just to be wasteful and ineffective (Mostert 2001), but has resulted in the wrongful conviction of parents for the sexual abuse of their children and led to the separation of children from their families. We cannot assume that well-intended treatments are always helpful, neutral or harmless. In the absence of good evidence to support particular interventions we should be cautious about offering them to people with learning disabilities who may have difficulty in resisting them.

How many people with learning disabilities experience mental health problems?

Given the difficulties in identifying mental health problems in people with learning disabilities discussed earlier, you won't be surprised to find that research on the rates of mental health problems in this population is patchy and inconsistent, with prevalence rates varying between 10 and 80 per cent (Borthwick-Duffy 1994). Higher rates (40 per cent upwards) are reported if challenging behaviour is included as a mental health problem or if the population studied was referred for psychiatric evaluation (e.g. Bouras and

---

Exercise 27.5

What proportion of people with learning disabilities and the general population do you think will experience the following mental health problems?

Depression

Anxiety

Psychosis/schizophrenia

Substance misuse

Dementia

What were the reasons behind your guesses?

Drummond 1992). Low prevalence rates (15 per cent downwards) are reported by studies using general case notes to identify mental health problems (e.g. Borthwick-Duffy and Eyman 1990). Studies of general populations of people with learning disabilities using screening instruments or psychiatric evaluation to identify cases tend to report prevalence rates between these two extremes, usually between 20 and 40 per cent (e.g. Lund 1985; Taylor *et al.* 2004a). This compares to a prevalence rate of approximately 25 per cent for similar mental health problems in the general population (Goldberg and Huxley 1980).

Separate to mental health problems there are issues of recognized diagnosis. Evidence on specific diagnoses experienced by people with learning disabilities is patchy:

- *Depression*: reported prevalence rates for depression vary widely (Stavrakaki 1999), although studies focusing on depressive symptoms typically report very high rates from 44 per cent (Marston *et al.* 1997) to 57 per cent (Meins 1995). People with mild/moderate learning disabilities display the range of depressive symptoms found in the general population, although the validity of the 'atypical' symptoms reported for people with severe/profound learning disabilities is questionable (Ross and Oliver 2003a).

- *Anxiety*: the little research evidence available suggests high levels of anxiety disorders in adults with learning disabilities (e.g. 27 per cent; Stavrakaki and Mintsioulis 1997), although the validity of diagnoses of anxiety is particularly questionable for people with severe/profound intellectual disabilities (Matson *et al.* 1997).

- *Psychosis*: there is some evidence that rates of psychosis are substantially higher among people with learning disabilities (Lund 1985; Turner 1989; Doody *et al.* 1998), although estimated rates of psychosis vary from 2 to 6 per cent. Once again, the absence of reliable self-report makes the diagnosis of psychosis in people with severe/profound intellectual disabilities difficult.

- *Substance misuse*: general research suggests low levels of alcohol and drug use among adults with learning disabilities (e.g. Lund 1985), although alcohol use may be higher in more independent living circumstances (Robertson *et al.* 2000b).

- *Dementia*: the prevalence of dementia is much higher among older adults with learning disabilities compared to the general population (21.6 vs. 5.7 per cent aged 65+; Cooper 1997). People with Down's syndrome are at particularly high risk of developing dementia, with an age of onset 30–40 years younger than the general population (Holland *et al.* 1998).

- *Anger and aggression*: studies conducted across three continents using broadly similar designs and methods have found the prevalence of aggression among people with learning disabilities to be between 10 and 16 per cent in community populations, and 35 to 47 per cent in institutional and specialist service settings (see Taylor 2002; Taylor and Novaco in press for reviews). Lindsay and Law (1999) found that the assessed rate of clinically significant anger problems among clients referred to a specialist community learning disability service in Scotland was 66 per cent. Recent epidemiological research suggests that the prevalence of anxiety and conduct disorders may be much higher among children and youths with learning disabilities, although rates of depression are similar (Linna *et al.* 2000; Tonge and Einfeld 2000; Emerson 2003).

Assessing mental health problems in people with learning disabilities

The beginning of any effective intervention for a person's mental health problems must be accurate, timely and regular assessment:

- accurate in terms of reliable and valid assessment tools to ensure that people's mental health problems are not being missed, but also that people are not being given unnecessary labels;

- timely to ensure that people experience distressing and debilitating mental health problems for as short a period as possible;

- regular to ensure that any mental health problems are recognized, but also to ensure that people do not acquire a permanent label of dual diagnosis when their mental health problem may have been resolved.

The development of reliable and valid mental health screening measures for people with learning disabilities is in its early stages, with a proliferation of measures and little evidence on the reliability or validity of any of them (Deb *et al.* 2001; Beail 2004; Dagnan and Lindsay 2004; Novaco and Taylor 2004). Different measures vary according to whether they are:

- developed for the general population and then used or adapted for people with learning disabilities, or whether they are specifically designed for people with learning disabilities;

- designed as self-report measures to be completed by people with learning disabilities (almost always in an interview format), or whether they are designed to be completed by informants about the person with learning disabilities (in either a questionnaire or interview format);

- designed primarily for people with mild/moderate learning disabilities, people with severe/profound learning disabilities, or the whole range of people with learning disabilities;

- designed to act as a screen across a wide range of mental health problems, or whether they focus in more detail on a particular mental health problem;

- offered with training and knowledge of mental health issues and how to use the measure;

- able to be undertaken in a reasonable time by the professional, the person with learning disabilities and/or the informant.

A wide range of mental health measures are presented in Tables 27.1 and 27.2, together with some information on their characteristics and purposes. When working in more depth with a person, it can also be useful to develop individual measures for the most important aspects of that person's experience (Stenfert Kroese *et al.* 1997; Finlay and Lyons 2001; Dagnan and Lindsay 2004; Taylor *et al.* 2004b).

Case study: *Joan*

In addition to detecting and describing the mental health problems of clients, good clinical assessment is required to enable the clinician to carry out case formulations of complex problems and to make decisions about appropriate interventions and salient treatment targets. In this case study the use of different assessment approaches to guide formulation and treatment planning is illustrated with a particularly complex mental health case.

At the time of assessment Joan was a 45-year-old woman with mild learning disabilities (WAIS full scale IQ = 59). She was compulsorily detained under the Mental Health Act 1983 for treatment in an acute mental health ward of a specialist learning disability hospital service. Joan was the youngest of six siblings, and though she was a twin, her twin sibling died at birth. Her mother died of cancer when Joan was 4 years old. Joan attended a special school due her learning difficulties, but on leaving school she got a job in a factory that she enjoyed. She married her first husband in her early twenties and had a child soon after. Her husband was violent and sexually abused their daughter. They had two more children together, but after nine years of marriage Joan separated from her husband. She remarried, but this marriage lasted for only a few months. Thereafter Joan was supported by her family, and in particular her older brother.

Joan had a long history, starting at the age of 16, of contact with mental

Table 27.1 Assessment measures: multiple mental health problems

Measure	General population measure or specific for people with learning disabilities?	Areas assessed	Completed with person with learning disabilities?	Completed with informant?	Details of measure
Screening tools for multiple mental health problems					
Reiss Screen for Maladaptive Behavior (Reiss 1998a, 1998b)	Specific	Total Aggressive behaviour Psychosis Paranoia Depression (behavioural signs) Depression (physical signs) Dependent personality disorder Avoidant behaviour Autism	No	Yes	36 items Adequate reliability Adequate sensitivity Questionable specificity (Sturmey and Bertman 1994)
Diagnostic Assessment for the Severely Handicapped (DASH) (Matson et al. 1991)	Specific	Total Anxiety Depression Mania Autism Schizophrenia Stereotypies/tics Self-injury Elimination disorders Eating disorders Sleep disorders Psychosexual disorders Organic syndromes Impulse control/miscellaneous	No	Yes	Designed for people with severe learning disabilities 83 items Adequate reliability Unknown sensitivity or specificity

(continued)

Table 27.1 (continued)

Measure	General population measure or specific for people with learning disabilities?	Areas assessed	Completed with person with learning disabilities?	Completed with informant?	Details of measure
Psychopathology Instrument for Mentally Retarded Adults (PIMRA) (Matson et al. 1984; Senatore et al. 1985)	Specific	Total Schizophrenic disorder Affective disorder Psychosexual disorder Adjustment disorder Anxiety disorder Somatoform disorder Personality disorders	Yes	Yes	56 items Adequate reliability Questionable sensitivity and specificity (Sturmey et al. 1991)
PAS-ADD Checklist (Moss et al. 1996c)	Specific	Total Affective/neurotic disorder Organic condition Psychotic disorder	No	Yes	29 items Adequate reliability Reasonable sensitivity Questionable specificity (Moss et al. 1998; Taylor et al. 2004a)
Mini PAS-ADD (Prosser et al. 1998)	Specific	Total Anxiety & phobia Depression Expansive mood Obsessions & compulsions Psychoses Dementia Autistic features	No	Yes	86 items Good reliability Good sensitivity Some specificity (Prosser et al. 1998; Deb et al. 2001)

Measure	General population measure or specific for people with learning disabilities?	Areas assessed	Completed with person with learning disabilities?	Completed with informant?	Details of measure
Symptom Checklist 90 (revised) (SCL-90-R) (Derogatis 1983; Kellett *et al.* 1999)	General (adapted)	Global severity index Positive symptom distress index Positive symptom total Somatization Obsessive-compulsive Interpersonal sensitivity Depression Anxiety Hostility Phobic anxiety Paranoid ideation Psychoticism	Yes	No	Adapted by using an assisted completion format 90 items Good reliability Adequate sensitivity and specificity (Kellett *et al.* 1999)
Brief Symptom Inventory (Derogatis 1993; Kellett *et al.* 2003, 2004)	General (adapted)	Global severity index Positive symptom distress index Positive symptom total Somatization Obsessive-compulsive Interpersonal sensitivity Depression Anxiety Hostility Phobic anxiety Paranoid ideation Psychoticism	Yes	No	Adapted by using an assisted completion format 53 items Good reliability Adequate sensitivity and specificity (Kellett *et al.* 2003, 2004)

(continued)

Table 27.1 (continued)

Measure	General population measure or specific for people with learning disabilities?	Areas assessed	Completed with person with learning disabilities?	Completed with informant?	Details of measure
Detailed diagnostic assessments for multiple mental health problems					
Psychiatric Assessment Schedule – Adults with Developmental Disability (PAS-ADD) (Moss et al. 1997)	General (adapted)	To *ICD-10* criteria Schizophrenia Depression Phobic anxiety disorders Other anxiety disorders Autism screen	Yes	Yes	Comprehensive adaptation of Schedules of Clinical Assessment in Neuropsychiatry (World Health Organization 1992) Extensive rewording and redesign for use with both person with learning disabilities and an informant Uses *ICD-10* standard psychiatric classification system for diagnosis (World Health Organization 1993) Semi-structured interview; core 145 questions Adequate reliability and validity (Moss et al. 1996a, 1996b, 1997; Costello et al. 1997; Deb et al. 2001)

Table 27.2 Assessment measures: specific mental health problems

Measure	General population measure or specific for people with learning disabilities?	Areas assessed	Completed with person with learning disabilities?	Completed with informant?	Details of measure
Zung Depression Scale (Zung 1965; Kazdin et al. 1983; Prout and Schaefer 1985; Lindsay et al. 1994; Dagnan and Sandhu 1999)	General (adapted)	Depression	Yes	No	20 items Original measure used (Prout and Schaefer 1985) Adapted with wording changes and fewer response options (Kazdin et al. 1983; Lindsay et al. 1994; Dagnan and Sandhu 1999) Good reliability and validity
Beck Depression Inventory (Beck et al. 1961)	General (adapted)	Depression	Yes	No	21 items Original measure used (Prout and Schaefer 1985) Adapted with wording changes and fewer response options (Kazdin et al. 1983; Helsel and Matson 1988; Nezu et al. 1995) Good reliability and validity

(continued)

Table 27.2 *(continued)*

Measure	General population measure or specific for people with learning disabilities?	Areas assessed	Completed with person with learning disabilities?	Completed with informant?	Details of measure
Glasgow Depression Scale (Cuthill et al. 2003)	Specific	Depression	Yes	Yes – carer supplement	20 items Carer supplement 16 items Good reliability Good sensitivity and specificity (Cuthill et al. 2003)
Mental Retardation Depression Scale (Meins 1995, 1996)	Specific	Depression	No	Yes	9 items Adequate reliability and validity (Meins 1995, 1996)
Zung Self-Rating Anxiety Scale (Zung 1971; Lindsay et al. 1988, 1994)	General (adapted)	Anxiety	Yes	No	20 items Adapted with wording changes and fewer response options (Lindsay et al. 1994) Adequate reliability and validity
Beck Anxiety Inventory (Beck and Steer 1990; Lindsay and Lees 2003)	General (adapted)	Anxiety	Yes	No	21 items Adapted (Lindsay and Lees, 2003) Unknown reliability and validity

Measure	General population measure or specific for people with learning disabilities?	Areas assessed	Completed with person with learning disabilities?	Completed with informant?	Details of measure
Glasgow Anxiety Scale (Mindham and Espie 2003)	Specific	Anxiety	Yes	No	27 items Good reliability Good sensitivity and specificity (Mindham and Espie 2003)
Mood Interest & Pleasure Questionnaire (Ross & Oliver 2002, 2003b)	Specific	Mood: Interest and pleasure	No	Yes	Designed for people with severe learning disabilities 25 items Good reliability, adequate validity (Ross and Oliver 2002, 2003b)
Positive & Negative Syndrome Scale (PANSS) (Kay et al. 1989; Hatton et al. under review)	General	Psychotic experiences: positive symptoms, negative symptoms, general symptoms	Yes	No	28 items Good reliability Good validity on positive symptoms and general symptoms, inadequate validity on negative symptoms (Hatton et al. under review)
Psychotic Rating Scales (PSYRATS) (Haddock et al. 1999; Hatton et al. under review)	General	Psychotic experiences: auditory hallucinations, delusions	Yes	No	17 items Good reliability Good validity on auditory hallucinations, unknown validity on delusions (Hatton et al. under review)

(continued)

Table 27.2 (continued)

Measure	General population measure or specific for people with learning disabilities?	Areas assessed	Completed with person with learning disabilities?	Completed with informant?	Details of measure
Novaco Anger Scale (NAS) (Novaco 2003; Novaco and Taylor 2004)	General (adapted)	Anger: disposition and experience in the cognitive, arousal and behavioural domains	Yes	No	48 items Original measure (Novaco 2003) Adapted for people with mild-borderline learning disabilities and to be administered as a structured interview (Novaco and Taylor 2004) Good reliability and validity
Provocation Inventory (PI) (Novaco 2003; Novaco and Taylor 2004)	General (adapted)	Anger: reactivity across a range of potentially provoking situations	Yes	No	25 items Original measure (Novaco 2003) Adapted for people with mild-borderline learning disabilities and to be administered as a structured interview (Novaco and Taylor 2004) Good reliability and validity

Measure	General population measure or specific for people with learning disabilities?	Areas assessed	Completed with person with learning disabilities?	Completed with informant?	Details of measure
Ward Anger rating Scale (WARS) (Novaco 1994; Novaco and Taylor 2004)	General	Anger: a two-part scale regarding (a) verbal and physical behaviours associated with anger and aggression and (b) anger attributes displayed during the previous seven days	No	Yes	25 items Original measure (Novaco 1994). Part B has good reliability and validity with men with LD (Novaco and Taylor 2004)
Imaginal Provocation Test (IPT) (Taylor et al. 2004b)	General (adapted)	Anger: an idiographic measure of anger reactivity in terms of emotional and behavioural responses and attempts to regulate these	Yes	No	10 items (administered in two parallel forms) Original measure (Novaco 1975) Adapted for use with people with LD Good reliability and validity and sensitive to change following intervention (Taylor et al. 2004b)

health and learning disability services due to difficulties with coping with life stressors, self-injury and suicide attempts. During the previous few years, one of Joan's sisters died of cancer and her oldest sister emigrated. Her brother remarried and her father became frail. In this context of dwindling support, Joan's most recent contact with mental health services followed her overdosing on prescribed medication because she felt unable to cope with her children. She had a period of inpatient treatment, during which she reported experiencing sexual abuse from another patient. Her children were taken into care and Joan was eventually discharged home. Unfortunately, shortly after this Joan set fire to her house in a further attempt to kill herself because she felt unable to cope once more. These events precipitated her admission to her current placement where she had been for 18 months.

In the past Joan had been treated with ECT and was currently pre-scribed antipsychotic medication which she disliked taking because of its side-effects. Joan presented a number of challenges to the team working with her including frequent agitation and aggression, and occasional violence. She also reported, almost continuously, a range of negative and distressing beliefs and fears such as 'I'm dead', 'I'm brain-dead', 'I'm dying', 'I'm being poisoned', 'No one loves me', 'They [staff] hate me' and 'They [staff] don't believe me'. Joan was referred for an assessment and formulation of these problems to help with treatment planning. The assessment was carried out jointly by psychology and nursing colleagues over an eight-week period and included clinical assessment to gain information from Joan and staff working with her directly, as well as formal assessment and a case-note review.

During the first few weeks, regular sessions were held with Joan to build some rapport and trust in order to facilitate engagement in the assessment process. This involved listening to her concerns and fears uncritically, with-out challenging any of the assumptions underlying them, and slowly intro-ducing the rationale for formal assessment procedures to help her with her problems. The formal assessments conducted included the Mini-Mental State Examination (MMSE; Folstein *et al.* 1975). This indicated that, taking her learning disability into account, Joan was grossly cognitively impaired. She was significantly disorientated in relation to time and place, her simple recall was poor, and her visuo-spatial planning and organization was impaired. Joan's performance on the Autobiographical Memory Inventory (AMI; Kopelman *et al.* 1990) showed that she had very significant problems with ordering and recalling details of significant events in her life, with memory for recent events being even more compromised than for those from earlier in her life. For example, she could not recall or even estimate with any degree of accuracy her youngest child's date or year of birth. The Psychiatric Assessment Schedule – Adults with Developmental Disabilities (PAS-ADD; Moss *et al.* 1997), conducted with the client and an informant, indicated that Joan was experiencing a 'severe depressive episode with mood congruent psychotic symptoms'. The assessment of Joan's situation also suggested that the staff team were inconsistent in their responses to and management of her problems and distress.

A formulation of Joan's problems was developed using a psychological model of mental health whereby interrelated biological, environmental and social factors are mediated by psychological processes before being expressed as mental health problems. In Joan's case, predisposing biological factors possibly included cognitive deficits and information processing difficulties associated with her learning disability. The environmental context included frequent experiences of abuse and loss of important family members, and more recently placement in an environment with carers who were confused about how to support her needs. Salient social factors included the repeated loss and breakdown of close supportive relationships leading to isolation, and currently antagonism and hostility with primary carers. It was proposed that these previous events, along with current stressors, impacted adversely on Joan's psychological functioning and were experienced by her as feelings of guilt, worthlessness and low self-esteem, along with acute anxiety and fear that important others would reject and abandon her. At times of high stress and arousal these feelings could be experienced intensely as depressive and negative automatic thoughts that she was useless, worthless, unloved and unlovable. As she may as well be dead, she felt dead (or 'brain dead') and her self-injury and suicide attempts were linked to this belief system. She dealt with her acute fear of abandonment and loss by alienating those around her so that they were unable to get close enough to harm or reject her. Carers' responses to Joan's aggression were interpreted by her as malevolent and expressed as paranoid ideation that others were trying to harm or kill her.

The treatment plan recommended for Joan based on this assessment and formulation included the following sequential but overlapping interventions:

1   Training and support for direct care staff working with Joan to help them better understand her problems and develop more consistent approaches to the behavioural expression of these difficulties. It was hoped that this would help Joan to feel safer and more secure in her current placement.

2   Psychological intervention, utilizing a modified cognitive behavioural approach, to gently explore whether Joan could be encouraged to test some of her assumptions about herself and her environment and slowly begin to undermine the negative beliefs and schema that resulted in her feelings of depression, worthlessness and paranoia.

3   During Joan's short periods of relative remission, meaningful activities (and eventually occupation) could be encouraged and supported to counteract feelings of boredom and worthlessness, and to begin to build self-esteem and confidence.

4   In the longer term, depending on progress with the above measures, helping Joan to remember and order the important events in her life so that she might deal with unresolved issues and place them in context could be considered using a life story book type approach.

Promoting good mental health in people with learning disabilities

---

Exercise 27.6

Imagine a person with a particular mental health problem.

What interventions might work for this person?

How would you decide which intervention(s) to try?

If this was a person with mild learning disabilities, would the range of possible interventions be different? Why?

What adaptations, if any, would you have to make to an intervention to make it work for a person with mild learning disabilities? Why?

Identifying and accurately assessing potential mental health problems in a person with learning disabilities is a necessary first step in trying to promote mental health. Once this has been achieved, what can be done to actively promote good mental health? As with mental health interventions for the general population, interventions with people with learning disabilities can be broadly put into three categories:

1   Biological interventions, typically medication.
2   Psychological interventions, typically behavioural approaches, cognitive behavioural therapy and psychodynamic psychotherapy.
3   Social interventions, which may involve changing the life circumstances of the person and working with families and staff systems.

Before discussing particular mental health interventions, it is important to note that evidence for the effectiveness of any intervention for people with learning disabilities is sparse and very rarely at the level of well-designed randomized controlled trials. For any professional engaged in a mental health intervention with a person with learning disabilities, creativity is needed in designing and conducting interventions, and rigour is required in assessing the effectiveness of the interventions for the individual.

Biological interventions

Although there is a large evidence base concerning the effectiveness of psychotropic medications (medication designed to alter some aspect of psychological functioning) in the general population, there is very little systematic evidence concerning their use with people with learning disabilities (Matson *et al.* 2000; Thompson *et al.* 2004). In the absence of systematic evidence, clinical recommendations suggest using similar medication strategies for people with and without learning disabilities, particularly in terms of prescribing specific medications for specific, diagnosed mental health problems (Berney 2000; Rush and Frances 2000). However, there is substantial evidence showing that particular psychotropic medications are often overprescribed for people with learning disabilities, inappropriately prescribed for challenging behaviours rather than diagnosed mental health problems and prescribed in complex and dangerous combinations (Robertson *et al.* 2000a):

- *Antipsychotic medication*: older, neuroleptic antipsychotics are frequently prescribed for people with learning disabilities (25–57 per cent of people living in NHS settings; 20–50 per cent of people living in community-based residential services; 10 per cent of people living independently or with family members; Robertson *et al.* 2000a). These antipsychotics are most often prescribed to reduce challenging behaviour, despite strong evidence that they have no specific impact on such behaviour beyond sedation and have long-term and irreversible side-effects (Robertson *et al.* 2000a; Thompson *et al.* 2004). There is very little evidence concerning the use of newer, atypical antipsychotics with people with learning disabilities. Although some studies suggest they may reduce some aggression and self-injury, there are conflicting findings and associated side-effects such as sedation and weight gain (Thompson *et al.* 2004).

- *Antidepressant medication*: rates of antidepressant prescriptions for people with learning disabilities are much lower (14 per cent in NHS settings; 6 per cent in community-based residential services) and more closely associated with diagnoses of depression (Robertson *et al.* 2000a). However, older antidepressants such as monoamine oxidase inhibitors and tricyclics are reported to be mixed in their effectiveness with dangerous side-effects (Thompson *et al.* 2004). Newer selective serotonin reputake inhibitors (SSRIs) have been reported to be effective in small studies of people with learning disabilities and depression (Thompson *et al.* 2004).

- *Antiepileptic medication*: rates of epilepsy are high among people with learning disabilities, and antiepileptics are frequently prescribed (46 per cent in NHS settings; 36 per cent in community-based residential services; Robertson *et al.* 2000a). However, in the general population some antiepileptic drugs have also been shown to be effective in stabilizing mood among people with bipolar disorder (manic depression), although there is only case study evidence concerning people with learning disabilities (Thompson *et al.* 2004).

- *Hypnotic and anxiolytic medication*: a wide range of medications can be used to reduce symptoms of anxiety and panic, although their use is not widespread among people with learning disabilities (11 per cent in NHS settings; 9 per cent in community-based residential services; Robertson *et al.* 2000a) and there is little evidence concerning their effectiveness with people with learning disabilities (Thompson *et al.* 2004).

- *Medication to change behaviour*: two types of medication have received attention for their potential to control specific challenging behaviours.

The first are stimulants, increasingly prescribed to control hyperactivity in children; there is substantial evidence concerning both the effectiveness and the side-effects of these medications for children with learning disabilities (Thompson *et al.* 2004). The second are opioid antagonists, which have been shown to be effective in reducing certain types of self-injury shown by people with learning disabilities (Thompson *et al.* 2004).

Clearly, many people with learning disabilities are regularly prescribed inappropriate and sometimes dangerous psychotropic medication with no clear rationale or evidence of effectiveness. If a person is prescribed any psychotropic medication, it is vital to ensure that:

- any psychotropic medication prescription is accompanied by a clear rationale for its use;
- there are regular medication reviews by a person with the authority to alter prescriptions;
- there is ongoing regular assessment of a person's mental health status and behaviour, so as to review the effectiveness of medication regimes;
- there is consideration of the latest available evidence concerning both the effectiveness and the side-effects of psychotropic medications;
- wherever possible, attempts are made to reduce both the dosages and the number of psychotropic medications prescribed; research evidence shows that the antipsychotics of 50 per cent of people with learning disabilities can be reduced or withdrawn without any adverse impact on mental health or behaviour (Ahmed *et al.* 2000).

Psychological interventions

Research evidence concerning the efficacy of psychological interventions for people with learning disabilities and mental health problems is equally sparse, although some general reviews are beginning to appear (Hatton 2002; Beail 2003; Prout and Nowak-Drabik 2003; Sturmey 2004). Existing evidence consists of a small number of case studies using behavioural interventions with symptoms of mental health problems, a larger body of case series and occasional trials using cognitive behaviour therapy for a range of mental health problems, and uncontrolled trials using psychodynamic psychotherapy with mental health problems. While it is clear that people with learning disabilities can benefit from psychological interventions (Hatton 2002; Prout and Nowak-Drabik 2003), it is unclear how many people could benefit or what approaches work best for whom (Beail 2003). Specific assessments of the skills required for particular therapeutic approaches rather than assessments of general ability are likely to be more clinically useful in guiding which intervention to use (Beail 2004; Dagnan and Lindsay 2004).

Psychological interventions have typically focused on five domains of mental health problem: depression, anxiety, psychosis, anger and offending:

- *Depression*: a small number of case studies and a case series of routine practice have investigated cognitive behaviour therapy with people with mild/moderate learning disabilities and depression, and reported improvements in self-reported depressive symptoms and behaviour (Lindsay *et al.* 1993; Dagnan and Chadwick 1997; Lindsay and Olley 1998), with improvements maintained at two- to six-month follow-up (Lindsay 1999).

- *Anxiety*: again, a small number of case studies and a case series have demonstrated the potential feasibility of cognitive and behaviour therapies in reducing anxiety among people with learning disabilities. Behavioural interventions such as relaxation appear to be effective in reducing anxiety and improving cognitive performance among people with mild, moderate and severe intellectual disabilities (Lindsay and Baty 1986; Lindsay *et al.* 1989; Morrison and Lindsay 1997). Anxiety management training (e.g. Lindsay *et al.* 1989) and behavioural and cognitive behavioural interventions for specific phobias (e.g. Dixon and Gunary 1986; Lindsay *et al.* 1988) have been shown to be effective in isolated reports. Case studies and a case series of cognitive behaviour therapy have shown reductions in self-reported anxiety and embarrassment (Lindsay *et al.* 1997), maintained at six-month follow-up (Lindsay 1999).

- *Psychosis*: little evidence is available concerning psychosocial interventions for people with learning disabilities and psychosis. Two case study reports of behavioural treatments with four people with mild to severe learning disabilities and psychosis have demonstrated reductions in the display of 'psychotic speech' (Stephens *et al.* 1981; Mace *et al.* 1988). A single case study and a case series of five people with mild learning disabilities and psychosis, using cognitive behavioural and psychosocial approaches, resulted in improvements in psychotic symptoms and other outcomes (Leggett *et al.* 1997; Haddock *et al.* 2004). Kirkland (2004) adapted an established cognitive behavioural formulation model for use with three men with mild learning disabilities who experienced auditory hallucinations and/or paranoid delusions. An accessible diagrammatic approach to shared formulations helped these clients understand their symptoms better and test out their beliefs, and resulted in some subjective relief from their distressing symptoms.

- *Anger*: more intervention studies have been conducted concerning cognitive behavioural interventions to reduce anger in people with learning disabilities, mainly using adaptations of the Novaco (1975, 1993) approach to anger management. Taylor (2002) and Taylor and Novaco (in press) have reviewed numerous case and case series studies, and a small number of uncontrolled group studies involving individual and group therapy formats that have yielded reductions in levels of anger and aggression that were maintained at follow-up. In addition there have now been three small outcome studies that have established the effectiveness of group cognitive behavioural anger treatment over waiting list control conditions with clients with learning disabilities and anger and aggression problems living in community settings (Rose *et al.* 2000; Willner *et al.* 2002; Lindsay *et al.* 2004a). The Lindsay *et al.* (2004a) study is noteworthy in that it was conducted over a period of ten years. Consistent with other studies, the treatment group improved significantly when compared to the waiting list control group and improvements were maintained for up to 15 months. In addition, these authors compared the experimental and the control groups for the percentage of participants who were physically assaultive over an equivalent time period. They found that significantly fewer of the experimental group physically assaulted others (14 vs. 45 per cent respectively) and concluded that this was a result of the anger management intervention. Case series of cognitive behavioural anger treatment have also been shown to be effective with female and male participants who were classified as forensic cases or who were convicted offenders (Allan *et al.* 2001; Lindsay *et al.* 2003). Taylor *et al.* (2002a, 2004a, in press a) reported on a series of three concatenated controlled studies that involved male offenders with mild to borderline learning disabilities receiving intensive individual and formulation-guided cognitive behavioural anger treatment in secure inpatient settings. The treatment groups improved significantly on self-reported measures of anger disposition, anger reactivity and anger control compared to the control groups. Staff ratings of study participants' anger disposition converged with clients' self-reports but did not reach statistical significance. Improvements in observed behaviour are not inevitable, often due to a low base rate phenomenon, and the multi-faceted nature of these interventions makes it difficult to evaluate which elements of this treatment approach are most effective.

- *Offending*: Lindsay *et al.* (2004b) have comprehensively covered the field of offending by people with learning disabilities. Further, there have been a number of reviews of psychological interventions with offenders with learning disabilities (e.g. Clare and Murphy 1998; Lindsay 2002; Taylor 2002; Lindsay and Taylor in press). These interventions are often delivered as a condition of diversion from the prison system and may take place in community or secure settings under probation orders or mental health act sections respectively. Cognitive behaviour therapy focusing on the attitudes of sex offenders with mild to moderate learning disabilities (see Lindsay 2002 for a review), including offences against women and children, has been reported to be successful in changing attitudes in uncontrolled trials of six (Lindsay *et al.* 1998a) and 24 (Lindsay 1999) sex offenders with learning disabilities (see also Lindsay *et al.* 1998c), although treatment has to be of sufficient duration to influence reoffending rates (Lindsay and Smith 1998). A preliminary report of a group intervention for sex offenders with learning disabilities showed some success in reducing reoffending rates, and a case study of two stalkers with learning disabilities showed mixed success (Lindsay *et al.* 1998d). A single case study has reported a successful cognitive behavioural intervention for a man with mild learning disabilities convicted of setting fires (Clare *et al.* 1992) and in a complex offending case (Clare and Murphy 1998). In a pre-post group study design, Taylor *et al.* (2002b) reported significant improvements on fire-specific and associated clinical measures for 14 male and female convicted arsonists with mild to borderline learning disabilities who received a broadly cognitive behavioural group intervention in a low secure hospital setting. Using the same treatment approach, a case series of four males with mild learning disabilities who set fires were found to benefit clinically from this intervention (Taylor *et al.* 2004c), while five women with mild to borderline learning disabilities and chronic histories of setting fires had not set any fires two years after completing this treatment (Taylor *et al.* in press b).

Psychodynamic psychotherapeutic interventions

There have been several suggestions that psychodynamic psychotherapy can be useful for people with learning disabilities and mental health problems (Beail 2003, 2004). Recent UK uncontrolled trials of routine clinical practice have demonstrated promising results for psychodynamic interpersonal therapy with adults with mild to moderate learning disabilities, including adults referred for 'behaviour problems' (Frankish 1989; Beail 1998), adults with mental health problems (Beail and Warden 1996; Beail 2000) and adult offenders (Beail 2001).

Case study: *James*

As mentioned in the introduction to this chapter, one possible reason that people with learning disabilities have not historically been offered psychological therapies to help with their mental health problems is the belief that these approaches would not be effective as clients are not clever enough to understand or engage in talking therapies. This issue has been raised in connection with cognitive behavioural therapy generally (e.g. Stenfert Kroese 1998) and the cognitive component of cognitive behavioural anger treatment for people with learning disabilities specifically (Rose *et al.* 2000; Willner *et al.* 2002). So, can people with learning disabilities successfully engage in work on the content of thoughts/cognitions that play a role in maintaining mental health problems?

James is a 22-year-old man with mild learning disabilities (WAIS full scale IQ = 66) and borderline personality disorder. He has history of depression, self-injurious behaviour, sexually aggressive behaviour and physical violence. James attended special schools but was excluded on several occasions because of assaults on other students. As a 17-year-old James was sexually abused by an older male friend of his family. His mental health and behavioural problems deteriorated after this time. The frequency of James' self-injury increased and he complained of mood swings and difficulty in controlling his temper. When he was 20 he was prescribed antidepressant medication for low mood, poor appetite, sleep problems and flashbacks to his own sexual abuse. Unfortunately, soon after this, James overdosed on his medication and was admitted to the acute mental health ward of a specialist learning disability hospital. After only a short time in this environment James was displaying sexually predatory behaviour towards less able patients, refusing his medication and being physically aggressive towards staff, and required physical restraint. Consequently he was sectioned under the Mental Health Act 1983 and transferred to a low secure forensic ward in the hospital.

James continued to be disturbed and aggressive and was assessed as a potential candidate for individual anger treatment. Self-rated anger assessments specially modified for clients with learning disabilities were used to assess the level of James' anger problems and to guide the treatment. The Novaco Anger Scale (NAS; Novaco 1993) is a measure of anger disposition that assesses the cognitive, arousal and behavioural components of an individual's experience of anger. The Provocation Inventory (PI; Novaco 1993) is a measure of anger reactivity across a range of anger-provoking situations. James' scores on these assessments were significantly higher than the means for his reference group and his scores on the cognitive sub-scale of the NAS and the unfairness/injustice sub-scale of the PI were particularly elevated. The cognitive behavioural anger treatment used with James was developed especially for clients with mild learning disabilities and severe or chronic anger control problems (Taylor and Novaco in press). It incorporates cognitive restructuring, arousal reduction and behavioural skills training components in equal measures. James completed all 18 sessions of anger treatment (6 sessions preparatory phase and 12 sessions treatment phase) within the planned time period and without incident. His approach towards the treatment was positive and generally enthusiastic. His response to the different components of the intervention was also positive. James learned how to control the physiological component of anger arousal through a combination of breathing control, progressive muscular relaxation, distracting imagery and self-instructions. He was able to show limited ability to deal successfully with angry situations using role-play, although his coping skills in terms of problem-solving lagged behind his understanding of these issues, and this was reflected in ongoing difficulties outside the therapy sessions.

In terms of the cognitive component of the therapy, James was able to learn to identify the automatic thoughts (usually negative and unhelpful) that accompanied angry incidents. As the treatment progressed he was able to spontaneously generate alternative and more adaptive cognitions in response to such incidents. In treatment James engaged in cognitive restructuring with relative ease, and in so doing demonstrated an ability to take the perspective of others by putting himself in their position in relation to particular situations. Figure 27.1 provides an example, from within a treatment session, of how James was able to use an incident that occurred between sessions to generate alternative thoughts about a particular situation (being told that his behaviour programme was about to be changed).

THINKING DIFFERENTLY ABOUT ANGER SITUATIONS

Name: James

Date: 9 / 1 / 02

	Situation Where? What? Who? 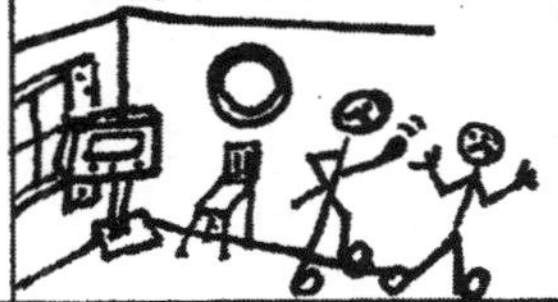	Thoughts About the Situation 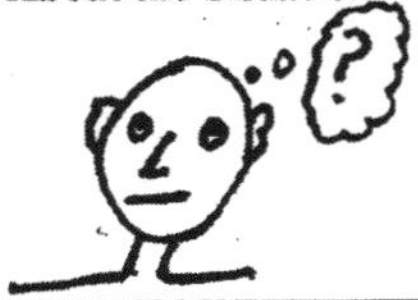	Emotional Feelings 0 – 10 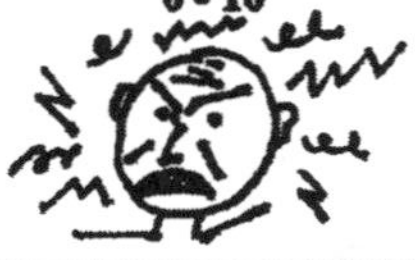	Physical Feelings 0 – 10 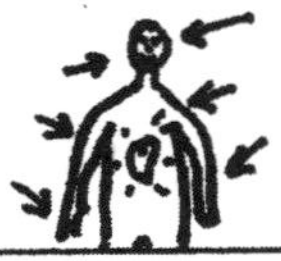	Reaction What did you Do/behave? 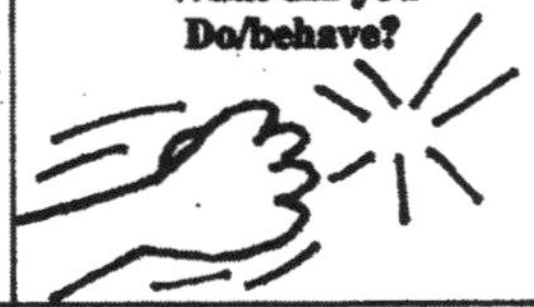
A C T U A L	I was in my room getting ready to go out. A member of staff came in and told me they were changing my behaviour programme	Why are they changing my programme? They are trying to make it harder for me; to get me into trouble. Its not right. They don't care!	Very angry 8/10	Really tensed-up. Tight chest and sore head	I shouted at the staff and swore at him. Called him names.
P O S S I B L E		• They are changing my programme to try to help me. • He is telling me this cos he thinks I'll be pleased	Not very angry – maybe a bit worried 2/10	More relaxed – less tense 2/10	I would talk to them nice and calm to find out why they want to change my programme

Figure 27.1 Generating alternative thoughts

He could see that thinking about this situation differently would lead him to feel less angry, be more in control and so react in a more adaptive and productive manner. The 'possible' or alternative thoughts-emotional feelings-physical feelings-reaction chain generated by James in response to the activating situation was then used in the session by James to practise coping more effectively with anger; first in imagination (using stress inoculation technique while relaxed) and then in practice (using role-play). James was then encouraged to practise thinking differently about situations between sessions using daily anger logs so that this skill was moved temporally closer to real situations.

It can be seen from this example that people with (mild) learning disabilities can make the link between cognitions/thoughts and feelings/reactions and unlink the automatic connection between events and feelings/reactions. Thus people with learning disabilities can engage in and benefit from the cognitive component of cognitive behavioural therapy. James' pre-post treatment and follow-up scores on the self-rated anger assessments support this view. The cognitive sub-scale of the NAS came down following treatment and remained lower at eight-month follow-up. James' scores on the unfairness/injustice sub-scale of the PI followed a similar pattern. While James' behaviour on the ward continued to cause staff concern, their staff-rated anger scores converged with James' self-ratings and reflected his progress in the anger treatment.

Social interventions

Given the life circumstances that put people with learning disabilities at potentially greater risk of developing mental health problems, it would be expected that social interventions would be developed to reduce social and environmental risk factors and increase resilience (Jenkins 2000). However, interventions at this level have very rarely been conducted with people with learning disabilities, beyond the involvement of broader interpersonal systems such as families or staff members around the person (e.g. Rose *et al.* 2000; Taylor *et al.* 2002a; Haddock *et al.* 2004). Interventions designed to improve people's living arrangements have rarely been designed with mental health as an outcome, and broader policy changes such as deinstitutionalization have rarely been evaluated in terms of their impact on mental health (Emerson and Hatton 1996). There is clearly a great potential for social interventions to improve the mental health of people with learning disabilities.

▌ Conclusion

As this chapter has shown, the picture concerning people with learning disabilities and mental health problems is changing, from one of almost total professional indifference to rapidly increasing professional interest and concern. However, some of the most basic issues concerning the conceptualization, assessment and management of mental health problems in people with learning disabilities have yet to be resolved. The social contexts within which people with learning disabilities live further complicate the picture. Taking mental health problems in people with learning disabilities seriously has the potential to liberate many people from debilitating distress and enable them to lead fulfilling lives. However, the history of services for people with learning disabilities teaches us that professional interest can be a mixed blessing; professional interest in mental health problems also contains the potential for unnecessary labelling, further stigma, restrictive service interventions and unnecessary medication. It is our responsibility to ensure that we work towards the former rather than being complicit in the latter.

Resources

Bouras, N. and Holt, G. (1997) *Mental Health in Learning Disabilities: Training Package* (2nd edn). Brighton: Pavillion.

Foundation for People with Learning Disabilities (2002) *Count Us In: The Report of the Inquiry into the Mental Health Needs of Young People with Learning Disabilities*. London: Foundation for People with Learning Disabilities.

Holt, G., Gratsa, A., Bouras, N., Joyce, T., Spiller, M.J. and Hardy, S. (2004) *Guide to Mental Health for Families and Carers of People with Intellectual Disabilities*. London: Jessica Kingsley.

Taylor, J.L. and Novaco, R.W. (in press) *Anger Treatment for People with Developmental Disabilities: A Theory, Evidence and Manual Based Approach*. Chichester: Wiley.

References

Ahmed, Z., Fraser, W., Kerr, M.P., Kiernan, C., Emerson, E., Robertson, J., Allen, D., Baxter, H. and Thomas, J. (2000) Reducing antipsychotic medication in people with a learning disability, *British Journal of Psychiatry*, 176: 42–6.

Allan, R., Lindsay, W.R., MacLeod, F. and Smith, A.H.W. (2001) Treatment of women with intellectual disabilities who have been involved with the criminal justice system for reasons of aggression, *Journal of Applied Research in Intellectual Disabilities*, 14: 340–7.

American Psychiatric Association (1994) *Diagnostic and Statistical Manual of Mental Disorders*, 4th edn. Washington, DC: American Psychiatric Association.

American Psychological Association (2002) *Ethical Principals and Code of Conduct*. Washington, DC: American Psychological Association.

Arscott, K., Dagnan, D. and Stenfert Kroese, B. (1999) Assessing the ability of people with a learning disability to give informed consent to treatment, *Psychological Medicine*, 29: 1367–75.

Bailey, N.M. and Cooper, S.-A. (1997) The current provision of specialist health services to people with learning disabilities in England and Wales, *Journal of Intellectual Disability Research*, 41: 52–9.

Beail, N. (1998) Psychoanalytic psychotherapy with men with intellectual disabilities: a preliminary outcome study, *British Journal of Medical Psychology*, 71: 1–11.

Beail, N. (2000) An evaluation of outpatient psychodynamic psychotherapy amongst offenders with intellectual disabilities, *Journal of Intellectual Disability Research*, 44: 204.

Beail, N. (2001) Recidivism following psychodynamic psychotherapy amongst offenders with intellectual disabilities, *British Journal of Forensic Practice*, 3: 33–7.

Beail, N. (2003) What works for people with mental retardation? Critical commentary on cognitive behavioural and psychodynamic psychotherapy research, *Mental Retardation*, 41: 468–72.

Beail, N. (2004) Methodology, design, and evaluation in psychotherapy research with people with intellectual disabilities, in E. Emerson, C. Hatton, T. Thompson and T.R. Parmenter (eds) *The International Handbook of Applied Research in Intellectual Disabilities*. Chichester: Wiley.

Beail, N. and Warden, S. (1996) Evaluation of a psychodynamic psychotherapy service for adults with intellectual disabilities: rationale, design and preliminary outcome data, *Journal of Applied Research in Intellectual Disabilities*, 9: 223–8.

Beck, A.T. and Steer, R.A. (1990) *Manual for the Beck Anxiety Inventory*. San Antonio, TX: The Psychological Corporation.

Beck, A.T., Ward, C.H., Mendelsohn, M., Mock, J. and Erbaugh, J. (1961) An inventory for measuring depression, *Archives of General Psychiatry*, 4: 561–71.

Bender, M. (1993) The unoffered chair: the history of therapeutic disdain towards people with a learning difficulty, *Clinical Psychology Forum*, 54: 7–12.

Bentall, R.P. (2004) *Madness Explained: Psychosis and Human Nature*. London: Penguin.

Berney, T.P. (2000) Methods of treatment, in M.G. Gelder, J.L. Lopez-Ibor Jr and N.C. Andreasen (eds) *New Oxford Textbook of Psychiatry*. Oxford: Oxford University Press.

Berrios, G.E. (1996) *The History of Mental Symptoms: Descriptive Psychopathology Since the Nineteenth Century*. Cambridge: Cambridge University Press.

Borthwick-Duffy, S.A. (1994) Epidemiology and prevalence of psychopathology in people with mental retardation, *Journal of Consulting & Clinical Psychology*, 62: 17–27.

Borthwick-Duffy, S.A. and Eyman, R.K. (1990) Who are the dually diagnosed? *American Journal of Mental Retardation*, 94: 586–95.

Bouras, N. and Drummond, C. (1992) Behaviour and psychiatric disorders of people with mental handicaps living in the community, *Journal of Intellectual Disability Research*, 36: 349–57.

Bouras, N. and Holt, G. (1997) *Mental Health in Learning Disabilities: Training Package*, 2nd edn. Brighton: Pavilion.

Bramston, P. and Fogarty, G. (2000) The assessment of emotional distress experienced by people with an intellectual disability: a study of different methodologies, *Research in Developmental Disabilities*, 21: 487–500.

Brown, G.W. (2000) Medical sociology and issues of aetiology, in M.G. Gelder, J.L. Lopez-Ibor Jr and N.C. Andreasen (eds) *New Oxford Textbook of Psychiatry*. Oxford: Oxford University Press.

Clare, I.C.H. and Murphy, G.H. (1998) Working with offenders or alleged offenders with intellectual disabilities, in E. Emerson, C. Hatton, J. Bromley and A. Caine (eds) *Clinical Psychology & People with Intellectual Disabilities*. Chichester: Wiley.

Clare, I.C.H., Murphy, G.H., Cox, D. and Chaplin, E.H. (1992) Assessment and treatment of fire-setting: a single-case investigation using a cognitive behavioural model, *Criminal Behaviour & Mental Health*, 2: 253–68.

Cooper, J.E. and Oates, M. (2000) The principles of clinical assessment in general psychiatry, in M.G. Gelder, J.L. Lopez-Ibor Jr and N.C. Andreasen (eds) *New Oxford Textbook of Psychiatry*. Oxford: Oxford University Press.

Cooper, S.A. (1997) High prevalence of dementia among people with learning disabilities not attributable to Down's syndrome, *Psychological Medicine*, 27: 609–16.

Cooper, S.A. (ed.) (2003) Diagnostic criteria for psychiatric disorders for use with adults with learning disabilities (DC-LD), *Journal of Intellectual Disability Research*, 47: Supplement 1.

Costello, H. (2004) Does training carers improve outcome for adults with learning disabilities and mental health problems? PhD thesis, King's College, University of London.

Costello, H., Moss, S., Prosser, H. and Hatton, C. (1997) Reliability of the ICD-10 version of the Psychiatric Assessment Schedule for Adults with Developmental Disability (PAS-ADD), *Social Psychiatry and Psychiatric Epidemiology*, 32: 339–43.

Cuthill, F.M., Espie, C.A. and Cooper, S.-A. (2003) Development and psychometric properties of the Glasgow Depression Scale for people with a learning disability: individual and carer supplement versions, *British Journal of Psychiatry*, 182: 347–53.

Dagnan, D. and Chadwick, P. (1997) Assessment and intervention, in B. Stenfert Kroese, D. Dagnan and K. Loumidis (eds) *Cognitive-Behaviour Therapy for People with Learning Disabilities*. London: Routledge.

Dagnan, D. and Lindsay, W.R. (2004) Research issues in cognitive therapy, in E. Emerson, C. Hatton, T. Thompson and T.R. Parmenter (eds) *The International Handbook of Applied Research in Intellectual Disabilities*. Chichester: Wiley.

Dagnan, D. and Sandhu, S. (1999) Social comparison, self-esteem and depression in people with learning disabilities, *Journal of Intellectual Disability Research*, 43: 372–9.

Dagnan, D. and Waring, M. (2004) Linking stigma to psychological distress: testing a social-cognitive model of the experience of people with intellectual disabilities, *Clinical Psychology and Psychotherapy*, 11: 247–54.

Deb, S., Thomas, M. and Bright, C. (2001) Mental disorder in adults with intellectual disability, I: Prevalence of functional psychiatric illness among a community-based population aged between 16 and 64 years, *Journal of Intellectual Disability Research*, 45: 495–505.

Department of Health (2001) *Seeking Consent: Working with People with Learning Disabilities*. London: Department of Health.

Derogatis, L.R. (1983) *SCL-90-R: Administration, Scoring and Procedures: Manual II*. Towson, MD: Clinical Psychometrics Research.

Derogatis, L.R. (1993) *Brief Symptom Inventory: Administration, Scoring and Procedures Manual*, 3rd edn. Minneapolis, MN: National Computer Systems.

Dixon, M.S. and Gunary, R.M. (1986) Fear of dogs: group treatment of people with mental handicaps, *Mental Handicap*, 14: 6–9.

Doody, G.A., Johnstone, E.C., Sanderson, T.L., Cunningham-Owens, D.G. and Muir, W.J. (1998) 'Pfropfschizophrenie' revisited: schizophrenia in people with mild learning disability, *British Journal of Psychiatry*, 173: 145–53.

Edelstein, T.M. and Glenwick, D.S. (2001) Direct-care workers' attributions of psychopathology in adults with mental retardation, *Mental Retardation*, 39: 368–78.

Einfeld, S.L. and Tonge, B.J. (1999) Observations on the use of the *ICD-10 Guide for Mental Retardation*, *Journal of Intellectual Disability Research*, 43: 408–13.

Elliott, J., Hatton, C. and Emerson, E. (2003) The health of people with learning disabilities in the UK: evidence and implications for the NHS, *Journal of Integrated Care*, 11: 9–17.

Emerson, E. (2001) *Challenging Behaviour: Analysis and Intervention in People with Severe Intellectual Disabilities*. Cambridge: Cambridge University Press.

Emerson, E. (2003) Prevalence of psychiatric disorders in children and adolescents with and without intellectual disability, *Journal of Intellectual Disability Research*, 47: 51–8.

Emerson, E. and Hatton, C. (1996) Deinstitutionalization in the UK and Ireland: outcomes for service users, *Journal of Intellectual and Developmental Disability*, 21: 17–37.

Emerson, E., Moss, S. and Kiernan, C. (1999) The relationship between challenging behaviour and psychiatric disorders in people with severe developmental disabilities, in N. Bouras (ed.) *Psychiatric & Behavioural Disorders in Developmental Disabilities & Mental Retardation*. Cambridge University Press: Cambridge.

Emerson, E., Hatton, C., Felce, D. and Murphy, G. (2001) *Learning Disabilities: The Fundamental Facts*. London: Foundation for People with Learning Disabilities.

Featherstone, K. and Donovan, J. (2002) 'Why don't they just tell me straight, why allocate it?' The struggle to make sense of participating in a randomised controlled trial, *Social Science & Medicine*, 55: 709–19.

Finlay, W.M. and Lyons, E. (2001) Methodological issues in interviewing and using self-report questionnaires with people with mental retardation, *Psychological Assessment*, 13: 319–35.

Folstein, M.F., Folstein, S.E. and McHugh, P.R. (1975) Mini mental state: a practical method for grading the cognitive state of patients for the clinician, *Journal of Psychiatric Research*, 12: 189–98.

Frankish, P. (1989) Meeting the emotional needs of handicapped people: a psychodynamic approach, *Journal of Mental Deficiency Research*, 33: 407–14.

Goldberg, D.P. and Huxley, P. (1980) *Mental Illness in the Community: The Pathway to Psychiatric Care*. London: Tavistock.

Goodey, C.F. (1996) The psychopolitics of learning and disability in seventeenth-century thought, in D. Wright and A. Digby (eds) *From Idiocy to Mental Deficiency: Historical Perspectives on People with Learning Disabilities*. London: Routledge.

Haddock, G., McCarron, J., Tarrier, N. and Faragher, E.B. (1999) Scales to measure dimensions of hallucinations and delusions: the psychotic symptom rating scales (PSYRATS), *Psychological Medicine*, 29: 879–89.

Haddock, G., Lobban, F., Hatton, C. and Carson, R. (2004) Cognitive-behaviour therapy for people with psychosis and mild intellectual disabilities: a case series, *Clinical Psychology & Psychotherapy*, 11: 282–98.

Hassiotis, A., Barron, P. and O'Hara, J. (2000) Mental health services for people with learning disabilities: a complete overhaul is needed with strong links to mainstream services, *British Medical Journal*, 321: 583–4.

Hastings, R.P., Hatton, C., Taylor, J.L. and Maddison, C. (2004) Life events and psychiatric symptoms in adults with intellectual disabilities, *Journal of Intellectual Disability Research*, 48: 42–6.

Hatton, C. (2002) Psychosocial interventions for adults with intellectual disabilities and mental health problems: a review, *Journal of Mental Health*, 11: 357–73.

Hatton, C., Haddock, G., Taylor, J.T., Coldwell, J., Crossley, R. and Peckham, N. (under review) The reliability and validity of general psychotic rating scales with people with mild and moderate intellectual disabilities: an empirical investigation, *Journal of Intellectual Disability Research*.

Helsel, W.J. and Matson, J.L. (1988) The relationship of depression to social skills and intellectual functioning in mentally retarded adults, *Journal of Mental Deficiency Research*, 32: 411–18.

Holland, A.J., Hon, J., Huppert, F.A., Stevens, S. and Watson, P. (1998) Population-based study of the prevalence and presentation of dementia in adults with Down's syndrome, *British Journal of Psychiatry*, 172: 493–8.

Jenkins, R. (2000) Public policy and environmental issues, in M.G. Gelder, J.L. Lopez-Ibor Jr and N.C. Andreasen (eds) *New Oxford Textbook of Psychiatry*. Oxford: Oxford University Press.

Kay, S.R., Opler, L.A. and Lindenmayer, J.P. (1989) The positive and negative syndrome scale (PANSS): Rationale and standardisation. *British Journal of Psychiatry*, 155 suppl. 7, 59–75.

Kazdin, A.E., Matson, J.L. and Senatore, V. (1983) Assessment of depression in mentally retarded adults, *American Journal of Psychiatry*, 140: 1040–3.

Kellett, S., Beail, N., Newman, D.W. and Mosley, E. (1999) Indexing psychological distress in people with intellectual disabilities: use of the Symptom Checklist-90-R, *Journal of Applied Research in Intellectual Disabilities*, 12: 323–34.

Kellett, S., Beail, N., Newman, D.W. and Frankish, P. (2003) Utility of the Brief Symptom Inventory in the assessment of psychological distress, *Journal of Applied Research in Intellectual Disabilities*, 16: 127–34.

Kellett, S., Beail, N., Newman, D.W. and Hawes, A. (2004) The factor structure of the Brief Symptom Inventory: intellectual disability evidence, *Clinical Psychology and Psychotherapy*, 11: 275–81.

Kendell, R.E. (1975) The concept of disease and its implications for psychiatry, *British Journal of Psychiatry*, 127: 305–15.

Kirkland, J. (2004) Cognitive-behaviour formulation for three men with learning disabilities who experience psychosis: how do we make it make sense? *British Journal of Learning Disabilities*, 32: 1–6.

Kopelman, M., Wilson, B. and Baddeley, A. (1990) *Autobiographical Memory Inventory*. Bury St Edmonds: Thames Valley Test Company.

Kutchins, H. and Kirk, S.A. (1997) *Making Us Crazy: DSM – The Psychiatric Bible and the Creation of Mental Disorders*. London: Constable.

Leggett, J., Hurn, C. and Goodman, W. (1997) Teaching psychological strategies for managing auditory hallucinations: a case report, *British Journal of Learning Disabilities*, 25: 158–62.

Lindsay, W.R. (1999) Cognitive therapy, *The Psychologist*, 12: 238–41.

Lindsay, W.R. (2002) Research and literature on sex offenders with intellectual and developmental disabilities, *Journal of Intellectual Disability Research*, 46(suppl. 1): 74–85.

Lindsay, W.R. and Baty, F.J. (1986) Behavioural relaxation training: explorations with adults who are mentally handicapped, *Mental Handicap*, 14: 160–2.

Lindsay, W.R. and Law, J. (1999) Outcome evaluation of 161 people with learning disabilities in Tayside who have offending or challenging behaviour. Presentation to the BABCP 27th annual conference, University of Bristol, July.

Lindsay, W.R. and Lees, M.S. (2003) A comparison of anxiety and depression in sex offenders with intellectual disability and a control group with intellectual disability, *Sex Abuse*, 15: 339–45.

Lindsay, W.R. and Olley, S. (1998) Psychological treatment for anxiety and depression for people with learning disabilities, in W. Fraser, D. Sines and M. Kerr (eds) *Hallas' The Care of People with Intellectual Disabilities*, 9th edn. Oxford: Butterworth Heinemann.

Lindsay, W.R. and Smith, A.H.W. (1998) Responses to treatment for sex offenders with intellectual disability: a comparison of men with 1- and 2-year probation sentences, *Journal of Intellectual Disability Research*, 42: 346–53.

Lindsay, W.R. and Taylor, J.L. (in press) A selective review of research on offenders with developmental disabilities: assessment and treatment, *Clinical Psychology & Psychotherapy*.

Lindsay, W.R., Michie, A.M., Baty, F.J. and MacKenzie, K. (1988) Dog phobia in people with mental handicaps: anxiety management training and exposure treatments, *Mental Handicap Research*, 1: 39–48.

Lindsay, W.R., Baty, F.J., Michie, A.M. and Richardson, I. (1989) A comparison of anxiety treatments with adults who have moderate and severe mental retardation, *Research in Developmental Disabilities*, 10: 129–40.

Lindsay, W.R., Howells, L. and Pitcaithly, D. (1993) Cognitive therapy for depression with individuals with intellectual disabilities, *British Journal of Medical Psychology*, 66: 135–41.

Lindsay, W.R., Michie, A.M., Baty, F.J., Smith, A.H.W. and Miller, S. (1994) The consistency of reports about feelings and emotions from people with intellectual disability, *Journal of Intellectual Disability Research*, 38: 61–6.

Lindsay, W.R., Neilson, C. and Lawrenson, H. (1997) Cognitive-behaviour therapy for anxiety in people with learning disabilities, in B. Stenfert Kroese, D. Dagnan and K. Loumidis (eds) *Cognitive-behaviour Therapy for People with Learning Disabilities*. London: Routledge.

Lindsay, W.R., Marshall, I., Neilson, G., Quinn, K. and Smith, A.H.W. (1998a) The treatment of men with a learning disability convicted of exhibitionism, *Research in Developmental Disabilities*, 19: 295–316.

Lindsay, W.R., Overend, H., Allan, R., Williams, C. and Black, L. (1998b) Using specific approaches for individual problems in the management of anger and aggression, *British Journal of Learning Disabilities*, 26: 44–50.

Lindsay, W.R., Neilson, C.Q., Morrison, F. and Smith, A.H.W. (1998c) The treatment of six men with a learning disability convicted of sex offences with children, *British Journal of Clinical Psychology*, 37: 83–98.

Lindsay, W.R., Olley, S., Jack, C., Morrison, F. and Smith, A.H.W. (1998d) The treatment of two stalkers with intellectual disabilities using a cognitive approach, *Journal of Applied Research in Intellectual Disabilities*, 11: 333–44.

Lindsay, W.R., Allan, R., MacLeod, F., Smart, N. and Smith, A.H.W. (2003) Long-term treatment and management of violent tendencies of men with intellectual disabilities convicted of assault, *Mental Retardation*, 41: 47–56.

Lindsay, W.R., Allan, R., Parry, C., Macleod, F., Cottrell, J., Overend, H. *et al.* (2004a) Anger and aggression in people with intellectual disabilities: treatment and follow-up of consecutive referrals and a waiting list comparison, *Clinical Psychology and Psychotherapy*, 11: 255–64.

Lindsay, W.R., Taylor, J.L. and Sturmey, P. (eds) (2004b) *Offenders with Developmental Disabilities*. Chichester: Wiley.

Linna, S.L., Moilanen, I., Ebeling, H., Piha, J., Kumpulainen, K., Tamminen, T. and Almqvist, F. (2000) Psychiatric symptoms in children with intellectual disability, *European Child & Adolescent Psychiatry*, 8: 77–82.

Lord Chancellor's Department (1999) *Making Decisions: The Government's Proposals for Making Decisions on Behalf of Mentally Incapacitated Adults*. London: The Stationery Office.

Luckasson, R.A., Scchalock, R.L., Spitalnik, D.M., Spreat, S., Tasse, M., Snell, M.A., Coulter, D.A., Borthwick-Duffy, S.A., Alya-Reeve, A., Buntinx, W.H.E. and Craig, P.A. (2002) *Mental Retardation: Definition, Classification, and Systems of Supports*, 10th edn. Washington, DC: American Association on Mental Retardation.

Lund, J. (1985) The prevalence of psychiatric morbidity in mentally retarded adults, *Acta Psychiatrica Scandinavia*, 72: 563–70.

Mace, F.C., Webb, M.E., Sharkey, R.W., Mattson, D.M. and Rosen, H.S. (1988) Functional analysis and treatment of bizarre speech, *Journal of Behavior Therapy & Experimental Psychiatry*, 19: 289–96.

Marston, G.J., Perry, D.W. and Roy, A. (1997) Manifestations of depression in people with intellectual disability, *Journal of Intellectual Disability Research*, 41: 476–80.

Matson, J.L., Kazdin, A.E. and Senatore, V. (1984) Psychometric properties of the Psychopathology Instrument for Mentally Retarded Adults, *Applied Research in Mental Retardation*, 5: 881–9.

Matson, J.L., Gardner, W.I., Coe, D.A. and Sovner, R. (1991) A scale for evaluating emotional disorders in severely and profoundly mentally retarded persons: development of the Diagnostic Assessment for the Severely Handicapped (DASH) Scale, *British Journal of Psychiatry*, 159: 404–9.

Matson, J.L., Smiroldo, B.B., Hamilton, M. and Baglio, C.S. (1997) Do anxiety disorders exist in persons with severe and profound mental retardation? *Research in Developmental Disorders*, 18: 39–44.

Matson, J.L., Bamburg, J.W., Mayville, E.A., Pinkston, J., Bielecki, J., Kuhn, D., Smalls, Y. and Logan, J.R. (2000) Psychopharmacology and mental retardation: a 10 year review, *Research in Developmental Disabilities*, 21: 263–96.

Meins, W. (1995) Symptoms of major depression in mentally retarded adults, *Journal of Intellectual Disability Research*, 39: 41–5.

Meins, W. (1996) A new depression scale designed for use with adults with mental retardation, *Journal of Intellectual Disability Research*, 40: 220–6.

Mindham, J. and Espie, C.A. (2003) The Glasgow Anxiety Scale for people with an Intellectual Disability (GAS-ID): development and psychometric properties of a new measure for use with people with mild intellectual disability, *Journal of Intellectual Disability Research*, 47: 22–30.

Morrison, F.J. and Lindsay, W.R. (1997) Reductions in self-assessed anxiety and concurrent improvements in cognitive performance in adults who have moderate intellectual disabilities, *Journal of Applied Research in Intellectual Disabilities*, 10: 33–40.

Moss, S., Prosser, H. and Goldberg, D. (1996a) Validity of the schizophrenia diagnosis of the psychiatric assessment schedule for adults with developmental disability (PAS-ADD), *British Journal of Psychiatry*, 168: 359–67.

Moss, S., Prosser, H., Ibbotson, B. and Goldberg, D. (1996b) Respondent and informant accounts of psychiatric symptoms in a sample of patients with learning disability, *Journal of Intellectual Disability Research*, 40: 457–65.

Moss, S.C., Prosser, H., Costello, H., Simpson, N. and Patel, P. (1996c) *PAS-ADD Checklist*. Manchester: Hester Adrian Research Centre, University of Manchester.

Moss, S., Ibbotson, B., Prosser, H., Goldberg, D., Patel, P. and Simpson, N. (1997) Validity of the PAS-ADD for detecting psychiatric symptoms in adults with learning disability (mental retardation), *Social Psychiatry and Psychiatric Epidemiology*, 32: 344–54.

Moss, S., Prosser, H., Costello, H., Simpson, N., Patel, P., Rowe, S., Turner, S. and Hatton, C. (1998) Reliability and validity of the PAS-ADD Checklist for detecting psychiatric disorders in adults with intellectual disability, *Journal of Intellectual Disability Research*, 42: 173–83.

Mostert, M.P. (2001) Facilitated communication since 1995: a review of published studies, *Journal of Autism and Developmental Disorders*, 31: 287–313.

Nettleton, S. and Gustafsson, U. (2002) (eds) *The Sociology of Health and Illness Reader*. Cambridge: Policy Press.

Nezu, C.M., Nezu, A.M., Rothenberg, J.L. and Dellicarpini, L. (1995) Depression in adults with mild mental retardation: are cognitive variables involved? *Cognitive Therapy and Research*, 19: 227–39.

Novaco, R.W. (1975) *Anger Control: The Development and Evaluation of an Experimental Treatment*. Lexington, MA: D.C. Heath.

Novaco, R.W. (1993) *Stress Inoculation Therapy for Anger Control: A Manual for Therapists*. Unpublished manuscript, University of California.

Novaco, R.W. (1994) Anger as a risk factor for violence among the mentally disordered, in J. Monahan and H. Steadman (eds) *Violence and Mental Disorder: Developments in Risk Assessment*. Chicago: University of Chicago Press.

Novaco, R.W. (2003) *Novaco Anger Scale and Provocation Inventory (NAS-PI)*. Los Angeles, CA: Western Psychological Services.

Novaco, R.W. and Taylor, J.L. (2004) Assessment of anger and aggression in male offenders with developmental disabilities, *Psychological Assessment*, 16: 42–50.

Parker, I., Georgaca, E., Harper, D., McLaughlin, T. and Stowell-Smith, M. (1995) *Deconstructing Psychopathology*. London: Sage.

Porter, R. (1990) *Mind-forg'd Manacles: A History of Madness in England from the Restoration to the Regency*. London: Penguin.

Prosser, H., Moss, S.C., Costello, H., Simpson, N. and Patel, P. (1998) *The Mini PAS-ADD: A Preliminary Assessment Schedule for the Detection of Mental Health Needs in Adults with Learning Disabilities*. Manchester: Hester Adrian Research Centre, University of Manchester.

Prout, R. and Nowak-Drabik, K.M. (2003) Psychotherapy with persons who have mental retardation: an evaluation of effectiveness, *American Journal on Mental Retardation*, 108: 82–93.

Prout, H.T. and Schaefer, B.M. (1985) Self-reports of depression by community based mildly mentally retarded adults, *American Journal of Mental Deficiency*, 90: 220–2.

Quigley, A., Murray, G.C., McKenzie, K. and Elliot, G. (2001) Staff knowledge about symptoms of mental health in people with learning disabilities, *Journal of Learning Disabilities*, 5: 235–44.

Reed, J. and Clements, J. (1989) Assessing the understanding of emotional states in a population of adolescents and young adults with mental handicaps, *Journal of Mental Deficiency Research*, 33: 229–33.

Reiss, S. (1988a) *Reiss Screen for Maladaptive Behavior*. Worthington, OH: IDS.

Reiss, S. (1988b) The development of a screening measure for psychopathology in people with mental retardation, in E. Dibble and D. Gray (eds) *Assessment of Behavior Problems in Persons with Mental Retardation Living in the Community*. Rockville, MD: National Institute of Mental Health.

Reiss, S., Levitan, G.W. and McNally, R.J. (1982) Emotionally disturbed mentally retarded people: an underserved population, *American Psychologist*, 37: 361–7.

Robertson, J., Emerson, E., Gregory, N., Hatton, C., Kessissoglou, S. and Hallam, A. (2000a) Receipt of psychotropic medication by people with intellectual disability in residential settings, *Journal of Intellectual Disability Research*, 44: 666–76.

Robertson, J., Emerson, E., Gregory, N., Hatton, C., Turner, S., Kessissoglou, S. and Hallam, A. (2000b) Lifestyle related risk factors for poor health in residential settings for people with intellectual disabilities, *Research in Developmental Disabilities*, 21: 479–86.

Rojahn, J., Lederer, M. and Tasse, M.J. (1995a) Facial recognition by persons with mental retardation: a review of the experimental literature, *Research in Developmental Disabilities*, 16: 393–414.

Rojahn, J., Rabold, D.E. and Schneider, F. (1995b) Emotion specificity in mental retardation, *American Journal of Mental Retardation*, 99: 477–86.

Rose, J., West, C. and Clifford, D. (2000) Group intervention for anger in people with intellectual disabilities, *Research in Developmental Disabilities*, 21: 171–81.

Ross, E. and Oliver, C. (2002) The relationship between mood, interest and pleasure and 'challenging behaviour' in adults with severe and profound intellectual disability, *Journal of Intellectual Disability Research*, 46: 191–7.

Ross, E. and Oliver, C. (2003a) The assessment of mood in adults who have severe or profound mental retardation, *Clinical Psychology Review*, 23: 225–45.

Ross, E. and Oliver, C. (2003b) Preliminary analysis of the psychometric properties of the Mood Interest and Pleasure Questionnaire (MIPQ) for adults with severe and profound learning disabilities, *British Journal of Clinical Psychology*, 42: 81–93.

Royal College of Psychiatrists (2001) *DC-LD: Diagnostic Criteria for Psychiatric Disorders for Use with Adults with Learning Disabilities/Mental Retardation* (Occasional Paper OP 48). London: Gaskell.

Rush, A.J. and Frances, A. (eds) (2000) Expert consensus guidelines series: treatment of psychiatric and behavioural problems in mental retardation: special issue, *American Journal on Mental Retardation*, 105: 159–226.

Sandifer, M.G., Hordern, A. and Green, A.M. (1970) The psychiatric interview: the impact of the first three minutes, *American Journal of Psychiatry*, 126: 968–73.

Scull, A. (1993) *The Most Solitary of Afflictions: Madness and Society in Britain 1700–1900*. New Haven, CT: Yale University Press.

Senatore, V., Matson, J.L. and Kazdin, A.E. (1985) An inventory to assess psychopathology in mentally retarded adults, *American Journal of Mental Retardation*, 89: 459–66.

Sims, A. (1988) *Symptoms in the Mind: An Introduction to Descriptive Psychopathology*. London: Bailliere Tindall.

Stavrakaki, C. (1999) Depression, anxiety and adjustment disorders in people with developmental disabilities, in N. Bouras (ed.) *Psychiatric & Behavioural Disorders in Developmental Disabilities & Mental Retardation*. Cambridge: Cambridge University Press.

Stavrakaki, C. and Mintsioulis, G. (1997) Anxiety disorders in persons with mental retardation: diagnostic, clinical, and treatment issues, *Psychiatric Annals*, 27: 182–9.

Stenfert Kroese, B. (1998) Cognitive-behavioural therapy for people with learning disabilities, *Behavioural and Cognitive Psychotherapy*, 26: 315–22.

Stenfert Kroese, B., Dagnan, D. and Loumidis, K. (eds) (1997) *Cognitive-behaviour Therapy for People with Learning Disabilities*. London: Routledge.

Stephens, R.M., Matson, J.L., Westmoreland, T. and Kulpa, J. (1981) Modification of psychotic speech with mentally retarded patients, *Journal of Mental Deficiency Research*, 25: 187–97.

Sturmey, P. (1999) Classification: concepts, progress and future, in N. Bouras (ed.) *Psychiatric & Behavioural Disorders in Developmental Disabilities & Mental Retardation*. Cambridge: Cambridge University Press.

Sturmey, P. (2004) Cognitive therapy with people with intellectual disabilities: a selective review and critique, *Clinical Psychology and Psychotherapy*, 11: 222–32.

Sturmey, P. and Bertman, L.J. (1994) Validity of the Reiss Screen for maladaptive behaviors, *American Journal of Mental Retardation*, 99: 201–6.

Sturmey, P. and Gaubatz, M. (2002) *Clinical and Counselling Psychology: A Case Study Approach*. Boston, MA: Allyn & Bacon.

Sturmey, P., Reed, J. and Corbett, J. (1991) Psychometric assessment of psychiatric disorders in people with learning difficulties (mental handicap): a review of the measures, *Psychological Medicine*, 21: 143–55.

Sturmey, P., Taylor, J.L. and Lindsay, W.R. (2004) Research and development, in W.R. Lindsay, J.L. Taylor and P. Sturmey (eds) *Offenders with Developmental Disabilities*. Chichester: Wiley.

Taylor, J.L. (2002) A review of the assessment and treatment of anger and aggression in offenders with intellectual disability, *Journal of Intellectual Disability Research*, 46(suppl. 1): 57–73.

Taylor, J.L. and Novaco, R.W. (in press) *Anger Treatment for People with Developmental Disabilities: A Theory, Evidence and Manual Based Approach*. Chichester: Wiley.

Taylor, J.L., Novaco, R.W., Gillmer, B. and Thorne, I. (2002a) Cognitive-behavioural treatment of anger intensity in offenders with intellectual disabilities, *Journal of Applied Research in Intellectual Disabilities*, 15: 151–65.

Taylor, J.L., Thorne, I., Robertson, A. and Avery, G. (2002b) Evaluation of a group intervention for convicted arsonists with mild and borderline intellectual disabilities, *Criminal Behaviour & Mental Health*, 12: 282–93.

Taylor, J.L., Hatton, C., Dixon, L. and Douglas, C. (2004a) Screening for psychiatric symptoms: PAS-ADD Checklist norms for adults with intellectual disabilities, *Journal of Intellectual Disability Research*, 48: 37–41.

Taylor, J.L., Novaco, R.W., Guinan, C. and Street, N. (2004b) Development of an imaginal provocation test to evaluate treatment for anger problems in people with intellectual disabilities, *Clinical Psychology & Psychotherapy*, 11: 233–46.

Taylor, J.L., Thorne, I. and Slavkin, M. (2004c) Treatment of fire-setters, in W.R. Lindsay, J.L. Taylor and P. Sturmey (eds) *Offenders with Developmental Disabilities*. Chichester: Wiley.

Taylor, J.L., Novaco, R.W., Gillmer, B.T., Robertson, A. and Thorne, I. (in press a). Individual cognitive behavioural anger treatment for people with mild-border-line intellectual disabilities and histories of aggression: a controlled trial, *British Journal of Clinical Psychology*.

Taylor, J.L., Robertson, A., Thorne, I., Belshaw, T. and Watson, A. (in press b) Responses of female fire-setters with mild and borderline intellectual disabilities to a group-based intervention, *Journal of Applied Research in Intellectual Disabilities*.

Thompson, T., Zarcone, J. and Symons, F. (2004) Methodological issues in psycho-pharmacology for individuals with intellectual and developmental disabilities, in E. Emerson, C. Hatton, T. Thompson and T.R. Parmenter (eds) *The International Handbook of Applied Research in Intellectual Disabilities*. Chichester: Wiley.

Tonge, B. and Einfeld, S. (2000) The trajectory of psychiatric disorders in young people with intellectual disabilities, *Australian & New Zealand Journal of Psychiatry*, 34: 80–4.

Trent, J.W. Jr (1994) *Inventing the Feeble Mind: A History of Mental Retardation in the United States*. Berkeley, CA: University of California Press.

Turner, T.H. (1989) Schizophrenia and mental handicap: an historical review, with implications for further research, *Psychological Medicine*, 19: 301–14.

van den Hout, M., Arntz, A. and Merckelbach, H. (2000) Contributions of psychology to the understanding of psychiatric disorders, in M.G. Gelder, J.L. Lopez-Ibor Jr and N.C. Andreasen (eds) *New Oxford Textbook of Psychiatry*. Oxford: Oxford University Press.

Willner, P., Jones, J., Tams, R. and Green, G. (2002) A randomised control trial of the efficacy of a cognitive behavioural anger management group for clients with learning disabilities, *Journal of Applied Research in Intellectual Disabilities*, 15: 224–35.

World Health Organization (1946) Constitution of the World Health Organization, *Official Record of the World Health Organization*, 2: 100.

World Health Organization (1992) *Schedules of Clinical Assessment in Neuropsychiatry, Version 1*. Geneva: World Health Organization.

World Health Organization (1993) *ICD-10 Classification of Mental and Behavioural Disorders*. Geneva: World Health Organization.

World Health Organization (1996) *ICD-10 Guide for Mental Retardation*. Geneva: World Health Organization.

Wong, J.G., Clare, I.C.H., Gunn, J. and Holland, A.J. (1999) Capacity to make health care decisions: it's importance in clinical practice, *Psychological Medicine*, 29: 437–46.

Wright, D. and Digby, A. (1996) *From Idiocy to Mental Deficiency: Historical Perspectives on People with Learning Disabilities*. London: Routledge.

Zung, W.K. (1965) A self-rating depression scale, *Archives of General Psychiatry*, 12: 63–70.

Zung, W.K. (1971) A rating instrument for anxiety disorders, *Psychosomatics*, 12: 371–9.

28

Making a life in the community
Is intensive personalized support enough?

Gordon Grant and Paul Ramcharan

Introduction

Over the last decade there has been a mushrooming interest in participatory research with people with learning disabilities though critiques of the politics, processes and outcomes of such research are still rare (see Walmsley and Johnson 2003; Ramcharan *et al.* 2004; and Chapter 34, this volume). Accounts which feature the voice of people with learning disabilities do however point to creative, rewarding and quite independent lives. They can also demonstrate that assumptions about people being 'non-contributing' do not hold (Alderson 2001). However, obtaining useful data from the person's own perspective is easier said than done (Prosser 1989; Wight-Felske 1994) and can take a considerable amount of negotiation, commitment, creative endeavour and support. Early studies in the ethnographic mould have tended to concentrate on people with whom communication does not pose 'a problem' for researchers and this research presupposes a dialogue between user and researcher (Edgerton 1984; Langness and Levine 1986). There have however been some fascinating attempts to represent the lives of people with profound and complex disabilities that also show up people's hidden capacities and contributions (Goode 1994). As it is with the research relationship, so too are there issues surrounding support by formal services and the community.

This chapter is based on the experiences of two people with a learning disability who have been living in the community for some time. The two people involved were selected on the basis of the intensive work required of both key workers and support workers in efforts to sustain their independence and quality of life in ordinary community settings. It will be seen that each person had made considerable progress in certain domains of their lives. Despite the intensive personalized support work from which they have each benefited, disabling barriers created by services and society still prevent them from realizing their expressed needs and wants. The chapter therefore ends with an analysis of these problems.

The two stories we report here emerged from early experiences of implementing individual planning systems in Wales (Felce *et al.* 1998) before the advent of person-centred planning (see Chapter 24). They nevertheless highlight some of the contemporary issues to be faced when seeking to work in individualized and person-centred ways.

The research (Ramcharan *et al.* 1997) aimed to be as creative as possible in seeking to elicit people's views. Interviews, prompt cards, informal conversations and lengthy periods of participant observation were used to build up a picture of people's everyday lives, the challenges they faced, how they endeavoured to meet them and how their experiences were mediated by services and the wider environment.

Names have been changed to preserve anonymity.

About the two individuals

Both people were viewed as 'high priorities' on the caseloads of their key workers, one because of his social isolation and history of mental illness (Mark) and one because of the uncertainties about the appropriateness of her present housing (Jo). Both were middle-aged and lived in council housing. They were each quite practised at expressing themselves and in making their needs and demands known to others.

Below we use the term 'community' rather than 'case' study both to move from the notion of 'ownership' of 'cases' by services and to set the criteria against which we will discuss efforts at individualized support.

Mark: a community study

Mark is a middle-aged man who has spent much of his time in institutions and at other times has drifted around the country. Details of his past life are unclear but he appears to have spent time in at least six institutions. For the past four years he lived by himself in a one-bedroomed council flat. He had basic cooking skills and was able to look after himself with support from the community learning disability team. Mark is a very caring individual, concerned about the problems of others as well as himself. He is able to use public transport and knows his way around the statutory and voluntary agencies that support him. He is articulate, although his conversation shows something of a preoccupation for certain aspects of his life such as the inadequacy of his welfare benefits. This can make it difficult for others to move beyond these subjects in their conversations with him.

Mark's problems in living independently stem from his inability to read, write or handle money, and he can be exploited financially because of his generous nature. He will readily give much of his money away with little appreciation of its value. When the current key worker and community nurse, Jim, began working with him, Mark's main problem was a history of mental illness which led to his aggressive outbursts, sometimes 'ranting and raving' in the office when more funds were not forthcoming. He has also been subject to hysteria attacks which occurred on a weekly basis. Mark describes these as, '. . . not a fit, it's hysteria. My body goes stiff and my tongue goes stiff and I'm crying'. At this time, about three and a half years ago, he was seeing a consultant psychiatrist weekly, having regular injections to alleviate his aggression as well as taking other medication three times a day. Since Jim assumed responsibility there has been a striking improvement in Mark's behaviour, which Jim attributes to the relationship he has built up with Mark with clear and firm guidelines while allowing Mark as much control over his life as possible. In addition two family aides and a nurse support worker from the community team are involved in supporting him.

Tom, a family aide, comes on Mondays and takes Mark out. They often end up in a café. Jim would like to see Tom doing more practical things aimed at skills training but Mark sees Tom's role as befriender and confidant. On Tuesdays and Thursdays the nurse support worker comes in for two hours to encourage self-help skills, particularly cooking. A second family aide visits on Wednesdays. Mark comments that, 'She cooks sometimes, stuff I can't cook and does things in the flat. She does shopping.' As far as helping decide what to buy, Mark says that, 'I'm supposed to but I don't because I don't like doing it, I get muddled. Sometimes they do cleaning. It's not part of their job but they do it for me. Washing because I can't.'

Tom took Mark to art therapy which he very much enjoyed. Even while off sick, Tom had taken Mark on a day's outing and helped him with his Sunday dinner. Although a relaxation tape provided by the psychologist had not proved helpful ('It drives me potty') the contact was appreciated: 'She helped me with my panic attacks.'

Jim visits Mark at home at least weekly. He strongly believes in a holistic approach to his work. The range of services with which he has provided Mark is very broad. 'He gives me injections every month now. Every month so that's good' (i.e. reduced from fortnightly). 'I used to have four tablets, down to three. Sometimes if he asks for me, the specialist [psychiatrist], I go up to the hospital but Jim has seen the specialist for me. He writes to charities for me, different charities. He got me a holiday in Spain, that was nice. Once I didn't have the money for a TV licence. He got it for me from the League of Friends'. Other people besides Jim have worked at raising money for Mark's holiday in Spain. In addition, Jim has cut Mark's hair, procured a refrigerator and washing machine, provided practical help like getting the washing machine plumbed in, emotional support and a structured approach to Mark's behavioural problems, which appears to have been successful. His aggressive behaviour has dramatically reduced, his panic attacks are occurring now only about twice a year and his contact with the psychiatrist, mediated by Jim, is now rare.

Jim suggests that the improvement in behaviour is partly because Mark now gets attention for doing good rather than bad things. Mark had been banned from the Department of Social Security office and job centre in another town. He had also been banned from county hall but recently a member of the staff from county hall phoned to comment on the enormous change in his appearance and manner. The easy access to support must also help: 'If I have a problem and I can't cope with it, I go to Jim or one of the family aides. I'm really tensed up you know.'

Mark is receiving a high level of support from services with some contact every weekday. Indeed, with Mark's frequent visits to the community team office he is known to all team members. All went to his flat for his birthday celebration. Mark clearly values Tom, the family aide, as a friend. Mark is a member of a local quality assurance group which gives him a feeling of status. He is said to make useful contributions and is an ardent advocate of the service. Jim is seen as 'a brother'. Some of Mark's other social contacts are also mediated by service providers. He calls in at a MIND drop-in centre two or three times a week where 'you can have a talk, chat, you know, watch videos, play cards, everything'. Jim had to persuade the drop-in centre to accept Mark at a time when they were understaffed but this has proved to be a much valued refuge. Mark sometimes has tea at a local group home but only when a certain member of staff is on duty. Visits to the Red Cross provide sound support as well: 'I go in there sometimes, have a talk and they give me clothes.' Mark has strong religious beliefs and he was for a time absorbed into a local church. This included joining a visit to Lourdes.

Outside this agency network Mark is known in local shops and cafés. Asked about friends apart from the care assistant, he cited a woman and her son with whom he had once lodged and an elderly lady he visits sometimes. When Mark first moved into the flat he had problems with some teenagers who threw eggs at his windows, resulting in one being broken. This hostility is no longer in evidence. Mark gets on well with a neighbour who has done a lot for him although he can be jealous of her other visitors. He avoids Gateway, a social club organized around the interests of people with learning disabilities, because he feels it labels him: 'I don't like that. I want to be treated as an adult.'

The quality of Mark's life is affected by his dependence on welfare benefits. He is very conscious of struggling financially and states that he cannot afford the food he wants or leisure activities. He spends a lot of money on cigarettes which he says he needs to relax. He has a lot of good clothes but these are mainly second-hand from a variety of sources, including the community team. The lack of new clothes is something about which he is ambivalent; he wants them but likes getting good-quality items free. Mark is unwilling to work for less than a proper wage and will not attend the training centre, which he sees as exploitative. He says he has worked in the past as a kitchen porter. Jim believes he would fit in well as a care assistant's assistant but feels that with his history of aggression neither health nor social care agencies would be willing to take him on, even as a volunteer.

Despite frequent contact with professionals and some outside social contacts, Mark expressed feelings of loneliness, particularly during evenings and weekends: 'I listen to tapes, I listen to the television, to foreign affairs and things like that.' Mark does not go out in the evenings and often goes to bed in the early evening. Jim bought him a canary for company: 'I tell my problems to the bird and sometimes he helps.' However, Mark does not want to live in a group home and values the privacy of his current living arrangements. Jim believes he would be better living in some situation offering oversight and company.

Summary about Mark

Because of his long history of hospitalization and treatment for mental illness, Mark has been supported intensively by Jim, his key worker. Jim's preparedness to work with any of Mark's needs and concerns has allowed him to develop a close and trusting relationship with Mark. This appears to have paid significant dividends, particularly in the amelioration of Mark's aggression and in a reduction of his medication. That Mark lives alone has been another factor in Jim's regular pattern of visiting. It is one, however, that has served to avert crises. Mark is without a paid job and he refuses to attend the training centre. There appear to be no work, education or training alternatives available to him. He is dependent on welfare benefits and finds life a struggle financially. He would like to buy new clothes for himself but cannot afford them. Mark's situation illustrates how, despite close and intensive support from his key worker, family aide and nurse support worker, and contact with voluntary agencies, he tends to lead a rather socially isolated life. This is even more pronounced during evenings and at weekends. Most importantly, he lacks family contact and the level of his contact with the neighbourhood and other members of the local community are weak. The reliance on services is huge and Jim and Tom are committing a substantial amount of their time to Mark, sometimes outside of work hours. If, indeed when, they move on the personalized support and its very nature are likely to substantially alter Mark's experience of life 'in the community'.

Exercise 28.1

Given more recent developments in supporting people for employment (see Chapters 20 and 26), what employment training and preparation options might you suggest to Mark? What might you do to help Mark with his sense of loneliness?

Jo: a community study

Jo is a middle-aged woman living in a two-bedroomed council flat with another woman, Jane. The two women knew each other before moving in to their flat, but Jo cannot remember having been asked whether she would choose to live with Jane, or whether she chose to live in this flat. She used to live in a hostel. The home support worker, Zoe, does not think they were given a choice about whether they wanted to live together. Jo's key worker, Mo, says that they were given a choice, that they had been living in a house with one other person, but that they chose to move without the other woman. Jo remembers spending a lot of money on furniture, pictures and other household items when she moved into the flat. She was involved from the start in choosing these with Jane and enjoyed that experience. Shown a seven-runged ladder Jo indicated that she had reached rung four in terms of the best place she could live. She pointed to the bottom rung in terms of the hostel where she used to live, explaining that she could not do the things or go to places she wanted to when there. Jo would love to live on her own nearer to town but she says she has not told anyone because she is afraid they will take the flat away from her. Jo gets on well with Jane most of the time, but they have occasional disagreements.

Mo believes that Jo cannot live on her own. She feels that because Jo does not have a family carer, she must herself take that role in the least interventionist way possible. She sees her role as making Jo as independent as possible. This means helping with budgets, shopping and independent living skills such as using community amenities. She aims to do this while at the same time giving Jo choice-making options. Much of Mo's role has been in supervising the support staff to facilitate Jo and Jane in these skills. There are sometimes conflicts. For example, Jo wants to know why she cannot have more money. The support staff and key worker make such responses as, 'Well I'm sorry Jo, but that's the reality of it', commenting, 'Jo finds that difficult to cope with'.

The two women have a total of 20 hours support from two home support workers. Zoe says that Jo thinks she is more independent than her support package suggests and that she still requires help with shopping, budgeting and personal hygiene. Zoe often cooks for the women for the weekend, as she worries that they will not cope as happened once before. Zoe keeps Jo's money in a locked box and gives her a certain amount each week. Jo would like control of her money and to be taught about budgeting. Zoe says that this training has been tried several times, but has failed. If she had more money Jo says she would spend it on clothes and put the rest in the bank.

Jo would like less time from the support workers. The support workers feel that their hours have been reduced already and that they need to spend more time with Jo and Jane, not less. Mo agrees but says that her requests to the team's budget-holder have failed because of the varying demands of people for whom the team has to make provision. The home support workers go shopping with Jo and Jane, taking them to a café for lunch once a week. They have also been on day trips together. Once a week Jo meets with other people and with a physiotherapist for gentle exercise to aid her manual dexterity and body movement. The key worker has also helped Jo to join the local library and Zoe reads with her sometimes.

Mo believes that there were a lot of health problems for Jo because she was overweight. Jo had also contracted chest infections which had put her in hospital twice, on both occasions as a result of her smoking. Mo's GP had advised Mo to encourage Jo to give up smoking and go on a diet. Mo therefore arranged for a psychologist to make an assessment and implement a plan for cutting down on her smoking, and for more healthy eating. Jo did not feel too committed to stopping smoking, but she went along with this for a while. Things have reverted to her original smoking pattern recently, although she is now on a low-tar brand. One of the home support workers who smokes was encouraged by the psychologist not to do so in front of Jo.

In the evenings Jo likes to watch 'the soaps', listen to her radio and sometimes knit. She goes out on a Tuesday and Wednesday evening, catching the bus with Jane to two different clubs. Both are segregated activities. At one they play bingo and at the other, games. Most of the people at this club are middle-aged and have a lot in common in terms of their past experiences. They talk a lot about the past and support each other with present problems. Jo mentioned that one of the group had recently lost a relative, and that the group had arranged a card and sent someone to attend the funeral. The other club has a younger crowd, mostly from the training centres. They listen to music, and Jo takes her knitting along. They sometimes have a disco which Jo loves. On other nights Jo says she sometimes gets bored and goes to town, walks around and sometimes goes to a café for tea. At the weekends she does some tidying as well as watching TV.

During the week Jo has to get to town by bus two mornings a week for a cleaning job. On the other mornings she goes to a training centre where she usually sits in the smoking area and knits. She is not very happy about this. What she would really like to do is to work with children. Zoe thinks Jo is too old to be contemplating this. More recently the key worker, Mo, found another voluntary job for Jo in an old people's home, and Jo is delighted at this development. Again Jo is being paid a small amount for this work. As a result she spends one day less per week at the training centre.

There is a house meeting every fortnight with Jo and Jane's key workers and the home support workers. This has a problem-solving focus. There was also an individual planning meeting recently to discuss Jo's wish to get a job, go to college and have more control of her life. It was decided that Jo would apply for some voluntary jobs and that she should eventually stop going to the local training centre. Her link worker at the individual planning meeting was fully in agreement with this proposal. It was decided that Jo was too old for college but that there were ways around getting her involved in computing which she had expressed a desire to learn. The result of the individual plan to date is that Jo is now spending an extra day at work with elderly people.

Zoe has also become worried about Jo's memory and has liaised with Mo about this. A psychological assessment of memory has recently been undertaken. Other formal assessments have been done for cooking skills, and a plan implemented at a local agency to teach Jo these skills. However, this has now ceased. Otherwise the fortnightly meetings are the forum in which most of the planning takes place. Liaison between the workers involved in Jo's life therefore takes place regularly and their assessments tend to be made on the basis of their observations when with Jo.

Mo is of the opinion that Jo and Jane are not well suited to living together, and that it should be a long-term aim to find someone to move in who is more suited to Jo. She considers that Jo would be lonely living on her own. Mo takes the view that, in order to extend her independent living skills, Jo needs help to go out more, and perhaps to get away for a break or a holiday. This needs a further input from the support workers which again is not Jo's stated wish. It is also difficult because of a lack of resources. Finally, Mo feels that a suitable form of employment which would not affect Jo's welfare benefits would also be desirable.

Summary about Jo

Jo is living in ordinary housing and knows her neighbours. When living in the hostel Jo was unable to make choices about what to eat, and she had less choice about what to watch on TV and less opportunity to choose what she could do in the community. In comparison she is now using public transport freely, going into town on her own and using cafés, shops and the local library. In addition she is going on a number of day trips with her home support worker.

Through the efforts of her key worker, Jo has now obtained two part-time, voluntary jobs. Although she uses two segregated clubs, one of these is highly valued for the friendships that she has fostered and maintained for a number of years.

The balance between Jo's wish for independence as opposed to Mo's and Zoe's assessment about things that Jo cannot do for herself remains a problem. The balance between risk-taking and overprotection requires negotiation but at the very least both 'sides' are aware that this is the case. The implementation of an assessment of memory for example might be construed as a means of assessing to what extent Jo is capable of extending her choices. Absent budget management skills have however meant that there are things that Jo cannot do for herself.

The limits to Jo's community participation are considered by staff to be a product of her disabilities as well as of resource shortfalls. The change from the hostel to the flat has increased Jo's independence and choice, as has the input of the support workers and staff now involved in her life.

Like Mark, Jo's life is in many ways supported through the input of formal services and meetings concerned with her 'needs' are top-heavy with professionals. It is hard to see how other members of a support network independent of services could be used in developing over time a plan to meet Jo's wishes. Indeed, knowing Jo, she would not want more people 'interfering' in her life.

Exercise 28.2

What factors would you take into account in striking a balance between risk-taking and over-protection in supporting Jo? Were Jo to move into a place of her own rather than shared accommodation, what would you regard as the main risks?

Some reflections

Using stories collected as part of a research study we have commented above on the efforts made by key workers and support workers to maintain or facilitate the independence and quality of life of Mark and Jo. By the standards of many people with whom we spent time as part of the research Mark and Jo have substantial service supports and inputs. Indeed, although they were not living with family and had little or no contact with them, they were independent enough to be able to move about relatively freely in the community. In this sense their presence in the community was not reliant upon services or other support. Despite this there remain gaps in their lives. Below we review these gaps and deficiencies more closely.

Life at home

It is interesting that there was no desire expressed by either of the individuals to move back to forms of accommodation that had been experienced in the past. They each rated their present living arrangement very highly and equated their present circumstances with new freedoms, increased opportunities to make decisions for themselves and self-evident improvements in their independence. For Mark, who had spent a considerable amount of his life in one or more institutions, living in the community was considered to be an achievement in itself. It served to disprove the predictions of staff from the institutions who could not see this dream as ever succeeding. In this respect it was for Mark an important factor in his self-image and esteem, especially as he lived on his own. For Jo, the dream was to have her own home in the city, 'near to the action'. She did not, however, want to share this with her staff for fear of losing her present accommodation. In Jo's case her expectations about living by herself were somewhat at odds with the view taken by her key worker and support workers, but then this discontinuity was something that all the support workers were committed to bridging through their joint work with Jo.

Both Mark and Jo had their own house keys, could decide when to go out or return home, when to retire to bed and, for the most part, what to do at home. However, while Mark had literally the free run of his home, Jo had to bear Jane's needs and interests in mind. This had on more than one occasion led to a team meeting to resolve differences. The support worker almost continually worked to ensure that both Jo and Jane respected each other's space. This was never easy since 'don't leave your knitting on the settee' was seen as interfering by Jo. Many such interactions gave a sense that there was a figure independent of Jo and Jane 'mothering' them incessantly.

Participating in the community

One of the undoubted benefits enjoyed by Mark and Jo was the freedom to make connections in the community. They both enjoyed travel and being able to use public transport. They each also revelled in taking us as researchers to see where they usually 'hang out'.

Spending time with Mark and Jo, and especially going out with them in their communities, made us very much aware of the extensive social networks which they were capable of developing. However, it was also very clear for Mark that the majority of his social contacts were in the form of passing acquaintances. This was mirrored for Jo except in so far as she visited her friends, all with a learning disability, at a club on a weekly basis. Like many such clubs it remained insular and there was little opportunity for contact with the wider community.

Despite having regular haunts, both Jo and Mark had a lot of 'free time'. Jo spent much of her time sitting in front of the TV and had resisted attempts by staff to get her to a leisure centre to swim. The staff saw this as one way of controlling her weight but Jo was resolute in resisting the proposal. Mark chose to fill this time by going into town, window shopping and spending time in cafés. It was a kind of liminal world in which he remained and was likely to remain a passive participant. At his age this perhaps presaged the lifestyles of older people with learning disabilities whose lives feature almost incessantly painful 'placements' in a series of unwelcoming 'settings' (Grant *et al.* 1995).

So, Mark had become well known within his local community where local people and shopkeepers would stop to talk or acknowledge him. In this respect there was definitely a supportive or protective function served by this diffuse network of social contacts. However, figures in this network were not confidants, and neither did they provide practical support or relationships strong or close enough to Mark to be enjoined in person-centred planning. There was also the negative side of being in the community: both Mark and Jo had occasionally experienced verbal abuse. It is not hard to see with their lack of understanding about money that this might leave them open to financial exploitation by unscrupulous persons.

Friendships based on meaningful reciprocities with ordinary people were not usually in evidence for Mark and Jo. Like many people with learning disabilities, not least those who have spent much of their lives in institutional care, social contacts with surviving family members were often not capable of being exploited, either because parents and siblings had died or lost interest. Confiding relationships with individuals not labelled by virtue of disability or with support staff were rare.

This lack of social inclusion was most pronounced in Mark's case where it surfaced as loneliness. Making relationships was difficult for Mark and Jo, especially when they presented behaviours that were difficult for others to understand or to cope with. Both had unnatural amounts of 'free time' on their hands and it was not easy to build relationships if other people were 'busy' doing other things like working, studying or looking after their families.

Another factor influencing participation in the community was relative poverty. We found this in a substantial number of the 56 people with learning disabilities with whom we spent time as part of this study. All were dependent on welfare benefits, something about which they were patently aware. Mark and Jo were typical of other service users in this respect and both complained about not having enough money to buy the things they liked. There was also evidence that Mark went without the kind of food or leisure activities he liked though it was difficult to judge how far this was as a result of the amount of money he spent on cigarettes. Neither were in full-time employment so they did not have the benefit of a salary or wage. It is important not to underestimate the significance of the autonomy that money can buy for individuals, especially when considered against images in the media of 'hedonistic' spending, a fact that does not escape those who have sufficient time to find the TV a 'close friend'.

The social world of Mark and Jo was one in which they involved themselves in both segregated and non-segregated community activities. However, family aides had played a key role in effecting a shift towards use of ordinary facilities within the community and both looked forward to going out with them. Mark was trying to shed his association with Gateway because of his aversion to anything connected with 'learning disability'. He still frequents the MIND drop-in centre however. Jo, on the other hand, particularly values holidays and day trips with her support worker. However, from these 'forays into the community' neither has built any lasting relationships. Given the paucity of close contact with members of the community, it is not surprising that Mark and Jo saw their closest friends as being service workers.

In short, they had a community presence but, despite all they had to offer, they remained on the periphery (Dowson 1997) with clear obstacles to their participation in the labour market, to transferring out of segregated services and to involvement with community groups.

Work and employment

Neither Mark nor Jo were in full-time paid work and they were not receiving any kind of employment training. Jo had some remunerated employment in the form of part-time cleaning jobs which paid her a small amount of money each week. Both Mark and Jo had negative attitudes about 'traditional' day services and about the places where they had lived before.

Although Jo also attended the local training centre during the mornings when she was not doing her part-time jobs, she disliked going there and usually spent her time smoking and knitting in one of the rooms. Mark refused to attend the training centre as he regarded it as exploitative. There appeared to be no planned realistic employment training, alternative day activities, further education or open employment opportunities for Mark and Jo. Work was a black hole in their lives and this had a profound impact upon their lifestyles. Indeed, squeezes on local authority spending were causing some of the further education opportunities to be closed down. Moreover, Jo's support worker set expectations low enough to ensure that any earnings would not affect Jo's benefits.

Finding appropriate employment, employment training or further education openings for Mark and Jo was therefore not easy. Service systems were not geared to employment as a central objective, but there were also some individual factors involved. Mark had openly rejected the training centre and his employment prospects were blighted by his outbursts of aggression towards other people. Jo, meanwhile, had two small part-time jobs and it was not proving easy to dovetail other activities around these. Although Jo was still of an economically active age she considered herself 'too old' for further education. For Jo, payment was limited to the earnings limit so that her benefits would not be affected.

Individualized support

Even from the brief descriptions provided here it will be evident that Mark and Jo had been receiving intensive and continuous support from their key workers. Moreover, the relationships that had developed as a result were close and personal. This appeared to account for the way in which they looked upon their key workers as friends as much as professional supporters. They knew that their key workers knew them as people with interesting and valued identities. It should be noted that both were seen as a priority by services and that our study found many people were receiving little or no service input (Grant *et al.* 1994). In this light, Mark and Jo represented perhaps the 'best case scenario' in terms of a test of whether individualized support really could work.

One of the important ingredients in this individualized approach was the close working relationship of key workers and support workers with Mark and Jo, together with her housemate Jane. The support workers often knew their clientele very well. They engaged in practical and, for the most part, valued activities with individuals in a way that nobody else did. Informed work from key workers was in this sense dependent on the 'particularistic' knowledge of support workers about each person.

Unlike many people with learning disabilities, Mark and Jo were able to speak for themselves and therefore represent a group whose wishes and aspirations should be most readily known. In the research we found it common for support workers (or families) to have worked out methods of communicating with individuals, either by signing, by having come to recognize the special language used by individuals, or by using other facilitated communication techniques. Individualized work was particularly impressive when it was able to draw upon these channels of communication (see Chapter

13). However, it also left us pondering why greater responsibility for individual planning could not be taken by individuals in support worker roles. If person-centred care in present policy is to succeed, questions were also raised about how it might be possible to extend the 'search for dreams' to others in the community. The paucity of real relationships outside of services left us feeling that for many people the link to services as the prime movers in supporting community life would also maintain the continued dependence on these services, a form of transinstitutionalization – i.e. transfer from one institution to another. We have also found in another study (Ramcharan *et al.* 2004) that for many living on the margins there is not a 'community who cares'.

Service-oriented approaches meant that the balance between risk-taking and protection remained a high priority and could sometimes be stifling (see Chapters 7 and 24). Despite the view that individuals had the right to self-determination, the focus on risk assessment could lead to unemployment (Mark); to financial difficulties (Mark and Jo); and to closer relations with service personnel as friends (Mark and Jo), all being a function of over-protection. Support workers were in the front line in seeking to mediate and monitor these processes, pointing again to the necessity of their close work with key workers. Where the risks were high, as in Mark's case, key workers tended to visit very frequently.

Although we do not report here key worker perspectives about the organizational and professional factors bearing upon their work, it should be mentioned that this intensive involvement could only be sustained in a few cases because of workload pressures. It meant that other individuals and their families were denied visits or support for lengthy periods. Deciding workload priorities was never easy and inevitably left hard-pressed key workers feeling guilty about having to overlook some people's needs in favour of others. There are issues therefore about how many people key workers could sustain relationships with that were to the depth and level required to give a truly person-centred input.

Perhaps the most important observation of Mark and Jo's lives was that it was hard to see how to fashion links sufficiently strong to develop a 'circle of friends' who would want to be involved in their lives and whose relationships would allow for this to be meaningfully the case. Outside of services we found nobody who could occupy the role of confidant, special friend or a member of a 'circle of support' (see Chapter 24). This also raises questions about the place others can legitimately play in the lives of people with learning disabilities, and the extent to which this is out of choice, an issue discussed in Chapter 29.

Conclusion

Jo and Mark can be distinguished from many people with learning disabilities by being a priority for their local services. These services have put in place substantial support and sought to make the care as 'seamless' as possible by creating close links between the different parts of the services involved. As cases of 'individualized care' they therefore represent the 'cream of the crop'. Despite this, when weighed against the changes in experience for Jo and Mark, personalized support comes out wanting on a number of counts.

The two community studies of Mark and Jo show that there are no easy recipes for developing individualized support packages and that needs-driven, individualized support committed to a valued life philosophy is a continuous process that must be handled carefully. Much had been attained with Jo and Mark living independently and having intensive and continuous support, in having more choices and freedom to experience different things, and in securing opportunities for them to demonstrate their capacities, interests and gifts.

However, resource shortfalls and poor service designs left individuals with only a toehold in the community. Despite living reasonably independent lives, Mark and Jo were still forced either to use segregated day services or to exercise their right to withdraw themselves from such settings. This frequently left them with little or nothing constructive to do during the day but to wander around their local community or, in the case of others because of limitations to mobility, restricted them to a life within the walls of their own home. An integrated policy for employment, employment training and leisure was conspicuously lacking. As a result, key workers had an uphill struggle to locate meaningful day activities for individuals. Though supported employment opportunities had taken root, they were far from universally available. While supported employment schemes will suit some individuals they are not a panacea and can still fail to enable people to achieve social inclusion (Wistow and Schneider 2003).

The disadvantages individuals experienced were in these respects more a function of economic and social deprivation and service deficiencies than of their learning disabilities, as has been found in other ethnographies (Traustadottir and Johnson 2000). It is in this sense that the economics of the care relationship can be seen as disadvantaging, disempowering and disabling.

Valuing People (Department of Health 2001) places great store in the work of Partnership Boards to provide the necessary structures for day services and employment designed to meet individual needs. It is unknown as yet whether they can deliver what people want or whether there is the capacity to generate the resources to make visions a reality.

At another level, current policy in England in relation to person-centred planning (see Chapter 24) implies a shift towards the empowerment of circles of support. These circles are envisioned as groups made up of those who care about and love the person as well as professionals who might provide practical help and support. The move to 'self-sufficiency' within each person's community is, however, dependent upon that community being in place and willing to be involved.

The formation of close and friendly relationships with key workers, support workers and others has already been noted. The establishment of such relationships is one of the undoubted keys to the success of individual work with individuals and families. Yet it has been argued that the 'service worker as friend' results in disappointment when personnel move on; it acts as no substitute for long-term community friendships (Ramcharan *et al.* 1997). Most people with a learning disability have few friends (see Chapters 23 and 29) of their own who are not paid (e.g. key workers or categories of support workers like family aides).

Lessening the dependency on 'paid' helpers and friends and enabling individuals to establish genuine reciprocal relationships with other people who may become their friends remains a major developmental challenge. We share the view that the service system has so far paid insufficient attention to methodologies for helping users and families to build supportive and non-paid relationships with others (Dunst *et al.* 1989). Given that the long-term survival of individuals with even quite mild forms of learning disability appears to depend on a variety of paid and unpaid roles (Edgerton 1984; Edgerton and Gaston 1991), striking a balance between the two appears to be vital.

Mark and Jo's stories also raise some important questions about who has the right to intervene in the lives of people with learning disabilities. Despite valiant efforts from key workers and others, there were 'background figures' in the service system controlling access to needed services and supports that seemed to work against people's best interests. System economics and wholesale gaps in service systems also undermined intensive, individualized support work.

In among these hidden systems of power over care and economic survival, Mark and Jo nevertheless showed huge resilience and constantly strove to make and maintain contacts that were or would be meaningful to them. Mutual helping was also in evidence. Through people's peer networks we witnessed mutual aid with things like shopping, making meals and even decorating. Person-centred planning that seeks to build on mutual aid between people, and is based on an understanding of an individual's social network, is expected to assist in these endeavours but hard evidence is still awaited. The issues surrounding such 'communities of interest' that people with learning disabilities develop and maintain will therefore be vital to their success in the community. In the following chapter there is further discussion about just these community ties.

References

Alderson, P. (2001) Down's Syndrome: cost, quality and value of life, *Social Science and Medicine*, 53: 627–38.

Department of Health (2001) *Valuing People: A New Strategy for Learning Disability for the 21st Century*. London: Department of Health.

Dowson, S. (1997) Empowerment within services: a comfortable delusion, in P. Ramcharan, G. Robert, G. Grant and J. Borland (eds) *Empowerment in Everyday Life: Learning Disability*. London, Jessica Kingsley.

Dunst, C.J., Trivette, C.M., Gordon, N.J. and Pletcher, L.L. (1989) Building and mobilising informal family support networks, in G.H. Singer and L.K. Irvin (eds) *Support for Caregiving Families: Enabling Positive Adaptation to Disability*. Baltimore, MD: Paul H. Brookes.

Edgerton, R.B. (ed.) (1984) *Lives in Process: Mildly Retarded Adults in a Large City*. Washington, DC: AAMD.

Edgerton, R.B. and Gaston, M.A. (1991) *'I've Seen It All': Lives of Older Persons with Mental Retardation in the Community*. Baltimore, MD: Paul H. Brookes.

Felce, D., Grant, G., Todd, S., Ramcharan, P., Beyer, S., McGrath, M., Perry, J., Shearn, J., Kilsby, M. and Lowe, K. (1998) *Towards a Full Life: Researching Policy Innovation for People with Learning Disabilities*. Oxford: Butterworth Heinemann.

Goode, D.E. (1994) *A World Without Words: The Social Construction of Children Born Deaf-Blind*. Philadelphia, PA: Temple University Press.

Grant, G., McGrath, M. and Ramcharan, P. (1994) How families and informal supporters appraise service quality, *International Journal of Disability, Development and Education*, 41(2): 127–41.

Grant, G., McGrath, M. and Ramcharan, P. (1995) Community inclusion of older people with learning disabilities, *Care in Place: The International Journal of Networks and Community*, 2(1): 29–44.

Langness, L.L. and Levine, H.J. (eds) (1986) *Culture and Retardation*. Dordrecht: Reidel Publishing.

Prosser, H. (1989) *Eliciting the Views of People with a Mental Handicap: A Literature Review*. Manchester: Hester Adrian Research Centre, University of Manchester.

Ramcharan, P., McGrath, M. and Grant, G. (1997) Voices and choices: mapping entitlements to friendships and community contacts, in P. Ramcharan, G. Robert, G. Grant and J. Borland (eds) *Empowerment in Everyday Life: Learning Disability*. London: Jessica Kingsley.

Ramcharan, P., Whittell, B. and Grant, G. (2004) *Advocating for Work and Care: The Experience of Family Carers Seeking Work*, a report to the Community Fund. Sheffield: University of Sheffield.

Traustadottir, R. and Johnson, K. (eds) (2000) *Women with Intellectual Disabilities: Finding a Place in the World*. London: Jessica Kingsley.

Walmsley, J. and Johnson, K. (2003) *Inclusive Research with People with Learning Disabilities: Past, Present and Futures*. London: Jessica Kingsley.

Wight-Felske, A. (1994) Knowing about knowing: margin notes about disability, in M. Rioux and M. Bach (eds) *Disability Is Not Measles: New Research Paradigms in Disability*. North York, Ontario: Roeher Institute.

Wistow, R. and Schneider, J. (2003) Users views on supported employment and social inclusion: a qualitative study of 30 people in work, *British Journal of Learning Disabilities*, 31(4): 166–74.

29 Engaging communities of interest

Paul Ramcharan and Malcolm Richardson

Introduction

Think about the friendships, acquaintances, work, leisure, spiritual, service, professional and other relationships in your life. How close are each of the people with whom you have contact for these purposes? How close are they geographically or how close in terms of the things you share and in terms of how close you feel to them? Now do Exercise 29.1.

Exercise 29.1

Think about the people around you, those with whom you share time or with whom you do things. Now ask what role each of these people play in your life and why they are important to you.

In this exercise you will have thought about the people in your life and their importance to you. You might be able to put these into concentric circles representing how close and how important the relationship with each person is, as shown in Figure 29.1.

Exercise 29.2

Using Figure 29.1, think about a person with learning disabilities living in a family home and one living independently with support. How do these compare to your relationships? Are there any differences?

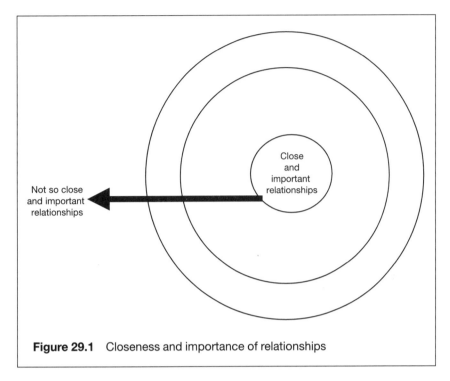

Figure 29.1   Closeness and importance of relationships

In undertaking Exercise 29.2 you may have found in your comparisons a number of things that recur in the literature on relationships and people with learning disabilities: a paucity of friendships (e.g. Firth and Rapley 1990; Emerson and McVilly 2004); being present in the community but not being part of it (Todd *et al.* 1990; Dowson 1997; Myers *et al.* 1998); differences in the extent and nature of relationships with services dependent upon the residential setting (Ramcharan *et al.* 1997; Emerson and McVilly 2004); and having a smaller number of supportive networks or having a lack of 'distributive competence' (Booth and Booth 1998; Jenkins 1998).

There are several ways of looking at the nature of the relationships that you have just thought through in the exercises, not least that outside of affective or loving relationships it is often common interests (i.e. communities of interest) that tie people to each other in their relationships. Current UK policy states that 'People with learning disabilities are often socially isolated . . . Good services will help people with learning disabilities develop opportunities to form relationships' (Department of Health 2001: 81). But what sort of relationships? And how might such good services operate? In what follows we will examine the ways in which such relationships fill 'fundamental needs', how they have been measured and their 'ecology'. Having done this we will then examine how these ideas have been reflected in policy and what implications this may have for your practice.

The nature of social relationships

Many of the chapters in this volume (e.g. see Chapters 8, 11, 23, 26 and 31) consider in more detail some of the ways in which families, support services, neighbourhoods, self-advocacy groups and other arenas provide the loci within which the social relationships of people with learning disabilities are acted out. We will not look in detail at these in what follows but, rather, offer an opportunity to understand a little more the nature of relationships and the intentions of service personnel who seek to develop and maintain them.

Fulfilling fundamental human needs

In considering the nature of relationships, Bayley (1997) reviews the literature on the ways in which such relationships fulfil differing fundamental needs. He hypothesizes that, 'For people with learning difficulties to lead fulfilled lives they need to experience a range of relationships in order to meet the range of basic human emotional and cognitive needs' (p. 31). Following on from Weiss (1975, 1979) and latterly Bulmer (1987), a number of such needs are identified:

- attachment and intimacy where feelings can be expressed freely;
- social integration where people share common concerns and aims;
- nurturance, denoting a close relationship allowing development and growth within the confines of a special relationship;
- reassurance of worth in which people feel some sense of accomplishment and self-esteem;
- reliable assistance in which the structures and resources are made available to meet other needs;
- guidance derived from respect for others.

Drawing on O'Brien and Lyle's (1987) five accomplishments, Bayley also argues that many people with learning disabilities do not have the opportunity to make choices unless supported to do so. The element of choice is therefore an important seventh category to be included in the above typology.

Exercise 29.3

As a person who will be providing a support service to people with learning disabilities, consider which of the above categories you feel you might fulfil.

One of the abiding features of relationships is that though they wax and wane they provide some consistency in a person's life. In contrast, service personnel are likely to be transient, making replication of naturally existing relationships rather more difficult. There are also key issues about the closeness and intimacy elements that are implied in the areas of 'attachment and intimacy' and 'nurturance'. Professional values imply, moreover, that there is a need to establish some degree of 'aloofness' and that becoming too involved or being too close is potentially problematic.

On the other hand there are ways in which service workers are in a position to provide the conditions in which people with learning difficulties as clients may become more socially integrated in local groups, in sustaining a sense of self-worth and self-esteem through guidance and in offering reliable assistance. Facilitating choice is exceptionally important in this regard since people with learning disabilities often need to be supported to exercise choice out of experiences of different options. For example, in a study of the experiences of people living in a learning disability hospital Ramcharan (1998) found that those people who could not move around on their own were less likely to be involved in day activities, socialize more widely and so forth. It was also found that this group was likely to have higher self-care needs and was less able to communicate verbally. The picture was one of a disempowered group who had high support needs and who were therefore unable to foster or sustain relationships without support. This placed service workers in an exceptionally important 'facilitative' role in terms of supporting the relationships that are fundamental to experiencing a good quality of life.

Margaret Flynn, describing a one-off visit to a respite facility (Flynn *et al.* 1994), relates that she had received two marriage proposals by the time she had left later that afternoon. Bayley (1997) refers to 'relationship vacuums': where existing relationships are unable to fulfil fundamental human needs a vacuum is created. Such vacuums can be filled inappropriately as with Flynn's experience outlined above. More importantly, a lack of relationships sufficient to fulfil the fundamental needs we have as sentient social beings leads to isolation, loneliness and lack of self-esteem or self-identity.

In other chapters in this book consideration is given to the home and family life, work, education, leisure, social, spiritual and service experiences of people with learning disabilities. It is clear from these chapters that as a matter of 'lifecourse' the nature of the relationships we have and the needs they fulfil will differ over that lifecourse. Services are there not to replace these relationships but to ensure that, as far as is possible, naturally occurring networks exist that can provide the conditions in which people experience the range of choices that might at any point in their lives fulfil their fundamental needs. To do this requires an understanding of social networks and identity.

Relationships and networks

Exercise 29.4

In Figure 29.1 you are likely to have people in each concentric circle for yourself and the two people with learning disabilities. Now link together the people by drawing a line between those who have contact with one another. What you have produced should look a little like a net, or a social network to be more precise.

Wenger (1996) has pointed to a number of different ways in which social networks can be categorized, studied and understood. As she argues, 'Support networks have been shown to vary in terms of size, density, linkages, content and composition and to be affected by gender, marital status, social class and state of health' (Wenger 1992: 6). However, for many people with learning disabilities both social and support networks have been widely reported to be impoverished. Early social network studies examined network size, density composition (family, friends others), geographical spread, intensity or frequency of contact and the nature of network relations. However, a second approach focuses on the specific purposes served by the network (e.g. care networks or political networks). As Wenger has suggested, understanding these types of 'purposive network' has been particularly useful in the context of social support and social policy because they have 'demonstrated a clear relationship between network characteristics, levels and types of informal help and support received and help seeking behaviour' (1996: 64). Links have also been made between network typologies and outcomes, for example quality of life and the experience of isolation and loneliness and feelings of stress and social malaise (see Lunsky and Benson 2001; Odom *et al.* 2004). In other words, the relationships we have are vitally important to our sense of self, well-being and fulfilment.

Our sense of self or identity is reliant upon a number of factors. Renblad (2002) has recently shown how the networks of people with learning disabilities will differ dependent upon their history and where they live, work or have their leisure. This article also highlights how important other people are in supporting a range of experiences in different environments. As will be shown later, this network is essential to the present person-centred planning (PCP) framework in the UK. But for now it is worthy of note that our sense of self may be a product of our socialization, of the environments in which we operate or the social relationships that we have. For many people with learning disabilities this sense of identity is an 'excluded' identity (Borland and Ramcharan 1997). In other words, from the very earliest of ages, children with learning disabilities are separated from the mainstream. They go to special schools, attend segregated day services and are very much less likely later on in life to be in paid employment or living in their own homes.

The experiences of such separation therefore prepare them for a life of 'being different' or being 'excluded'.

Castells (1997) proposes that identity therefore takes place within a context marked by power relations where the dominant institutions of society impose their will structurally in the development of identity. This fits in well with the experience of many people with learning disabilities of the 'excluded identity' and is very much anathema to the central tenets of contemporary UK learning disability policy based on rights, independence, choice and inclusion (Department of Health 2001). Castells proposes that for many stigmatized groups there are ways in which they will build a 'resistance identity' to the dominant model in fighting for their rights. We have seen how this might operate in Chapter 8 which considered the self-advocacy movement and the ways in which it seeks to speak up for people with learning difficulties.

Castells also identifies the 'project identity' in which people build a life for themselves outside of the disability identity ascribed to them, thereby taking on new forms of inclusive identities. People with learning disabilities who have managed this border crossing (Peters 1996) between an excluded to an included identity are as yet few and far between despite inclusion as a concept being implicitly about making this transfer.

In summary, for professionals working to support people with learning disabilities there is a need to consider

- those areas in which they have a role in maintaining relationships and, if so, what type;
- how best to facilitate and set the conditions through which natural relationships that meet fundamental human needs can be fulfilled;
- the extent to which their inputs lead to an 'included identity' and to 'border-crossing'.

Exercise 29.5

Knowing the two people with learning disabilities as you do, consider how you might best accomplish the three objectives set out above. Then list all the problems that you may have to overcome in order to accomplish this aim.

The ecology approach to communities of interest

Above we intimated that the nature of social relationships and support networks is central to the ways in which people seek to fulfil their fundamental human and social needs. At its worst, institutions such as the learning disability hospitals, 'total institutions' as Goffman (1962) called them, have sought to appropriate all aspects of people's lives – home, leisure, social, health and medical and so forth. In this ecological milieu, social relationships are (or were) highly controlled. Thus for example the separation of the sexes between wards prevented as far as possible the chance of intimate relationships (see Chapter 4). The structures and timetables led to a fixed number of relationships and very limited scope for choice or for extending social interaction beyond the confines of those dictated by such structures. And yet, despite this, a huge number of personal histories and other accounts are pointing to the valued social relationships, friendships and intimate relationships that flourished despite institutionalization (e.g. Deacon 1982; Barron 1989; Potts and Fido 1991; Lundgren 1993; Cooper 1997).

In short, the will to have friendships and relationships transcends even the most stringently applied institutional structures and rules. But these structures do mean there are limits on the numbers of people with whom all needs might be satisfied. Hence, people may have to make do with relationships that might be structured differently in different environments.

The situation 'in the community' may also be problematic. For example, it has been pointed out that people with learning disabilities are in the community but that they pass through it in their buses to segregated settings and are, as such, not part of that community (Dowson 1997). In this view, the likely social relationships are still broadly made and sustained with other people with learning disabilities rather than with others in the community or neighbourhood. Ramcharan *et al.* (1997) have also shown that a substantial proportion of parents have a 'handicapped orientation' to their children with learning disabilities, so that parental choices about the events to which they might go are limited to segregated activities only. The same study also found that in supported living arrangements a lack of funds often meant that people were unable to move about freely in the community and that many saw their support staff as their friends. As Todd (2000: 613) says: 'Without any voluntary movement from within the community itself, or more adequate preparation and conceptualization of the processes of social participation, people with intellectual disability will continue to depend on staff to foster those opportunities'.

In each of the above cases there are seen to be limits to which it is possible to overcome all the negative elements associated with institutionalization, even where people with learning disabilities live with their parents or in independent living situations. Since their relationships are a product of both their history and of the support they receive in fashioning their lives we therefore have to ask how an 'inclusive identity' and 'shared interests with others' can be developed and maintained. This is by no means an easy thing to do and certainly it is not easy for staff who support people with learning difficulties. Indeed, it has been argued that 'When community is an experience rather than a location, space or a legal structure, then inclusion cannot only be a space by changing institutional roles. It must also, and even primarily, be a matter of sharing one's life with other people ... This is where the limitations of using public policy as a major vehicle for change appear' (Reinders 2002: 2).

So how then is policy seeking to manage these issues?

Policy and theory dimensions

Recent policy in relation to health and social care has almost entirely been based upon notions of the assessment of individual needs and provision to the individual. For example, the NHS and Community Care Act 1990 and the associated White Paper *Caring for People* (Department of Health 1989) in the UK are based upon a care management model in which 'A practitioner is allocated to assess the needs of the individual . . . in a way that also recognize[s] their strengths and aspirations' (Social Services Inspectorate 1991: 9).

Valuing People (Department of Health 2001), the present policy in England in relation to people with learning disabilities, proposes that 'Person-centred planning is a mechanism for reflecting the needs and preferences of a person with a learning disability and covers such issues as housing, education, employment and leisure' (p. 49). PCP is considered in Chapter 24. However, for the moment the point to be made is that the assessment by professionals under the NHS and Community Care Act remains based around the individual. It remains part of the process of gaining access to services under *Valuing People* though exhortations are made for commissioners and purchasers to make their decisions on the basis of the person's wishes as identified in the PCP process. *Valuing People* talks about improving access to mainstream leisure facilities and about proposing that 'good services will help . . . develop opportunities to form relationships' (p. 81). But note here that all of the emphasis resides within support and funding for the individual. The difference with the PCP approach is in using a circle of support to discover the person's dreams and wishes and to seek to develop 'community' through their own efforts and through those of the services they can access. In this sense there has been a movement towards seeing the circle (close friends, family and advocates) as 'responsible for' developing both community presence and inclusion.

The present policy backdrop is therefore far removed from the proposals of the Seebohm Report (1968) and Barclay (1982), with their emphasis on a 'community development model'. In this model one of the tasks of service workers was to both resource and actively support the development of communities. This was no easy thing to achieve. Seebohm recognizes that 'community' as a concept is often related to locality, for example rural communities or communities of reciprocal interest such as those outlined in the seminal work of Willmott and Young (1960) in the East End of London. However,

> although community has traditionally rested upon geographical locality, and this remains an aspect of many communities, today different members of a family may belong to different communities of interest as well as the same local neighbourhood. The notion of a community implies the existence of a network of reciprocal social relationships, which

among other things ensure mutual aid and give those who experience it a sense of well-being.

(Seebohm Report 1968: 147)

Seebohm therefore saw the role of services as being part of a network of local services to the community at the same time as being dedicated to developing communities, neighbourhoods and working with voluntary and other organizations to develop capacity locally. In this way the 'ecology' of this approach is one tied to mutual interests forged within communities for their own common welfare. This approach to collectives differed in ethos to individualized approaches to community inclusion.

The work of Philip Abrams (see Bulmer 1986) is perhaps best associated with ideas about 'neighbourhoodism' though it does not feature in the learning disability literature very strongly. Abrams argued that forms of care can differ dependent upon the personnel involved and on what setting the care is provided. So, for example, professional care in institutions leads to an 'institutional treatment' model whereas care by non-specialists will involve an 'institutional care' model. In contrast, in the community, professional care will yield a 'community treatment' model and lay or non-specialist inputs will produce 'community care' – i.e. care by the community, something alluded to earlier (Reinders 2002). For Abrams it was absolutely vital to transfer as much care to the community as possible, to deprofessionalize relationships and set people free of service dependency, and to work in building communities. The point here is not to dismiss 'professional knowledge' but to make sure that knowledge is used to maintain independent living and a high quality of life.

In Abrams' view, the likely means through which such community care might be developed was through such approaches as neighbourhood groups, good neighbour schemes, participation of people in local voluntary organizations and via the running of 'communities of interest'. There are problems with this model, not least the oft-cited ones of identifying the 'community that cares' and the mammoth task involved in community redevelopment. However, such community development approaches play second fiddle in contemporary policy to the centrality of PCP and the artful use of the circle of support in making and sustaining the appropriate community contacts. Where better to start than by drawing together family, friends, advocates and others (of the client's own choosing) as the engine that seeks to extend their community contact and fulfil their dreams and aspirations? So although individual assessment remains it is not solely services that are charged with 'community inclusion'. Rather, the circle of support has been given primary responsibility to establish from the person's aspirations what involvement they would like and to become 'providers' alongside formal services. In this model no responsibility is placed on the service sector to develop the communities or neighbourhoods themselves. You will note that the different models therefore have markedly different implications for the roles and tasks of health and social care workers.

Exercise 29.6

Think about the two people with learning disabilities whose networks you outlined earlier. Undertake an assessment of their individual needs using a PCP model (see Chapter 24). What does this tell you about how best to fulfil their fundamental needs? Now repeat the exercise but using a community development approach. What are the pros and cons of each approach?

Below, using the present policy context relating to individual assessment, we provide an extended example of how the development of communities of interest and community inclusion might be coordinated and managed.

Communities of interest: the PCP model

In the review above Weiss's (1979) work points to the importance of the 'unit relationship' (i.e. who interacts with whom) and the relationship between this unit and fulfilling 'fundamental human needs'. At a broader level, the 'social network' has also been identified as being a 'natural' one which tends to pre-exist services: a 'supportive' network which develops out of naturally occurring networks who help and support, or a 'purposive' network geared towards a specific target or goal. It was suggested, using Abrams' work, that where services seek to develop a service delivery model through networks, they represent a community treatment model and that this contrasts with 'community care' in which the locus of interest is the community itself rather than the service system. Finally it was argued that the ecology of care was vital. Institutional care produced what Castells sees as an excluded identity and this could just as easily apply to pervasive services in the community (i.e. to the transinstitutionalization of care). For Castells, resistance and finally an identity outside of services was the goal and this might be viewed in terms of the ecology or location of care, whether family, neighbourhood and friends or the wider community.

A number of assumptions are therefore implicit in any approach to 'community' and to 'communities of interest'. This is no less true of the policy of PCP than it is of any other model. Below we aim to disentangle some of these assumptions and, in doing so, identify alternative approaches to the 'community of interest' that is chosen by and serves people with learning disabilities.

In a recent study of carers seeking work (Ramcharan *et al.* 2004) it was found that their ability to work was dependent upon the extent to which they could share the care among other formal and informal supporters in such a way as to release them to enter employment and balance work with care. Under the principle of 'less eligibility', benefits are likely to be lower than payment for employment. The state is therefore likely only to be funding alternative care arrangements at a minimal level even though the recent Carers Equal Opportunities Bill in the UK places a duty on local authorities to assess whether a carer works or wants to work. It is therefore more likely that carers seeking work will have to look for informal, neighbourhood and community support in place of statutory services. However, as the report goes on to say, 'Unless there is some form of exchange, there does not seem to be much informal help available . . . Systems of exchange exist only to the degree that the exchange is seen as being manifestly equal . . . Help is therefore constructed as a "good" or a "service", i.e. something generated out of a materialist mentality' (p. 38). One can immediately see the relevance of this to PCP where there is an assumption that somehow there will over time be a circle of support ready and willing to engage with the interests of a person with learning disabilities in an ongoing plan about their future. Read the following example where PCP has been undertaken.

Case study: *Jane*

Jane is in her fifties. She has shared a house near the town centre for over 15 years with her sister, her boyfriend and two other people. All had previously resided in a hospital for people with learning difficulties. Jane and the other residents share the same named nurse but each has had a different personal support worker throughout these years. Jane has a degenerative eye condition and the home is adapted for her visual impairment. A 'typical week' in Jane's life involves going to the leisure centre on Monday morning with her sister for a health and fitness class held in the swimming pool; attending the local church on Wednesday mornings; Thursday afternoon at the library and a women's support group and attending a day centre at other times where she enjoys painting, yoga, relaxation and horse-riding. The evenings vary depending what Jane and her companions have chosen to do: some evenings are spent watching Jane's favourite soaps on TV either in her room or in the shared TV lounge. Sometimes the residents collectively decide to order a takeaway meal or rent a video. The weekends include spending time with her boyfriend on Saturday and going to the shops while Sunday can involve a visit to her eldest sister or sharing Sunday lunch with other residents (see Figure 29.2 for a summary).

Jane's life is full (see Richardson 2000) and she puts this down to the assistance and support of the people around her. These include a nurse, a personal support worker, other staff she has known for years, an older sister, her boyfriend and some other friends. Although friends and staff have moved on there had been a stability of support that helped this circle of friends. The circle had supported her to try out different activities, plan ahead, make new friends, contact old friends, plan events, move from hospital, decorate her room, and many other things. As outlined in Chapter 24, the circle of support has undertaken all the elements of PCP, including a

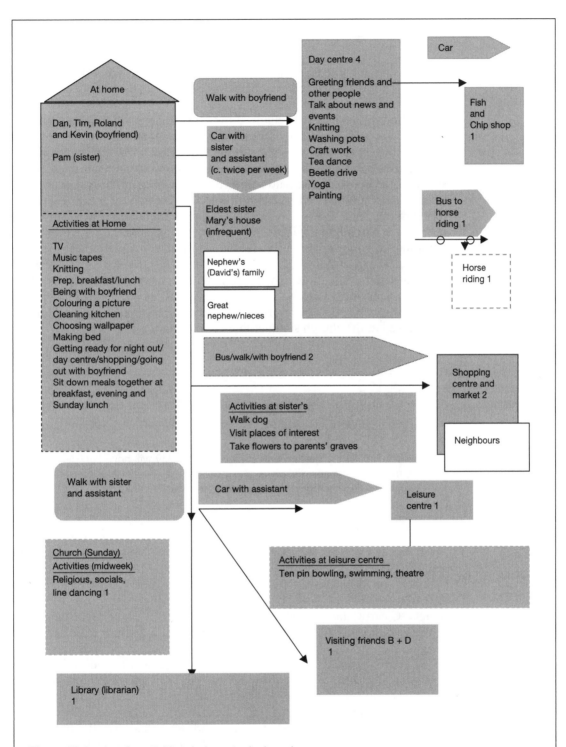

Figure 29.2 Jane's activities during a typical week

Note: This is an extract from a social network and community map made with Jane. The numbers in the boxes indicate how many times per week Jane undertook an activity. So, for example, it can be seen that Jane used a day centre four days per week, went horse-riding once a week and went out on the bus with her boyfriend twice a week.

'relationship mapping' exercise, identifying dreams and aspirations, looking for clues about what the person really wants, celebrating strengths and planning and 'planning a personal future'.

Although the circle has changed over time the people in it have made a huge difference to Jane's life. For example, it took some time for her to drum up the courage to ask why she couldn't do paid work like some of her friends. After Jane had identified that she wanted a paid job the support staff assisted her to obtain paid employment, washing up for two hours each week at a community centre. In addition, with the help of a member of the local church, Jane was able to continue church attendance after leaving the institution. Attending the local church with her sister would have been quite daunting, so her special interest person arranged for Jane to meet the local preacher. She in turn introduced Jane and her sister to a weekly dance evening and social events. In this way the large congregation got to know Jane and her sister and vice versa through a series of introductions and smaller activities over a period of several weeks. It is commonplace now for Jane to be involved in the church summer fayre and to have a brilliant time.

Exercise 29.7

Can you recognize any assumptions about who will be involved in a person's PCP?

Is it likely that every person with a learning disability will have sufficient contacts to make a meaningful circle of support as did Jane? What are the likely difficulties of developing community contacts where a person has none?

It can be seen that Jane's circle of support was extensive, committed and stable, including friends and staff with whom she had long-standing, reciprocal relationships. Circle members were also able to give of their time and were motivated to support Jane in harnessing contacts in the community. Clearly, staff played a vital role in this PCP. The circumstances for others may not be quite so propitious. If you look at Figure 29.2 you can imagine that for some people the network will be very small indeed.

It seems likely that for those with profound learning disabilities the nature of 'community life' will differ as will their past contacts with the community and the nature of their future contacts. Moreover, the degree of support often required means that there are additional problems with the systems of exchange outside of family and very close friends. For others with smaller circles the workload for practitioners may be even larger, leaving questions about how staff might provide meaningful support.

It was argued at the start of this chapter that where no system of exchange or reciprocity was in place there was a chance that circles of support would be impoverished. Calls to 'distribute competence' (Booth and

Booth 1998; Jenkins 1998) by extending the support network around the person assume that developing and sustaining such reciprocal relationships is non-problematic. Moreover, it should be noted that the form of planning implied above is based on 'individual interests' that have held hegemony within the social policy field at least since the 1980s. Thus we have assessments of the needs of person with learning disabilities alongside a separate assessment for their family carer.

The PCP 'revolution' transfers the onus for 'community care' to the interested community itself and away from the statutory services. It therefore involves assumptions about the ability to initiate, develop and sustain community relations that are reciprocal and can be maintained over time for all individuals with learning disabilities. It assumes a sharing community of interest alongside the individualization of care. If as suggested earlier there is very little evidence of the community that cares then how can that community be generated? Fortunately, the development of communities of interest is not new and has been the focus of much social care work in the past. Below we outline some of these approaches and the sense in which they occupy a different place to the PCP model.

Approaches to supporting and developing communities of interest

The majority of people with learning disabilities still live with their families although for adults this is changing over time. Despite this, many still remain in contact with family. The PCP system assumes that the unit of interest is the individual, but families are made up of more than just the person with a learning disability. The interests of the parents, siblings and sometimes others are often of vital importance to the resilience and success of the family as a unit. For many, the family represents the central unit for decision-making. This has several important implications.

Firstly, the unit of interest may not be that of the person with a learning disability but rather the family unit. Bringing people together to form a circle of support is likely to be time-intensive and for many families may be beyond their resources to do. In this sense there is a transfer of the 'locus of control' to another group. The 'locus of interest' as the person with learning disabilities may also detract from or conflict with the interests of the family unit. At its most extreme a focus on one person at the expense of others may lead to what Roberts (1997) has termed 'abusive normalization' where the interests of one person are represented to the exclusion of others. In so doing the approach can undermine the central unit for problem-solving, decision-making and surviving.

There are also assumptions in the PCP model about the extent to which relationships within a circle are interchangeable. One only has to think about how parents seek to support their (adult) children and the sense of love within families that is hard to find appropriately elsewhere. Similarly, 'good' neighbours (according to Abrams' seminal work reviewed earlier) are friendly, helpful but distant, seeking at all times to maintain privacy despite the contact with others. In this sense they are likely to be able to fulfil only particular roles in community support and in meeting fundamental needs associated with relationships. The idea of the circle of support itself seems to sacrifice this privacy for the benefits that accrue to the person with a learning disability, though it is by no means clear that the expectation is for all circle members to be similarly as frank about their own lives. In other words, there are, as argued earlier (Weiss 1979), some areas in which it remains very difficult to reproduce relationships. Where such relationships are required, external to those closest to the person, there is often a need to build this capacity over time. This is quite a 'specialist' task.

Dunst *et al.* (1989), in their 'family systems model', recognize that 'non-contingent giving' (i.e. giving without returning), is not likely to be the best form of exchange within communities, though it is better sustained within families. This may explain the earlier observation about the lack of informal community support found in the study of carers seeking work. To expect 'non-contingent giving' can lead to the dependence of one party, to systems of patronage and ownership by those who give without expecting anything in return and to loss of self-esteem for those parties who feel they have not contributed to the system of exchange. At worst, service interests may begin to outweigh the interests of the 'functioning' family unit where the PCP process becomes overly tied to service ideals and interests. This is likely to lead back to a community treatment rather than a community care ethos.

For families in which there is a person with a learning disability the likely 'coinage' of such exchange is missing: they don't attend the same schools as other children and adults; don't use the same transport; don't have the same needs in simple exchanges where families care for each other's children; and may be accompanied by such large socioeconomic differences that these undermine systems of equality between the parties in any exchange of support. Not surprisingly then, it is the artful use of promoting social support exchanges that is the expectation placed on families, a position that is hugely problematic for families caring for a disabled relative. In addressing some of these issues, the 'family systems' perspective features elements of 'human ecology . . . social support and social network theory . . . and help-seeking and help-giving theory' (Dunst *et al.* 1989: 125), very much those that were the interest of the earlier sections of this chapter.

In a project called SHaRE (Source of Help Received and Exchanged) Dunst *et al.* (1989) examined a system of shared and reciprocal relations set up between families caring for a relative with a learning disability. In this project the focus was on empowering families, developing strengths and capacities and extending contacts through an arranged system of networking. In this view, developing communities of interest is geared not around the person with a learning disability but around the family unit or, to be more precise, around the functioning unit of support. This will clearly differ dependent upon what that functioning unit is. So in Jane's case, long-term staff, friends from the past and relatives formed a sensible base for their work. But consider how the same might apply in the next case study.

Case study: *Clara*

Clara is 23 and suffers fits several times a day. She has what has been described as 'autism'. Her parents with whom she still lives are getting old and would like to see Clara living somewhere where they can be confident about her getting the love and care she needs, especially when they are too old to look after her. They live on a city estate and have not found supportive neighbours to share aspects of Clara's care.

From the earliest of ages Clara has found it very difficult to make friends. She grows attached to one or two people and loves having a hug with them. However, despite several efforts to help her make friends and develop such relationships with her peer group Clara has not done so. There have been real problems in the past two years in Clara's move from the special school. She now has two days at a training centre and two at a further education college where she is doing literacy and numeracy. The move has affected the family since her mother has had to give up one day of work and this has made their economic situation more fragile. More importantly, Clara has been having temper outbursts and has become withdrawn. It is clear she misses her teacher at school with whom she had a special relationship and she has not yet forged such a relationship among peers in her new day opportunities. The family are not clear about how to move forward and have nobody locally to whom they can turn for help.

Exercise 29.8

How would you use a circle of support where the person does not like crowds? What network of support can be forged for Clara in the community? What will the problems be?

Both Clara and her family are isolated. There is no natural network of support and little prospect that without many years of planning Clara will manage to form relationships close enough with others to make her happy and comfortable living and/or working elsewhere. The systems of support for the family and for Clara are difficult to build and to sustain.

Dunst *et al.* (1989: 136) report having worked to develop the skills of families in enhancing their 'competencies' as a means of creating a coinage for exchange and sharpening their 'network mobilization skills': 'A large number of project participants . . . learned the benefits of using informal exchanges . . . using the principles of reciprocal obligations and contingent helping . . . with neighbors, friends and relatives. These exchanges became part of their day-to-day activities'. In a family systems model it is therefore likely that much of the focus on Clara and her family would be on developing the capacity among *the family* to make contact with a community who share their interests. It would involve supporting a system of mutual exchange so that the parties felt comfortable with the arrangement. These contacts might extend the opportunities for Clara to build lasting relationships. Now it is not the case that a PCP approach does not or cannot do this, but rather that the emphasis is different.

A further product of the family systems approach may be self-help and self-health groups (see Wilson 1997) which have been extraordinarily important in establishing common interests and systems of mutual inter-dependence and exchange. As such they represent one way in which to formalize mutual exchange. Similarly, citizen advocacy (see Chapter 8) has been used as a means of developing both an instrumental and emotional relationship that lasts over a 'lifetime' and in which the person is partnered with an ordinary member of the community. However, such schemes have found recruiting a sufficient number of advocates very difficult (Ramcharan 1995).

Exercise 29.9

Think about when you do things for friends, neighbours and others. Is there a system of exchange? How did this system of exchange come about?

Do you undertake any 'non-contingent giving'? If so, to whom and why?

How might you work with families in which one member has a learning disability to develop systems of exchange?

The social systems model shares some interesting parallels and contrasts to PCP. Like the PCP system the role of staff is seen less as sole providers and more as empathetic listeners, resources, consultants, mobilizers, enablers and mediators. However, the family systems model starts with the centrality of families or the 'functioning unit' as the place where non-contingent giving is likely to best survive. It also recognizes the concerns of other communities of interest to the extent that a system of reciprocal exchange exists. The PCP approach does not problematize relationships in this way and does not see the family or the 'functioning unit' as the central unit of interest.

However, the idea of community development may be conceived even more broadly. In the 'ecological' approaches outlined earlier it was proposed that neighbourhoods and communities were an important focus as well as either the individual or the family. Emerging in the 1960s and 1970s there have been a number of attempts to address poverty and exclusion through community development initiatives. The early Community Development Projects (CDPs) had both a strong research focus but also one that sought to create and foster the development of local services and self-help (Lees and Smith 1975). Thomas (1983) identifies five strands of the 'community work' orientation. These involve:

- *community action* which seeks to develop collective action among public and private bodies in local decision-making;

- *community development* which emphasizes self-help, mutual support-building, neighbourhood integration and bringing collective action to bear in local politics;

- *social planning* which is concerned with assessing the community's needs and setting goals;

- *community organization* which is about linking community and welfare organizations;

- *service extension* which involves extending services into the community in an integrated and coordinated way.

More recent incarnations of the community work approach involve what has been termed 'capacity building' and have been applied to urban and rural renewal as well as to neighbourhood renewal schemes and to health and social care. Recently, arguments have been made about the ways in which 'community capacity building' has the potential to address health inequalities (Gibbon *et al.* 2002; Attree 2004). The community capacity approach is one that occupies a central place in the government's social exclusion initiatives and has led to a number of area-based initiatives such as health action zones, healthy living centres, Sure Start and New Deal for Communities (Social Exclusion Unit 1998: Department of Health 1999).

Communities of interest are, in this model, likely to be developed over time by community workers liaising with non-governmental organizations, self-advocacy groups, campaigning groups, local businesses and local decision-makers. The approach might also develop neighbourhood support schemes right through to pump-priming for local employment initiatives, as in the case study below.

Case study: *Antur Waunfawr*

Antur Waunfawr provides work for people with learning disabilities in a village with the same name in north Wales. It started with a gardening service and has diversified into making garden furniture, providing a recycling service, having a café and making a nature trail and sensory garden for visitors. It has become a well-known and intrinsic part of the community and local people not only use its well-priced services but have become involved. It also attracts visitors from outside the area and brings in tourist revenue. Antur is an invaluable part of the community and an essential part of the local economy which it helped regenerate after the decline of local slate mining (see www.anturwaunfawr.org/index.html).

In the broadest sense, community capacity-building may not represent a panacea for the needs of people with learning disabilities and their families. As a minority group their voice may be less likely to be heard. Hence, communities have a responsibility to support those who are most excluded and disadvantaged. As Bronfenbrenner says, 'The availability of supportive settings is . . . a function of their existence and frequency in a given culture or sub-culture' (1979: 7). What community development approaches do is work to develop the capacity of the community to provide such supportive settings. It would be of no use whatsoever to Jane or Clara to have a wonderful circle of support but not have a community primed and geared to support that circle. It seems ironic that 'partnership' is a key word across governmental sectors but not one that plays a major role in learning disability policy, especially given the potential benefit such collaborations might have within those communities that have been primed to share interests with learning disabled people and their families.

Exercise 29.10

How easy is it to know what supports are available in terms of friends, neighbours and community resources for Clara and Jane? Knowing Clara, Jane and other people with learning disabilities living in their area, how might you seek to build community capacity locally? What are the problems with such an approach?

Conclusion

Although we await systematic studies of the outcomes of PCP, there are accounts by people with learning disabilities on some websites that describe the processes clearly and indicate successes (e.g. www.circlesarounddundee. org.uk/pcp/). However, because PCP relies on the artful development of the plan it is easy to make misjudgements about what constitutes a PCP. There needs to be some critical attention paid to PCP initiatives that:

- expect too much of members of a circle and imply relationships that may be inappropriate;
- undermine the 'functioning unit', usually the family;
- represent a 'community treatment' approach with a service focus rather than a 'community care' approach based on community relationships;
- control rather than support the individual and impinge upon his or her privacy and that of the family;
- ignore the potential within communities to share the interests of people with learning disabilities.

Frequently the outcomes of PCP initiatives will be more or less good, occasionally disastrous and sometimes stupendously successful. Assisting people with learning difficulties, some of whom may not have spoken language with which to articulate their likes, wants, needs and aspirations, to explore and articulate what these are, and try to make them happen, is just as worthy an exercise as establishing the aspirations of the rest of humanity (see Chapter 13). And perhaps we should anticipate that the outcomes may be just as varied.

None of our futures are fixed. We are, all of us, in a process of becoming, finding out about the world and ourselves within it. PCP is not, therefore, a destination. It is a process aimed at enabling people to develop lives rich in activities and relationships and at putting the person in control of what happens in their life. In this chapter we have identified some additional approaches to supporting the development and longevity of 'communities of interest' by subjecting the assumptions of the PCP framework to critical analysis. In the earlier part of the chapter we also spoke of the extent to which it is necessary to work with the local community in order to make it more accepting. While PCP approaches do promote community presence and participation there remains much to be done to develop the accepting community and to build structures and mechanisms within the community to support people with learning difficulties as people first.

We have considered the lives of two individuals, each with their very particular circumstances. Jane's profile reveals how a widening network of support has enabled her to enjoy living in her local community and develop a wide range of relationships and activities. The significant factor underpinning this seems to be the stability of Jane's network and the readiness of her service providers to back off from control while delivering consistent and stable support. By contrast, Clara's network is heavily reliant upon her immediate family.

The basis of reciprocity and exchange means that people who are most disadvantaged are likely to have less resources to offer as exchange. Strengthening the family's ability to survive may be one additional option as posited in the family systems model. Moreover, it is great to have a circle of support to seek the contacts and experiences that lead to community inclusion. However, the community's capacity to absorb such demands may be limited. In such circumstances the development of community initiatives seems a vital parallel strategy, though not one actively supported by UK policy.

The family systems approach and the community development approach each take stances based on developing reciprocities and a system of exchange within the community. In contrast the PCP system relies on the members of the circle to make the most of their community and to keep motivated and committed over time. Although PCP remains the centrepiece of present UK policy this chapter has pointed to other approaches likely to confer over time upon Clara the potential benefit that accrues from having the continuity and stability that a wider network (like Jane's network) can deliver.

References

Attree, P. (2004) It was like my little acorn, and it's going to grow into a big tree: a qualitative study of a community support project, *Health and Social Care in the Community*, 12(2): 155–61.

Barclay, P. (1982) *Social Workers: Their Roles and Tasks*. London: Beresford Square Press.

Barron, D. (1989) Locked away: life in an institution, in A. Brachin and J. Walmsley (eds) *Making Connections: Reflecting on the Lives and Experiences of People with Learning Disabilities*. London: Hodder & Stoughton.

Bayley, M. (1997) *What Price Friendship? Encouraging the Relationships of People with Learning Difficulties*, Wooton Coutenay: Hexagon Publishing.

Booth, T. and Booth, W. (1998) Risk, resilience and competence: parents with learning difficulties and their children, in R. Jenkins (ed.) *Questions of Competence: Culture, Classification and Intellectual Disability*. Cambridge: Cambridge University Press.

Borland, J. and Ramcharan, P. (1997) Empowerment in informal settings, in P. Ramcharan, G. Roberts, G. Grant and J. Borland (eds) *Empowerment in Everyday Life: Learning Disabilities*. London: Jessica Kingsley.

Brofenbrenner, U. (1979) *The Ecology of Human Development: Experiments by Nature and Design*. Cambridge, MA: Harvard Universty Press.

Bulmer, M. (1986) *Neighbours: The Work of Philip Abrams*. Cambridge: Cambridge University Press.

Bulmer, M. (1987) *The Social Basis of Community Care*. London: Allen & Unwin.

Castells, M. (1997) *The Information Age: Economy, Society and Culture, vol II: The Power of Identity*. Oxford: Blackwell.

Cooper, M. (1997) Mabel Cooper's life story, in J. Atkinson, M. Jackson and J. Walmsley (eds) *Forgotten Lives: Exploring the History of Learning Disability*. Kidderminster: BILD.

Deacon, J.J. (1982) *Tongue-Tied: Fifty Years of Friendship in a Subnormality Hospital*. London: Royal Society for Mentally Handicapped Children and Adults.

Department of Health (1989) *Caring for People in the Next Decade and Beyond*. London: HMSO.

Department of Health (1999) *Reducing Health Inequalities: An Action Report*. London: Department of Health.

Department of Health (2001) *Valuing People: A New Strategy for Learning Disability for the 21st Century*. London: Department of Health.

Dowson, S. (1997) Empowerment within services: a comfortable delusion, in P. Ramcharan, G. Roberts, G. Grant and J. Borland (eds) *Empowerment in Everyday Life: Learning Disabilities*. London: Jessica Kingsley.

Dunst, C.J., Trivette, C.M., Gordon, N.J. and Pletcher, L. (1989) Building and mobilizing informal family support networks, in G.H.S. Singer and L.K. Irving (eds) *Support for Caregiving Families*. Baltimore, MA: Paul H. Brookes.

Emerson, E. and McVilly, K. (2004) Friendship activities of adults with intellectual disabilities, in *Journal of Applied Research in Intellectual Disabilities*, 17(3): 191–7.

Firth, H. and Rapley, M. (1990) *From Acquaintance to Friendship: Issues for People with Learning Disabilities*. Kidderminster. BIMH Publications.

Flynn, M. with Liverpool self advocates (1994) *Taking a Break: Liverpool's Respite Services for Adult Citizens with Learning Disabilities*. Manchester: National Development Team.

Gibbon, M., Labonte, R. and Laverack, G. (2002) Evaluating community capacity, *Health and Social Care in the Community*, 10(6): 485–91.

Goffman, E. (1962) *Asylums: Essays on the Social Situation of Mental Patients and Others*. Harmondsworth: Penguin.

Jenkins, R. (ed.) (1998) *Questions of Competence: Culture, Classification and Intellectual Disability*. Cambridge: Cambridge University Press.

Lees, R. and Smith, G. (1975) *Action-Research in Community Development*. London: Routledge & Kegan Paul.

Lundgren, K. (1993) *Ake's Book*. Sweden: Orebo Bokforlaget Libris.

Lunsky, Y. and Benson, B.A. (2001) Association between perceived social support and strain, and positive and negative outcome for adults with mild intellectual disability, *Journal of Intellectual Disability Research*, 45(2): 106–13.

Myers, F., Ager, A., Kerr, P. and Myles, S. (1998) Outside looking in? Studies of community integration of people with learning disabilities, *Disability and Society*, 13: 389–414.

O'Brien, J. and Lyle, C. (1987) *Framework for Accomplishment*. Decatur, GA: Responsive Systems Associates.

Odom, S.L., Klingerman, K. and Jakowski, M. (2004) Investigating inclusion: a review of research methods for individuals with intellectual disability, in E. Emerson, C. Hatton, T. Thompson and T.R. Parmenter (eds) *The International Handbook of Applied Research in Intellectual Disabilities*. Chichester: Wiley.

Peters, S. (1996) The politics of identity, in L. Barton (ed.) *Disability and Society: Emergent Issues and Insights*. Harlow: Addison Wesley Longman.

Potts, M. and Fido, R. (1991) *A Fit Person to be Removed*. Plymouth: Northcote House.

Ramcharan, P. (1995) Citizen advocacy and people with learning disabilities in Wales, in R. Jack (ed.) *Empowerment in Community Care*. London: Chapman & Hall.

Ramcharan, P. (1998) *Fostering a Culture of Civil Rights in a Learning Disability Hospital. A Report to the Gwynedd Community Trust, Learning Disability Services*. Bangor: University of Wales, Bangor, Centre for Social Policy Research and Development.

Ramcharan, P., McGrath, M. and Grant, G. (1997) Voices and choices: mapping entitlements to friendships and community contacts, in P. Ramcharan, G. Roberts, G. Grant and J. Borland (eds) *Empowerment in Everyday Life: Learning Disabilities*. London: Jessica Kingsley.

Ramcharan, P., Whittell, B. and Grant, G. (2004) *Advocating for Work and Care: The Experience of Family Carers Seeking Work*. Sheffield: University of Sheffield.

Reinders, J.S. (2002) The good life for citizens with intellectual disability, *Journal of Intellectual Disability Research*, 46(1): 1–5.

Renblad, K. (2002) People with intellectual disabilities: activities, social contacts and opportunities to exert influence (an interview study with staff), *International Journal of Rehabilitation Research*, 25(4): 279–86.

Richardson, M. (2000) How we live: participatory research with six people with learning difficulties, *Journal of Advanced Nursing*, 32(6): 1383–95.

Roberts, G. (1997) Empowerment and community care: some of the legal issues, in P. Ramcharan, G. Roberts, G. Grant and J. Borland (eds) *Empowerment in Everyday Life: Learning Disabilities*. London: Jessica Kingsley.

Seebohm Report (1968) *Report of the Committee on Local Authority and Allied Personal Social Services*. London: HMSO.

Social Exclusion Unit (1998) *Bringing Britain Together: A National Strategy for Neighbourhood Renewal*. London: The Stationery Office.

Social Services Inspectorate (1991) *Care Management and Assessment: Manager's Guide*. London: HMSO.

Thomas, D. (1983) *The Making of Community Work*. London: George Allen & Unwin.

Todd, S. (2000) Working in the public and private domains: staff management of community activities for and the identities of people with intellectual disability, *Journal of Intellectual Disability Research*, 44(5): 600–20.

Todd, S., Evans, G. and Beyer, S. (1990) More recognised than known: the social visibility and attachment of people with developmental disabilities. *Australia and New Zealand Journal of Developmental Disabilities*, 16(207): 18.

Weiss, R.S. (1975) The provisions of social relationships, in Z. Rubin (ed.) *Doing Unto Others*. Englewood Cliffs, NJ: Prentice-Hall.

Weiss, R.S. (1979) The fund of sociality, *Transaction/Society*, 6(9): 36–43.

Wenger, G.C. (1992) Bangor longitudinal study of ageing, *Generations Review*, 2: 6–8.

Wenger, G.C. (1996) Social network research in gerontology: how did we get here and where do we go next? in V. Minichiello, N. Chappell, H. Kendig and A. Walker (eds) *Sociology of Aging: International Perspectives*. Melbourne: International Sociological Association.

Willmott, P. and Young, M. (1960) *Family and Class in a London Suburb*. London: Routledge & Kegan Paul.

Wilson, J. (1997) Self-help groups as a route to empowerment, in R. Jack (ed.) *Empowerment in Community Care*. London: Chapman & Hall.

PART FIVE

Ageing and end of life issues

In this final part of the book we consider ageing and end of life issues. Not so long ago, three score years and ten was a stage in life that very few people with severe learning disabilities would reach. How things have changed. Indeed a 'good old age' is something to be enjoyed by increasing numbers of people, but the chapters in this section demonstrate that it is a life stage full of creative challenges for health and social care practitioners.

In common with the last four parts of the book, Chapter 30 presents us with some more narratives, this time about older people with learning disabilities. The reader should be aware that narrative accounts of older people with learning disabilities are still relatively rare. In the right hands, such narratives offer incredibly important insights into personal histories, telling us much about the ways in which society has moulded people, what people have in turn contributed to the world around them, and how they have made sense of their lives.

Kelley Johnson shows us that life in old age can indeed be a fruitful and rich picking, for some people more meaningful than earlier life stages. It need not be marked by an inexorable physical, psychological and social decline, though losses and disabling consequences do occur. Memories and reminiscences become an increasing part of people's lives, while hopes and dreams are ever present. The experience of later life fuses the past, present and future, as if to remind us not to reduce the complexities of old age to what people are able to utter or to their typical behaviour, important though these may be. There are also reminders in this chapter about not slipping into further stereotypes about ageing. The narratives demonstrate that everyone has a story to tell, and none are the same. They provide the reader with an appreciation of:

- different explanations for reactions to earlier traumatic events in people's lives;

- the importance of mementoes to people as ways of linking the past with the present;
- long-term consequences of losses in people's lives;
- evidence of forms of resistance to challenges and deprivation that can lead to resilience;
- the importance of dreams and aspirations in later life.

Christine Bigby in Chapter 31 tells us about ways in which older people with learning disabilities adapt as they age. She focuses on the active engagement and participation of older people, demonstrating that social inclusion, one of the aims and principles of *Valuing People*, is realizable for people in later life. Drawing on a template from gerontological research, she draws attention to social relationships and subjective perceptions where belonging, continuity and purpose are critical ingredients. The chapter reminds us that an understanding of later life in people with learning disabilities can be improved by knowledge of developments in mainstream gerontology. The chapter will help the reader to understand:

- ageing and diversity in older people with learning disabilities;
- the functions of informal support for older people;
- impacts of retirement policies;
- heuristics for enriching the social relations of older people;
- ways of engaging older people more meaningfully in plans and decision-making about their own lives.

Bereavement and end of life issues are the subjects of Chapter 32. Through a series of case studies, Sheila Hollins and Irene Tuffrey-Wijne depict experiences of death, loss and bereavement in the lives of older people with learning disabilities, their families and care workers. Taboos about death and dying, often involving conspiracies of silence, are identified that can prevent older people from securing the help they need. It is shown that with sensitive, timely and coordinated support, older people with learning disabilities can be assisted to work through these challenges, as long as they are kept at the centre of decision-making. The chapter helps the reader towards an understanding of:

- the complexities of end of life decision-making;
- ethical issues that can arise in relation to consent, risk and quality of life;
- involving and informing people about their personal health and illnesses;
- acting on the presumption of capacity in decision-making;
- issues faced by all those principally involved – people with learning disabilities, families and practitioners.

Chapter 33 addresses the subject of healthy and successful ageing. Taking a cue from Chapter 31, Gordon Grant reviews ideas and theories from the gerontological literature that may help to inform a better understanding of healthy and successful ageing in people with learning disabilities. Paradoxically, it is shown that accessing health services remains problematic for many older people, and that services have much to accomplish in 'getting closer' to older people in everyday practice. Determinants of health in old age and how people make sense of their lives in later life are discussed. The practice implications of supporting healthy and successful ageing are also considered. The chapter seeks to provide the reader with an appreciation of:

- theories about healthy and successful ageing;
- the importance of life history and life span influences on later life adaptation;
- challenges for achieving 'person-centredness' in supporting older people;
- determinants of physical and mental health in later life;
- personal experiences of older people with learning disabilities.

Chapter 34, the last in this book, is quite different from all the others. Deliberately positioned at the very end, it represents an *envoi* or concluding word as well as a watershed. We have therefore left the last word to Jan Walmsley to say something about the evolution of the inclusive research agenda and how this may shape the search for knowledge in the future. It raises big questions about the ways we research the everyday lives of people with learning disabilities, and whether and how inclusive research can help to liberate people. Written at a time when agencies that fund research are seeking more meaningful ways to place research at the service of people with learning disabilities, the chapter can indeed be seen as a kind of watershed between old and new ways of thinking about the relations between research, the production of knowledge and the everyday lives of people with learning disabilities. In this chapter the reader is guided towards an understanding of:

- the genesis and evolution of inclusive research with people with learning disabilities;
- effects of the social model of disability on the development of inclusive research;
- differences between participatory and emancipatory research;
- necessary alliances in research between people with learning disabilities, academics and others.

30

A late picking
Narratives of older people with learning disabilities

Kelley Johnson

> A late picking – the old man sips his wine
> And eyes his vineyard flourishing row on row.
> Ripe clusters, hanging heavy on the vine,
> Catch the sun's afterglow.
>
> (Hope 1975)

Introduction

Sometimes the best wine comes late in the season. And for some older people with learning disabilities life may reach its fullness and its strength later in life (Bigby 2000). Of course as with wine this is not always so. It is a mistake to believe that the lives of all people with learning disabilities follow a similar trajectory. For some people increasing age may lead to a fragility that is not only physical but involves a disruption to the very foundations of their former lives (Allen *et al.* 2005a, 2005b). However, the narratives in this chapter do suggest that for some people with learning disabilities who are entering later years this period of their lives is indeed experienced as a 'late picking'. They also show the diversity of people's lived experience even when the broader context in which it occurs is similar.

As an author I feel somewhat uncomfortable about writing a chapter which documents the life narratives of people with learning disabilities. Surely they can speak for themselves? Many can. However, access to editors, to publishers and to the written word remain problematic for many people with learning disabilities who have a story to tell. This may be particularly true for older people who have sometimes had less access to formal education and fewer opportunities to be heard. Others find articulating their experience in spoken or written ways very difficult or impossible. This chapter provides a space for some of these voices to be heard. It also provides a place where questions can be asked about people's lives and where the role of a researcher who works with people with learning disabilities can be explored and made subject to questions.

Where do the narratives come from?

The life narratives which make up a substantial part of this chapter have been contributed by three different people with whom I have worked over the past ten years. It is important to explore how they were written and in what circumstances, and in particular the role which I played in their production. The position of the writer in what are originally largely oral narratives is important because it can shape the way people's stories are told and the way in which they are documented. Each of these narratives is accompanied by a short commentary and by a series of questions for reflection. One of the narratives in this chapter is essentially a case study while the others are autobiographical accounts or autobiographies (Walmsley and Atkinson 2000). They come from two different research studies which are briefly described below.

Deinstitutionalizing women

'In the early 1990s I spent 20 months in a locked unit in a large Australian institution for people with learning disabilities' (Johnson 1998a, 1998b). Twenty-one women lived in the unit and all had been labelled as having learning disabilities and challenging behaviour. They ranged in age from early twenties to 72 years old and they had had very diverse life experiences. However, it was difficult to find ways to discover or to tell their life narratives. Many of them were not able to tell their stories directly, others remembered only fragments.

Lena Johnson's narrative which is included in this chapter was developed by talking with her over time, reading her files, observing what her life was like in the locked unit and talking with staff about her. Lena found it difficult to talk about her life in any extended way but did make very clear some of the things she had done and the nature of her preferences. Unlike some of the other women I was not able to talk with her family as they were banned from seeing her. I did not show Lena the account I wrote of her life because it was completed after she had left the institution and because it would have been very difficult for her to make sense of a narrative presented in this fashion. I continue to feel somewhat uncomfortable about this. The words in Lena's story are mine although I use quotes from her and from her institutional files to develop what is essentially a case study.

Living safer sexual lives

This was a large action research study in which 25 people with learning disabilities talked with researchers over an extended period of time about their lives (Johnson *et al.* 2000; Harrison *et al.* 2002; Frawley *et al.* 2003; Walmsley and Johnson 2003). The study had a strong focus on relationships and sexuality and the narratives in this chapter reflect this emphasis, but we were committed to a view that these issues were part of people's lives and needed to be seen within the context of how they lived. A total of 13 women and 12 men agreed to contribute their stories. I met with the woman whose narrative is included in this chapter for several hours at her home over three different visits. We talked together about her life and with her permission I taped our discussion. At the end of each session I transcribed the tape and talked with a colleague about it. I then reflected on the experience and used this to start the next discussion. At the conclusion of the sessions the transcribed tapes were written into a story using only Margaret's own words.

The story was necessarily shortened. It was taken back to Margaret and read to her. She did not want to make changes to it and was happy for it to be published. She had the right at any time up to the final approval of the story to withdraw it and she was encouraged to make any changes that she might want to in relation to it. The same process was used by the man who worked with men with learning disabilities who were involved in the project. The third narrative in this chapter was contributed by one of the men in the study.

Exercise 30.1

Developing narratives which are not the direct written words of the person concerned is always problematic because the writer's attitudes, views and concerns may determine what is included. Reflect on the two ways in which narratives were gathered for this chapter. What differences might you expect to see in the style and content that might be due to the way they are gathered?

Narratives usually exclude people who are not able to tell their story. Consequently we often only hear directly from some people and not at all from others. What kinds of method can be used so that people who are not able to converse with others can also be heard?

The position of the researcher and writer is important. I am an Anglo-Australian woman in my middle years. I work as an academic and as an advocate with people with disabilities. How might these characteristics influence the way I collaborate with people with learning disabilities who are contributing narratives? Think about yourself. What characteristics might impact on work you might do with people with learning disabilities either in direct service provision or in research?

Some people with learning disabilities feel very strongly about the 'ownership' of information about them. How far do you think these narratives are owned by

> the people who contributed them in one way or another? How far do you think that they are really 'my' stories as the writer?

Lena Johnson: 'Lena is all ready'

'Lena's probably always been like this and she's too old to change' (staff member in the locked unit).

Lena lived in a locked unit within a large institution when I met her. She was aged 72. She was a short sturdy woman who was extremely physically fit. Each day she would arrive in the room where the women spent most of their days, carefully dressed, most often in a pleated skirt and a matching grey and red jumper. Her short grey hair was always carefully combed. She sat primly on the vinyl couch with her feet together and her hands in her lap. Unlike the other women in the unit, her front teeth had not been removed. She was a very sociable woman with a loud voice and a constant flow of conversation that referred to herself always in the third person. ('Lena is all ready. She has her good clothes on.') Until she was 64 she had lived with her mother in the wider community. She spoke often of her mother who was 100 years old and lived in a nursing home where Lena visited her on a fortnightly basis. Sometimes she talked about her former home and the vegetable garden, her visits to the races and the card games with her mother's friends. She was highly skilled, could cook, clean, ride a bicycle and knew the basics of driving a car (though she did not have a licence).

When Lena's mother became ill she was sent to the institution on the doctor's advice. At first she was in an open unit with other older women. Although staff recorded that she was kind to these women for the first few months she had little in common with them. All were frail, many could not speak and none had her kinds of skills. After some time there were staff reports that Lena was attacking the other women in the unit and that she had 'dirty habits'. As a result she was moved to the locked unit where she lived for four years. She had very limited capacity within the locked unit to exercise any of her skills although sometimes she assisted staff in folding the clean clothes. Lena very much enjoyed knitting but staff only allowed her to do this on rare occasions because she had attacked some other women in the unit with the knitting needles. There were no books or magazines in the unit. She could not go outside except on twice-weekly walks in the grounds. She had no friends in the unit.

In the locked unit, she would frequently climb through the windows in an effort to escape. Staff would watch her in amusement and then go out to fetch her back. She collected small items from other women in the unit or from staff and hid them carefully, in her bed, her clothes and her shoes. Sometimes she left a neat pile of faeces behind the couch in the day room.

In the years since her admission to the institution she had been on large doses of largactil and melleril which had been stopped by staff in the locked unit. She was now the only woman there who was not on some form of tranquillizer. During the closure of the institution there was much discussion about Lena's future.

There was general consensus among staff in the locked unit that she should go into the community. However, regional staff who would be responsible for supporting her there refused to accept her and she was matched to a large metropolitan institution. Advocacy by one staff member and myself prevented this and she was eventually matched to a community residential unit in the country where there was less demand for places. The locked unit was closed relatively early in the institutional closure process and Lena with other women was moved to another unit with different staff and additional residents. At this time her mother died unexpectedly.

Lena attended the funeral and then visited her former home for the last time. Staff who accompanied her helped her to dig up some rhubarb roots as a lasting memory of her former life. She had no photographs and no other mementoes. The house was sold.

Commentary

Becoming older inevitably means loss of many different kinds: relationships, work and sometimes home. In the space of eight years, Lena had lost a whole way of life, her family, the less restricted lifestyle in the open unit and then what passed as her home within the locked unit. Finally her mother died.

Lena's reactions to these traumatic life events were interpreted by those around her as due to her intellectual disability and 'challenging behaviour'. Another way of looking at her reactions may be to see them in terms of a grief-filled response to very traumatic life events by someone who was not able to articulate her emotional reactions in words and who had nobody who understood her feelings (Sinason 1992).

A different perspective again may be to regard her behaviour as one form of resistance to the position in which she had been placed. Her behaviour can then be seen as a way of attempting unconsciously or consciously to change the situation in which she found herself and as a way of escaping from it (Nind and Johnson unpublished).

For all of us, but particularly for many older people, the memories of a past life, reminiscences and the presence of photographs and mementoes are important ways of linking present and past experience. Lena had nothing. Her 64 years in the community were negated and did not impact on decisions about her future life in which she had little decision-making power.

Unlike many other older people with learning disabilities, Lena had spent most of her life in the community. With brief exceptions, when she was admitted to respite care, she had lived with her mother and had had a relatively 'ordinary life'. However, once her mother became ill and old, institutional care was seen as the only solution for her living arrangements. In her case it was a large institution. However, other older people with disabilities may find themselves placed in nursing home care or at constant risk of reinstitutionalization (West 2000; Allen *et al.* 2005b). Once she was labelled as having challenging behaviours it was very difficult for Lena to leave the institution even though it could be argued that these may have been in part a result of her institutionalization.

Exercise 30.2

The professional training we receive provides us with ways of seeing the world. Sometimes this can lead us to ignore or neglect important aspects of people's lives that lie outside our professional focus. How do you think the professional training of the people working with Lena may have limited their ability to relate to her?

If you were working with Lena, what changes would you have wanted to make to her life circumstances that might have enabled her to have a better quality of life?

What strategies would you use to work with someone on loss issues, particularly if they found it difficult to tell you about them?

Margaret Crowley: 'I wanted it real nice . . . not sex like that'

I'm 57. I live in Broadmeadows. I live by myself. I do cooking and that. Cleaning up a bit and all that. I do it on my own. Sometimes Tim comes over and helps me.

He lives down at Altona. I've been in this flat since October. Before that I've been all over the place. I couldn't share with anybody any more because things happen. I couldn't share with people because they used to get upset or things like that or eat my food off my plate. And wear my clothes.

I go out to work at the neighbourhood house. Part-time job cleaning. I'm on the committee. I go out and teach about legal rights and I'm on the board of an advocacy group. I do art and I do reading and writing. I'm going to be involved with Stepping Out, a new advocacy group. That will be next year probably. We're going to have a conference. I'm always out.

Dad went to war and mum couldn't look after us. I didn't know she had a disability. He came back from the war. But I thought he went to war and didn't come back. I only remember him when he used to come back from war. He used to lift me up in the air. I was taken away when I was two years old. Two years old I was taken away. We all got split up. Tim, me, Pearl, Maree, Jimmy, May. I went into a convent and I was only there for a little while and then I got sent away from my sister and I went to the Manor House. And I went to school there.

It was alright. We used to have dates, Irish dancing, the bishop came.

We had parties and all that. We had a holiday house down at the beach. And we used to have stars. Stars, like if you were tidy or things like that or you did it good. You got a star and then you got a prize. And then we used to have church and say the rosary and all that.

I knew I had a mother but I used to cry every night and all that. I had jobs. I couldn't keep jobs. I used to mind children, two children and clean up the place and things like that. I used to come out and go to this lady's place. And the lady said 'Oh you're a good worker.' But I was getting sick, I was getting tired. I used to lay on the bed and go to sleep. I was only a teenager, 16 or 17. I was crying and bumping my head against the wall. And the nuns said, 'Oh you're playing up.' And I used to never go to bed. I used to sleep on the floor and the next morning I used to get up and all that. I used to run down the paddock with no shoes on.

And I was starting to get sick. 'Cause I wanted me mum. She didn't visit me until I was about 14. We all went into this big party and I didn't know my mum was there and two brothers. Big brother and little brother. And I didn't know. And she came over and I remember that it was me mum and all that. And then I went over to one of the nuns, 'That's my mum, that's my mum.' And I threw my arms around her and started to cry. And then dad, my stepfather was there. My stepfather said, 'Come on, come on come and sit by me.' And all the girls were sitting around looking and all that and we were talking and he gave me a kiss on the head. And then it was time to go. So we all went separate ways and I turned back and start looking and all that. They had gone. And then I started to get sick.

At the Manor House I used to work in the kitchen and things like that. The nuns put me away. Because I just wanted me mum. Because I was running away. From the Manor House. Going to people's places. I run to a shop and the lady said, 'Oh where do you come from?' I said I came from the Manor House and so she gave me a drink of water and rang the Manor House up. The nuns came and I went back with them.

They didn't tell me they were going to put me in Hillside [an institution for people with intellectual disabilities]. They put me in this infirmary. And it was small with about four beds. And I used to sleep on the floor. I wouldn't sleep on the bed. I used to sleep on the floor. And the doctor came and said why is she sleeping on the floor. 'Oh she wants to.' And the doctor gave me a needle in the leg so I wouldn't run away and I had to have a shower and they packed my case. Some of the clothes in it wasn't belonging to me. And so they packed my case and didn't tell me where I was going. And we got in, I think it was a taxi. I can't remember. And one nun sat on one side and one on the other side so I wouldn't jump out. How can I jump out because I was all dopey?

I went to Stony Glen [psychiatric hospital] and the two nuns went inside and I was sitting out in reception. The two nuns came out and said, 'Oh good-bye good-bye' and left me. And left me there. And I had to go in this big dormitory and I was crying. I had to get undressed. And they were having supper. And I was crying. And the doctor came and I wouldn't look at him. I was under the blankets and wouldn't look at him. And the doctor asked me a few things.

'Oh what . . . oh do you hear voices?' I said 'No I don't hear no voices. I miss my mum.' So after that he went off. And the next morning I had to have shock treatment. Shock treatment. 'Cause I was doing all these things and that. Laying down and running away and laying on the ground. So after that I had shock treatment, not all at once, now and again. I was getting a lot better.

The nuns only came to see me about twice that's all and then they didn't come back. They didn't want me back. So then the doctors said, 'You're going to a nice ward you're going to Hillside. Going into a nice ward. Going into an open ward.'

And so I went in the bus and that. And they said, 'Look over there. You're going right up on that hill.' So I went there and I had to go and see all these doctors and they asked me questions and things like that and I had to go to the receiving ward. I was there for a couple of months. I can't remember how long. And then I stayed down there and they decided to shift me. To F28. That was up the top [of the hill]. I was upset I wouldn't eat me meals and wouldn't come inside for the staff. I used to lay out in the yard and six or more staff used to drag me inside. I used to go right out in the yard but I wouldn't move and this staff sister said, 'Well get her inside.' I wouldn't come inside. So I didn't have no food. But when the sister came out I used to go in for her. I wouldn't go in for the nurses. And then when she didn't come on duty they used to drag me inside and shove the food in my mouth and things like that. I used to tear my clothes up. Smash windows and all that. Smash windows and tear clothes. And they used to put me, drag me in a single room and no clothes on and there was a bar thing on the window.

Then I started to get better. Because me mum started to come. She started visiting me. Because she used to visit Tim my brother. But I didn't know. I didn't know he was there.

She didn't know that I was up there. And the sisters and nurses didn't tell her, didn't tell me mum. So Pearl me sister was up there too. And she had a boyfriend. And that's how I got to know how my brother was there. Pearl had a boyfriend and over the fence we used to talk to the boys. So that's how I found out. And then I called out, 'Are you really my brother?' And he said 'Yes.' So I had this long dress on; no shoes on.

My hair wasn't done properly and that. Then he went back and told the staff. And the staff must have rung up the ward that I was in. And they said yes there is two Crowleys. And then she started coming.

I was in Hillside for 25 years. I worked there. I worked there, scrubbed floors, made beds, swept floors, scrubbed all the skirting boards. If it wasn't done properly you had to do it again. Things like that. We didn't get paid for work. If you gave someone a meal you got punished. A nurse lost her ring and we all got punished. Weren't allowed to talk in the day room. Weren't allowed to go to bed.

I went and saw the social worker and said I want to get out. I was scared at first. So I had a lot of chances to go out. I didn't take them. Then this lady came and she said do you want to go to Mayberry House and I said, 'Oh yeah I want to go to Mayberry House.' It was a halfway house and all that. So I wanted to go. I was a bit nervous and they said goodbye and all that. Tim was there. He was out. Tim was out at the time. I was sitting there thinking 'what am I going to do?' Sitting down and me brother came in. 'What am I going to do?' 'Do you want to go out?' And I said, 'Oh yes I want to go out.' Live it all up. I was drinkin'. Tim used to work and things like that. We used to have big jugs of beer and all that.

We used to be upset. We come out of Hillside. I mean we used to drown our sorrows. We used to drink and all that. We hadn't done it before and things like that. And Mayberry House was terrible. Oh I was sick. I had to see what do you call it a psychiatrist. He didn't say much. I was scared of him. I was scared of this lady on the staff. Oh she used to bang on the table and all. Oh she shouted at me. She didn't hit people. She used to dope me up and things like that.

After Mayberry House I went to some people from Hillside. I used to look after them and feed them cause they couldn't do that. I thought I wasn't going to look after them. I didn't want to. I said, 'I'm not going to stay here.' So we all went to our separate house. I went by myself. I went by myself with this other girl. She had psych problems. She got this carving knife. She nearly hurt me. I said, 'I'm not going to stay here. I'm not staying here.'

One minute she was all right and the next minute she was orf. So I never used to come home. I used to go out and I didn't come back. I lived in lots of different places. Now I live on my own.

I was in Stony Glen and they had dances and things like that in Stony Glen. And I went over by myself to the dance and met this boy and that and then he took me over to the dance, went behind the tree I was scared. He put his thing, you know his penis, out and I got scared and I ran away. And I said, 'Oh oh' and I ran back and I told the staff and staff said, 'Don't go there any more.' Down to the dance.

I must have been about 18. I didn't really know what he wanted. I was scared 'cause it was my first time 'cause I was in the convent. I knew nothing about sex. Because I came from the convent. And came out and didn't know.

Staff didn't talk to us about sex. But like when I was in Hillside I can't remember now but they showed a video about babies, babies coming out and all that. The staff used to get off with other residents up there. It was awful. Well I was working in the laundry and one of the staff said to me, 'Come on, come into my car and we'll go . . .' But I didn't get into his car.

Well at Hillside I went down the paddock, down the paddock, I went down the paddock. With a bloke who lived in one of the other units. First we went to the dance. At Hillside. You were allowed to dance with him and that. We went down there to the paddock. 'Cause you didn't have any privacy. Weren't allowed to go in people's rooms. He took me clothes off. He took me clothes off and things like that and I said, 'Oh geez.' And I went looking down looking to see if anyone was coming. 'Cause I got scared. So then the bloke was laying on top of me. And he wouldn't get off me. He wouldn't get off. I said, 'Get off me. Get off me.' I started putting me clothes back on. He wouldn't get off me. I wanted it real nice but not sex like that. So I told him you know get off me. But he wouldn't get off me. I saw him after that. I was dancing with him and that. I didn't really want to dance with him.

The other bloke I met. He was quite nice. He lived at Hillside too. He was quite nice. We went into the toilet and we had condoms. He had it on. He went to do it and it snapped. So he said, 'I'm not going to do it again.' So we didn't do it any more. He got scared. And then another time I went into his room we had sex. He got scared of the staff. So I got into bed but we didn't do anything because of the staff. I writ a letter, stupid me writ a letter to him and the staff got it. We weren't allowed to see each other any more. He said to me 'cause he was getting out he said to me, 'Oh can you get out 'cause I'm getting out.' He said, 'Well you don't ask you'll be in there forever.' That's what he said and that. But I didn't go out.

When I got out I met this man in Carlton. We got engaged. And everything was going all right. He used to come to Mayberry House and see me. I had an engagement party. Things like that. I was going to get married. I was looking forward to it. He was going to move out of that place and go to a cleaner place. Then a dreadful thing happened. Part of it was I didn't know what I was doing. It was another bloke, and me boyfriend and they got stuck into me. They didn't rape me. I can't remember now it was so long ago. I got sick and things like that. They didn't beat me up. They did sex to me. I was so upset. I was drunk. They were gentle.

And then the boyfriend said, 'Oh you knew all about that didn't you?' I didn't see him any more. I felt terrible. And I wasn't engaged any more.

Later I got engaged again you know. He was all right. But he went off with me flatmate. I don't think he loved me very much. Well he didn't sit by me he didn't sit next to me at the train. He sat somewhere else. He didn't hang on to me hand.

And things like that. He didn't give me a bed. He made me sleep on the floor. Yeah on the floor, on the couch. He didn't give me his bed. We had intercourse a couple of times. We had a good relationship. He used to come over for weekends and things like that.

I wanted somebody like I've got now, like I've got now. A nice one now. And we go out together and he stays here for weekends and all things like that. He touches me first and things like that. See the blokes I go with you know. They just want sex I think. Dave's all right. But the others yeah.

I met Dave down at Coburg. Near the station and he asked me. To be his you know girlfriend. And I said, 'Yes.' I thought I'd chance it. He was on his bike. I thought I'd give him a chance. I don't want it to be like the others. He cares about me. He helps with housework. Sometimes he'll cook for me. And I'll cook for him and we'll share. We didn't have intercourse straight away. We have intercourse now and again. I won't have it without a condom and he says that's all right. I want to get married. We want to get married in the gardens. I'm just thinking about getting married. We've been together nearly seven weeks I think. He stayed the last week. The weekend. It was all right. He helped me cook and that and those things were good.

I couldn't have children. Too old. Must have been about 39 or something. 'Cause I got out of Hillside then. I didn't have children I didn't have a chance to and I love children. I used to look after children in Hillside. Taught them how to sweep the floor how to make the beds when they were small.

Commentary

Supporting Margaret to tell her story was a very emotional experience for me. At many levels her story is bleak. The losses of relationships and lifestyle that many of us experience as we get older happened for her in early life. This was true for many people with learning disabilities who experienced early institutionalization. The loss of her family, particularly her mother, wounded her deeply and this experience has left scars that she still carries into her later years. For Margaret this loss explains much of her later behaviour which was interpreted by those around her as either 'mad' or 'challenging'. Like many women with learning disabilities Margaret was denied any of the stereotypical roles of adult women, as worker, lover or mother (Asch and Fine 1988, 1992; Johnson and Traustadottir 2000). Yet in some ways her life was also a distorted mirror of the lives of often poor women in the wider community: hard unpaid (or poorly paid) work, caring for children (though not her own) and those in need, and few opportunities for creative leisure. However, for her there were not the intimate adult relationships, the links with family and friends that other women may find as part of their lives. For her these came later. Bleak though her story is, there is also a resilience in her resistance to her negative life experiences and a real joy now in her later life. A flat of her own, peace and meaningful activities. These things are accompanied by a hope that the future may offer a loving relationship. It is as if the expectations of early adulthood have been pushed into older life: a late picking indeed.

Exercise 30.3

Margaret's story is rich in detail and memory. Her life is an important whole for her as she gets older. Yet in many instances we fail to take account of the memories and experiences of people with learning disabilities. What difference does it make to our perceptions of people if we see them as having a past and memories?

How do we balance the understanding of the person that comes from knowing their past, their memories and their dreams with the need for them to have privacy?

What interventions if any would you have wanted to make to Margaret's life to support her in leading 'an ordinary life' in her younger years?

Derek Housemann: 'I would have been a different person'

I have three brothers and sisters. I'm the youngest. I still keep in touch with them. They ring me up now and then at home and have the odd conversation and normal routine things, see if everything is okay. My dad went to the war. So I didn't see him at all. He never made it home.

I went to a home when I was only a small boy, about 5 or 6 or maybe 8 or 9. Mother was very fragile, very old and she had got to the stage where she couldn't look after me any more. And not only that. I became ill one night and she couldn't look after me. I needed a lot of training. I needed a lot of training and supervision. And I needed a lot of looking after. I couldn't do nothing for myself.

And I had trouble dressing myself, showering myself, making my bed. And I couldn't provide my meals and do dishes and things like that.

I went to Bridgestone Boys Training Centre [an institution for people with learning disabilities] in the country. Then they got me some more skills and some more training sort of thing. I was one of the youngest of the lot. Ah Bridgestone, well I'd hope that a lot of things would have improved a lot really, there was a lot of bullying that went on there. But it happened during the night, not during the day. Bullying means when you're being treated badly, like you've got more than one boy involved. You've got one guy punching you, another guy kickin' you and another guy pullin' your hair out. They didn't do it to anyone else. It was about sexual issues with men. And I was the one who copped it all and I didn't like that treatment. I thought 'this is ruining my life, what the hell is goin' on?' I sort of had to stand up. They thought the best way for me is not stay there any more because they didn't like the way I was being treated. So I had to move from there to Hillside [another institution for people with learning disabilities].

I lived in Hillside for nine years. I tried to get away. Because of the treatment I was coppin'. Bullyin' and the meals I didn't like. But I didn't have any luck. I was brought back. Some [of the staff] were good and some were bad. But I think the only time they were good to you was when you cooperated with them.

At Hillside males weren't allowed to hang around the female wards. If they were caught they would be punished. And the punishment would be [to be] doped up with medicine every night, locked in a single room, a vacant room. Even if you went to the pictures at night, like they used to have pictures in the concert hall of a night time, the males weren't allowed to go there on their own. They had to go in a group with about two staff members. And when they got to the concert hall all females had to sit on one side and males the other. They weren't to be trusted during the movies.

At Hillside there's a mortuary where they keep the dead bodies right. Behind that mortuary there's an old shack. Behind that old shack was another old building. Myself and a female went for a walk one day down behind there and we started talking. She told me a little bit about how she'd got into this relationship when she was young. I told her mine. She took a liking to me you know and we became good friends and then she started rubbing my back. She touched several parts of my body and she said I'd like you to have a sexual relationship with me . . . we got caught. Well she got locked up as punishment and the same thing applied to me. Never saw her again. I was very annoyed because I felt they were taking our rights away. When you moved out of the institution you had to be careful because moving out from an institution to the outside community and living in a private accommodation place like that you had to respect the needs of other people.

After I left Hillside I moved around a bit. Now we live on our own in a house. Me and another disabled person and we do things to help one another.

I would have been a different person had I not been put away in those institutions. I wouldn't have done a lot of different things. I had no say in those things. It was a bit heartbreaking but I just couldn't do nothing about it. But over the last couple of years it's been a new ball game, there's been a big improvement and things. There's been a lot of change. In people's attitudes, people's sense of humour, people's manners.

I work for a self-advocacy group that helps promote the rights of people with learning disabilities. It's great work and I've been involved with lots of issues and I've been out and about in country areas and spread the word on learning disability.

I have heaps of friends. I'd try and forget the past if I could. Leave all that behind me and just keep thinking of the future. Hope that one day I might become a father. Maybe move into a house on the Gold Coast. Settle down, maybe pick up a young lass, start all over again. But I would do different things. It wouldn't be so hectic or heavy. I would do different things that I would be able to do like say I'm a father now, I've got my own children. I would concentrate on the children, the house, the wife, the family. But as far as jobs are concerned no. It wouldn't be as important.

Commentary

For Derek, as for the other two people in this chapter, institutionalization played an important part in shaping how he sees himself and also how he now views the world around him. Not all older people with learning disabilities had this experience. Like Lena, many lived with their parents in the community and some managed to sustain relatively independent lives even without services to support them. However, my work with older people with learning disabilities over the past ten years suggests that institutions were a feature in many of their lives, either because they had lived in them or because there was a possibility of doing so. Derek does not have very much to say that is positive about institutional life. His experiences of sexual and physical abuse reflect research which reveals that men and women with learning disabilities have high rates of the experience of sexual abuse (McCarthy 1999, 2000). Derek is articulate about his experience in institutions. While he comments that some staff were good, his perception is that this was conditional on compliance by the residents in the institution. He expresses regrets about both a missed life and also actions for which he was responsible. He is clear and definite about seeing institutionalization as the main reason for these regrets.

Independence and meaningful work are important for Derek as he gets older. He is experiencing a 'late picking' in which his life is more open and interesting and he is experiencing a positive change in attitudes towards him by other community members. He sees this as important. Part of his late picking is the dreaming of other life possibilities. These dreams are an important part of his life. They are dreams which are easily recognizable by all of us: intimate and loving relationships, a nice place to live and children to love and care for. Yet they are the dreams for many people of a younger adulthood. Both Derek and Margaret are experiencing them in later life.

Exercise 30.4

What differences and similarities do you find between Derek's experience and that of Margaret and Lena? How important do you think gender is in shaping the way these people have lived their lives?

'Tread softly for you tread on my dreams': how can we support people to turn dreams into reality? What is our responsibility when working with them to know about these dreams and to help achieve them?

What do you think these people learned from institutional life? In what ways were these experiences the same or different to their lives in the community?

Conclusion

A late picking. For some people with learning disabilities later life can be richer and more meaningful than their earlier lives. This is particularly true for those people who are now entering later life. The hope is that the dreams and hopes that they are carrying into their older years are ones that can be achieved more readily by younger people now.

The narratives in this chapter reveal how important the personal construction of a life is as we get older. Margaret and Derek speak from within their lives. There are memories, dreams, hopes and wounds. They see their lives as ordinary. They are not victims to themselves but people who are seeking meaning and love in their lives. In contrast, Lena's narrative comes from the outside. I did not know what motivated her nor what her dreams and fears were. I could make inferences about this; guess between the lines. As a result her narrative is less internal, less real. Yet many of us work with people who find it difficult to articulate their past and their dreams. We need to be aware constantly that 'not being able to say it' does not mean that the person's inner world does not exist. We need to act and relate always on the assumption that it is there.

As people grow older their experience of life also extends and memories and reminiscences become increasingly a part of their lives. A failure on the part of those around them to value or to learn about these things reduces the complexity of an individual to a snapshot of current behaviour. Nor should we assume that because people are growing older they are ceasing to dream of what might still be in their lives. For people who have been denied many of the experiences that those without a disability take for granted, such dreams may focus on newly-opened possibilities. For others the dreams may be different. To be aware of the reality of dreams for individuals can shift the way we work with them, making our responses more exciting and stimulating and changing the way we see both 'older people' and those with disabilities.

Note

This project was funded by the Victorian Health Promotion Foundation and was undertaken at the Australian Institute for Sex Health and Society at La Trobe University, Melbourne. I would like to acknowledge the other principal researchers on this project: Dr Lynne Hillier and Dr Lyn Harrison.

References

Allen, T., Traustadottir, R. and Spina, L. (2005a) It's never too late, in K. Johnson and R. Traustadottir (eds) *In and Out of Institutions: Deinstitutionalisation and People with Intellectual Disabilities*. London: Jessica Kingsley.

Allen, T., Traustadottir, R. and Spina, L. (2005b) A home before I die? in K. Johnson and R. Traustadottir (eds) *In and Out Of Institutions: Deinstituionalisation and People with Intellectual Disabilities*. London: Jessica Kingsley.

Asch, A. and Fine, M. (1988) Introduction: beyond pedestals, in M. Fine and A. Asch (eds) *Women with Disabilities: Essays in Psychology, Culture and Politics*. Philadelphia, PA: Temple University Press.

Asch, A. and Fine, M. (1992) Beyond pedestals: revisiting the lives of women with disabilities, in M. Fine (ed.) *Disruptive Voices: The Possibilities of Feminist Research*. Ann Arbor, MI: University of Michigan Press.

Bigby, C. (2000) *Moving on Without Parents: Planning, Transitions and Sources of Support for Middle-Aged and Older Adults with Intellectual Disability*. Eastgardens: McLennan and Petty.

Frawley, P., Johnson, K., Hillier, L. and Harrison, L. (2003) *Living Safer Sexual Lives: A Training and Resource Pack for People with Learning Disabilities and Those Who Support Them*. Brighton: Pavilion.

Harrison, L., Johnson, K., Hillier, L. and Strong, R. (2002) Nothing about us without us: the ideals and realities of participatory action research with people with an intellectual disability, *Scandinavian Journal of Intellectual Disability Research*, 5(2): 56–70.

Hope, A.D. (1975) *A Late Picking*. London: Angus & Robertson.

Johnson, K. (1998a) *Deinstitutionalising Women: An Ethnographic Study of Institutional Closure*. Melbourne: Cambridge University Press.

Johnson, K. (1998b) Deinstitutionalisation: the management of rights, *Disability and Society*, 13(3): 375–87.

Johnson, K. and Traustadottir, R. (2000). Finding a place, in R. Traustadottir and K. Johnson (eds) *Women with Intellectual Disabilities: Finding a Place in the World*. London: Jessica Kingsley.

Johnson, K., Hillier, L., Harrison, L. and Frawley, P. (2000) *People with Intellectual Disabilities: Living Safer Sexual Lives*. Melbourne: Australian Research Centre in Sex, Health and Society, La Trobe University.

McCarthy, M. (1999) *Sexuality and Women with Learning Disabilities*. London: Jessica Kingsley.

McCarthy, M. (2000) Consent, abuse and choices, in R. Traustadottir and K. Johnson (eds) *Women with Intellectual Disabilities: Finding a Place in the World*. London: Jessica Kingsley.

Nind, M. and Johnson, K. (unpublished manuscript) *Listening not Labelling: Changing the Discourse of Challenging and Stereotyped Behaviour*.

Sinason, V. (1992) *Mental Handicap and the Human Condition: New Approaches from the Tavistock*. London: Free Association Books.

Walmsley, J. and Atkinson, D. (2000) Oral history and the history of learning disability, in J. Bornat *et al. Health Welfare and Oral History*. London: Routledge.

Walmsley, J. and Johnson, K. (2003) *Inclusive Research with People with Learning Disabilities*. London: Jessica Kingsley.

West, R. (2000) Finding a sister, in R. Traustadottir and K. Johnson (eds) *Women with Intellectual Disabilities: Finding a Place in the World*. London: Jessica Kingsley.

31

Growing old

Adapting to change and realizing a sense of belonging, continuity and purpose

Christine Bigby

Introduction

Increased life expectancy during the last 50 years means that ageing has become an integral part of the lifecourse for people with intellectual disability. The experience of ageing is shaped by each individual's unique biography, the historic time through which they have lived and their current social context. As knowledge about later life for people with intellectual disability increases, many of the individual changes and the altered social context and expectations should be anticipated. Responses and adaptations to ensure continued citizenship can be planned. Presently, however, some commentators suggest that old age is more likely to pose threats to an individual's sense of continuity, belonging and purpose rather than being celebrated as a valued achievement (Thompson 2002; Bigby 2004). The aim of this chapter is to consider why this might be so and how these tendencies might be countered.

The theme of this chapter is the continued active engagement and participation of older people with intellectual disabilities in social relationships and the achievement of a lifestyle in which the critical ingredients are a sense of belonging, continuity and purpose. While such domains are found in conceptualizations of the quality of life, the notion of achieving a 'sense of' is drawn from a framework developed by Nolan *et al.* (2001). This framework emphasizes the subjective and perceptual nature of experiences and what might constitute a 'good life' for an older person. I chose to focus on these aspects, not to downplay the critical role of health in the ageing process but to draw attention to the importance of social relationships and subjective perceptions in complementing good health in the achievement of well-being in later life.

Individuals derive their sense of belonging from meaningful relationships with family and friends and by being part of a neighbourhood or community of interest. A sense of continuity highlights an individual's connection with his or her past, the pre-existing and sometimes lifelong interests, relationships, health and lifestyle that accompany him or her on their journey into old age. A sense of purpose is achieved via opportunities to exercise choice and pursue one's own goals and chosen activities.

Belonging, continuity and purpose are subjective outcomes that stem from the principles of rights, independence, choice and inclusion that inform policy and guide a vision of aspirations for the lives of people with intellectual disabilities of all ages (Department of Health 2001). Interpreting and implementing these principles poses some different dilemmas at this latter stage of the lifecourse. This chapter examines these challenges and the changing social contexts – expectations, family roles and composition, service structures and policy directions – that impact on people with intellectual disability as they age.

Ageing and diversity

With the exception of people with Down's syndrome and those with profound and multiple disabilities, the life expectancy of people with intellectual disability is now more similar to that of the general population than ever before. Research in the USA suggests that the population life expectancy from birth is 70.1 years compared to 66.1 years for all groups with intellectual disability except those with Down's syndrome, for whom it is 55.8 years (Janicki *et al.* 1999). Unlike the general population, gender differences in life expectancy for people with intellectual disability have not been widely explored. A common stereotypical view is that people with intellectual disability age prematurely. This view stems from the widely acknowledged premature ageing processes experienced by people with Down's syndrome and the use by researchers of younger definitions to ensure that this group is not excluded from studies of ageing. A trend towards countering this stereotype of premature ageing is the adoption of the more conventional age of 60 years in relation to people with intellectual disability (Hogg and Lambe 2000; Grant 2001).

UK estimates suggest that 12 per cent of the population with severe intellectual disability is 60 years or over, approximately 25,000 people (Hogg and Lambe 2000; Department of Health 2001). In Australia, the proportion is generally smaller at around 6 per cent (Bigby 2004). Two demographic trends are clear:

- the number and proportion of older people with intellectual disability is increasing and will continue to do so until after the 'baby boomer' generation moves into later life;
- the absolute numbers of older people with intellectual disability are small, and they form a very small proportion of both the general older population and of those with intellectual disability.

If 60 years marks the start of old age, the years to come might be thought of as categories. For example, the 'younger old' are often differentiated from the 'old old' or the 'frail aged', or the 'third age' from the 'fourth age' (Laslett 1989). The third age, during the sixties and early seventies, is a period when people are more likely to be relatively fit and active and, having retired from work, seek other roles and activities to gain a sense of purpose. The fourth age, during the mid-seventies onwards is more likely to be characterized by fragility, declining health and consequent restrictions on activity and community participation. The majority of older people with intellectual disabilities are, at the moment, among the younger old rather than the old old group (i.e. the third rather than the fourth age category). Each cohort of older people will have lived through a different historic time and have been influenced by that unique combination of changing attitudes, policies and social conditions that characterizes their generation. The significance of cohort is highlighted for people with intellectual disabilities currently in their sixties, born between 1940 and 1950. They and their families have experienced remarkable shifts in attitudes and responses to disability, from a focus on segregation and protection to one of inclusion and community support. As the narratives in Chapter 30 illustrate, some of the current cohort of older people, unlike those born in the last two decades, will have spent much of their lives in large-scale congregate living, only moving out in mid and later life as institutions have been closed. Such experiences have a lasting impact on connections to family, community and to one's own life history. For example, people with intellectual disabilities who have remained at home with parents have stronger relationships with family members in later life than those who left home at an earlier age (Skeie 1989; Bigby 1997a). Moving from an institution can threaten an individual's sense of continuity unless the essence of both formal and informal institutional records and stories of their past life are captured and also transferred with them to the community. Various examples are found, however, where institutional closure has acted as a catalyst in reconnecting individuals to their past or in rediscovering family members (Green and Wunsch 1994; West 2000).

Older people with an intellectual disability are a diverse group, in regard to health, ability, connections with family and friends, service use patterns and the individual impact of the ageing process. Prevailing attitudes and the design of services will be influenced by culture as well as by nation-specific policies. Nevertheless, as a group, older people with intellectual disability have a number of things in common. They:

- age at a similar rate to the general population, and have a slightly reduced life span compared to the general population (there are however, some notable exceptional sub-groups such as people with Down's syndrome; Evenhuis *et al.* 2001);
- have high risk factors associated with ill health, particularly related to lifestyle such as exercise, diet and socioeconomic status (Rimmer 1997);
- have high rates of psychological disturbance, largely accounted for by a high rate of Alzheimer's disease among people with Down's syndrome (Cooper 1997);

- are less likely to be employed or attend a day service than their younger counterparts (Walker *et al.* 1996);
- are more likely to live in shared supported accommodation than in a private home with family members or friends (Emerson *et al.* 2001);
- have reduced access to specialist disability services (Bigby 2000; Thompson and Wright 2001);
- are less likely to have strong advocates and robust informal social networks than their younger counterparts (Bigby 2000);
- live on the margins of communities rather than being active participants (Grant *et al.* 1995);
- experience substantial discrimination on the basis of age (Walker and Walker 1998);
- are less likely to be resettled from institutions than their younger counterparts (Walker and Walker 1998);
- are expected by staff to have a lower potential for growth, development and acquisition of skills and greater levels of independence compared to their younger counterparts (Walker and Walker 1998; Bigby *et al.* 2001);
- have fewer choices and opportunities for active programming than their younger peers (Moss and Hogg 1989).

Yet in sharp contrast older people with intellectual disabilities as a group are the survivors of their generation and also have:

- a continuing ability to learn (Lifshitz 1998);
- less severe disabilities than their younger counterparts, being more skilled in relation to adaptive behaviour and functional skills (Moss 1991);
- greater competence than at any other stage of their lives (Edgerton 1994).

Stereotypes and age discrimination

The profile above reflects systematically low expectations, limited opportunities and poor access to support for older people with intellectual disabilities. Many of these aspects stem from age-related discriminatory societal attitudes and structures, or from ageism, rather than from inherent personal characteristics or the ageing process itself. Since its inception, research on this group has identified the multiple jeopardies they face. As members of multiple disadvantaged groups in society, 'the aged', 'the disabled', 'the poor' and 'women', the effects of discrimination on these older people can become magnified (MacDonald and Tyson 1988).

Negative views and low expectations held by workers become self-fulfilling prophecies and contrast sharply with evidence discussed in this chapter that older people can adapt to community living, become more independent, learn new skills, acquire new interests and lead more active lives.

Exercise 31.1

What images come to mind when you think of 'older people'? Do you think these images reflect negative stereotypes and if so how?

Think of an older person you know well and consider to what extent they conform to the stereotypical image of an older person.

Spend some time talking to an older person about their life history and their perception of themselves.

Do you think your views of growing old have changed as you have got older?

Countering ageism does not mean disregarding age but requires a more concerted focus on the individual, their needs and aspirations. The principles of equity and inclusion suggest that older people with intellectual disabilities should have opportunities to mix with people of all abilities and ages; should use generally available community facilities; and should be included in broader community groups, activities, organizations and a diverse social milieu. This does not ignore their need for age-related specialist support, or negate the legitimacy of groups or friendships based on age. Rather it emphasizes that individual needs, choice or common interest should be the basis of determining support or grouping people.

Informal social relationships

Informal relationships are as fundamental to inclusion and citizenship as formal rights (Reinders 2002). Inclusion requires connections to others; relationships with family, friends, neighbours and acquaintances. This implies more than just presence in a community. These relationships can help to foster a sense of continuity and belonging.

The majority of older people with learning difficulties do not have a spouse and children which means they do not have roles such as partner, grandparent or mother-in-law, although they might acquire new roles such as great aunt. When parents die, their closest relatives are likely to be siblings or more distant relations such as cousins, nieces, nephews, aunts and uncles. For some people the loss of their parents can signify a shift to an adult rather than child role and the opportunity for new intimate friendships.

As people age their networks are fluid and particularly vulnerable to shrinkage and disruption due to death, illness, house moves and retirement of network members. Many friendships of people with intellectual disabilities, particularly those with peers, are specific to a particular context such as accommodation or a day centre, and they seldom meet outside of this setting. The context-specific nature of friendships means that such relationships are vulnerable to disruption. For example, an Australian study found that none of the people who had retired from day services, or who had moved to aged care accommodation, retained contact with friends from previous settings. Neither did they retain contact with neighbours when they moved from the locality (Bigby 2000). This represents an abrupt cessation of important established social ties.

Qualitative research suggests that friendships between people with intellectual disability can have depth, richness and longevity (Knox and Hickson 2001). An emphasis on valued social roles can detract from recognizing or valuing friendships between people with intellectual disabilities (Chappell 1994). What is important, however, is to distinguish friendships from mere groupings of people where individuals, although proximate to each other, have no common bonds. More research is needed and attention paid to the meanings that people with intellectual disabilities themselves give to relationships.

Those people who have remained at home with parents for much of their lives are often strongly connected to family and share friendships with their parents. There is a danger for them that incidental contact with the extended family will be lost when parents die, and more effort is required from relatives to involve them in family gatherings, as they no longer live in the parental home where family events take place. In addition, although contact with shared family friends might be retained after the death of parents, such friends are likely to be from an older generation and to predecease them.

Being known in a locality or community of interest can be very important to a person's sense of belonging (see Chapters 23 and 29). Grant *et al.* (1995) found that older people with intellectual disabilities were more likely to have acquaintances than close friends. These might be unnamed individuals or groups of people who they see regularly, neighbours in the local area, supporters of a football club or other patrons at a café.

A defining characteristic of older people's informal networks in Bigby's study (2000) was a 'key person' who took responsibility for oversight of their well-being. Key people had a close long-term relationship with the older person, demonstrated considerable commitment to their well-being and played many 'caring about' roles. They were likely to be a sibling, more distant relative or long-term family friend who had been informally nominated by a parent to assume responsibility for the person following the parent's death.

Key people were the most stable element in older people's networks but as they are from the same or an older generation they may predecease the older person. In such cases some key people had planned their own succession to be replaced by another person, most often a niece or nephew. However, as people with intellectual disability aged, the chances of losing a key person and not having them replaced increased. This loss leaves some older people very vulnerable, as it means they have no one outside formal services who can protect their rights and oversee their well-being by proactively monitoring the quality of services and decision-making.

Informal relationships provide diverse types of support that can include:

- 'Caring for' functions or 'direct support':
    - provision of hands-on day-to-day care;
    - development of skills;
    - provision of backup or short-term replacement of other members;
    - emotional support;
    - listening;
    - advising.
- 'Caring about' or 'indirect support':
    - decision-making;
    - financial management;
    - adoption of formal or legal roles;
    - mediating, negotiating and advocating with service systems;
    - monitoring service quality;
    - supervision of medical needs;
    - coordinating support from other network members;
    - visiting and companionship.   (Bigby 2000)

Clearly, some types of informal support can be replicated by formal support services, and paid relationships can replace the informal without loss of quality. However, it is particularly difficult for formal organizations or paid relationships to have a long-term or sole commitment to an individual and thus take a long-term advocacy stance. Yet these tasks are critically important for people dependent on services to meet their day-to-day needs. The inability of formal services to substitute for some of the key roles fulfilled by informal network members emphasizes the vulnerability of those people who lack strong informal networks of support.

The question of retirement

Formal roles, such as paid or volunteer worker, or participation in formal programmes, such as adult training and support centres or colleges of further education, are important mechanisms that foster successful engagement and social inclusion. Forced retirement from the workforce at an early or fixed chronological age, though more flexibly applied in recent years, is still common. However, this notion potentially creates an arbitrary point for exclusion from formal roles or programmes and withdrawal of specialist support for individuals that threatens their continued engagement and inclusion. This is a matter that has been subject to much debate. Some have argued that retirement is irrelevant for people with intellectual disabilities who have not been in paid employment and that it will lead to social isolation and further devaluation. Others argue that they should have the same rights as other older people to retire, be it from services or work, and to lead a more relaxed lifestyle (Wolfensberger 1985; Sutton *et al.* 1992; Ashman *et al.* 1995; Heller 1999).

Retirement from services is sometimes justified on the basis of the changes that occur to people's needs as they age. Factors such as the declining skill level of older people, their reduced abilities, the increased time required to perform tasks, a need for a quieter and less boisterous environment, and incompatibilities with the interests of younger participants have been suggested as possible reasons for programme changes (Lambe and Hogg 1995; Bigby *et al.* 2001). For some people these assumptions are unfounded. For example, an Australian study found that despite evidence showing that a lower proportion of older than younger participants have high support needs, and that two thirds of the older group did not have health-related support needs, staff still considered that increased resources were required to take account of these same older people's higher support needs (Bigby *et al.* 2001).

Arguments are also put forward that day programmes for younger people and the staff who run them have neither the resources nor skills to respond to the needs of older people. Implicit in this position is the requirement for more flexible funding and specialist knowledge of both the ageing process and service systems to provide appropriate programmes for older people (Department of Health 1997; Department of Human Services 1999).

The nature of employment or day programmes people use as they age can be influential in shaping perceptions of the necessity to retire, or whether adaptation is a feasible alternative. For example, one of the drivers behind the development of retirement programmes in the US system was that their strong training/developmental focus was perceived as less appropriate as people aged (Moss 1993). Retirement may of course be used as a discriminatory mechanism for managing demand on other parts of the service system.

It can be argued, however, that if day programmes are based on person-centred planning (see Chapter 24) there is little reason why they should not be sufficiently flexible to adapt to age-related changes (Department of Health 1997). Underpinning this argument is the view that merely reaching a certain age should not be sufficient reason for retirement or to institute changes to a person's lifestyle and daytime activities.

Aspirations and realities

A fundamental consideration in debates about retirement is the views of people with intellectual disabilities themselves. Studies that have tapped people's views suggest that they value continued active engagement with their world, express the desire to continue working, continue learning, participate in more leisure activities, and place a high value on structured activities (Bigby 1992, 1997b; Ashman *et al.* 1995; Heller 1999). Bigby's (2000) study highlighted the opportunities relished by some older people who perceived later life as a period when they were free to pursue their own interests and relationships unrestricted by parental protectiveness. Older people with disabilities who are working seldom express the desire to retire and are concerned about loss of income and social isolation if they do so (Sutton *et al.* 1992; Ashman *et al.* 1995). One US study found that the majority of people who had retired wanted to return to work (Rogers *et al.* 1998). Edgerton's study (1994) suggests that as people aged they became less dependent on benefactors, more competent than at any other stage of their lives and wanted the freedom to choose what suited them, and to exercise control even if this meant opting out of day services. They also wanted the right to associate with their friends, however defined, whether disabled or not.

Much more research is required to understand how older people with intellectual disabilities perceive ageing and what constitutes 'the good life' as they grow older. However, the limited data available contrasts starkly with the many anecdotal stories that older people just want to 'stay at home and put their feet up' or that they are more likely to be 'observers than participants' (Bigby *et al.* 2001). It also contradicts the traditional view that successful ageing is about disengagement from the world (Cumming and Henry 1961).

A major concern is evidence that despite their aspirations for continuing inclusion, older people with intellectual disabilities experience few opportunities to participate in meaningful day and leisure activities of their choice (Bigby 1992, 1997b; Grant *et al.* 1995; Hawkins 1999). Rogers *et al.* (1998: 127) sum it up by suggesting that: 'retirees days were often filled with diversionary activity rather than leisure that was valued and meaningful to participants. Furthermore, they were not provided with opportunities to retain contact with previous friends or develop new social contacts'. Even involvement in day-to-day domestic household activities tends to drop off for the older age groups (Wilson 1998).

There is little evidence to suggest that day programmes developed specifically for older participants lead to better outcomes than age-integrated programmes. An Australian study found that staff did not have superior knowledge of ageing issues. Such programmes run the risk of reinforcing age stereotyping and reducing individual choice instead of addressing issues based on individual preference or interest (Bigby *et al.* 2001).

Evidence of poor-quality services for older people is found in the UK where considerable variation exists in the nature of service provision across different regions (Robertson *et al.* 1996; Department of Health 1997; Fitzgerald 1998). The majority of service users in a small qualitative study attended segregated day services that were considered to offer a limited choice of activities (Fitzgerald 1998).

Use of day support programmes available to all older people in the community may also be disadvantageous for older people. Substantial disparity between the quality and type of programmes available to older people using care services compared to those in receipt of disability services has been reported. In this study, disability services were found to offer more individualized and educational activities and participants were more involved in community and leisure pursuits (Moss *et al.* 1992). Similarly, research in Australia suggests that structured individualized activities are not available to older people with disabilities who attend generic aged day services (Bigby 1998).

As discussed earlier, older people with intellectual disabilities often have poor informal social networks that limit participation in social activities. Accordingly, many people are reliant on others to present opportunities, provide support to exercise choice and support participation in meaningful activities. However, contextual, financial, physical and attitudinal barriers have been reported as undermining such social support (Glausier *et al.* 1995; Hogg 1996; Fitzgerald 1998; Messant *et al.* 1999).

Carers often determine choice of activity based on imperatives such as management of group needs rather than individual preferences (Glausier *et al.* 1995; Rogers *et al.* 1998). The congregate nature of activities accentuates a lack of individual choice and residential staff have limited time available after undertaking mundane housekeeping and caring tasks (Bigby *et al.* 2002). Difficulties in accessing transport and the cost of activities are also common hurdles. Attitudes of the public, staff and other programme participants also restrict opportunities offered and obstruct access to community leisure facilities or generic programmes for older people, such as day centres (Glausier *et al.* 1995; Grant *et al.* 1995; LePore and Janicki 1997; Heller 1999). Individual characteristics such as poor motivation, choice, lack of skills, knowledge or preparedness, may also hinder participation in activities. However, structural and contextual elements such as the absence of staff support are considered to be more important than interpersonal factors (Hawkins 1999).

Ensuring a sense of purpose

The necessity for retirement should not be taken as a given but must be critically appraised and accompanied by the question, 'retirement to what?', with weight given to issues of replacement of support and compensation for roles, social relationships or activities that might be lost or disrupted as a result (Seltzer and Krauss 1987; Janicki 1990). The theory of 'selective optimization with compensation' proposed by Baltes and Baltes (1990) provides a useful framework for thinking about responding to the individual and social changes associated with ageing. Further theories and perspectives about successful adaptation and ageing can be found in Chapter 33. Selective optimization suggests that successful adaptation involves three core processes, all of which should be based on individual choice:

- greater selection of activity as physical capacity reduces;
- compensation for loss of either skill or function by internal and external adjustments (e.g. changes to behaviour, type of support provided, adaptation of the physical environment or use of aids);

- optimization, making the most of what you have, by engaging in behaviours and activities that maximize reserves and enrich life choices.

These three core processes must be located in an anti-discriminatory framework that actively seeks to counter negative stereotypical social attitudes and structures that might impact on the older person. Notions of adaptation and compensation highlight the multiple ways of responding to or compensating for the change or loss associated with ageing. Individual behaviour or patterns of activities may be altered and the external social or physical environment may be adapted, by increasing opportunities, changing support offered, or introducing supportive technological mechanisms. This approach emphasizes that older as well as younger people have personal goals, and require support to explore, decide and put in place opportunities and realize goals. The theory can also be used to inform planning processes by putting a focus on external as well as individual adaptations to changes that may be necessary to support individuals to realize goals.

Exercise 31.2

Can you provide examples of adaptations and compensations for loss or change associated with ageing? Think about this for: changes in individual behaviour; changes to physical environment; and changes to formal support.

Lifestyle support

Traditional frameworks for considering retirement support tend to pose the questions about whether new or specialized programmes should be designed for older people or whether they should utilize programmes for people with disabilities of all ages or for older people in the general community. Three models are generally considered:

- *Age integration*: including older people in programmes for younger people with disabilities. For example, continued attendance at a day activity centre for people with intellectual disability.
- *Generic integration*: including older people with disabilities in programmes for the general aged population. For example, attendance at senior citizens' centres, day centres for the frail aged.
- *Specialist programmes*: developing specialized activities for older people with disabilities. For example, day centres dedicated to older people with intellectual disabilities.

Another approach is to focus on the outcomes sought and the strategies necessary to achieve these. Key outcomes of effective lifestyle support to older people with intellectual disabilities that have been discussed in this chapter draw on the work of Nolan *et al.* (2001) and are: a sense of belonging, continuity and purpose. Strategic approaches to achieving these, which can be incorporated into a variety of programme models, are:

- provision of choice and person-centred planning;
- maintenance and strengthening of social networks;
- support for participation in the community;
- maintenance of skills;
- opportunities for self-expression and sense of self;
- promotion of health and a healthy lifestyle.

The following sections discuss these strategies further.

Provision of choice and person-centred planning

Person-centred planning focuses attention on the capacity and ability of an older person to pursue chosen goals, and provides a safeguard against a more global response to ageing that can result in the reduction or limitation of opportunities or activities (Sanderson 2000). Planning reinforces the importance of individuality or a sense of significance: that each individual has his or her own characteristics, needs, wishes and aspirations. Plans should reflect an individual's characteristics; health, abilities, interests and their social context; living situation; co-residents and social networks; and previous life experiences. The three narratives in Chapter 30 illustrate the very individual aspirations of each of the older people concerned.

Plans should be constructed collaboratively with the person and those who know them well, including those who provide everyday support. They should encompass all areas of life, taking account of all waking hours.

Case study: *Maurice*

Maurice is aged 62 and moved out of a large institution to a small shared house in the community several years ago. He has a terrific sense of humour and loves being around other people. During the season he attends the football matches that are held at his team's home ground. He understands much of what goes on around him but has limited speech and others find it difficult to understand what he is communicating. He has been attending a full-time day programme together with the four other residents in his house, but staff are suggesting he should start to think about retirement. The house has had several changes of supervisor and none of the current staff have a good sense of Maurice's history or the things he enjoys doing. His mother died several years ago and he continues to maintain regular contact with his father who lives on the family farm.

Exercise 31.3

If you were developing a person-centred plan for Maurice:

What else would you need to know about him? How might you find these things out?

What assumptions might you and others make about Maurice and how can these be avoided?

What age-related changes might Maurice be experiencing and what adaptations might be considered to take account of these?

When you have formulated a plan, what strategies might you use to ensure it is a living document and is used to guide the support provided to Maurice? How often would you review the plan?

Notions of person-centred planning and choice are embedded in current policies but the scope and breadth with which they are translated into practice varies considerably. It is too easy for choice to be within predetermined parameters and planning restricted to one segment of a person's life. For example, choice can sometimes mean 'a programme booklet is developed each year and the client and/or carers get to choose what programmes they will do each day' (Bigby *et al.* 2001). Even when plans are mandated or drawn up, quality and implementation have been major issues (Felce *et al.* 1998; Mansell and Beadle-Brown 2004).

In tandem with person-centred plans, organizations must also plan the use of resources, primarily support staff, to ensure that the visions encapsulated in the plans are implemented. Aims such as participating in daily domestic tasks or developing connections to family, friends and acquaintances are not achieved just by the availability of staff and their use of intuition. They require detailed and careful planning of staff time and strategies to ensure that both opportunity and effective support are provided.

Maintenance and strengthening of social networks

Support from social workers, case managers or direct care staff can foster development of informal relationships but also, through neglect and ignorance, the obstruction or disruption of these. A first crucial step is recognition of the value and range of informal relationships of each older person. The initial stage of planning should ensure each individual's network is actively mapped, and that the history and significance of relationships are understood. A proactive stance is then needed to take account of relationships and adapt support to deal with potential disruption when lifestyle changes, such as retirement, are proposed. Strategies can range from raising the awareness of staff about the importance of relationships, the reorientation of support to facilitate contact with friends or the implementation of more formal 'network-building programmes'.

Formal network-building programmes are based on the idea that participation in activities or taking on valued social roles are a means of developing individual relationships. Person-centered planning techniques are used by a 'community builder' to piece together a picture of the person with a disability and to explore the local community for potential sites and activities, where the person may play a role or contribute to community life. Once an activity is identified the community builder's role is to introduce the person, and seek out and foster the development of natural supports from among other participants. The degree to which friendships develop depends on attentive listening, strategy, persistent support and sometimes luck. Community builders can be employed as part of a specialist programme or such a role may be fulfilled by a case manager. Their success lies in the ability to take risks, and to be creative and flexible. This requires significant investment of time, intensive in the exploratory stage and less so but often continuing in the long term (see e.g. Kultgen *et al.* 2000; Harlan-Simmons *et al.* 2001).

As people age, maintaining family relationships may need more active support as relatives encounter mobility or health problems. The structure of day-to-day activities creates opportunities or obstacles to building friendships. Occasional outings in large groups to venues such as shopping centres or the cinema are unlikely to lead to the development of new relationships. Yet it is just these sorts of activity to anonymous public spaces in groups that occupy much of the time that people with intellectual disability spend in the community (Walker 1995; Bigby *et al.* 2002). The location, continuity, regularity, size of group and meaning of the activity to the individual are all key considerations in whether obstacles or opportunities are created in everyday lives for relationships to develop. People's lives are too often fragmented by programmes with residential staff being unaware of 'day programme' friends. This can mean that such friendships do not flourish or opportunities for shared evening or weekend activities are not supported.

Exercise 31.4

How would you build up a map of Maurice's informal social relationships? What are the different types of relationship he might have?

How might you ensure you have included long-term relationships with other residents from the institution where Maurice lived for many years and those with others who participate in his day programme?

What sorts of family relationships might an unmarried person of Maurice's age have? In what ways might the support that Maurice needs to maintain contact with his family and friends change as both he and they get older? What strategies could be pursued to provide opportunities for Maurice to form new relationships?

Support for participation in the community

Person-centred plans should explore strategies for community participation, which in turn are closely related to the maintenance and strengthening of social relationships. Identification of an individual's goals, strengths and interests should lead to an exploration of opportunities that might be available, such as volunteer work, or membership of clubs or organizations. This should be followed by strategies to negotiate and gain entry to an organization, and to provide ongoing support to enable continued participation. Too often community participation is understood to be the use of community facilities such as swimming pools or cinemas, or attendance at disability-specific and other aged care or community activities. This may not involve active social interaction or shared interests and experiences with other community members. Hallmarks of participation should be the sense of purpose to the individual and their active connection to a community of interest. As with planning, participation is variously translated into practice, with a notable difference between the people experiencing themselves as a contributing member of the community as opposed to mere physical presence in community settings.

Exercise 31.5

How would you describe differences for Maurice between participation in the community and merely being present?

What communities of interest might Maurice belong to?

What questions would you ask to be sure that the activities Maurice participates in are meaningful to him?

What strategies would you use to ensure that Maurice has a sense of continuity in his life?

Maintenance of skills

Support to maintain skills contributes to an older person's continuing sense of autonomy and independence and is particularly important in the context of age- or health-related changes. As with the other factors, a first step is the recognition that maintaining or developing skills is an important goal that may require planned strategies and creative adjustments to the environment and choice of activities to compensate for changes such as loss of physical or sensory capacities. For example, a person with Alzheimer's disease may slowly lose their motivation to participate in everyday activities or initiate interaction and will progressively require more frequent prompting and increasing levels of support to exercise their skills. Activities may have to be simplified or broken into smaller steps to compensate for cognitive change but support continued engagement. Action to maintain skills should occur in the informal domestic sphere as well as in the service context. Adaptation of teaching strategies and environmental modifications can compensate for cognitive and sensory changes: for example, allowing longer reaction times or the person to go at their own pace, excluding background noise, providing optimal lighting or using environmental cues such as pictorial representations, colour and texture.

Age-related assumptions or stereotypes are likely to be particularly prevalent and disadvantageous to individuals in connection to skill development. For example, an Australian study of different types of day service used by older people with intellectual disabilities found that maintenance of skills was not well met. Programmes generally had few ambitious individual goals in regard to skill development, and they often reflected a sense of gradual decline to passive rather than active pursuits. In some instances, resistance was found to any individual planning concerning skills or activities as it was seen as irrelevant because people were older (Bigby *et al.* 2001).

Opportunities for self-expression and sense of self

Opportunities for self-expression and connection to one's own life history are important in tackling some of the psychological tasks associated with later life. Erikson (1973), who adopts a stage theory of personality development, suggests that older people are confronted with achieving 'ego integrity versus despair'. This involves the acceptance that one's life has had a meaning whether or not it has been 'successful' and the acceptance of one's own mortality. Seltzer (1985) conceptualizes some of the developmental tasks of ageing for older people with intellectual disabilities as: adjustment to losses, restructuring of roles, reassessment of self-concept and acceptance of mortality.

Strategies for achieving these tasks include reminiscence and life review – opportunities for individuals to express how they feel about themselves and what is happening in their world. Avenues for self-expression and reflection may occur through drama, art, group or individual opportunities to tell personal stories or reminiscence, and use of photo albums and other memorabilia. For example, objects such as seashells can be used to bring back memories and discussions about past holidays that involved going to the sea. Where people have lost contact with families, lived in institutions or moved many times, compiling a record of their life story may be an important task. Life story work (see Chapter 1) can also be important in maintaining a connection with people with Alzheimer's and ensuring the continued engagement of informal network members with an older person. Such a strategy is being used by one of the major UK providers of residential care for people with disabilities (Grundy 2002). Work with older carers of middle-aged adults with intellectual disability has used life story books as a means to engage carers in thinking about the future and adopting a proactive approach to preserving a person's life history to inform those who may become involved in the person's life as they age. Various guides are available. For example, *My Life Book* was developed by the Sharing Caring Project

(1999) in Sheffield. Also important is active and appropriate support for coping with grief and loss (see Chapters 10 and 34).

Exercise 31.6

If you were Maurice's case manager, how important do you think it would be to ensure the staff that supported him every day were aware of his life history and significant events and people in his life? How might you ensure this occurred? What strategies might you put in place to provide Maurice with opportunities to connect with and reflect on his past?

Promotion of health and a healthy lifestyle

Physical health underpins almost all aspects of a person's life, and for people with intellectual disability it can be optimized by an approach that encompasses health promotion, health surveillance and health care (Moss *et al.* 1998). These issues are addressed in depth in Chapters 3, 12, 17, 18, 27, 32 and 33. It is important however not to compartmentalize notions of health but to incorporate health promotion into all aspects of a person's life. Of note too is that people with intellectual disability often embark on the ageing process from a very disadvantageous and unhealthy lifestyle, having led sedentary lives, with little exercise, poor diets and accompanying weight problems (Rimmer 1997; Janicki *et al.* 2002). A sense of the low level of physical activity and exercise among adults with intellectual disability is provided by Emerson who found that the inactivity rates of adults with intellectual disability living in a variety of supported residential settings in the UK were equivalent to those of non-disabled people over the age of 75 years (Emerson 2002).

Stereotypical views that lead to inaction on health-related issues can further disadvantage older people. For example, an Australian study found that while day programmes used by older people were sensitive to physical health issues, many accepted reduced fitness and poor health without accurate assessment. One staff member commented that 'too much emphasis [was placed] on the women's health as much of what they experienced was either just old age or common ailments' (Bigby *et al.* 2001).

Participation in structured exercise programmes, restructuring everyday life to extend the amount of physical activity and health education all have the potential to build a healthier lifestyle. Research has demonstrated the ability of older people with intellectual disability in the community to participate and enjoy structured exercise programmes (Heller *et al.* 2002). In a similar manner to that adopted for other older people, aspects of daily life can be structured to involve more physical activity, for example, dispensing with the automatic channel changer, using stairs instead of lifts, walking to the next rather the nearest bus stop, using a watering can instead of a hose.

Exercise 31.7

Key questions to ask about Maurice's lifestyle might be:

What exercise does he have in the course of a regular week and how could physical activity be built into his everyday routine?

If Maurice were to be confined to a wheelchair how could he continue to exercise?

What types of food should Maurice have in his diet and what should he be avoiding or eating in small quantities?

Who should take responsibility for ensuring Maurice has a healthy lifestyle?

Now go back through all the exercises. You should now have a series of 'best ideas' to support Maurice. Remember this still raises issues about who decides, who implements and who organizes. Once again the person-centred plan is the vehicle for these decisions.

Conclusion

This chapter has provided an overview of some of the issues associated with ageing for people with intellectual disabilities. It has highlighted the diversity of this population and the discriminatory social attitudes that can impact on older people. Achieving an individual sense of belonging, continuity and purpose are seen as some of the key outcomes that society in general and community care services in particular should be seeking for these older people. The chapter has considered debates about retirement and the need to critically consider its likely impact on an individual's social relationships and sense of purpose. Strategic approaches to supporting a purposeful lifestyle for older people with intellectual disabilities are proposed within an over-arching framework that emphasizes the importance of adaptation and compensation for individual and social changes associated with ageing. Finally, students should be mindful that the voice of people with intellectual disabilities is largely missing from much published research and debate about responses to ageing. The meaning of belonging, continuity and purpose for each individual will reflect their own unique perceptions and interpretation of their activities, experiences and relationships. The challenge lies in finding ways to uncover and bring these into focus, so that dreams and aspirations can be realized.

References

Ashman, A., Suttie, J. and Bramley, J. (1995) Employment, retirement and elderly persons with developmental disabilities, *Journal of Intellectual Disability Research*, 39(2): 107–15.

Baltes, P. and Baltes, M. (1990) Psychological perspectives on successful aging: the model of selective optimisation with compensation, in P. Baltes and M. Baltes (eds) *Successful Ageing: Perspectives from the Behavioural Sciences.* Cambridge: Cambridge University Press.

Bigby, C. (1992) Access and linkage: two critical issues for older people with an intellectual disability, *Australia and New Zealand Journal of Developmental Disabilities*, 18: 95–110.

Bigby, C. (1997a) When parents relinquish care: the informal support networks of older people with intellectual disability, *Journal of Applied Intellectual Disability Research*, 10(4): 333–44.

Bigby, C. (1997b) Later life for adults with intellectual disability: a time of opportunity and vulnerability, *Journal of Intellectual and Developmental Disability*, 22(2): 97–108.

Bigby, C. (1998) Shifting responsibilities: patterns of formal service use by older people with intellectual disability, *Journal of Intellectual and Developmental Disability*, 23: 229–43.

Bigby, C. (2000) *Moving on Without Parents: Planning, Transitions and Sources of Support for Older Adults with Intellectual Disabilities.* New South Wales: McLennan & Petty.

Bigby, C. (2004) *Aging with a Lifelong Disability: Policy, Program and Practice Issues for Professionals.* London: Jessica Kingsley.

Bigby, C., Fyffe, C., Balandin, S., Gordon, M. and McCubbery, J. (2001) *Day Support Services Options for Older Adults with a Disability.* Melbourne: National Disability Administrators Group.

Bigby, C., Frederico, M. and Cooper, B. (2002) *Not Just a Residential Move but Creating a Better Lifestyle for People with Intellectual Disabilities: Report of the Evaluation of Kew Residential Services Community Relocation Project 1999–2001.* Melbourne: Department of Human Services.

Chappell, A. (1994) A question of friendship: community care and the relationships of people with learning difficulties, *Disability and Society*, 9(4): 419–33.

Cooper, S. (1997) Epidemiology of psychiatric disorders in elderly compared with younger people with learning disabilities, *British Journal of Psychiatry*, 170: 375–80.

Cumming, E. and Henry, W. (1961) *Growing Old.* New York: Basic Books.

Department of Health (1997) *Services for Older People with Learning Disabilities.* London: HMSO.

Department of Health (2001) *Valuing People: A New Strategy for Learning Disability for the 21st Century.* London: Department of Health.

Department of Human Services (1999) *Day Services for People Ageing with a Disability.* Melbourne: Department of Human Services.

Edgerton, R. (1994) Quality of life issues: some people know how to be old, in M. Seltzer, M. Krauss and M. Janicki (eds) *Lifecourse Perspectives on Adulthood and Aging.* Washington: American Association on Mental Retardation.

Emerson, E. (2002) *Unhealthy lifestyles.* Paper presented at the inaugural European

International Association for the Scientific Study of Intellectual Disability Conference, Dublin, Ireland, June.

Emerson, E., Hatton, C., Felce, D. and Murphy, G. (2001) *Learning Disabilities: The Fundamental Facts*. London: Foundation for People with Learning Disabilities.

Erikson, E. (1973) *Childhood and Society*. New York: Norton.

Evenhuis, H., Henderson, C., Beange, H., Lennox, N. and Chicoine, B. (2001) Health ageing – adults with intellectual disabilities: physical health issues, *Journal of Applied Research in Intellectual Disabilities*, 14(3): 175–94.

Felce, D., Grant, G., Todd, S., Ramcharan, P., Beyer, S., McGrath, M., Perry, J., Shearn, J., Kilsby, M. and Lowe K. (1998) *Towards a Full Life: Researching Policy Innovation for People with Learning Disabilities*. Oxford: Butterworth Heinemann.

Fitzgerald, J. (1998) *Time for Freedom? Services for Older People with Learning Difficulties*. London: Values in Action.

Glausier, S., Whorton, J. and Knight, H. (1995) Recreation and leisure likes/dislikes of senior citizens with mental retardation, *Activities, Adaptations and Aging*, 19: 43–54.

Grant, G. (2001) Older people with learning disabilities: health, community inclusion and family caregiving, in M. Nolan, S. Davies and G. Grant (eds) *Working with Older People and their Families*. Buckingham: Open University Press.

Grant, G., McGrath, M. and Ramcharan, P. (1995) Community inclusion of older adults with learning disabilities, *Care In Place, International Journal of Networks and Community*, 2(1): 29–44.

Green, J. and Wunsch, A. (1994) The lives of six women, *Interaction*, 7(4): 11–15.

Grundy, P. (2002) This is your life, *Community Care*, 7(13): 40.

Harlan-Simmons, J., Holtz, P., Todd, J. and Mooney, M. (2001) Building social relationships through values roles: three adults and the community membership project, *Mental Retardation*, 39(3): 171–80.

Hawkins, B. (1999) Rights, place of residence and retirement: lessons from case studies on aging, in S. Herr and G. Weber (eds) *Aging, Rights and Quality of Life*. Baltimore, MD: Brookes.

Heller, T. (1999) Emerging models, in S. Herr and G. Weber (eds) *Ageing, Rights and Quality of Life*. Baltimore, MD: Brookes.

Heller, T., Hsieh, K. and Rimmer, J. (2002) Barriers and supports for exercise participation among adults with Down syndrome, *Journal of Gerontological Social Work*, 38(1/2): 161–78.

Hogg, J. (1996) Leisure, disability and the third age, *Journal of Practical Approaches to Developmental Handicap*, 18: 1.

Hogg, J. and Lambe, K. (2000) Stability and change in the later years: the impact of service provision on older people with intellectual disabilities, in D. May (ed.) *Transitions in the Lives of People with Learning Disabilities*. London: Jessica Kingsley.

Janicki, M. (1990) Growing old with dignity: on quality of life for older persons with lifelong disability, in R. Schalock (ed.) *Quality of Life: Perspectives and Issues*. Washington, DC: American Association on Mental Retardation.

Janicki, M., Dalton, A., Henderson, C. and Davidson, P. (1999) Mortality and morbidity among older adults with intellectual disability: health services considerations, *Disability and Rehabilitation*, 21(5/6): 284–94.

Janicki, M., Davidson, P., Henderson, C., McCallion, P., Teates, J., Force, L., Sulkes, S., Frangenberg, E. and Ladrigan, P. (2002) Health characteristics and health service utilisation in older adults with intellectual disability living in community residences, *Journal of Intellectual Disability Research*, 46(4): 287–98.

Knox, M. and Hickson, F. (2001) The meaning of close friendships: the view of four people with intellectual disabilities, *Journal of Applied Research in Intellectual Disabilities*, 14(3): 276–91.

Kultgen, P., Harlan-Simmons, J. and Todd, J. (2000) Community membership, in M. Janicki and E. Ansello (eds) *Community Supports for Aging Adults with Lifelong Disabilities*. Baltimore, MD: Brookes.

Lambe, L. and Hogg, J. (1995) *Their face to the wind: Service Developments for older People with Learning difficulties in Grampian Region*. Dundee: Enable.

Laslett, P. (1989) *A Fresh Map of Life: The Emergence of the Third Age*. London: Weidenfeld & Nicholson.

LePore, P. and Janicki, M. (1997) *The Wit to Win: How To Integrate Older Persons with Developmental Disabilities into Community Aging Programs*, 3rd edn. Albany, NY: NY State Office of Aging.

Lifshitz, H. (1998) Instrumental enrichment: a tool for enhancement of cognitive ability in adult and elderly people with mental retardation, *Education and Training in Mental Retardation and Developmental Disabilities*, 33(1): 34–41.

MacDonald, M. and Tyson, P. (1988) Decajeopardy – the aging and aged developmentally disabled, in J. Matson and A. Marchetti (eds) *Developmental Disabilities: A Lifespan Perspective*. San Diego, CA: Grune & Stratton.

Mansell, J. and Beadle-Brown, J. (2004) Person-centred planning or person-centred action? Policy and practice in intellectual disability services, *Journal of Applied Research in Intellectual Disabilities*, 17(1): 1–9.

Messant, P., Cooke, C. and Long, J. (1999) Primary and secondary barriers to physically active healthy lifestyles for adults with learning disabilities, *Disability and Rehabilitation*, 21(9): 409–19.

Moss, S. (1991) Age and functional abilities of people with mental handicap: evidence from the Wessex Mental Handicap Register, *Journal of Mental Deficiency Research*, 35: 430–45.

Moss, S. (1993) *Aging and Developmental Disabilities: Perspectives from Nine Countries*. Durham, NH: The International Exchange of Experts and Information in Rehabilitation.

Moss, S. and Hogg, J. (1989) A cluster analysis of support networks of older people with severe intellectual impairment, *Australia and New Zealand Journal of Developmental Disabilities*, 15: 169–88.

Moss, S., Hogg, J. and Horne, M. (1992) Individual characteristics and service support of older people with moderate, severe and profound learning disability with and without community mental handicap team support, *Mental Handicap Research*, 6(3): 3–17.

Moss, S., Lambe, L. and Hogg, J. (1998) *Aging Matters: Pathways for Older People with a Learning Disability*. Worcestershire: British Institute of Learning Disabilities.

Nolan, M., Davies, S. and Grant, G. (2001) Integrating perspectives, in M. Nolan, S. Davies and G. Grant (eds) *Working with Older People and Their Families*. Buckingham: Open University Press.

Reinders, J. (2002) The good life for citizens with intellectual disability, *Journal of Intellectual Disability Research*, 46(1): 1.

Rimmer, J. (1997) *Aging, Mental Retardation and Physical Fitness*. Arlington, VA: The Arc of the United States.

Robertson, J., Moss, S. and Turner, S. (1996) Policy, service and staff training for older people with intellectual disability in the UK, *Journal of Applied Research in Intellectual Disabilities*, 9(2): 91–100.

Rogers, N., Hawkins, B. and Eklund, S. (1998) The nature of leisure in the lives of older adults with intellectual disability, *Journal of Intellectual Disability Research*, 42(2): 122–30.

Sanderson, H. (2000) *Person-centred Planning: Key Features and Approaches*. York: Joseph Roundtree Foundation.

Seltzer, G. (1985) Selected psychological processes and aging among older developmentally disabled persons, in M. Janicki and H. Wisniewski (eds) *Aging and Developmental Disabilities: Issues and Approaches*. Baltimore, MD: Brookes.

Seltzer, M. and Krauss, M. (1987) *Aging and Mental Retardation: Extending the Continuum*, Washington: American Association on Mental Retardation.

Sharing Caring Project (1999) *My Life Book*. Sheffield: Sharing Caring Project.

Skeie, G. (1989) Contact between elderly people with mental retardation living in institutions and their families, *Australia and New Zealand Journal of Developmental Disabilities*, 15: 201–6.

Sutton, E., Sterns, H. and Roberts, R. (1992) Retirement for older persons with developmental disabilities, in E. Ansello and N. Eustis (eds) *Aging and Disabilities: Seeking Common Ground*. Amityville, NY: Baywood.

Thompson, D. (2002) Growing older with learning disabilities: the GOLD programme, *Tizard Learning Disability Review*, 7(2): 19–26.

Thompson, D. and Wright, S. (2001) *Misplaced and Forgotten: People with Learning Disabilities in Residential Services for Older People*. London: The Mental Health Foundation.

Walker, A. and Walker, C. (1998) Normalisation and 'normal' ageing: the social construction of dependency among older people with learning difficulties, *Disability and Society*, 13(1): 125–42.

Walker, A., Walker, C. and Ryan, T. (1996) Older people with learning difficulties leaving institutional care – a case of double jeopardy, *Ageing and Society* 16: 125–50.

Walker, P. (1995) Community based is not community: the social geography of disability, in S. Taylor, R. Bogdan and Z. Lukfiyya (eds) *The Variety of Community Experiences*. Baltimore, MD: Brookes.

West, R. (2000) Discovering a sister, in R. Traustadottir and K. Johnson (eds) *Women with Intellectual Disabilities: Finding a Place in the World*. London: Jessica Kingsley.

Wilson, C. (1998) Providing quality services for individuals who are aging in community based support settings: what are the issues for service providers? Paper presented at the 34th Annual Conference of the Australian Society for the Study of Intellectual Disability, Adelaide, SA, November.

Wolfensberger, W. (1985) An overview of social role valorisation and some reflections on elderly mentally retarded persons, in M. Janicki and H. Wisniewski (eds) *Aging and Developmental Disabilities: Issues and Approaches*. Baltimore, MD: Brookes.

32

Promoting healthy lifestyles

End of life issues

Sheila Hollins and Irene Tuffrey-Wijne

Introduction

Nowadays people with learning disabilities are increasingly likely to live into old age, and develop age-related illnesses such as cancer and Alzheimer's disease, of which they may eventually die (Tuffrey-Wijne 2003). A comprehensive review of the health of people with learning disabilities was recently commissioned by the Scottish Executive to consider the particular health risks faced by this group (Scottish Executive 2004). However, they still have a much shorter life expectancy overall than other people (McGuigan *et al.* 1995) and thus the experience of death among their contemporaries is also much commoner. Most of us associate death with older age, and young adults have typically only experienced death among their grandparents. This can lead to a false sense of one's own predicted longevity. Not so for adults with learning disabilities who are very likely to have lost friends through death in their school and college days and from among their friends in clubs and day centres. The causes of earlier death are well documented and include epilepsy, choking or silent aspiration of food, and accidents. The most frequently documented cause of death is respiratory conditions including the final common pathway – bronchopneumonia (Eymen *et al.* 1988; Evans and Alberman 1990; Mölsä 1994; Hollins *et al.* 1998). Despite this, people with learning disabilities are more likely to be 'protected' from knowledge of death or impending death. Many carers feel concern about their capacity to understand and cope with the finality of death, or do not recognize their need to be informed and included, and to grieve (Oswin 1991; Blackman 2003). If people with learning disabilities themselves face a life-threatening illness, this 'conspiracy of silence' often persists (Brown *et al.* 2002). The availability of choices regarding end of life issues, such as what treatment or care is to be provided and where, is crucial for the achievement of an optimal quality of life, yet this is difficult to achieve if the person concerned is not informed and involved. Providing appropriate and sensitive end of life support, whether this is early or late in life, presents a major challenge to family, support networks and services.

This chapter will explore end of life issues and bereavement. Through three case studies, it will highlight pertinent issues and best practice in providing appropriate end of life and bereavement care.

End of life issues

Case study: *Jennifer*

Jennifer Thomas was born ten weeks prematurely. She was the much longed-for third child of Joan and Brian Thomas, who already had Christopher, aged 2, and Sarah, aged 1. Jennifer had many health problems, including cerebral palsy, epilepsy and severe learning disabilities. Her parents were initially told that she would probably not survive more than a few weeks. She was in hospital for five months. When it became clear that, given intensive support, she might survive a couple of years, her parents were advised to move her into a long-stay hospital for people with learning disabilities. Joan and Brian were grief-stricken by the situation. They knew that they could not possibly care for Jennifer themselves. They had Christopher and Sarah to consider and insufficient community support was available. They felt that the best way to cope was by breaking off all contact with Jennifer. They did not tell their other children about her. They asked only to be contacted about Jennifer if there was a life-threatening situation.

Jennifer was transferred to Hollyfields, a large hospital for people with learning disabilities 350 miles away. For the next 26 years, she lived in a ward with 13 other residents. She was the most severely disabled person on the ward. She was unable to move her limbs and couldn't talk, although she had a lovely smile. She spent her life in a cot in one corner of the room. The nurses gave her intensive physical support, including night checks every 20 minutes. Jennifer had regular seizures day and night, which were promptly dealt with. During these 26 years, Jennifer's parents were telephoned 11 times; reasons for alarm included severe epileptic seizures, pneumonia and unexplained physical deterioration. They rushed to the hospital several times, and were deeply shocked and distressed by the sight of their daughter in an alien-looking environment, surrounded by severely disabled people. Each time, Jennifer pulled through. Brian and Joan did not visit Jennifer between these calls, nor did they maintain any other contact with the hospital.

When long-stay hospitals were beginning to close down, it was suggested that Jennifer be moved into a community home. After much negotiation, a potential home was found for her not far from where her parents lived. A social worker and a community psychiatrist went to talk to Joan and Brian, to find out how they felt about their daughter. They spent a number of long, difficult and tearful sessions with them. Joan and Brian felt that their family had never been really complete. They decided that they would like Jennifer to live nearby in an ordinary home, and that it was time to tell their other children about her. Christopher and Sarah were shocked by the news, but wanted to meet their sibling.

The nurses on the ward were extremely upset by the proposal of Jennifer's move. They felt that she belonged on the ward, it was her home, and although she could not communicate her wishes, she seemed happy enough. They also felt that a community home would not be able to provide Jennifer with the same level of care; their 20-minute night checks had saved Jennifer's life on a number of occasions. They argued that Jennifer should be allowed to stay in the hospital.

Joan, Brian and their grown-up children knew the risks involved. The proposed home would care for six severely disabled adults, but it was homely rather than hospital-like. There would be two sleeping staff at night, one of whom would have a nursing qualification and would be connected to residents' rooms through an intercom. Joan and Brian had always wanted to get to know their daughter, but felt unable to do so while she was in hospital.

The community psychiatrist and the social worker supported Jennifer's move. The hospital managers were keen to move out as many people as possible. The resident doctor thought that although Jennifer's needs were profound, with the right support she could live in a community setting. However, he recognized that this was not without risk: if Jennifer had a major epileptic seizure that was not promptly treated, she could die. In any case, her health could deteriorate at any time.

Exercise 32.1

What do you think is the best way forward in this situation? Should Jennifer stay in the hospital where she has lived all her life, and where her life has been saved on several occasions? Or should she be moved into a more homely environment, where her family could get to know her? If possible, get together with others to debate this issue, each taking on a different professional or parental role. You *must* reach a decision.

Outcome 1

Despite the protestations of the nurses on the ward, Jennifer was settled into her new home. Her parents and siblings visited her regularly, and were happy about the renewed contact. Two months later, Jennifer had a major epileptic seizure during the night and could not be resuscitated. Joan and Brian were sad about this, but felt happy that Jennifer was part of their family at the end of her life. Joan said she finally felt 'whole' as a mother and was grateful that she and her husband had been supported to be parents to Jennifer.

Outcome 2

It was decided that Jennifer would be allowed to stay on the ward. The nurses continued to care for her in the same way. They felt she was not unhappy, although it was impossible to be sure about this. Joan and Brian still got distressed by the hospital set-up, and never visited again. Neither did Jennifer's sister Sarah. Her brother Christopher came to see her three times over the next few years. Jennifer died seven years later of a chest infection.

Exercise 32.2

Having read these outcomes, how do you feel about the decision you proposed?

Do you think future outcomes alter the way decisions are perceived as right or wrong?

What if the outcomes were altogether different?

Outcome 3

As in Outcome 1, Jennifer was settled into her new home and was visited regularly by her family. It was difficult to tell whether she was happier than before, but her family were delighted with Jennifer's inclusion. Jennifer died seven years later of a chest infection.

Outcome 4

As in Outcome 2, Jennifer remained on the ward, and her family didn't visit. Despite the nurses' dedicated care, she died two months later following an epileptic seizure.

End of life decision-making

End of life decision-making means making choices that are likely to affect the quality of someone's remaining life, how long someone will live, and where they will live and be cared for. This is hardly ever straightforward, because it is usually difficult to predict exactly what will happen to someone's health, and what the consequences of any choices are. There are often no clear right or wrong answers. As in Jennifer's case, a number of salient issues need to be considered, including quality of life, communication and collaboration.

Quality of life

'Quality of life' is a key consideration in the provision of palliative care, and should inform all end of life decision-making. This is not as easy as it sounds. It is not unusual for health professionals to base the decision whether or not to provide active treatment on their own assumptions about the quality of another person's life. However, 'quality of life' is a very personal concept. It is the individual's satisfaction or happiness in life in domains he or she considers important (Flanagan 1978). While a healthy person may feel that their life would not be worth living if they could not walk and talk, someone like Jennifer (who has never known any different) may still be enjoying a good quality of life. When making treatment and care choices, it is therefore important to consider 'quality of life' from the other person's perspective. If the person cannot tell us what they value in their life, it can often still be determined by talking to those who know the person well.

Quality of life is affected by ill-health. Our priorities might change, and illness has an impact on the domains that are important to us for a good quality of life. Various tools have been developed to measure quality of life at the end of life (e.g. Cohen *et al.* 1995; Wilson 1995). Most of these look at a number of domains, such as physical, emotional, social, cognitive and spiritual; some include an assessment of symptoms and their impact. While it may not be possible to use such tools directly with people with learning disabilities, it can be useful to keep these domains in mind when thinking about someone's quality of life.

A focus on quality of life becomes particularly important if it is clear that someone's life expectancy is limited, and the personal cost of prolonging life may be considerable. Any proposed course of action that could be detrimental to someone's quality of life needs to be carefully discussed and agreed by all involved. If the person is able to make his or her wishes known, this should be the main consideration in the decision-making process. A further discussion of quality of life issues, including a longer version of the exercise, can be found in *Positive Approaches to Palliative Care* (listed in the further reading section of this chapter – see p. 703).

There can be a degree of risk involved in allowing someone to enjoy a good quality of life. In Jennifer's case, it could be argued that the risk of being less protective (not having her in her cot at all times and not observing her every 20 minutes) would be too great: she would probably die sooner. However, for Jennifer to live in a more stimulating environment and enjoy family relationships may be so valuable that it is worth taking the risk. Thinking about risk management, what level of risk would you be comfortable with? What personal reasons in your own life might influence your perspective?

Exercise 32.3

Think about the following questions:

What do you value most in your life? Can you name five things that contribute to your quality of life? (This could be anything, e.g. family, friends, health, work, skills, hobbies, faith, food, holidays . . .)

Think of one person with learning disabilities you know. What do you think this person values most in life? If you don't know, how could you find out? Could you ask the person? Spend time with him or her? Ask close carers, family, friends?

Communication and collaboration

When a person with learning disabilities reaches the end of life, those involved are affected in different ways. Let us look at some of the issues. First, those faced by the person with learning disabilities:

- *Changes in health*: the person is likely to notice that they are less able to do things, needing increased help with tasks of daily living. They may experience symptoms such as fatigue, pain, nausea, shortness of breath or others.

- *Worry and anxiety*: the person will probably be worried, especially if they are not helped to understand their situation. It can be particularly worrying if they receive conflicting messages, where one person says 'you are ill' and another says 'everything is just fine'.

- *Changes in circumstances*: the person may have to go to hospital, or move into a different setting altogether.

- *Communication problems*: it is likely that the person has difficulty in communicating their feelings, symptoms, fears or wishes. Their ways of communicating may be misinterpreted or disregarded.

Issues faced by the family include:

- *Involvement*: families who have not been particularly involved in a person's life may want or need more involvement now (as in Jennifer's case). While many care settings are excellent at including the family as important partners, others may resent the (sometimes sudden) emergence of family wishes. Many families, however, are very involved throughout the person's life, and often know the person better than anyone else. They need to be included in end of life care and decision-making.

- *Experience of services*: some families, particularly of older people, do not have an entirely positive experience of learning disability services. They may have had to struggle in the past to get the best possible care for their relative. Services have changed enormously over the past decades, and the way families have experienced this will affect their way of coping and communicating with the influx of new services at the end of life. Alternatively, if the family has been happy with the services provided, or if they feel that their relative is finally settled happily, it may be difficult to accept that a change of services is now necessary.

- *Anticipatory loss*: the family has to face an imminent bereavement. In addition to the general shock and sadness of loss faced by all of us, families of people with learning disabilities may re-experience feelings of loss and bereavement faced when a disabled child was born, or when their child or sibling left the family home. Some people will have feelings of guilt or anger.

Issues faced by carers include:

- *Lack of skills and resources*: daily caregivers may feel strongly that they do not have the skills and resources to support someone towards the end of life. This can be particularly difficult if the person lives in a residential home rather than with their family. Staff at the home may feel that they don't have enough staff to cope with physical illness, that they lack the facilities or they may have a philosophy of enabling independence rather than giving increased support.

- *Involvement*: many carers, including paid carers at residential homes, are highly committed to the people they support. Often, this involvement contributes to a good quality of life for the person. However, sometimes such involvement can be damaging, particularly if carers feel that they are the only ones who can support the person properly, to the exclusion of other services.

- *Lack of experience regarding death*: many carers in learning disability services are relatively young and may never have experienced death at close hand, leading to feelings of fear (Tuffrey-Wijne 1998).

Issues faced by services include:

- *The right place of care*: services have to decide whether the person can continue to be supported in their usual home. This depends on the level of support available in the home, either through the home's own staff or with additional support services (such as primary care). The person's wishes, and those of the family, need to be taken into account.

- *Profusion of services*: towards the end of life, a huge variety of professionals can become involved, including GPs, district nurses, hospital doctors, physiotherapists, chaplains, palliative care (or hospice) doctors and nurses, social workers and learning disability teams. It is not difficult to imagine a damaging lack of coordination among all these services.

The lists are not exhaustive, but they do give a flavour of the complexity of issues that may arise towards the end of someone's life. Everybody's experience and viewpoint is valid and needs to be acknowledged. In order to provide optimum support, it is crucial that all parties involved communicate among themselves and with each other. Studies have shown that people were most satisfied with services relating to life-limiting illness and end of life when there was a good partnership working between the different organizations involved, and a sharing of knowledge and information (Northfield and Turnbull 2001; Brown *et al.* 2002).

Feelings and emotions often run high when someone with learning disabilities faces a life-limiting situation. If you role-played Jennifer's situation, you may have realized how passionate people can become. It is crucial that any decision is taken with the best interests of the person with learning disabilities in mind. Looking back to the people involved in Jennifer's situation, they would have to ask themselves what their own interest was, and whether this would truly serve Jennifer best. There can often be no easy answers.

Case study: *Charles*

Charles Manning was a 62-year-old man with moderate learning disabilities. He lived in a flat with two friends, where a team of support workers took turns to come in during the day. Having lived in an institution when he was young, Charles was happy to have a degree of independence now, and particularly enjoyed going to the day centre. Charles' only relative was a brother in America who hadn't been in contact for 35 years.

When Charles noticed that he was having difficulty passing urine, he mentioned this to Mohammed, the support worker he was closest to. Mohammed took him to see his GP, who referred him to hospital for investigations. Charles found this difficult as he had a fear of hospitals, but he coped well. Cancer of the prostate was diagnosed, which was still in the early stages and had not spread to any other parts of the body.

The hospital consultant called Mohammed in to discuss the results. He explained that the best course of action was to 'wait and see'. Cancer of the prostate is usually slow growing, and in any case the consultant thought Charles would not be able to cope with the radiotherapy treatments. Mohammed did not know that prostate cancer in the early stages can often be cured by radiotherapy.

Exercise 32.4

What do you think of the proposed course of action? What do you think Mohammed should do? Should Charles be told about his diagnosis and any possible treatments? Consider what could happen next.

Outcome 1

Mohammed did not know much about cancer, and assumed that the doctor would give him the best possible advice. He reported back to his manager that the hospital had said Charles didn't need any treatment. The team of support workers assured Charles that everything was OK. Charles coped with his urine difficulties as best he could. After three years, he started complaining of painful legs. Mohammed had left by then, and the new support worker didn't think it was anything serious, so initially Charles didn't see a doctor. Over the next six months, the pain got progressively worse. When Charles finally went to the GP, he was sent into hospital immediately, and it was found that the cancer had spread to his bones. Charles was given painkillers. He was never told his diagnosis. He became increasingly weak and died of metastatic prostate cancer a year later.

Outcome 2

Mohammed felt uncomfortable about not telling Charles, but he didn't think he knew enough about cancer to talk to Charles himself. He asked his manager for help, who called the local learning disabilities team for advice. Dianne, the learning disability nurse, contacted the hospital consultant and questioned him about his decision not to treat Charles. She discovered that the consultant would have treated other people with the same cancer as Charles, but that he didn't think that Charles could give his informed consent to treatment. Dianne called together a case conference and it was agreed that she would explain everything to Charles, and try to establish his wishes. Using a picture book (*Getting On With Cancer*, see further reading), Dianne talked to Charles about his cancer and explained the possibility of having curative radiotherapy. Charles understood this and decided he would have the treatment because he didn't want things to get worse. He went into hospital ten times for radiotherapy. Dianne and Mohammed supported him when his fear of hospitals took over, helping him again and again to understand why he needed to go. They also helped him to take things easy when he was tired from the treatments. Five years later, scans confirmed that the cancer had not returned, and Charles enjoyed a good quality of life for many more years.

Exercise 32.5

With others, role-play the following scenarios:

The consultant tells Mohammed the test results. Mohammed asks questions, and disagrees with the consultant; he thinks Charles should be told.

Dianne or Mohammed (or both) explain everything to Charles.

What was it like to act out these roles? If you were in Mohammed's position, what support would you need? What do you think Charles needs?

This case has highlighted a number of difficult issues that often arise when someone develops a life-threatening illness. These include consent to treatment, talking about the illness and choice-making. Let us look at these issues more closely.

Consent to treatment

Charles' consultant made the assumption that Charles wouldn't be able to give consent to treatment. It should never be assumed that people are not able to make their own decisions simply because they have learning disabilities. The laws on consent to treatment vary. Scotland led the way with the Adults with Incapacity (Scotland) Act, which took effect in 2000 (HMSO 2000). Under this Act, doctors are ultimately responsible for making health care decisions if a person is not capable of giving consent. It gives them clear guidelines on how to assess capacity, starting from the principle that all adults (including those with learning disabilities) are presumed capable of taking health care decisions. However, the Act recognizes that the capacity of an individual may vary, depending on time, circumstances and types of decision. In England and Wales, a Draft Mental Incapacity Bill was published in 2003 (Department for Constitutional Affairs 2003). This Bill aims to bring clarity and certainty to the decisions that have to be made by both health and social care workers for the people they support. So far, it has been common law that where someone cannot consent to treatment it is the duty of the health professional (usually the doctor) to act in the person's 'best interest'. In other words, professionals have to do 'what is right' for their patient. As in Scotland, the new Bill recognizes that adults may be able to take some decisions, even if they are not able to consent to others. Professionals will have to argue much more clearly why they think someone cannot take a particular decision. For the moment, comprehensive advice on consent can be found in a guidance document titled *Seeking Consent: Working with People with Learning Disabilities* (Department of Health 2001a).

So let us look more closely at Charles' situation. In order to be able to give valid consent, Charles needs to be competent (in other words, capable of taking that particular decision); he should not be pressured into a decision; and he should be provided with enough information to enable him to make the decision. In order to assess his capacity to decide about having treatment, he must be able to comprehend and retain information about the treatment, understand the consequences of not having the treatment and use this information to make his decision.

In this case Charles was capable enough to decide whether to have radiotherapy treatment or not. But what if he was not capable? Would the consultant then be right not to treat him? It can be argued that the consultant would be denying Charles potentially life-saving treatment, which he would have given if Charles didn't have learning disabilities. This lack of treatment could be seen as negligent. The consultant would have to decide what was in Charles' best interest, and to do this he would have to sit down with Charles' carers, advocate and (if he had any) his family. On the face of it, it seems that Charles' interest would be best served by giving him life-saving treatment. There would need to be a strong consensus to decide the opposite (e.g. if Charles' hospital phobia made having treatment more or less impossible).

Talking about the illness

Most people in our culture want to know about their illness. Even if they do not want to know all the details, or are happy to let the doctor decide what treatment is best, they want their questions answered honestly. For many years health care and palliative care professionals have advocated openness and honesty as the best way to help people cope with terminal illness, although they recognize that this needs to be done sensitively (Seale 1991). There is no reason to believe that this should be any different for people with learning disabilities. However, in the authors' experience, people with learning disabilities are often shielded from knowledge about their diagnosis. Family and carers are often closest to the person and have developed effective ways of communicating. While most will probably work from the principles of choice and respect, they themselves may be unfamiliar with talking openly about illness and death, and feel very anxious about these taboo subjects. Health professionals are used to truth-telling, but they may be at a complete loss about how to communicate with people with learning disabilities, or they may think that others will tell the person about their illness. The only way forward is for everyone to work closely together.

People with learning disabilities need to have their illness and any (proposed) medical procedures explained to them in very concrete, practical terms. Exactly what is happening now? What will happen next? Doctors and nurses (e.g. a Macmillan nurse) can help family and carers with this. Time needs to be taken to explain, with the help of demonstrations or pictures if necessary. A series of picture books has been designed for this purpose (the 'Books Beyond Words' series, see further reading). It is important that everyone involved knows what information has been given, and conflicting messages are avoided. It is not unusual for one person to answer questions honestly while another person says that everything will get better. This can only add to someone's confusion and distress.

Choice-making

Towards the end of life, and particularly if there is a life-threatening illness that can no longer be cured, any decisions and choices about the person's life should be aimed at achieving the best possible quality of life. We have already considered the many variables that can contribute to someone's quality of life. Choices need to be made, not only about the big issues (treatments, wills and funerals) but also about the day-to-day issues that may be of more immediate importance to the person with learning disabilities. Here are some examples of end of life choices:

- 'My mum is coming to visit, but I get so tired now from the day centre that I won't enjoy her visit. Maybe I can stay at home on the day when she visits.'

- 'I want to be free of pain, but the painkillers make me feel sleepy and I don't like that. Are there any other ways to cope with the pain?'
- 'I know that the chemotherapy makes me live longer, but I hate it so much. Do I have to have it?'
- 'Who do I want to look after me when I get more ill? I like it here at home, but I'm not sure my mum can manage.'
- 'They say that I shouldn't smoke but I like it and I want to.'

There are many different ways to help someone make choices, and such help needs to be highly individualized and culturally sensitive. One idea could be to create a life story book, with pointers to the important people, events and values in someone's life. For a more in-depth discussion of choice-making at the end of life, see *Positive Approaches to Palliative Care.*

Religion, culture and end of life

The choices people make in terms of the end of life and after-death practices are strongly influenced by their religion and culture. Religion and culture give many people the values, attitudes and beliefs that are important in their lives. Religion is linked to a spiritual faith, which usually has a set of practices and rituals, including death rituals. Culture is determined by the environment people grew up in. For example, in some cultures it is normal behaviour to express feelings of distress by crying, while in others this would be seen as a sign of weakness and 'not coping'. Cultures can vary even from family to family. It is important never to make assumptions, as cultural and religious practices can vary widely. For example, it is not enough to know that someone grew up in the West End of London and belongs to the Muslim faith. You would need to find out what particular elements from a specific culture or religion someone embraced. You can only do this by communicating closely with the person involved, their family and their close friends.

It takes a team to support someone at the end of life. The team consists of the person with learning disabilities themselves, their close friends and family and their carers and advocates. It can include the learning disabilities team, the primary care team, the hospital and specialist teams and the faith community: the list is potentially very long. Working and living with death and dying is never easy, but if everyone works together and the person with learning disabilities is fully included, it can be an enriching life experience for everyone involved.

Bereavement issues

Case study: *Kumar*

Kumar Parikh had Down's syndrome and was the only child of Saroj and Gyan Parikh. His mother, Saroj, was his main carer until her health deteriorated. His father, Gyan, was a businessman who travelled a great deal during his working life until his late sixties, so had relied on his wife to make decisions about family matters. Saroj died of heart failure after a long illness when she was 73, and Kumar was just 40. During her illness, which included many hospital admissions, Gyan began to play a bigger part in supporting Kumar each day. He was now 74 years old and fully retired. He enjoyed quite good health but was aware that Kumar was likely to outlive him.

Kumar had always lived at home and, as an only child with a busy father, had been used to being the centre of his mother's attention. When his father retired there were some upsetting battles as Gyan began to assert more authority at home, and the family requested advice and help from the community learning disability team at this time. When Saroj was admitted to hospital the team arranged for Kumar to have two weeks of respite care. This soon became a pattern, with Kumar having respite, if it was available, whenever his mother was admitted. During her last illness, the period of respite was longer than usual and Kumar was in respite when his mother died.

Exercise 32.6

What do you think is the best way forward in this situation? Should Kumar stay in the respite unit until the funeral is over or should his father be supported to take Kumar home so that he can be involved in the Hindu funeral rituals and grieve with his father and other family members and friends (see Raji *et al.* 2003)? Should he stay in the respite unit until a decision has been made about where he will live in the future? Or should he be able to go home and make plans for his future over the next few months when he and his father have had time to come to terms with Saroj's death? If possible, get together with others to debate this issue, each taking on a different role. You *must* reach a decision.

Outcome 1

It was decided that Kumar should stay in the respite unit and the manager agreed with Gyan that Kumar would not attend the funeral as they thought he would not fully understand what was happening. Although it is traditional for male relatives to participate fully in Hindu funeral rites, children and women do not and people with learning disabilities are also often excluded. Kumar went to the day centre as usual on the day of the funeral and did not see his father for some days, although some of the relatives who came to the funeral did visit him in the unit. The family suggested to Gyan that it would be too difficult for him to have Kumar back home, but they were all worried about what would happen to Kumar. Gyan's sister thought that there was a risk that Gyan would be left to cope on his own and was worried what would happen if he became ill or died. Gyan decided to say that Kumar couldn't come home. The community team social worker started to look for a new home for him and found an adult family placement with a Hindu family in another part of town. Gyan was able to visit him and invited him to come home for a meal once a month. Kumar seemed to settle although he was very quiet and became incontinent, and would become very angry if anyone mentioned his mother. His father died three years later and the family home was left to his sister.

Outcome 2

It was decided that Kumar should go home as soon as possible and social services agreed to pay for a one-to-one worker to provide several hours of support each day. They agreed that the support would be reviewed in six weeks' time, and adjusted if necessary, but the social worker reassured Gyan that it would not be withdrawn until Kumar had his own person-centred plan with the support he needed in place. The social worker also said that he would have the choice of Direct Payments so that he could purchase care that was culturally sensitive and flexible to meet his particular needs. An agency support worker was found who came from the Hindu community and was able to support Kumar in the immediate period after his mother's death. Another worker soon joined him and they took it in turns to support Kumar in his personal care, and in resuming his daytime occupation. Kumar made it clear that he wanted to stay at home with his father, but his behaviour and mood became difficult when it was suggested to him that he should move into a group home. His father was worried that the support being offered now might not be sustained in the longer term and realized that he needed a great deal of financial advice before being able to decide whether to leave his house to Kumar in his will (see Harker and King 2002). He was put in touch with a housing adviser and decided to set up a family trust. He decided that he wanted Kumar to stay in the house he had lived in for his whole life. He made arrangements for his care to be managed by the trust and made appropriate provision in his will. Gyan died three years later and Kumar stayed at home with increased support. A friend of Kumar's came to live with him and through the Supporting People finance available in each local authority they were able to afford to have a support worker sleeping in the house every night. Kumar missed his father and initially hid all the photos of his parents. A support worker referred him to the local bereavement counselling service, and he saw a counsellor for several months, which helped him a great deal.

Exercise 32.7

Having read these outcomes, how do you feel now about the decision you proposed?

Do you think future outcomes alter the way decisions are perceived as right or wrong?

What if the outcomes were altogether different?

Outcome 3

As in Outcome 1 Kumar settled into his new home, but one of his new 'family' died suddenly and Kumar was immediately moved back into respite.

Outcome 4

As in Outcome 2 Kumar stayed at home with his father but the support agency appointed a worker who later exploited Kumar by 'borrowing' money from him when he went with him to the bank.

The impact of a bereavement

Grief following the death of a close relative or friend is a normal and common reaction. The following responses are described by many bereaved people: feeling fear and panic; numbness and disbelief about what has happened; feeling out of control; being under- or overactive; losing appetite for food; being unable to sleep; having a poor memory; hearing the voice of the dead person; wanting to talk to them; forgetting they have died; being cross with other people; crying a lot; being unable to think or work. For someone with a learning disability the same reactions may be expressed behaviourally rather than in words. Disturbances of sleep and appetite are relatively easy to notice, but unexplained anger towards people or objects, or self-harm may be harder to understand (Hollins and Sireling 1999).

Exercise 32.8

Think about the following questions:

In Exercise 32.3 you were asked to name five things that contribute to your quality of life. You may have chosen family, health, work, skills, hobbies, faith, food, holidays . . . What would it be like for you to lose one, two, or even all of these five things, for example following a bereavement?

Think of one person with learning disabilities you know who has been bereaved. What do you think this person values most in life? How many of these things were lost when they were bereaved? Is there anything anyone could do to restore some of these things to the person now? If you don't know, how could you find out? Could you ask the person? Spend time with him or her? Ask close carers, family or friends?

Communication and collaboration

When a person with learning disabilities is bereaved, those involved are affected in many different ways. Let us look at some of the issues. First, those *faced by the person with learning disabilities*:

- *Changes in skills*: grief can lead us all to lose some skills, usually temporarily, and this may be because of our preoccupation with our loss or because of the unexpected additional skills we need to acquire to cope without the person who has died. For example, people with learning disabilities may become incontinent, less articulate, or forget the way home from a familiar activity.

- *Worry and anxiety*: the person may not understand about the finality of death. Worry about where the deceased person has gone may lead to searching behaviour. Carers may describe this as wandering or repetitive behaviour, not recognizing what the person is looking for. For example, the person who did not attend her father's funeral and was told that he had 'gone away', kept asking, 'Where's Dad?' over and over. Staff saw this as inappropriate when it was still being asked three years later, but having missed the opportunity to include her in the funeral rituals, nobody had found a way to explain his death to her. The emotional experience of being a chief mourner, and the way in which the different senses help us to understand the finality of death, had been denied to her.

- *Changes in circumstances*: sometimes the person who died was the main carer or the only person who really understood the speech or signs used by the bereaved person. Often someone will lose so much more than the person who has died. They may lose their home, their familiar routines, the experience of being understood, their neighbours, visiting tradespeople – the list is endless. Unfamiliar people, places and routines replace these losses, and initial moves are usually temporary. Oswin (1991) described how some people might be moved several times in the months following the death of their last surviving parent.

- *Communication problems*: just as with the end of life issues discussed above, it is likely that the person has difficulty in communicating their feelings, fears or wishes. Their way of communicating may be misinterpreted or disregarded.

Issues faced by the family include:

- *Involvement*: many families are very involved throughout the person's life, and often know the person better than anyone else. They need to be included in important decision-making at times of transition. Family members, including siblings, who have not been recently involved in a person's life may want or need more involvement now. The bereavement their relative is experiencing may be a shared bereavement with their own grief, affecting their response to the family member with a learning disability. While many care managers and care settings are excellent at including the family as important partners, others may resent the (sometimes sudden) emergence of family wishes. Recent government policy on learning disability recognized that family carers were often not fully involved in decision-making, and strongly advocated more family involvement (Department of Health 2001b).

- *Experience of services*: families who have continued to care for their relative at home may find the sudden involvement and influence of social workers or learning disability professionals rather difficult, particularly if they have been used to doing their own problem-solving within their own informal networks. They may be confused by the gap between the reality of the service response to their family bereavement, and the aspirations in *Valuing People* or the plans being discussed by their local Partnership Board. Alternatively they may be familiar with more traditional segregated service provision and find newer ideas about person-centred planning bewildering.

Issues faced by carers include:

- *Lack of skills and resources*: daily caregivers may think that they have the skills and resources to support someone who has been bereaved, but in practice find that it is an area of human experience with which they are unfamiliar. This can be particularly difficult if the person lives in a residential home rather than with their family. Staff at the home may feel that they cannot cope with changes in behaviour or mood and are unable, due to staffing, to offer any increased support for someone's emotional needs at such a time.

- *Involvement*: many carers, including paid carers at residential homes, are highly committed to the people they support, perhaps to the extent of not wanting to use other supports which are available to all community members. Sometimes this may still result in a good outcome for the person. However, sometimes if carers feel that they are the only ones who can support the person properly, they miss out when carers do not have all the skills required. A recent study found that bereaved people with learning disabilities were able to benefit from referral to volunteer bereavement counselling services when their carers had the foresight to recognize the specialist skills of trained bereavement counsellors (Dowling *et al.* 2003).

- *Lack of experience regarding death*: many carers in learning disability services are young and may never have experienced bereavement at close hand, leading them to avoid talking about the person who has died.

Issues faced by services include:

- *The right place to live*: services may have to consider how to continue supporting the person in their usual home. This depends on the level of support available at home, which will be particularly pertinent if the person who died was the main carer. The person's wishes, and those of the family, need to be taken into account. There may be pressure on services to make decisions immediately after the bereavement. However, it is not a good idea to assess somebody's skills and wishes at this time for reasons discussed above.

- *Profusion of services*: at any time of transition there can be a large number and variety of professionals and others involved, including support workers, GPs, social workers and learning disability teams as well as family members, advocates and concerned neighbours or friends. There is a risk that some of the professionals will communicate well with each other, leaving other key people out including both formal and informal supporters. Sometimes, despite a relative lack of service availability, responses to bereavement can be over-professionalized, and fail to mobilize more ordinary personal and community support.

Each bereavement is different and the points raised here will not apply in every situation, but they do reflect issues that have recurred many times in the authors' own experiences. It is crucial that the person themselves remains at the centre of any response made by families and professionals, and that they are supported to remember their deceased friend or family member. This may require special attention to their understanding of the meaning of death. Readers are encouraged to use the bereavement titles in the 'Books Beyond Words' series of picture books for adults with learning disabilities, of which one author is the series editor.

Conclusion

When someone with learning disabilities approaches the end of life, they and their family, carers and services face a wide range of complex issues. Many people with learning disabilities are denied access to the same end of life care as the rest of the population. Issues regarding disclosure and consent can be particularly pertinent. Bereavement can be equally complex. Death, loss and bereavement are difficult areas of life, and for many people they are still taboo.

It is possible to provide sensitive and timely support, but this can only be achieved if everyone involved works closely and actively together, and if the person with learning disabilities is kept firmly in the centre of any choice and decision-making.

Further reading

Books Beyond Words series. This is a series of picture books written for and with people with learning disabilities, edited by Sheila Hollins. Relevant titles include:

Donaghey, V., Bernal, J., Tuffrey-Wijne, I. and Hollins, S. (2002) *Getting On With Cancer*. London: Royal College of Psychiatrists. This book tells the story of Veronica, a woman with Down's syndrome who has cancer. She has surgery, radiotherapy and chemotherapy. The book deals honestly with the unpleasant side of treatment.

Hollins, S. and Sireling, L. (1994) *When Mum Died* and *When Dad Died*. London: Royal College of Psychiatrists. These books tell the story of the death of a parent in a simple but moving way. They take a straightforward and honest approach to death and grief in the family.

Hollins, S., Dowling, S. and Blackman, N. (2003) *When Somebody Dies*. London: Royal College of Psychiatrists. This book shows people with learning disabilities that they need not be alone when they feel sad about someone's death, and that talking about it to a friend or to a counsellor can help them get through a difficult time.

All Books Beyond Words titles are available at £10 each from the Royal College of Psychiatrists, 17 Belgrave Square, London SW1X 8PG, tel. 020 7235 2351, ext. 146. Online orders: www.rcpsych.ac.uk/publications.

Hollins, S. and Sireling, L. (1999) *Understanding Grief*, 2nd edn. Brighton: Pavilion. This is a staff training pack about the experience of grief and bereavement for people with learning disabilities. *Available from the Department of Mental Health, St George's Hospital Medical School, Cranmer Terrace, London SW17 0RE.*

Jones, A. and Tuffrey-Wijne, I. (2004) *Positive Approaches to Palliative Care*. Kidderminster: British Institute for Learning Disabilities. This is an interactive study workbook for carers in learning disability services. It deals extensively with supporting a person with learning disabilities through terminal illness and bereavement. It is part of the Learning Disabilities Awards Framework, and can be accredited to Levels 2 and 3. *Available from the British Institute of Learning Disabilities, Campion House, Green Street, Kidderminster, Worcestershire DY10 1JL, tel. 01562 723010, email enquiries@bild.org.uk.*

Keywood, K., Fovargue, S. and Flynn, M. (undated) *Best Practice? Health Care Decision Making by, with and for Adults with Leraning Dsiabilites. Available from the National Development Team, Albino Wharf, Albion Street, Manchester M1 5LN, tel. 0161 2287055.*

Resources

Organizations to contact for help and advice

CancerBACUP, 3 Bath Place, London E2A 3JR. Telephone helpline: 0808 800 1234. Website: www.cancerbacup.org.uk. *CancerBACUP provides information about cancer and support to people with cancer, their families and friends.*

Cruse Bereavement Care, Cruse House, 126 Sheen Road, Richmond, Surrey TW9 1UR. Telephone helpline: 0870 1671677. *Offers free bereavement counselling, support and information to anyone bereaved by death.*

Macmillan Information Line, 89 Albert Embankment, London SE1 7UQ. Telephone helpline: 0845 601 6161. *Provides information about Macmillan services and other cancer organizations and support agencies.*

National Network for the Palliative Care of People with Learning Disabilities, St Nicholas Hospice, Macmillan Way, Hardwick Lane, Bury St Edmunds IP33 2QY, tel. 01284 766133. *Encourages and contributes to the development of good practice in the palliative care of people with learning disabilities.*

Video

A Billion Seconds. This video shows a 40-minute performance by the Strathcona Theatre Company. Acted by people with learning disabilities, it deals with issues concerning cancer, including bereavement. The video is suitable for people with learning disabilities, carers and professionals, and includes a booklet. *Available from the British Institute for Learning Disabilities, Campion House, Green Street, Kidderminster, Worcestershire DY10 1JL, tel. 01562 723010, email enquiries@bild.org.uk.*

References

Blackman, N. (2003) *Loss and Learning Disability*. London: Worth Publishing.

Brown, H., Burns, S. and Flynn, M. (2002) Supporting people through terminal illness and death, in Foundation for People with Learning Disabilities, *Today and Tomorrow, the Report of the Growing Older with Learning Disabilities Programme*. London: Mental Health Foundation.

Cohen, S. *et al.* (1995) The McGill Quality of Life Questionnaire: a measure of quality of life appropriate for people with advanced disease. A preliminary study of validity and acceptability, *Palliative Medicine*, 9: 207–19.

Department for Constitutional Affairs (2003) *Draft Mental Incapacity Bill*. London: The Stationery Office.

Department of Health (2001a) *Seeking Consent: Working with People with Learning Disabilities*. London: Department of Health.

Department of Health (2001b) *Valuing People: A New Strategy for Learning Disability for the 21st Century*. A White Paper. London: Department of Health.

Dowling, S., Hubert, J. and Hollins, S. (2003) Bereavement interventions for people with learning disabilities, *Bereavement Care*, 22(2): 19–21.

Evans, P.M. and Alberman, E. (1990) Certified cause of death in children and young adults with cerebral palsy, *Archives of Disease in Childhood*, 65: 325–9.

Eyman, R.K., Borthwick-Duffy, S.A., Call, T.L. and White, J.F. (1988) Prediction of mortality in community and institutional settings, *Journal of Mental Deficiency Research*, 32: 203–13.

Flanagan, J. (1978) A research approach to improving your quality of life, *American Psychology*, 33: 138–47.

Harker, H. and King, N. (2002) *Renting your Own Home: Housing Options for People with Learning Disabilities*. Kidderminster: British Institute of Learning Disabilities.

HMSO (2000) *Adults with Incapacity (Scotland) Act 2000*. London: The Stationery Office.

Hollins, S. and Sireling, L. (1999) *Understanding Grief*, 2nd edn. Brighton: Pavilion.

Hollins, S., Attard, M.T., von Fraunhofer, N., McGuigan, S. and Sedgwick, P. (1998) Mortality in people with learning disability: risks, causes, and death certification findings in London, *Developmental Medicine and Child Neurology*, 40: 50–6.

McGuigan, S., Hollins, S. and Attard, M. (1995) Age-specific standardised mortality rates in people with learning disability, *Journal of Intellectual Disability Research*, 39(6): 527–31.

Mölsä, P.K. (1994) Survival in mental retardation, *Mental Handicap Research*, 7: 338–45.

Northfield, J. and Turnbull, J. (2001) Experiences from cancer services, in J. Hogg, J. Northfield and J. Turnbull (eds) *Cancer and People with Learning Disabilities*. Kidderminster: British Institute of Learning Disabilities.

Oswin, M. (1991) *Am I Allowed to Cry? A Study of Bereavement Amongst People who Have Learning Disabilities*. London: Souvenir Press.

Raji, O., Hollins, S. and Drinnan, A. (2003) How far are people with learning disabilities involved in funeral rites? *British Journal of Learning Disabilities*, 31: 42–5.

Scottish Executive (2004) *Health Needs Assessment Report: People with Learning Disabilities in Scotland*. Glasgow: Health Scotland.

Seale, C. (1991) Communication and awareness about death: a study of a random sample of dying people, *Social Science and Medicine*, 32(8): 943–52.

Tuffrey-Wijne, I. (1998) Care of the terminally ill, *Learning Disability Practice*, 1(1): 8–11.

Tuffrey-Wijne, I. (2003) The palliative care needs of people with intellectual disabilities: a literature review, *Palliative Medicine*, 17(1): 55–62.

Wilson, I. (1995) Linking clinical variables with health-related quality of life: a conceptual model of patient outcomes, *Journal of the American Medical Association*, 273(1): 59–65.

33

Healthy and successful ageing

Gordon Grant

Introduction

Earlier chapters in this last section of the book have illustrated that survival to and beyond national retirement age has become increasingly common among people with learning disabilities, at least in post-industrial societies. Recent statistics from developed countries like the USA, Canada, Australia and the UK suggest that there is now but a handful of years that separate the life expectancy of people with learning disabilities from the population at large (Bigby 2004). However, life chances are significantly reduced when environmental factors like living conditions, poverty and world region are taken into account in addition to personal factors like gender and degree/ complexity of disability. By far the most significant among these are the environmental factors. This is once again a reminder that environmental factors are the source of major inequalities in the lives of people with learning disabilities as they reach old age, something that has been on the agenda of the World Health Organization (2001) for some years now. People with learning disabilities living in the world's poorest regions, for example, have a life expectancy that is just half that of those in more prosperous nations, a situation no doubt fuelled by systems of global economic and political governance that perpetuate a gulf between the world's richer and poorer nations.

This chapter concerns: ideas and theories that help to inform an understanding of healthy and successful ageing in people with learning disabilities; how people with learning disabilities talk about and make sense of ageing; and implications for practice.

Healthy and successful ageing – ideas and theories

Ageing is a process, not an event. How successfully individuals age depends on many factors including lifestyle, life history, informal and formal support from earlier years, genetic dispositions, and environmental constraints and opportunities. Many older people with learning disabilities age in a similar way to the general population so it is worth briefly introducing generic theories of successful ageing as most of these are equally applicable to people with learning disabilities. This applies just as well to their health status in later life. Indeed, healthy ageing is integral to successful ageing, and it is quite difficult to separate the two. In this section therefore ideas and theories about successful ageing are introduced before considering some of the exceptional or additional needs and circumstances of older people with learning disabilities, especially with regard to their health, and how these can be understood.

Brandstadter and Grieve (1994) place an emphasis on the ability of older people to maintain a sense of personal continuity and meaning in the face of different kinds of losses that accompany the ageing process. In order to achieve this they argue that three sets of complementary processes need to be invoked:

- *assimilation*: defines efforts people make to realize their original goals and aspirations; most useful when problems are reversible and can be easily compensated for;

- *accommodation*: when assimilation is not possible, it may be necessary to reshape goals, activities and priorities consistent with available resources;

- *immunization*: this occurs when individuals selectively interpret demands that threaten core components of an individual's identity that need to be protected, requiring either a reinterpretation of the significance of demands or a readjustment of individual performance.

All three processes are linked and integral to positive adaptation. If goals and aspirations remain consistent with realistic options then successful ageing is likely. People with learning disabilities might be expected to struggle more than most with the types of cognitive coping implied by the above strategies, but this remains a hypothesis yet to be tested.

Atchley's (1999) continuity theory suggests that over time individuals display remarkable consistency in patterns of thinking, living arrangements, social relationships and activity profiles. Similar to Branstadter and Grieve (1994), Atchley also stresses the importance of life history and biography to an understanding of experiences in later life. Reminiscence therapy in people with dementia is premised on such thinking. However, it serves to remind us that the present generation of older people with learning disabilities may have past lives punctuated by gaps and confusions about their identities, family and social relations as a result of the segregated and institutionalized conditions in which they used to live (see Chapters 1 and 30), making later life adjustment more difficult.

In their theory of 'selective optimization with compensation' Baltes and Carstensen (1996) suggest that three core processes are involved in successful ageing: greater selection of activity and function as physical activity reduces; compensation for loss or skill or function by using alternative means to achieve goals; and optimization by making the most of personal reserves to support selection and compensation. This line of thinking is useful in emphasizing that, like their younger counterparts, older people have goals, agency (capacity), the ability to discriminate and make choices, and the prospect of making accommodations and adjustments in the face of demands and challenges.

Meanwhile, in their cross-cultural study involving developed and developing nations, Fry *et al.* (1997) have shown that a good old age was associated with reliable physical health and functioning, material security, family and kinship networks and 'sociality'. Reliable physical health and functioning includes the capacity to take part in activities of one's choice, together with the energy, strength and vitality to continue in these. Material security refers to money, entitlements and resources sufficient to sustain a given level of living. Family and kinship networks define the immediate social structures to which older people are connected that provide them with support and care, advice and information, reassurance and worth. 'Sociality' has to do with life domains that allow people to receive positive feedback about themselves, as reflected in things like being and feeling part of the community and communities of interest, having the freedom to choose what to do and, by association, the ability to exert a sense of control over things that matter in one's life.

Activity theory proposed long ago by Lawton and Nahemow (1973) suggests that successful ageing depends upon maintaining activity in later life, a readiness to replace old roles with new ones, and a continuing involvement in the community and in social relations. Lawton *et al.* (1995) subsequently went on to demonstrate that activity alone is not enough and that cognitive challenges are required that allow older people to demonstrate competence and mastery. These are in turn likely to be important to positive self-image. Nahemow's (1990) subsequent ecological theory suggests however that in later life people need environments that are neither too demanding nor too devoid of stimulation.

For Coleman (1997) however, further development and empirical testing of theories of ageing is still necessary, especially in regard to:

- the importance of life history and life span influences on later life adaptation;

- development in later life with a focus on ordinary as opposed to exceptional ageing;

- understanding individual differences;

- a better appreciation of the existential challenges of frailty.

Coleman reminds us that in concentrating on successful ageing there is of course a danger of overlooking the impairments and chronic illnesses that can accompany the ageing process and how these are experienced. The onset and course of impairments and illnesses, and their implications for individuals, are real and inescapable. Hence, people in later life may be facing significant restrictions and declines in some areas of their lives while continuing to experience development and growth in others. This conceptualization is a far cry from the position taken up many years ago by Cumming and Henry (1961) in which it was claimed that as they age older people gradually withdraw from society, giving rise to what they labelled as 'disengagement theory'. This has come to be regarded as over-simplistic, unduly pathological and in any case contrary to the weight of contemporary gerontological evidence.

These generic theories and ideas about successful ageing have some clear implications for practice:

- If personal continuity and meaning are important in understanding how people age successfully, there is a need to be sensitive to factors that can give rise to discontinuities across the lifecourse (see Chapter 11) and how these can be predicted, prevented or ameliorated.

- Helping people to face and come to terms with biographical gaps or disruptions in their past lives may be difficult and even traumatic for individuals, as for example in the case of people who were previously institutionalized or the many older women with learning disabilities who have had their children taken away from them.

- Resourcefulness and resilience in individuals do not disappear just because they have reached a good old age. Rather, these attributes need to be respected and nurtured since they are integral to helping people to maintain a positive self-image.

- Commitment to the support of successful ageing is likely to require a balanced attention to people's strengths as well as to their needs, including an understanding of the internal processes individuals use to make accommodations as they age.

Exercise 33.1

Think of a close relative, perhaps a parent, that you know well who is aged 60 years or more. Then try to identify examples of assimilation, accommodation and immunization from the way your relative talks about managing things in later life. Consider which if any of these strategies seems to be most important to them.

According to Bigby (2004), some theories of successful ageing appear to be beyond the reach of many older people with learning disabilities. For example, writers such as Jorm *et al.* (1998) and Rowe and Kahn (1998) define successful ageing in terms of criteria that would be hard to reach such as absence of disease and disability, high cognitive skills and productive activity.

In relation to people with learning disabilities, Heller (2004) describes a support-outcomes model of successful ageing which emphasizes the importance of the environment and individualized supports in influencing outcomes. Outcomes are considered in relation to independence, quality of life, physical and emotional well-being and community inclusion. Interactions between personal and environmental factors are depicted as influencing these outcomes. Personal factors are described in terms of capabilities such as competence and attributes that help individuals to function in society. Environmental factors comprise the demands and constraints of everyday life. Desirable environments are seen to possess three main characteristics: opportunities for fulfilling people's needs; possibilities for fostering physical, social, material and cognitive well-being; and prospects for realizing a sense of stability, predictability and control. Supports may come from a variety of sources including people, technology and services.

Case study: successful ageing?

Maria is 61 years of age. She lives in a group home with two of her long-standing friends, Freda and Susan. The three women have known each other for decades, dating back to the time when they were all residents in a long-stay hospital. The home is managed by a local voluntary organization and the three women all hold tenancies.

Maria's parents died years ago though she had long since lost contact with them when she was a long-stay hospital resident. The circumstances surrounding this loss of contact are still rather cloudy. Maria compares her present living situation very favourably to that when she was living in a hospital. She likes the creature comforts of having her own room, a key to come and go when she pleases, and close friends in Freda and Susan with whom she shares much of her life. Maria had to leave the local day centre when she was 60. It is based on the other side of town so she rarely sees friends and companions that she knew there. Her home is based conveniently for local shops and amenities, but though she can walk to most places she has mobility difficulties due to having cerebral palsy. When she has been out on her own she has once or twice fallen and had to be taken to the accident and emergency department at the local hospital.

Because of her appearance and gait, over the years Maria has experienced many jibes and taunts from members of the public, usually gangs of young boys. Though she tries to ignore these comments they still affect her deeply. Maria has limited vocabulary and finds it difficult to defend herself against the offensive behaviour of other people. Like one or two of her friends she has tried to join the local physically handicapped and able bodied

(PHAB) club, but been rejected, apparently on the grounds that her learning disability disqualified her. This really hurt her. Her care manager has been trying to resolve this situation with the club, thus far without success.

Maria considers herself to be quite healthy though she admits to not having the energy she once had. Risk of falling and the avoidance of anti-social behaviour from gangs of young people have made her even more wary about being out by herself. Beyond her immediate friends, Freda and Susan, Maria does not really have a wider social circle. Since her retirement from the day centre her life has become even more home-based. As a result, she spends a lot of time listening to the radio or reading magazines in her own room or watching TV with Freda and Susan in the lounge. Maria has conservative expectations for material possessions, probably the by product of a life lived dependent upon financial support from the state.

Maria seems quite aware of her own mortality and is becoming increasingly concerned about the failing health of her two friends, Freda and Susan, both more frail than her.

Exercise 33.2

Thinking of Maria, consider what features of her environment enhance her well-being and what features undermine it.

Make a note of the features of Maria's social relations that have some influence on her well-being.

Thinking of the successful ageing model described by Heller (2004), what are the consequences for Maria of seeking a more stable and predictable lifestyle?

Accessing health services in later life

We are still a long way from knowing about all the factors that govern the health status of older people with learning disabilities. One of the reasons for this is that we do not know where many older people with learning disabilities are, so little or nothing is known of their circumstances. Older people with mild learning disabilities have probably long since successfully 'disappeared' in mainstream society and are no doubt managing their lives quite adequately, without specialist learning disability services. This is an assumption still in need of testing. Even for those with high support needs, many are 'lost' from specialist learning disability services, having retired from day services, moved into generic or elder care services, or managed somehow to get lost in the system because of a lack of active case finding or integrated case records linked by a 'cradle to grave' philosophy. This also makes it difficult, even impossible, to produce an accurate estimate of the number of older people with learning disabilities in most localities. Because this can leave individuals with less than appropriate support, it can easily result in unnecessarily restricted lifestyles (Foundation for People with Learning Disabilities 2002).

Even when people are known to services, there are barriers that continue to make it difficult for them to access appropriate health care. In their searching review about physical health issues involved in healthy ageing Evenhuis *et al.* (2001) for example have described many factors that mediate access to health services. These can be split for convenience into two groups: person-specific and environment-specific.

Person-specific

The limited articulacy of people with severe cognitive impairments is one of the main difficulties. This can inevitably lead to a significant masking of the ability of individuals to disclose how they are feeling, placing a high premium on those with close personal knowledge of the individual to make judgements on such matters, with all the risks this can entail. Similar challenges arise in the case of people with multiple disabilities where one condition can confuse or compromise patterns of symptomatology associated with another, thereby increasing the risk of inappropriate diagnosis and treatment. Imagine for example a deaf or hard of hearing person who is also aphasic (unable to understand or express speech because of brain damage) and unable to make use of a recognized signing system. Examples like this are quite common.

Environment-specific

Many more barriers to appropriate health care are created by the very environments in which people find themselves. Medical history-taking can take a long time and is largely dependent on observations of staff and family members who know the person well. Staff turnover is a complicating factor here, as also is the death, migration or incapacity of family members where important biographical and life history details can quickly disappear. Consent procedures and associated concerns, while necessary to protect the health and welfare of individuals, can protract medical history-taking even further.

Behavioural difficulties constitute an additional potential barrier. Individuals commonly find themselves being assessed in unfamiliar health care environments like accident and emergency departments, drop-in centres, community centres or GPs' surgeries, by people not well known to them. As a consequence they may have difficulty cooperating with examinations, tests and questions, primarily because of their fears and confusion associated with unfamiliar environments and people. Consent to treatment and compliance with treatment may therefore become problematic. There is plenty of evidence suggesting that many health care providers still lack the skills and sensitivities to deal with these situations in helpful ways.

Case complexity represents a further barrier to effective health care.

People often require access to a variety of medical and other specialists, placing a high premium on case management, case coordination and person-centred planning (see Chapter 24). The jury is still out on how well such systems work (Mansell and Beadle-Brown 2004).

Exercise 33.3

Think of an older person with learning disabilities well known to you who is at least 50 years of age. In regard to their ability to access generic health services, list all the personal factors that appear to act as barriers, then list all the environmental factors that seem to inhibit or bar access. Consider what should be done to deal with these barriers.

Getting closer to the person in everyday practice

These considerations raise interesting challenges for the types of knowledge likely to be necessary in helping people to negotiate access to services and more particularly in 'getting closer to the person' in professional practice. Drawing on the work of Liaschenko (1997) and Mead and Bower (2000), these can be summarized as follows: case knowledge, patient knowledge, communicative knowledge and person knowledge.

- *Case knowledge* refers to disembodied biomedical knowledge – that is, a knowledge of aetiology, clinical symptoms and prognoses. It is this knowledge that most clearly differentiates professional and clinical workers (as people with authority and power) from patients, families and others.

- *Patient knowledge* refers to a person's social circumstances and support relevant to contextualizing case knowledge. To some extent, health care workers will have access to such knowledge through case files and medical records.

- *Communicative knowledge* has to do with how people convey intent, meaning and understanding. This is especially important for older people with learning disabilities as for many such people their verbal competencies are severely impaired, making non-verbal communication, assistive communication technologies, allies and advocates important. In the use of these complementary communication systems people with learning disabilities are often more expert than those they are seeking to consult.

- *Person knowledge* comprises dimensions of agency, temporality and space. Agency refers to an individual's capacity to initiate meaningful action; temporality refers to how their life patterns are shaped by developmental, social and cultural clocks; while space here refers to how individuals relate to physical, social and political environments.

Person knowledge and communicative knowledge are domains in which the person with learning disabilities and their families have superior insights and relevant knowledge than professional and clinical workers. It is also the domain in which professionals are least knowledgeable. Patient knowledge, as defined above, is also a domain in which the person will in most circumstances have superior knowledge to other stakeholders, though this may also depend on their 'mental capacity'. Case knowledge, finally, is the most obvious domain in which practitioners will have superior knowledge.

In the present policy climate where such a great emphasis is placed on the forging of partnerships between doctors, health and social care workers, patients and families, all of these types of knowledge have to be brought into the equation. A dependency on case knowledge simply will not do as it reinforces traditional power relations and fails to capture the other types of knowledge mentioned that are central to understanding and empowering people. Though an oversimplification, Table 33.1 suggests that most of the relevant knowledge lies with the person, and to some extent their families, not the professional worker. This leaves a huge onus of responsibility with professionals to draw upon all these sources of knowledge if they are to stand a chance of 'getting close to the person' in helping to ensure that the person gets the support and help they need.

It remains ironic that one of the most long-standing barriers directly affecting access to appropriate health care in the UK for people with learning disabilities in general is that many are still not registered with GPs. Bringing registration up to 100 per cent was one of the targets of *Valuing People* (Department of Health 2001) that was to have been achieved by June 2004. That it has to be set as a target at all is an indictment for a developed country like the UK that has had a national health service, free at the point of access for everyone, for almost 60 years. Clearly, without such basic access there is not even a chance that professional and clinical workers will have an opportunity to develop case knowledge, and in the context of a typical ten-minute GP consultation there is little chance of patient, communicative or person knowledge being developed. It remains to be seen whether the new arrangements for health action planning or person-centred planning envisaged by *Valuing People* can deliver in these particular respects.

The recent *Health Needs Assessment Report* about people with learning

Table 33.1   Knowledge, the person, the family and the practitioner

Type of knowledge	Person as expert	Family as expert	Practitioner as expert
Case knowledge	Low	Low	High
Patient knowledge	High	Medium	Medium
Communicative knowledge	High	High	Low
Person knowledge	High	High	Low

disabilities in Scotland (NHS Health Scotland 2004) reaffirms some of these points by suggesting that there is a basic lack of health promotion, under-identification of ill health and a deficit in meeting those health needs specific to people with learning disabilities.

Determinants of health in old age

Physical health

Access to health care services aside, older people with learning disabilities experience rates of common adult and older age-related conditions compar-able to the general population. These seem to reflect the same connections between hereditary disposition and environment present in older people. For some conditions, rates are higher in older people with learning dis-abilities compared to age-related peers without learning disabilities, for example obesity, dental disease, gastro-oesophageal reflux and oesophagitis, constipation and gastrointestinal cancer. Further examples are reported to include heart disease, mobility impairments, thyroid disease, osteoporosis, pneumonia and psychotropic drug problems (Evenhuis *et al.* 2001).

It is important when considering the physical health of older people with learning disabilities that syndrome-specific conditions and associated conditions arising from central nervous system compromise are taken into account. The weight of evidence about these matters is developing very quickly now but there is insufficient space to detail it here.

It is thought that for people with milder learning disabilities there is the possibility that increased lifestyle choices may result in potential for risky behaviours, for example tobacco and substance abuse, violent behaviour and high-risk sexual behaviour. Poor diet and inappropriate caring practices are thought to have contributed to high rates of periodontal disease in adults with learning disabilities. Sedentary lifestyles, lack of exercise and work environments that fail to stimulate people are all implicated as environ-mental factors shaping poor health. Permissive attitudes that have too often led to the exclusion of people with learning disabilities from health screening programmes should no longer be allowed to hold sway.

However, there is no evidence that preventative health practices recom-mended for the general population should be withheld from people with learning disabilities. Evenhuis *et al.* (2001) in fact suggest that lifestyle issues should be targeted specifically because these may well result in substantial gains in longevity, improved functional capacity and quality of life in old age. In particular it is thought that special programmes targeted at safe sex practices, avoidance of tobacco and other harmful substances, oral hygiene, exercise and diet, and fire safety education are all in need of devel-opment and evaluation.

Mental health

Compared to younger adults, older people with learning disabilities are much more likely to have accompanying psychiatric disorders, especially depression, generalized anxiety disorder and dementia (Cooper 1997). Past history of affective disorder is also reported to be present in a larger proportion of the older group. As people with learning disabilities age their need for psychiatric services appears to increase.

The increased prevalence of psychiatric disorders in adults is associated with social, biological and medical factors, life events and specific syndromes (Cooper 1997; Tyrell and Dodd 2003). Among social factors are lack of education, institutionalization at an early age, limited social networks, loss of close and confiding relationships, bereavement, lack of valued roles (e.g. paid work, marriage/partnership, parenthood), low income and relative poverty, service breaks and transitions and shifting patterns of interdependence with parents during the life cycle. All these factors are thought to impact on personality and predispose individuals to mental health problems in later life. Abuse and neglect can have long-term consequences for individuals and their families (O'Callaghan *et al.* 2003) but it is difficult to gauge from the available evidence whether and how this may manifest itself in later life.

Biological factors are also important. The presence of a behavioural phenotype can heighten risk. For example, Down's syndrome can predispose to an increased risk of dementia of the Alzheimer's type. According to Prasher's (1995) findings for example, dementia in people with Down's syndrome grows from 2 per cent for those aged 30–39 years, to 9.4 per cent for those aged 40–49 years, 36.1 per cent for those aged 50–59 years and 54.5 per cent for those aged 60–69 years. This is substantially higher than in the general population. Conditions associated with compromise to the central nervous system such as cerebral palsy and epilepsy add further layers of dependency as the person ages (see Chapter 12).

Case study: premature ageing

Albert is 47 years old. His parents died several years ago so he now lives with his sister and brother-in-law, Kath and Jim. They live together on a small-holding in the rural hinterland of a popular coastal resort. Albert has Down's syndrome.

Albert used to attend the local day centre where he had many friends but he has not been there for a long time. Consequently he has lost touch with many of them. He was never the most regular attender as his parents were content to look after him at home. Subsequent to his parents' deaths he used to like going out with Jim to the local market, sometimes dropping in to the pub, where they would meet and have a banter with many of Jim's friends, but he now no longer does so. Kath regarded herself as having a close sisterly relationship with Albert and she unquestioningly took over responsibility for his support following her parents' deaths. Earlier in life Albert was sociable, helpful around the house and took an interest in things.

According to Kath and Jim, Albert's behaviour began to change before his parents died, making his parents even more indulgent towards him. Looking back they were unaware of the scenario that was to unfold.

Albert was displaying many of the characteristics of early onset dementia typical of a sizeable proportion of his age-related peers with Down's syndrome. It was some time before the reasons for this were understood. Understandably, Kath and Jim looked initially for environmental factors that may be behind Albert's behaviour changes – anticipation of his parents' deaths, cumulative effects of medication – before coming to realize that there was more to it than that. Albert's behaviour and personality had in fact been changing gradually but increasingly, turning him into an apparently different person. He was becoming withdrawn, taciturn, unresponsive, reclusive but also provocative. During the early stages of these changes, Kath and Jim tended to 'blame' Albert for acting in these ways, presuming his behaviour to be intentional or deliberate. Even now, with the full weight of a clinical diagnosis of his dementia of the Alzheimer's type, it is still difficult for them to accommodate Albert's persistent lack of cooperation.

Kath and Jim have different coping strategies. Kath somehow manages most of the time to displace her frustrations by telling herself that the dementia is masking the real Albert and that things beyond his control, his dementia, are the triggers behind his behaviour. Jim by contrast still personalizes Albert's behaviour and reacts angrily to what he sees as wilfully disruptive displays from Albert. On many occasions the bath water has been switched on and left running, gates have been left open allowing pets and animals to escape, and facial grimaces have been directed at Jim which he thinks are designed to provoke him. Given the chance Albert wanders off. These difficulties have led Kath and Jim to limit shopping and other trips into the community with Albert. As a result Albert is now virtually a captive in his sister and brother-in-law's house.

Exercise 33.4

Using any of the theories of successful ageing as a guide, see if you can locate what is successful in Albert's case.

Repeat the exercise but this time listing the things you consider to be signs of unsuccessful ageing in Albert's situation.

Using the categories of knowledge depicted in Table 33.1, write down what information you would need to gather about Albert and his family as the basis for offering them advice.

What specific advice would you give to Kath and Jim about their strategies for coping?

Tyrell and Dodd (2003) report that side-effects of medications are more common in older people with learning disabilities because of slower hepatic metabolism and renal excretion, and in some cases because of altered brain anatomy. Medications for epilepsy may, over a period of years, lead to over-sedation and confusion. These authors also suggest that in later life sensory impairments such as hearing loss or cataracts can lead to increased risk of behaviour disturbance. Similarly, physical health problems associated with ageing can predispose to depression and anxiety.

Gender and health

As in earlier life stages it is important to be aware of the gendered nature of conditions that can affect people in later life, and of the particular needs of women and men. After years of neglect this has become a priority for the World Health Organization (1997) which has become increasingly involved in promoting:

- advocacy for women's health and gender-sensitive health care delivery;
- promotion of women's health and prevention of ill health;
- making health care systems more responsive to women's needs;
- gender equality;
- involvement of women in the design, implementation and monitoring of health policies and programmes.

The health needs and circumstances of older women with learning disabilities was the subject of study for the World Health Organization (Walsh *et al.* 2001). In regard to sexual health in later life, people with learning disabilities have been reported as finding their needs and circumstances being ignored both by family members and services. It is easy for people's sexual health needs to be trivialized because of presumptions about incapacity, thresholds for giving consent and even in some cases because of perceptions that older people with learning disabilities are asexual beings able to live a fulfilling life without a sexual appetite. Such misplaced attitudes can lead to people being denied access to advice, education and support about safe sex and about all the range of reproductive health issues. Sadly some men and women with learning disabilities find themselves victims of sexual abuse that can leave them prone to sexually transmitted diseases, HIV and AIDS but these can go unrecognized for lengthy periods. Telling others about such abuse can be complicated because of a lack of knowledge, poor communication skills, fear and confusion.

At the time of writing little is known about the effects of the menopause on women with learning disabilities, though it is recognized that early onset is associated with particular syndromes like Down's and fragile-X.

Arrangements for screening women for breast cancer and cervical cancer, and similarly prostate cancer in men, frequently operate under such economic pressures that the extra time and resources required to explain and implement the procedures become barriers to participation.

Gender issues and health over the life span for people with learning disabilities are high on the national and international research agenda at this time. Narrative accounts that throw further light on these issues are now beginning to emerge, as we will see in the next section.

How people make sense of ageing

The first chapter in this last section (Chapter 30) of the book sheds important light on the personal and social world of older people. The narratives described there remind us that in later life people do indeed have stories to tell, memories to share, as well as hopes and dreams that they can articulate. However, some people have difficulties accomplishing this in ways that others can understand, which can lead us to think, erroneously, that they do not have important things to share and insights to offer.

Erickson *et al.* (1989) have shown that older people with learning disabilities display considerable insights into age-related changes in their personal and social lives. They were shown to have quite varied perceptions about growing older. Some wished to dissociate themselves from ageing while others had more concrete concerns about it, ranging from sedentary lifestyles, changes in employment status and loss of mobility to reduced social contacts, fears about incipient ill-health and a recognition that ageing ultimately heralds death. Some people were more optimistic than others about their future lives, especially about their anticipated use of leisure time. When considering the aspirations and anxieties of older people with learning disabilities it is clearly important to avoid stereotyping.

Edgerton *et al.* (1994), in their qualitative studies, have similarly shown considerable diversity in reports by older people with learning disabilities about their own health. There were nevertheless some consistent threads in people's experiences. Few attempted to exercise on a regular basis, even when enrolled on rehabilitative programmes. Only one person consistently avoided a high fat, high sugar diet. As a consequence many were reported to be overweight. Despite the best advice of relatives and care workers, many smoked cigarettes, possibly a legacy of years spent in institutionalized settings. Little drug or alcohol dependency was in evidence however. Few had any understanding of the links between smoking, diet, exercise and health. Only a handful of people could provide basic information about their own ailments or worries. All were reported to have problems determining when they were in need of health care, communicating their needs to others and understanding how to cooperate in treatment plans.

In the same study it was found that doctors often relied on informed guesswork about medications needed by individuals, and they were unaware of the drug hoarding habits of some individuals. Several serious cases came to light where doctors had overlooked medical and surgical procedures that individuals required.

In a recent study involving 18 countries, Walsh and LeRoy (2004) uniquely brought together accounts from 167 older women with learning disabilities about their experiences of ageing. In regard to well-being in later life, it was found that many of the women spoke of issues mirrored by population-wide studies of older women. Health, home, employment and financial security were commonly reported when they talked about their own well-being. For some of the women, religion was important. Pets were a source of comfort and company for others. Although a third of the women claimed that they had no worries, the rest pointed to familiar themes that were a source of anxiety to them: disability, family members, health, finances, the future, global threats and a host of more specific things. Fears about the death and poor health of family members were quite prevalent, and there were some anxieties about just 'getting on' with family members. Interestingly, we can see here that some of the big issues – especially health, family/home and finances – could be sources of well-being *or* of worry and concern. These were mixed blessings, and depended very much on individual circumstances. The case studies described in this chapter reaffirm this in some respects.

The women in Walsh and LeRoy's study were depicted as being relatively happy and composed, but nonetheless aware of lost opportunities. Many still yearned for marriage and intimacy. A few desired wistfully to bear children, despite awareness that this was no longer a realistic option for them. When asked about the worst event of the past year, many pinpointed fearful events such as robbery, falls, injuries and unpleasant health treatments (cervical smears, tooth extraction, ear operations and so on), once again demonstrating an awareness of rather more unpleasant things beyond their personal control. The majority of the women, however, retained realistic hopes and dreams for the future, some modest in nature such as continuing to live in the same familiar surroundings, and others more ambitious, hoping for a safer and more peaceful world.

Overall these women had achieved considerable life satisfaction and resilience (see also Chapter 15), while retaining an awareness of their own mortality and of environmental factors that contribute to or constrain their well-being. Life's 'late pickings' (see Chapter 30) show that people with learning disabilities can have many things to look forward to in later life. Their dreams are the dreams of ordinary people who have often lived extraordinary lives. Helping them to realize those dreams requires, on the part of those in support roles, a commitment to engaging with the constellation of personal and environmental factors that shape them.

Conclusion

Hopefully this chapter has shown that older people with learning disabilities can age successfully and have lots to look forward to in later life. Healthiness is integral to successful ageing and older people with learning disabilities have identified this themselves.

A number of theories about successful ageing have been introduced in order to sensitize the reader to ways of thinking about the psychological processes involved, and how these are shaped by individual and environmental factors. What virtually all these theories share in common is a presumption that older people with learning disabilities will be able to share the 'good life' in old age. While prospects for decline in cognitive and physical functioning may accompany ageing, much as it does in the general population, there are typically compensations to be found in other domains of people's lives.

It is important to point out however that these remain theories, and to date there have been few attempts to test them on populations of older people with learning disabilities. Perhaps the best way to think about them is as possible heuristics for glimpsing and making sense of the personal and social worlds of older people.

At a more pragmatic level it has been shown that older people with learning disabilities face some formidable barriers in gaining proper access to health services. With health being so integral to successful ageing, it is high time that the evident defects in the design and delivery of health services that complicate or obscure access to these older people are put right. There are undoubtedly parallel problems for people needing to access social care services too but evidence about that lies beyond the scope of this chapter.

Epidemiological studies, biomedical studies, surveys, intervention studies and qualitative research studies about the lives of older people with learning disabilities have received lots of impetus from interest shown by the World Health Organization in recent years. There is a considerable volume of research going on now into the challenges and opportunities of ageing in people with learning disabilities, an increasing amount involving the poorer nations of the world, and peoples reflecting different ethnicities and cultural traditions. We already know a lot about the biological, biographical and environmental determinants of health as people with learning disabilities age, and a growing amount about how people themselves make sense of what they experience in the process. Some of that evidence is reported in these pages. A key question for practitioners then is whether they are prepared to act on what we already know in enabling older people with learning disabilities to age successfully. For politicians and policy-makers, the question is whether they have the political will to create the conditions in which this group of older people can enjoy the same rights to health, social inclusion and citizenship as other older people.

References

Atchley, R. (1999) *Continuity and Adaptation in Aging: Creating Positive Experiences.* Baltimore, MD: Johns Hopkins University Press.

Baltes, M. and Carstensen, L.L. (1996) The process of successful ageing, *Ageing and Society*, 16(4): 397–422.

Bigby, C. (2004) *Ageing with a Lifelong Disability: A Guide to Practice, Program and Policy Issues for Human Service Professionals*. London: Jessica Kingsley.

Brandstadter, J. and Grieve, W. (1994) The aging self: stabilising and protective processes, *Developmental Review*, 14: 52–80.

Coleman, P. (1997) The last scene of all, *Generations Review*, 7(1): 2–5.

Cooper, S.A. (1997) Epidemiology of psychiatric disorders in elderly compared with younger adults with learning disabilities, *British Journal of Psychiatry*, 170: 375–80.

Cumming, E. and Henry, W. (1961) *Growing Old*. New York: Basic Books.

Department of Health (2001) *Valuing People: A New Strategy for Learning Disability for the 21st Century*. London: Department of Health.

Edgerton, R.B., Gaston, M.A., Kelly, H. and Ward, T.W. (1994) Health care for aging people with mental retardation, *Mental Retardation*, 32(2): 146–50.

Erickson, M., Krauss, M.W. and Seltzer, M.M. (1989) Perceptions of old age among a sample of ageing people with mental retardation, *Journal of Applied Gerontology*, 8(2): 251–60.

Evenhuis, H., Henderson, C.M., Beange, H., Lennox, N. and Chicoine, B. (2001) Healthy ageing – adults with intellectual disabilities: physical health issues, *Journal of Applied Research in Intellectual Disabilities*. 14: 175–94.

Foundation for People with Learning Disabilities (2002) *Today and Tomorrow: The Report of the Growing Older with Learning Disabilities Programme*. London: Mental Health Foundation.

Fry, C.L., Dickerson-Putnam, J., Draper, P., Ikels, C., Keith, J., Glascock, A.P. and Harpending, H.C. (1997) Culture and the meaning of old age, in J. Sokolovsky (ed.) *The Cultural Context of Aging: Worldwide Perspectives*. Westport, CT: Bergin & Garvey.

Heller, T. (2004) Aging with developmental disabilities: emerging models for promoting health, independence and quality of life, in. B.J. Kemp and L. Mosqueda (eds) *Aging with a Disability: What a Clinician Needs to Know*. Baltimore, MD: Johns Hopkins University Press.

Jorm, A., Christensen, H., Henderson, S., Jacomb, P., Korten, P. and Mackinnon, A. (1998) Factors associated with successful aging, *Australasian Journal on Aging*, 17(1): 33–7.

Lawton, M. and Nahemow, L. (1973) Ecology and the aging process, in C. Eisensdorfer and M. Lawton (eds) *Psychology of Adult Development and Aging*. Washington, DC: American Psychological Association.

Lawton, M., Moss, M. and Dumanel, L. (1995) The quality of life among elderly care receivers, *Journal of Applied Gerontology*, 14(2): 150–71.

Liaschenko, J. (1997) Knowing the patient, in S.E. Thorne and V.E. Harp (eds) *Nursing Praxis: Knowledge and Action*. Thousand Oaks, CA: Sage.

Mansell, J. and Beadle-Brown, J. (2004) Person-centred planning or person-centred action? Policy and practice in intellectual disability services, *Journal of Applied Research in Intellectual Disabilities*, 17(1): 1–10.

Mead, N. and Bower, P. (2000) Patient-centredness: a conceptual framework and review of literature, *Social Science and Medicine*, 51: 1087–110.

Nahemow, L. (1990) The ecological theory of aging: how has it been used? Paper presented to the American Psychological Association, Boston Symposium on Environment and Aging.

NHS Health Scotland (2004) *Health Needs Assessment Report – Summary: People with Learning Disabilities in Scotland*. Glasgow: NHS Health Scotland.

O'Callaghan, A., Murphy, G. and Clare, I.C.H. (2003) The impact of abuse on men and women with severe learning disabilities and their families, *British Journal of Learning Disabilities*, 31(4): 175–80.

Prasher, V.P. (1995) Age-specific prevalence, thyroid dysfunction and depressive symptomatology in adults with Down syndrome and dementia, *International Journal of Geriatric Psychiatry*, 10: 25–31.

Rowe, J. and Kahn, R. (1998) *Successful Aging*. New York: Random House.

Tyrell, J. and Dodd, P. (2003) Psychopathology in older age, in P.W. Davidson, V.P. Prasher and M. Janicki (eds) *Mental Health, Intellectual Disabilities and the Aging Process*. Oxford: Blackwell.

Walsh, P.N. and LeRoy, B. (2004) *Women with Disabilities Aging Well: A Global View*. Baltimore, MD: Paul H. Brookes.

Walsh, P.N., Heller, T., Schupf, N. and van Schrojenstein Lantman-de Valk, H. (2001) Healthy ageing – adults with intellectual disabilities: women's health and related issues, *Journal of Applied Research in Intellectual Disabilities*, 14: 195–217.

World Health Organization (1997) Gender as determinant of health, in *The World Health Report*. Geneva: WHO.

World Health Organization (2001) Healthy ageing – adults with intellectual disabilities: summative report, *Journal of Applied Research in Intellectual Disabilities*, 14: 256–75.

34

Research and emancipation

Prospects and problems

Jan Walmsley

Introduction

In this chapter the contribution of disability research to the field of learning disabilities is discussed. This exploration seeks to illuminate the interconnections between developments in disability studies and the evolution of policy, research and practice in learning disability.

The chapter begins by describing recent developments in thinking about disability, in particular the social model of disability. This is contrasted with what are called more traditional approaches to researching disability (including learning disability). The influence these developments in thinking about disability have had in learning disability is then discussed with a focus on three areas:

- the way policy has developed, using the recent English policy document *Valuing People* and its implementation as an example;

- the way research has developed, with particular reference to the degree to which the current English Learning Disability Research Initiative follows the principles of 'emancipatory research';

- the extent to which people with learning difficulties acknowledge a disabled identity.

Two recent developments have influenced disability research – the 'social model' of disability and what are loosely called 'social constructionist' approaches. There is no question that these ideas, in particular the social model, have been influential in learning disability, but it is by no means a straightforward story, for, as a number of commentators have said, the disabled people's movement has had an uneasy relationship with learning disability, more often than not ignoring its existence. Furthermore, relatively few people involved in learning disability – whether they be researchers, policymakers, practitioners or service users themselves – have acknowledged the significance of the influence of disability studies. Only a few people, including the present author, all associated with learning disability, have attempted to theorize connections between the two (Aspis 2000; Chappell *et al.* 2001; Walmsley 2001). Had we been writing this book 30 years ago it is highly unlikely that this issue would have been thought worthy of consideration. For until the 1990s, when the term 'learning disability' was adopted by the UK government, the links with the disability movement were relatively insignificant. The word 'mental' in 'mental handicap' linked more directly to the area of mental illness, and indeed the legislative framework of the 1959 Mental Health Act applied both to mental illness and to 'subnormality', as learning disability was then called. It is a connection which lingers in the public mind, but legislators are very clear – the *Valuing People* White Paper (Department of Health 2001) could not be more different to its equivalent in mental health. But then, it is not as closely aligned to legislation prompted by disability rights, such as the Disability Discrimination Act 1995. In the past generation, then, the position of learning disability in the pantheon of social policy has shifted, from an alignment with mental illness to an alignment with disability. The realignment is far from perfect – the disability movement continues by and large to conceptualize impairment as physical rather than mental, while learning disability, with its own White Paper, sits in a solitary place, as much influenced, I will argue, by normalization/social role valorization as it is by the social model of disability. But links there are, particularly conceptual, and these, along with their implications, will be explored here.

The social model of disability

One could argue that the social model of disability is one of the most significant influences on the philosophical landscape in social policy of the late twentieth century. Its influence on thinking in relation to oppressed and excluded groups is profound. As Mike Oliver commented, with reference to Tony Blair's stated determination to remove barriers to people fulfilling their potential, 'we are all social modellists now' (Oliver 2004: 7)!

The social model of disability defines disability as the societal response to impairment. As Tom Shakespeare summed it up, 'People are disabled by social barriers and failures of provision, not by their bodies' (Shakespeare 2003: 28). The contrast with more traditional definitions of disability are sharp. Whereas the social model locates problems in society – barriers to full participation by people with a variety of impairments – the traditional (often called 'medical') model locates the problem in the individual. To put it very crudely, rather than telling someone 'you can't do that job because you are blind' (the traditional or medical model), the social model puts the onus on society – in the case of employment, the employer – to make it possible for a person with visual impairments to carry out the job.

Exercise 34.1

Consider the case of a person with visual impairment applying to do your job. What adaptations would need to be made to make it possible?

Comment

As an academic I have had direct experience of this. A woman with a visual impairment did do a very similar job to me. She had a number of aids to assist her – a reading service which put papers onto tape for her, a magnifying glass, a change in our habits to ensure we explained what was on an overhead projector slide or handout. However, she also commented that time was a major factor. The bad practice of circulating papers just before a meeting often meant she could not use her reading service. The sheer weight of work to do at, for example, exam time, in a very short space of time, really taxed her and made it hard to carry out the job to the same standard a person with adequate sight could do without working ridiculously long hours.

Although the idea of 'barriers' appears quite straightforward, and in some cases is, the example above shows that barriers need not be just physical. Barriers can be physical, such as inaccessible buildings; they can be attitudinal, such as the belief that people with impairments cannot do certain things; they can be environmental, such as the way meetings are carried out; or they can be structural, built into the very fabric of society. The time issue my visually impaired colleague cited is a good example of just how much needs to change if people with visual impairments are to work on equal terms. We would, for instance, have to alter students' expectations that they would get their marks back in a relatively short time!

What about learning disability? We come to that later, but here it is worth pausing to note that Tom Shakespeare specifically refers to 'bodies' not 'brains' or 'minds' in his definition. This is not insignificant – people who write about the social model do not always consider impairments which are located in the brain rather than the body. As a consequence, our understanding of the barriers people with learning difficulties experience is far less well developed.

To understand the social model requires a distinction to be made between impairment and disability. Impairment is defined as 'lacking all or part of a limb. Or having a defective limb, organ or mechanism of the body' (UPIAS 1976: 14). Disability is defined as: 'The disadvantage or restriction of activity caused by a contemporary social organisation which takes little or no account of people who have physical impairments and thus excludes them from participation in the mainstream of social activities. Physical disability is therefore a particular form of social oppression' (UPIAS 1976: 14).

According to the social model, people are disabled because they encounter barriers to full participation in society, not because they individually have an impairment. Again, it is important to note that in these UPIAS definitions it is physical bodily impairment that is conceived. In 1976, as now, intellectual impairments were at best marginal to social model thinking.

In order to fully understand the idea of barriers it is helpful to categorize the types of things which are seen as barriers within the social model. French (2001) identifies three categories:

- *Structural barriers*: the underlying norms, practices and ideologies of society which are predicated upon a false notion of normal. This is well illustrated by reference to societies where a particular impairment is relatively common, such as Martha's Vineyard, New England, where a high proportion of deaf islanders appears to have led to an expectation that everyone be bilingual in sign language and spoken English, meaning that deaf people are neither excluded nor significantly disadvantaged (Groce 1985). The social model posits that the underlying assumptions of society are that everyone is an able-bodied autonomous adult – everyone else is therefore at a disadvantage.

- *Environmental barriers*: physical obstacles such as steps and narrow doorways, as well as assumptions – for example, about how meetings are run (with reference to written papers) or the time allowed to carry out particular tasks.

- *Attitudinal barriers*: beliefs that because people have an impairment they are unable to do certain things.

Exercise 34.2

Consider the barriers experienced by people with learning disabilities. Try to think of an example of each of the following:

Structural barriers

Environmental barriers

Attitudinal barriers

Comment
Structural barriers: the time allocated for certain tasks can be regarded as a structural barrier. In my own work, bids for research funding are often given very short timescales which make it impossible to fully include people with learning disabilities, and enable them to understand and contribute to the bid.

Environmental barriers: the way bus and train timetables are displayed. They rely on people having good reading skills and good eyesight. But they could be delivered via a voice system if there was a will to install such mechanisms at bus stops and railway stations.

Attitudinal barriers: have you ever taken someone with rather odd behaviour into a shop or a restaurant? If so, you'll know that at best you get stares and at worst you might be asked to leave.

The social model was a radical paradigm shift, with highly significant impact on individuals, on academic thinking and on policy. At a practical level, it was social model thinking which led to the conceptualization of independent living as a goal for disabled people, to be achieved by employing appropriate personal assistance (Morris 1993). It was, at least in part, campaigning by disabled people which led to legislation which made it mandatory for local authorities to make Direct Payments available so that assistance was under the direct control of disabled people, rather than mediated through care managers (Shakespeare 2003).

Perhaps as important has been the impact on disabled people's self-confidence. Numerous individuals testify to the importance of the social model as a vehicle for empowerment and liberation. Liz Crow, for example: 'For years now the social model of disability has enabled me to confront, survive and even surmount countless situations of exclusion and discrimination' (1996: 207). A perception that the impairment itself is not the problem, that it lies in societal structures and attitudes, has been tremendously liberating for many disabled people. It has led to developments like disability arts and music, and to the re-adoption of particular terms, such as cripple (Mairs 1986), to express defiance at the world. It has also inspired remarkably successful direct action, one factor leading to the passage of anti-discriminatory legislation in the UK during the 1990s (Shakespeare 2003).

It is, however, important to acknowledge that the social model is not adopted by everyone with impairments. Wendell (1996: 70) usefully reminds us that '[it is] important not to assume that people with disabilities identify with all others who have disabilities or share a single perspective on disability (or anything else), or that having a disability is the most important aspect of a person's identity or social position'. Nevertheless, the social model has undoubtedly contributed to a radical shift in the way disability, and disabled people, are viewed. The extent to which this radical shift applies to people with learning difficulties is an important issue and is explored further below.

The social model and learning disability

In this section I consider the extent to which social model thinking has influenced learning disability. Just to recap, salient features of the social model are:

- a distinction between disability (oppression created by society) and impairment (the missing or defective part of the body);
- an emphasis on barriers – environmental, attitudinal, physical and structural;
- pride in being disabled, assertion of a positive disabled identity;
- independent living, supported by assistance, controlled by disabled people, as the key to social inclusion and citizenship.

How far have ideas associated with the social model influenced learning disability? As indicated in the introduction this is approached through consideration of three areas:

- *implementing policy change*: the example of the UK White Paper *Valuing People*;
- *research*: the UK Learning Disability Research Initiative;
- *practice*: the extent to which people with learning difficulties and the organizations controlled by them have adopted the social model and the ideas associated with it.

Implementing policy change

In order to consider the influence of disability studies on policy change, I have chosen to focus on the UK where *Valuing People*, published by the Department of Health in 2001, was the first learning disability White Paper (signalling a major policy shift) since *Better Services for the Mentally Handicapped* in 1971. It is a useful benchmark by which to consider how far ideas developed in disability studies have influenced learning disability policy.

The key principles enunciated in *Valuing People* are:

- rights;
- independence;
- choice;
- inclusion.

All of these ideas, but especially rights and independence, are associated with the social model. We can usefully compare *Valuing People* with ideas developed by people who espouse the social model through considering *The Disability Manifesto*, published in the UK in the year *Valuing People* was published. The *Manifesto* summarizes the aspirations of the UK disabled people's movement at the beginning of the twenty-first century. It sets out the disability movement's view of independent living, and what is needed to achieve it:

> Independent living means enabling disabled people – regardless of age, impairment or where they live – to achieve the same rights and independence as non-disabled people. Independence is not about doing everything for yourself. Nobody does that. It is about having choices about what happens to you ... The cornerstone of independent living for the many disabled people who need support with aspects of daily life is personal assistance.
>
> (Campbell and Hasler 2001: 11)

The authors, Jane Campbell and Frances Hasler, set out what this might mean for community services:

- involvement of disabled people in drafting eligibility criteria;
- Direct Payments mandatory;

- end to charging for non-residential services, such as day centres;
- end to charging for social care services.

As Means *et al.* (2003: 163) point out, the *Manifesto*, although not at first sight revolutionary, implied a 'radical challenge to community care as currently organised' because it implied a change to the locus of control of what is provided, and how, from care services to individuals.

Valuing People, although it voiced some of the aspirations implicit in the *Manifesto*, did not go as far as identifying personal assistance as the key to realizing rights, independence, choice and inclusion. Rather, it continued to emphasize the importance of improving both specialist learning disability and mainstream services of all kinds – health, housing, support to carers, education – and of developing the workforce through training and partnership working. The nearest the White Paper approaches to social model ideas is in Chapter 4 entitled 'More choice and control for people with learning disabilities', where reference is made to advocacy (including self-advocacy), involvement in decision-making, accessible information and communication, Direct Payments and the role of the Disability Rights Commission in helping individuals enforce their rights.

However, the main emphasis in the White Paper is on service improvement. The key tool for achieving this at an individual level is not personal assistance as such, but person-centred planning (already now abbreviated to PCP): 'a mechanism for reflecting the needs and preferences of a person with a learning disability . . . such issues as housing, education, employment and leisure' (Department of Health 2001: 49). Person-centred planning has subsequently been the subject of special guidance issued by the English government, directing services to adopt person-centred approaches which start with the person and their capacities rather than their deficits. Although the need for personal assistance may be the outcome of a person-centred plan, the thrust is a service-based process, rather than an emphasis on the right to the type of assistance an individual needs to achieve his or her goals.

Reference also needs to be made to Partnership Boards, identified in the White Paper as responsible for implementing already-existing Joint Investment Plans and for developing local action plans. Partnership Boards are required to have representation from people with learning disabilities and carers who should be 'fully involved in the process' (Department of Health 2001: 116).

Although at first sight the principles of *Valuing People* seem to owe much to the rights-based approaches developed in disability studies, the mechanisms for achieving the principles are heavily dependent on the type of service development most closely associated with normalization/social role valorization. Barriers are not much mentioned, and the solutions are those developed by people associated with normalization/social role valorization through service improvement. Person-centred planning had been on the agenda since at least the mid-1980s, developed via 'individual person planning' by Roger Blunden (1980), refined by Brechin and Swain

(1986) as 'shared action planning' and further developed in the 1990s by Helen Sanderson as personal futures planning (Open University 1996). What was new was the adoption of such approaches as the answer, to be taken up by services throughout England, and managed as part of care management. One might see this as the bureaucratization of an idea!

Partnership Boards became the key tool for implementation of local improvements to service delivery. Although they have representation from 'users and carers', they remain under the control of the statutory services – a far cry from giving power to people with learning disabilities to determine their own futures. Key issues in *The Disability Manifesto*, particularly control over personal assistance, are minor refrains in the *Valuing People*; faith is still placed in the ability of services, albeit modernized and more responsive, to achieve the principles.

The relatively limited influence of disability rights ideas in *Valuing People* is not surprising. Not only are governments unlikely to easily relinquish the control over sizable budgets which *The Disability Manifesto* implies, the aspirations of the drafters of the *Manifesto* are not necessarily transferable to people with learning disabilities without significant amendment. For many people with learning disabilities, it is difficult to visualize a world in which they have the capacity to manage personal assistance without considerable help from families or advocates, whereas many people whose impairments are primarily physical may readily take on the role of employer.

Research

The impact of the social model of disability on research has been considerable. Here I set out the salient features of both traditional and social model research, and then discuss the extent to which its principles have been applied in learning disability research.

The social model of disability and research

If the social model defines disability as the societal response to impairment, it follows that research should shift from the 'problems' created by impairment to changing society in order to increase disabled people's opportunities for full inclusion. People who embrace the social model have been very critical of traditional or medical model research which is characterized as:

- research in which experts set the agenda, and decide what questions to ask;
- research in which disabled people are subjects whose problems are examined by non-disabled experts;
- research which assumes that the problem lies within the individual and his or her impairments, not within society;
- research which claims to be objective;
- research which does little to improve the lives of disabled people (Zarb 1992).

In a much-quoted exercise, disabled scholar Mike Oliver critiqued the Office of Population Censuses and Surveys 1986 *Survey of Disabled Adults*. He turned questions such as 'What complaint causes your difficulty in holding, gripping or turning things?' into 'What defects in the design of everyday equipment like jars, bottles and tins causes you difficulty in holding, gripping or turning them?' This simple exercise completely altered the locus of the problem (Oliver 1990: 7, 8). It demonstrated that a census, an apparently scientific and value-free activity, was actually rooted in a strongly medicalized, individualized perspective on impairment. This made the critique particularly powerful, showing how apparently objective research was actually rooted in a particular way of seeing the world.

Exercise 34.3

Change this traditional research question into one which reflects a social model approach: Does your health problem/disability prevent you from going out as often as you would like?

Social model theorists, led by Mike Oliver, Vic Finkelstein and Colin Barnes, pointed to three particular problems with traditional research:

- the focus was on the individual with impairments, not on their social relationships or the construction of society;
- it had failed to engage disabled people, except as passive subjects;
- it had not improved the quality of life of disabled people 'though it might have substantially improved the career prospects of researchers' (Oliver 1992: 63).

In arguing for change, leading social model proponents (e.g. Oliver 1992; Zarb 1992) identified 'emancipatory research' as the way forward. This built on the work of Paolo Freire (1986) who championed participatory action research, in which people in disadvantaged communities defined the problem, and then took action to address it. Disadvantaged people were thus in charge of the research agenda and how it was carried out. Freire argued that this was the liberating way forward if research was to really make a difference. Like Freire, supporters of the social model saw research as a tool for radical social change rather than merely an exercise in finding out more about particular phenomena. True achievement of emancipatory research requires drastic change in what Zarb called the 'material relations' of research. Key features are:

- research as a tool for improving the lives of disabled people;
- research commissioned and funded by organizations of disabled people;
- research in which disabled people have the opportunity to carry out the research;

- researchers accountable to the democratic organizations of disabled people;
- researchers 'on the side of' disabled people – no claim to objectivity.

Emancipatory research rapidly gained a position as the gold standard to which all right-thinking researchers in the disability rights camp aspired. For example, Mark Priestley, a non-disabled researcher, used the extent to which his work on the implementation of community care was emancipatory as a reference point throughout his account of it (Priestley 1999). It is difficult to point to many examples of research projects which fully meet the criteria 'emancipatory'. Indeed, both Finkelstein (1999) and Zarb (personal communication 2003) are on record as being pessimistic that the movement has lost its way. However, the aspiration has been immensely important, putting any researchers who are not themselves disabled in the position of needing to justify their stance, as Priestley did, and leading to a number of major funding bodies in the UK requiring that any academics aspiring to disability research must demonstrate how disabled people are engaged and involved – the Joseph Rowntree Foundation and the Big Lottery being prominent examples.

Emancipatory research and learning disability

So, 'emancipatory research' was the model advocated by leading scholars in disability research. This type of thinking is in marked contrast to traditional approaches in learning disability research which are based on experts scrutinizing people with learning disabilities as subjects (Kiernan 1999). A good example is the considerable body of research conducted during the 1980s and 1990s on deinstitutionalization from long-stay hospitals (see e.g. Mansell *et al.* 1987). On the whole this research relied upon an examination of the degree to which people were enabled to participate in society, using principles like O'Brien's five accomplishments (O'Brien and Lyle 1987) as a guide. There was very little consideration given to the idea that society needed to change to reduce people's barriers to participation. Rather, services were enjoined to try harder, to modify people's behaviour to make them more acceptable, to increase staffing levels so that people could take part in valued social activities (paid work, leisure), and to promote integration with 'valued people' – i.e. not people with learning difficulties (Chappell 1997). Chappell argues that this devalues people with learning disabilities by implying that associating with people with the same label is devaluing them.

The dominant philosophy here was normalization/social role valorization (Wolfensberger and Tullman 1989), a set of ideas which put much more emphasis on people changing to fit in, and on services adopting correct attitudes, than it did on barriers (Brown and Smith 1992; Emerson 1992). From the early 1990s research based on participatory principles began to emerge, in which people with learning disabilities joined with academic researchers as 'junior partners' (Walmsley 1994: 157), and the researchers themselves were sympathetic allies. This began to result in a different emphasis. For example, the book by Tim and Wendy Booth on parents with learning disabilities published in 1994 argued for a move away from the assumption of deficit to an acknowledgment that people struggle with parenting as much because of poverty, negative and unhelpful staff attitudes and practices, and lack of good role models as because of their impairments. Although the term 'barriers' was not used, this marked a departure from more traditional approaches. However, it did not acknowledge any direct influence from disability studies – Barnes, Oliver *et al.* do not feature in the bibliography – nor did it go anything like as far as an emancipatory stance would imply. In a paper published in 1994 I reflected upon what it would mean to apply emancipatory research thinking to the situation of parents with learning disabilities:

> Perhaps a group of parents getting together, deciding they wanted to find out why people like them were having such a hard time, raising some money, employing interviewers or doing it themselves, supervising the production of the report and finding someone to publish it. It is almost impossible to visualise such a scenario given the way things are at present; yet it is such a vision that application of the social model can create.
>
> (Walmsley 1994: 157)

The specific influence of the social model of disability on developments in research in learning disability began to be evident from the early 1990s onwards. This led some researchers to struggle to go beyond participation, to try to meet the more stringent demands of emancipatory research. In this form of research the researcher is the expert servant of disabled people who must put their knowledge and skills at the disposal of their research subjects, for them to use in whatever ways they choose (Oliver 1992: 111). This formulation goes beyond participatory research and transforms the long-standing role of the sympathetic ally into something more akin to an expert adviser to people with learning disabilities.

In research terms, the association with the social model of disability increased the demands on those who aspired to conduct research with people with learning disabilities, because true emancipatory research gives power and control of the research to disabled people. This raised the stakes considerably in terms of what some learning disability researchers began to demand of themselves and their work. The type of research characteristic of normalization-inspired models – that the research should demonstrate ways in which a 'normal life' could be promoted – was not enough. Somehow, the researcher was expected to find ways of giving control to people with learning disabilities, and of being accountable to them.

Townsley (1998: 78) cites emancipatory research principles in arguing for research to be made accessible: 'The field of disability research is currently making efforts to move towards a more emancipatory approach where the involvement of disabled researchers and consultants is central to the success of any research project'. Rodgers (1999) published a reflective piece on the extent to which her work with women on health issues met the demands of emancipatory research, and, while she concluded that it did not, indicated by her title, 'Trying to get it right', that it should have done!

Partly because the disabled people's movement has not embraced issues relating to learning disability or indeed mental health problems seriously (Beresford 2000), it has been difficult to explore its implications for people with learning disabilities. For example, the belief that access is vital, something subscribed to by all inclusive learning disability researchers (Townsley 1998), is less pressing in the disability field where it can safely be assumed that at least some physically disabled people can access complex theory. Physically impaired academics do not need plain text versions, Makaton or illustrated reports to be able to understand research, whereas most people with learning disabilities do (although they do need, sometimes, mechanical aids such as Braille versions, hearing loops, enlarged print etc.). Similarly, the assumption that, ideally, disabled people should carry out some research themselves is one that is more readily applied in the context of physical disability than it is for people with learning disabilities. At least some physically disabled people have access to higher education, the traditional training ground for researchers, far more readily than do people with learning disabilities. Even the ability to access research funds is easier for organizations of disabled people (though not as easy as it should be, perhaps) than it is for people with learning disabilities. These groups are likely to need human support in discovering what sources of funding are available, in completing a literature review and in filling in the forms.

Physically impaired scholars have the luxury of debating whether narrative research, the focus on individual experience, is a valid focus for research (Finkelstein 1996). However, if this position were adopted in learning disability, most of what has so far been published would not be permissible. The autobiography, life history and ethnographic traditions have led the field in inclusive learning disability research. There is little else other than service evaluations (Walmsley and Johnson 2003).

Parallels between people with physical impairments and people with learning disabilities are striking – but differences are also considerable. The equivalent to Braille, guide dogs, ramps and so on is not technological but human. For most research, people with learning disabilities need the assistance of non-disabled allies – and they are less amenable to control than technology.

To date, a wholesale migration to emancipatory research with people with learning disabilities has been considered but not implemented. Whether it could or should be are key issues, and are increasingly debated in the field. The slogan 'Nothing about us without us' challenges non disabled researchers to justify their right to even do research into learning disability, just as disabled activists have done. There is no question that some people with learning disabilities have adopted these ideas from the disabled people's movement (see e.g. Aspis 2000).

Exercise 34.4

Consider what 'emancipatory research' might mean for people with learning disabilities. What problems might there be in adopting this approach? Are there other ways of ensuring research does not exploit people with learning disabilities?

The Learning Disability Research Initiative

A brief examination of the Learning Disability Research Initiative, funded by the English Department of Health in the wake of *Valuing People*, will allow us to estimate how far ideas adopted from the disability movement have infiltrated learning disability research. The process by which research was commissioned is one area where a commitment to the involvement of disabled people is evident. Two people with learning disabilities were part of the commissioning panel. Eve Rank Petruzziello was one of these people. She reflected on the extent to which she and her colleague were able to influence the process to meet four principles:

- the extent to which projects included people with learning disabilities;
- inclusion from the very beginning of the research;
- the value of the research to people with learning disabilities;
- value for money (Holman 2003).

The connections with the principles of emancipatory research are evident in the first three of these principles. Rank Petruzziello reckoned that she had been able to influence decisions about what to fund to some extent, though she was critical of some of the practicalities – her involvement only began 'from the middle' (Holman 2003: 148) and the paperwork was late in arriving, giving her limited preparation time.

It is too early to say whether the principles she enunciated have been carried through into the projects themselves. A special issue of the *British Journal of Learning Disabilities*, published in 2003, gives progress to date. Space does not permit a detailed evaluation. However, the fact that in her evaluation of progress to date Noonan Walsh (2003) used questions such as, 'What is relevant?', 'Who should be involved?' and the degree to which dissemination guarantees accessibility to potential users of the research, including people with learning difficulties, shows that these questions, which are closely associated with emancipatory research, are very much on the agenda in current English government-funded research in learning disability. There has also been a commitment to producing accessible versions of research reports. The Learning Disability Research Initiative *Newsletter*, Issue 1 (2003) uses parallel texts to promote access. On one side of the page is the traditional prose text – on the other is an easy to read illustrated summary of the same information.

We must conclude that here, at least, the influence from disability research has been considerable. Although there is a long way to go before the 'material relations' of research production (Zarb 1992) are changed sufficiently to ensure people with learning disabilities have control of the funds, and the research itself, some of the principles associated with emancipatory research are firmly on the agenda in England.

Practice: disabled identity

I have considered the influence ideas about independent living have had on *Valuing People*, and the degree to which ideas about emancipatory research have impacted upon learning disability research. But what is probably a far more significant issue for people with learning disabilities is the degree to which they have been influenced by, and convinced by, the social model. Critics of normalization argue that it was imposed on people with learning disabilities by others (Chappell 1997). Arguably, the social model is equally external to people with learning disabilities. It is hard to locate a discovery of barriers in what are, admittedly, the quite limited writings by people with learning disabilities (an exception being Aspis 2000). This is a big subject, but if we return to the salient principles, we can focus on three of them:

- a distinction between disability (oppression created by society) and impairment (the missing or defective part of the body);
- an emphasis on barriers – environmental, attitudinal, physical and structural;
- pride in being disabled, assertion of a positive disabled identity.

The use of language is an area where the two groups have differed. The disability movement has insisted on use of the term 'disabled people' to convey the idea that disability is created by society. However, what has been called 'People First language'? Snow (2002) seeks to put the person first and the disability second. In this thinking, people with disabilities are people, first and foremost. As our society's language changes, as we talk about people first, it is argued that

- perceptions will change; and
- attitudes will change; and
- society's acceptance and respect for people with disabilities will increase; and
- an inclusive society will become a reality (Snow 2002).

This is reinforced by a number of studies (see e.g. Williams 2002) which show that people with learning disabilities reject labels. Indeed, the People First slogan 'label jars, not people' itself emphasizes this anti-labelling position. There is an obvious tension in establishing a self-advocacy group on the basis of belonging to the social category 'people with learning difficulties' and values which emphasize being part of an inclusive society (Simons

1992). Such a group reinforces the very category that people are seeking to downplay.

While people with learning difficulties and their allies have been trying to establish the principle of a common humanity, groups representing disabled people have been claiming the right to define and name themselves as a group with a distinctive separate identity. The disability movement promoted a much less ambiguous stance towards what some people would term 'segregation', by encouraging peer support, peer advocacy, disability arts, disability pride and disability culture.

The self-organization of disabled people challenged prevailing negative stereotypes and put forward the idea that disabled people were taking control of their own identity, confronting oppression and empowering themselves, especially through political activism. The development of disability culture in opposition to popular culture was a key strategy for promoting positive cultural conceptions of disability. The arts have been used a means of fighting back against the disabling dominant culture (Campbell and Oliver 1996).

Disabled people claim that if they do not define themselves, then others will continue to do it for them. Thus for many people, 'coming out' as a self-proclaimed disabled person has important political meaning (Wendell 1996). However, the extent to which people with learning disabilities have embraced their identity as a distinct social group is questionable. At the beginning of the 1990s Simons (1992) noted few connections between self-advocacy and disabled people's groups. It is only recently that social model ideas about pride in a separate identity have begun to impact on the self-advocacy 'movement', as have attempts to include people with learning difficulties in the disability movement. I have argued (Walmsley 1997) that when the social model of disability was being developed by disabled people, services for people with learning difficulties were largely influenced by a different family of ideas: normalization (Wolfensberger 1972); ordinary life (King's Fund 1980); social role valorization (Wolfensberger 1983); and the five accomplishments (O'Brien and Lyle 1987). The chief strategy for change that arises out of these service ideologies is for people with learning difficulties to 'pass' into the non-disabled group. In contrast, the more politicized lobby of disabled people draws upon the social model of disability to raise the consciousness of all disabled people, with the intention of tackling disadvantage through political action (Oliver 1990).

As noted already, the relationship that people with learning difficulties and self-advocacy organizations have with the disability movement is not straightforward. Aspis (quoted in Campbell and Oliver 1996) draws attention to the discrimination that people with learning difficulties have faced in the disability movement. People with certain impairments, including those with learning difficulties, are not always welcome. There have also been disagreements over language. Goodley (2002), for example, discusses criticisms of the term 'people with learning difficulties' made by those who prefer the term 'disabled people'. A degree of tension between people with learning difficulties and the disability movement is indicated in this statement from

Swindon People First: 'Disabled people without learning difficulties need to:

- respect us;
- listen to us;
- learn from us;
- not lecture us and tell us what we should think' (Swindon People First 2002: 100).

At present it is hard to assess what impact the social model of disability has had on people with learning difficulties and their organizations. Research that explores how such people perceive themselves suggests a very limited self-identification as 'disabled'. Davies and Jenkins (1997) found that only 28 per cent of their sample of people with learning difficulties included themselves in the social category of people with mental handicap/learning difficulties, and that 13 per cent of those discussed their identity in ways that were partial or unclear. Finlay and Lyons (2000) reported that it was hard to find evidence of a group identity, which they argue needs to be present if people with learning difficulties are to discuss and bring about change for themselves. The common assumption that people with learning difficulties experience a negative identity is hard to verify. There are a number of strategies which people may use to protect a 'threatened identity' (Breakwell 1986). Finlay and Lyons (2000: 47) suggested that 'It is not really possible to know for sure whether people do or do not really think they are group members but we cannot assume that just because researchers think the category is salient that the participants also see things this way'.

Certainly there are contradictions in the way people with learning difficulties relate to labels. There is plenty of evidence that they reject them – research carried out by self-advocates themselves points to at best an ambivalence about labelling (Palmer *et al.* 1999; Williams 2002). However, to stick with this rather lofty critical stance is perhaps to ignore the importance of opportunities to learn about the social model and mould it more specifically to the situation of people with learning difficulties. Simone Aspis, a self-advocate who acknowledges how she has been influenced by the social model, consciously chooses to describe herself as a 'disabled person with learning difficulties' (Aspis 2000). Louise Townson, a leading self-advocate, acknowledges how much she has learnt about the potential of the performing arts as a 'means of challenging negative perceptions through reviewing a book. However, the book taught me about the potential of performing arts for self-advocacy which was something I had no idea about' (Townson 2003: 836). This indicates that the power of social model ideas to help people with learning difficulties understand and challenge their situation has yet to be fully realized – exchange of information and the opportunities to learn would appear to be key issues here.

One might argue that people with learning difficulties are subject to internal oppression, in which they absorb the devalued position that they as a group have in society, and try to distance themselves from this negative identity. Recently, some disability scholars have adapted the social model to consider the idea of 'internal oppression': that the attitudes of disabled people may themselves be self-defeating. Eddie, interviewed for a book, recalled how hard it was for him to accept that he was disabled – denial was a strategy both he and his family used to deal with his difference:

> I was brought up believing I was the same as my brothers ... [My family] have come to accept the fact that I'm the same as everyone else, can do as well as anyone else which has its advantages which was not being molly coddled ... I was normal like everyone else and I had the opinion that I was better than disabled people and I wasn't disabled ... I knew I was disabled but I just couldn't accept it.
>
> (Shakespeare *et al.* 1996: 50)

It is not difficult to recognize that attitudes from parents may contribute to this denial of difference for people with learning difficulties also. Todd and Shearn (1997) identified strategies used by parents to shield people from knowing that they were the possessors of a 'toxic identity'. It may be worth considering the possibility that people with learning difficulties need the opportunity to learn about the social model before one concludes that it is an alien concept, imposed from afar.

Exercise 34.5

How far do you think the idea of 'internalized oppression' explains the failure of people with learning difficulties to develop a pride in being different?

Conclusion

It is beyond doubt that ideas developed in the disability movement have influenced thinking in learning disability also. Academics, policy-makers, practitioners and some people with learning difficulties have clearly been influenced by the disability movement's big idea. It is perhaps regrettable that the powerful thinking that has revolutionized thinking about physical impairment has not been brought to bear on the situation of people with learning difficulties also. Although disabled people should be natural allies of people with learning difficulties, given that they share experiences of impairment and oppression, in fact, in the UK at least, relationships have been patchy, and much disability research assumes that impairment is of the body rather than of the mind. A barriers approach has a great deal to offer the learning disability field. It is incredibly liberating to begin to think of barriers as being in society rather than as unmovable aspects of an individual.

It is, however, necessary to recognize that a direct translation of action developed for people with physical impairments is too crude a tool to deliver real and lasting changes for people with learning difficulties. More hard thinking is needed if policy and practice are usefully to adapt the social model for people with learning difficulties, but an important start has been made.

References

Aspis, S. (2000) Researching our history: who is in charge? In L. Brigham, D. Atkinson, M. Jackson, S. Rolph and J. Walmsley (eds) *Crossing Boundaries: Change and Continuity in the History of Learning Disabilities*. Kidderminster: BILD.

Beresford, P. (2000) What have madness and psychiatric system survivors got to do with disability and disability studies? *Disability and Society*, 15(1): 167–72.

Blunden, R. (1980) *Individual Plans for Mentally Handicapped People: a Draft Procedural Guide*. Cardiff: Mental Handicap in Wales Applied Research Unit, University of Wales College of Medicine.

Booth, T. and Booth, W. (1994) *Parenting under Pressure: Mothers and Fathers with Learning Difficulties*. Buckingham: Open University Press.

Breakwell, G.M. (1986) *Coping with Threatened Identities*. London: University Paperbacks.

Brechin, A. and Swain, J. (1986) Shared action planning, in *P555 Mental Handicap Patterns for Living*. Milton Keynes: The Open University.

British Journal of Learning Disabilities, special issue (2003) *Valuing People – The Interface with Research*. 31(4).

Brown, H. and Smith, H. (eds) (1992) *Normalisation: A Reader for the Nineties*. London: Routledge.

Campbell, J. and Hasler, F. (2001) *The Disability Manifesto*. London: Scope.

Campbell, J. and Oliver, M. (1996) *Disability Politics: Understanding our Past, Changing our Future*. Leeds: Disability Press.

Chappell, A. (1997) From normalization to where? in L. Barton and M. Oliver (eds) *Disability Studies Past Present and Future*. Leeds: Disability Press.

Chappell, A., Goodley, D. and Lawthorn, R. (2001) Making connections: the relevance of the social model of disability for people with learning difficulties, *British Journal of Learning Disabilities*, 29: 45–50.

Crow, L. (1996) Including all of our lives, in J. Morris (ed.) *Encounters with Strangers: Feminism and Disability*. London: Women's Press.

Davies, C.A. and Jenkins, R. (1997) She has different fits to me: How people with learning difficulties see themselves, *Disability and Society*, 12(1): 95–109.

Department of Health (2001) *Valuing People: A New Strategy for Learning Disability for the 21st Century*. London: Department of Health.

Emerson, E. (1992) What is normalization? in H. Brown and H. Smith (eds) *Normalisation: a Reader for the Nineties*. London: Routledge.

Finkelstein, V. (1996) The disability movement has run out of steam, *Disability Now*, February: 11.

Finkelstein, V. (1999) Doing disability research (extended book review), *Disability and Society*, 14(6): 859–67.

Finlay, W.M.L. and Lyons, E. (2000) Social categorisations, social comparisons and stigma: presentations of self in people with learning difficulties, *British Journal of Social Psychology*, 39: 129–46.

Freire, P. (1986) *Pedagogy of the Oppressed*. Harmondsworth: Penguin.

French, S. (2001) Living in the mainstream, in *K202 Care Welfare and Community, Workbook 2, Theories and Practice*. Milton Keynes: The Open University.

Goodley, D. (2002) What's in a label? *Community Living*, 15(3): 2.

Groce, N.E. (1985) *Everyone Here Spoke Sign Language*. Cambridge, MA: Harvard University Press.

Holman, A. (2003) In conversation: Eve Rank-Petruziello, *British Journal of Learning Disabilities*, 31(4): 148–9.

Kiernan, C. (1999) Participation in research by people with learning disability: origins and issues, *British Journal of Learning Disabilities*, 27(2): 43–7.

King's Fund (1980) *An Ordinary Life*. London: King's Fund.

Mairs, N. (1986) On being a cripple, in *Plaintexts: Essays, 9–20*. Tucson, AZ: University of Arizona Press.

Mansell, J., Felce, D., Jenkins, J., de Kock, U. and Toogood, S. (1987) *Developing Staffed Housing for People with Mental Handicap*. Tunbridge Wells: Costello.

Means, R., Richards, S. and Smith, R. (2003) *Community Care: Policy and Practice*, 3rd edn. London: Palgrave.

Morris, J. (1993) *Community Care or Independent Living*. York: Joseph Rowntree Foundation in association with Community Care.

Noonan Walsh, P. (2003) A courtly welcome: observations on the research initiative, *British Journal of Learning Disabilities*, 31(4): 190–3.

O'Brien, J. and Lyle, C. (1987) *Framework for Accomplishments: A Workshop for People Developing Better Services*. Decatur, GA: Responsive System Associates.

Oliver, M. (1990) *The Politics of Disability*. London: Macmillan.

Oliver, M. (1992) Changing the social relations of research production, *Disability, Handicap and Society*, 7(2): 101–14.

Oliver, M. (2004) Introduction, in M. Oliver, C. Barnes, J. Swain and S. French (eds) *Disabling Barriers: Enabling Environments*, 2nd edn. London: Sage.

Open University (1996) *Learning Disability: Working as Equal People*. Milton Keynes: The Open University.

Palmer, N., Peacock, C., Turner, F. and Vasey, B. supported by Williams, V. (1999) Telling people what you think, in J. Swain and S. French (eds) *Therapy and Learning Difficulties*. London: Butterworth Heinemann.

Priestley, M. (1999) *Disabled Politics and Community Care*. London: Jessica Kingsley.

Rodgers, J. (1999) Trying to get it right: undertaking research involving people with learning difficulties, *Disability and Society*, 14(4): 421–33.

Shakespeare, T. (2003) Having come so far, where to now? *Times Higher Education Supplement*, 7 November: 28.

Shakespeare, T., Gillespie Sells, K. and Davies, D. (1996) *The Sexual Politics of Disability: Untold Desires*. London: Cassell.

Simons, K. (1992) *'Sticking up for Yourself': Self Advocacy and People with Learning Difficulties*. York: Joseph Rowntree Foundation.

Snow, K. (2002) People First language. www.modmh.state.mo.us/Sikeston/people.htm.

Swindon People First Research Team (2002) *Journey to Independence: Direct Payments for People with Learning Difficulties*. Swindon: Swindon People First.

Todd, S. and Shearn, J. (1997) Family dilemmas and secrets: parents' disclosure of information to their adult offspring with learning disabilities, *Disability and Society*, 12(3): 341–66.

Townsley, R. (1998) Information is power: the impact of accessible information on people with learning difficulties, in L. Ward (ed.) *Innovations in Advocacy and Empowerment for People with Intellectual Disabilities*. Chorley: Lisieux Hall.

Townson, L. (with Chapman, R.) (2003) Review of disability arts against exclusion by D. Goodley and M. Moore, *Disability and Society*, 18(6), 835–6.

UPIAS (Union of the Physically Impaired against Segregation) (1976) *Fundamental Principles of Disability*. London: UPIAS.

Walmsley, J. (1994) Learning disability: overcoming the barriers? in S. French (ed.) *On Equal Terms*. London: Butterworth-Heinemann.

Walmsley, J. (1997) Including people with learning difficulties: theory and practice, in L. Barton and M. Oliver (eds) *Disability Studies: Past, Present and Future*. Leeds: Disability Press.

Walmsley, J. (2001) Normalisation, emancipatory research and learning disability, *Disability and Society*, 16(2): 187–205.

Walmsley, J. and Johnson, K. (2003) *Inclusive Research with People with Learning Disabilities: Past, Present and Futures*. London: Jessica Kingsley.

Wendell, S. (1996) *The Rejected Body*. London: Routledge.

Williams, V. (2002) *Being researchers with the label of learning difficulty: an analysis of talk carried out by a self-advocacy research group*, unpublished Ph.D. thesis, The Open University.

Wolfensberger, W. (1972) *The Principle of Normalisation in Human Services*. Toronto: National Institute on Mental Retardation.

Wolfensberger, W. (1983) Social role valorization: a proposed new term for the principle of normalization, *Mental Retardation*, 21(6): 234–9.

Wolfensberger, W. and Tullman, S. (1989) A brief outline of the principle of normalization, in A. Brechin and J. Walmsley (eds) *Making Connections: Reflecting on the Lives and Experiences of People with Learning Difficulties*. Sevenoaks: Hodder & Stoughton.

Zarb, G. (1992) On the road to Damascus: first steps towards changing the relations of disability research production, *Disability, Handicap and Society*, 7: 125–38.

Index

Page numbers in *italics* refer to tables; LD = learning disability; Acts of Parliament are listed under the heading legislation.

THE ART AND SCIENCE OF MENTAL HEALTH NURSING
A TEXTBOOK OF PRINCIPLES AND PRACTICE

Ian Norman and Iain Ryrie

Norman and Ryrie provide an integrative account of the discipline that accommodates many origins, influences and practices. I feel sure this book will be of considerable benefit to undergraduate nursing students and to qualified nurses engaged in professional development activities. I also believe the book is necessary reading for those who train our nursing workforce.

Andrew McCulloch, Chief Executive, The Mental Health Foundation

- What are the foundations of mental health nursing as a practice discipline?
- What interventions do mental health nurses draw upon?
- How can mental health nurses engage clients as partners in care and promote their recovery?

Mental health nursing is an art and a science; concerned with both the therapeutic relationship between nurse and client and the skills required for evidence-based practice. Nurses need to find ways of integrating both these elements to meet service users' demands and policy directives for mental health services.

This book provides an integrative account of mental health nursing, which incorporates its knowledge base and the practical skills required by nurses to meet the demands of national health care policy and service users' expectations.

Pedagogy to support readers includes chapter overviews and summary points, questions for reflection, annotated bibliographies, and fascinating case studies and service users' views to illustrate everyday clinical situations.

The Art and Science of Mental Health Nursing is essential reading for students, post-qualification mental health nurses and nurse lecturers.

Contributors

Peter Ashton, Robin Basu, Geoff Brennan, Daniel Bressington, Alison Carolan, Joe Curran, Jacqueline Curthroys, Philip Fennell, Richard Ford, Catherine Gamble, Lina Gega, Richard Gray, Kevin Gournay, Susan Gurney, Simon Houghton, John Keady, Cheryl Kipping, Steve Morgan, Ian Norman, Ian Noonan, Kingsley Norton, Steve Onyett, Leah Ousley, Shaun Parsons, Rachel Perkins, Hagen Rampes, Julie Repper, Paul Rogers, Iain Ryrie, Susan Sookoo, Marc Thurgood, Gill Todd, Janet Treasure, Keith Tudor, Andrew Wetherell, Phil Woods.

Contents

*Contributors – Preface – Foreword – **Part 1: Foundations** – The origins and expression of psychological distress – Mental health promotion – Mental health nursing: origins and orientations – The policy and service context for mental health nursing – Rehabilitation and recovery – Law and ethics of mental health nursing – **Part 2: Interventions** – Assessment and care planning – Assessing and managing risk – The therapeutic milieu – Psychosocial interventions – Pharmacological interventions and electro-convulsive therapy – Complementary and alternative therapies – **Part 3: Applications** – The person with a perceptual disorder – The person with a mood disorder – The person with an anxiety disorder – The person with an eating disorder – The person who misuses drugs or alcohol – Mental health problems in childhood and adolescence – The older person with dementia or other mental health problems – The person who uses forensic mental health services – The person with a personality disorder – **Part 4: Core Procedures** – Engaging clients in their care and treatment – Problems, goals and care planning – Behavioural techniques – Cognitive techniques – Medication management to concordance – Therapeutic management of aggression and violence – Therapeutic management of attempted suicide and self-harm – **Part 5: Future Directions** – Functional teams and whole systems – Reflections – Index.*

872pp   0 335 21242 5 (Paperback)   0 335 21588 2 (Hardback)

THINKING NURSING

Tom Mason and Elizabeth Whitehead

This major new textbook provides a unique one-stop resource that introduces nursing students to the disciplines that underpin nursing practice. The broad range of subjects covered includes Sociology, Psychology, Anthropology, Public Health, Philosophy, Economics, Politics and Science.

Written by nursing lecturers with nursing students in mind, this book enables nurses to grasp the principles behind these disciplines and apply the concepts to everyday health care practices. Each chapter offers:

- The theoretical background of the major tenets of each discipline
- A comprehensive discussion of how they relate to practice
- Cross-references to other relevant chapter sections
- Suggestions for further reading
- A glossary of key terms.

Practical advice is also available in a chapter dedicated to methods of research, planning and construction of written work. Moreover, the textbook is designed to encourage creative and lateral thinking beyond its use in planning and writing assignments.

Thinking Nursing is essential reading for nursing students on Common Foundation Programmes (both at diploma and degree level) and qualified nurses undertaking additional specialist training including masters degrees, as well as those involved in planning, designing and the implementation of educational courses for nurses.

Contents
Introduction – Thinking Sociology – Thinking Psychology – Thinking Anthropology – Thinking Public Health – Thinking Philosophy – Thinking Economics – Thinking Politics – Thinking Science – Thinking Writing – Conclusions – References – Index.

456pp   0 335 21040 6 (Paperback)   0 335 21041 4 (Hardback)

PSYCHOLOGY FOR NURSES AND THE CARING PROFESSIONS
SECOND EDITION

Jan Walker, Sheila Payne, Paula Smith and Nikki Jarrett

- In what ways does psychology contribute to health and health care?
- How can psychology be applied in different health and social care contexts?
- What are the current psychological approaches used in health and social care?

This book introduces students and practitioners to psychological knowledge and understanding, and helps them to apply sound psychological principles in clinical contexts.

The text retains the emphasis of the previous edition upon the application of fundamental psychological principles in health and social care settings but is extensively revised to give increased attention to the developing evidence base within the psychology of health and illness. New to this edition are:

- Key questions for each chapter
- Research-based applications to practice
- Inclusion of a family scenario, used throughout the book to focus on professional, patient and carer perspectives
- Revised glossary explaining important terms

The book provides clear and concise descriptions of psychological theories, research-based evidence, and practical examples of applications across the lifespan in different health and social care settings.

Psychology for Nurses and the Caring Professions is essential reading for all students undertaking diploma or degree level courses in nursing and health care, including nurses, midwives, occupational therapists, physiotherapists and radiographers. It is also a useful introduction to the application of psychology to health for professionals working in social care.

Contents
Series editor's preface – Preface – What is psychology? – The perception of self and others – Memory, understanding and information-giving – Learning and social learning – Development and change across the lifespan – Social processes in health care – Stress and coping – Psychology applied to health and well-being – Case study – Glossary – References – Index.

232pp   0 335 21462 2 (Paperback)   0 335 21501 7 (Hardback)

A SOCIOLOGY OF MENTAL HEALTH AND ILLNESS
THIRD EDITION

Anne Rogers and David Pilgrim

- How have sociologists theorized and researched mental health and illness?
- In what ways do sociologists approach this topic differently to those from other disciplines?
- How do we understand mental health problems in their social context?

This bestselling book provides a clear overview of the major aspects of the sociology of mental health and illness, and helps students to develop a critical approach to the subject. In this new edition, the authors update each of the chapters, taking into consideration recent relevant literature from social science and social psychiatry. A new chapter has been included on the impact of stigma, which covers an analysis of the responses of the lay public to mental health and illness and representations of mental health (particularly in the media) in a post-institutional context.

A Sociology of Mental Health and Illness is a key teaching and learning resource for under-graduates and postgraduates studying a range of medical sociology and health-related courses, as well as trainee mental health workers in the fields of social work, nursing, clinical psychology and psychiatry.

Contents
Acknowledgements – Introduction – Perspectives on mental health and illness – Stigma re-visited and lay representations of mental health problems – Social class and mental health – Women and men – Race and ethnicity – Age and ageing – The mental health professions – The treatment of people with mental health problems – The organization of mental health work – Psychiatry and legal control – Users of mental health services – References – Index.

272pp   0 35 21583 1 (Paperback)   0 335 21584 X (Hardback)

SOCIOLOGY AND HEALTH CARE
AN INTRODUCTION FOR NURSES, MIDWIVES AND ALLIED HEALTH PROFESSIONALS

Michael Sheaff

- Are patients 'customers'? What does this mean for the patient-practitioner relationship?
- What should the relationship be between expert knowledge and our own experiences when dealing with health and illness?
- Do people who are better off get better access to health care?

Debates about the future of health care bring questions about patient choice, paternalism and inequalities to the fore. This book addresses some of the sociological issues surrounding these questions including:

- The social distribution of knowledge
- The basis of professional power
- Sources of social inequalities in health
- The ability of health care services to address these issues

The book provides suggestions and examples of how sociological concepts and insights can be used to help think about important contemporary issues in health care. For that reason, it has a practical as well as academic purpose, contributing to improvement of the quality of interaction between patients and practitioners. The core themes running throughout the book are inequalities in health and the rise of chronic disease, with particular attention being given to psycho-social models of illness which locate individual experiences within wider social relationships.

Sociology and Health Care is key reading for student nurses and those on allied health courses, and also appeals to a wide range of professionals who are interested in current debates in health and social care.

Contents

256pp   0 335 21388 X (Paperback)   0 335 21389 8 (Hardback)

INCLUSIVE EDUCATION
READINGS AND REFLECTIONS

Gary Thomas and Mark Vaughan (eds)

Beautifully and meticulously crafted, this is a compelling commentary and collection of articles relating to the issue of inclusion . . . Thomas and Vaughan have set a new standard for books of this sort. Each selection is prefaced by well-argued explanations of its significance and all are assembled so that each logically leads to the next. This book will help those with the courage and determination to put the principle into practice. I just wish I had had it to hand over the past 20 years.

Tim Brighouse, writing in the *TES*

This book examines some of the key influences behind the moves towards inclusive education and inclusion in mainstream society. The first of its kind anywhere in the world, this important work features more than 50 extracts from key documents and classic texts, alongside illuminating commentaries by two experts in the field.

Inclusive Education: readings and reflections demonstrates that moves to inclusion have come from many directions: research; the imperative for greater social justice; calls for civil rights; legislation that prohibits discrimination; original, distinctive projects started by imaginative educators; and the voices of those who have been through special education. These sources are marshalled and organized in this book. It is essential reading for students on a range of courses in inclusive education and special educational needs, and for anyone wishing to understand the development of inclusive education, including teachers, head teachers, educational psychologists, and parents.

Contents
Part I: The context – rights, participation, social justice – Part II: Arguments and evidence against segregation – 1960s to today – Part III: Legislation, reports, statements – Part IV: Inclusion in action.

240pp   0 335 20724 3 (Paperback)   0 335 20725 1 (Hardback)

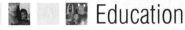 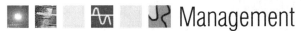
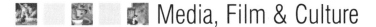
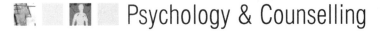
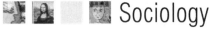
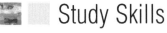
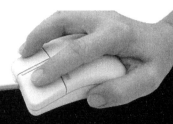
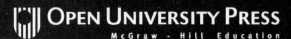